Telomeres

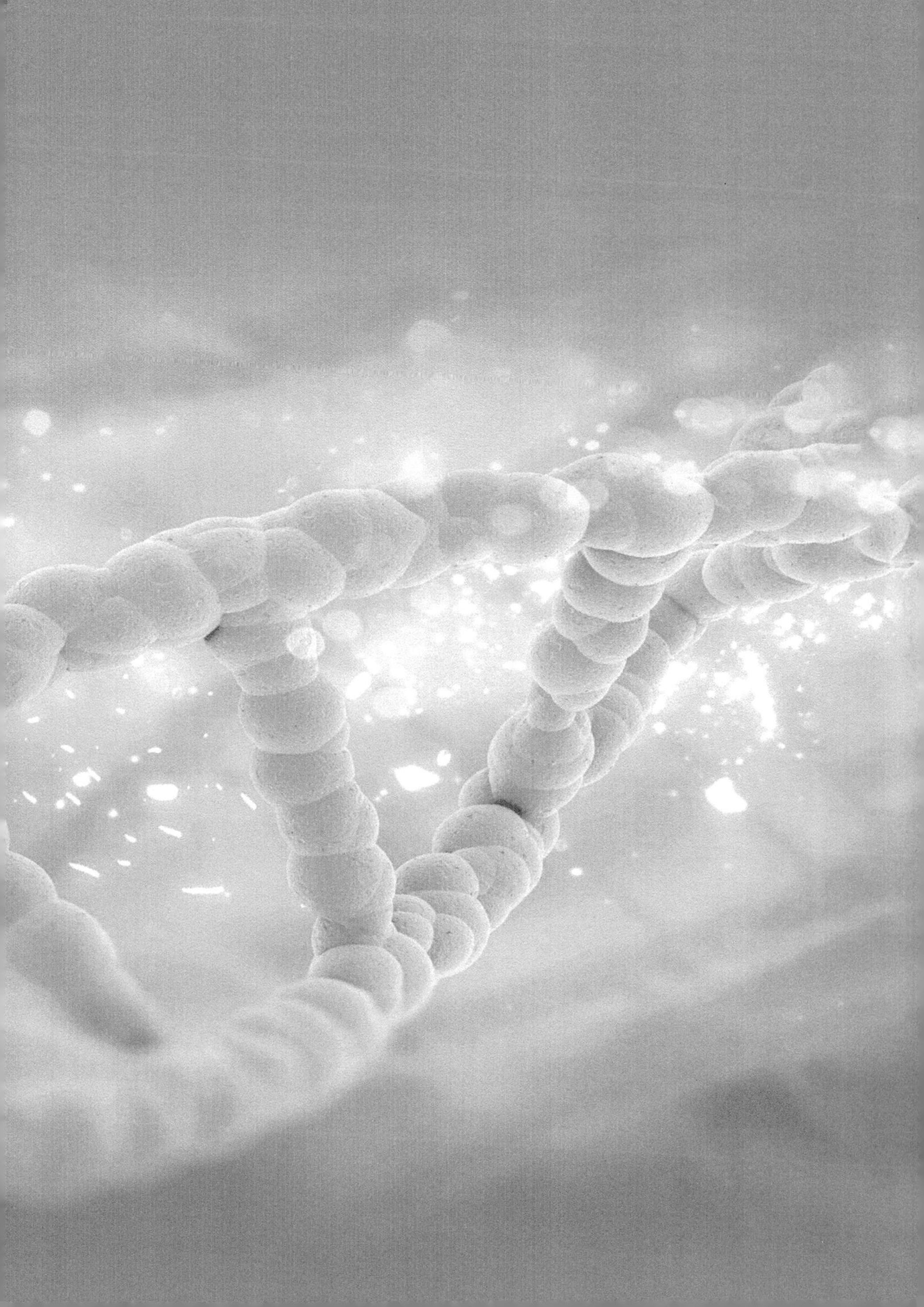

Telomeres

Biomarkers of a Healthy Life and Successful Aging

edited by

Aristidis Tsatsakis

JENNY STANFORD
PUBLISHING

Published by

Jenny Stanford Publishing Pte. Ltd.
101 Thomson Road
#06-01, United Square
Singapore 307591

Email: editorial@jennystanford.com
Web: www.jennystanford.com

British Library Cataloguing-in-Publication Data
A catalogue record for this book is available from the British Library.

Telomeres: Biomarkers of a Healthy Life and Successful Aging

ISBN 978-981-5129-49-6 (Hardcover)
ISBN 978-1-003-56809-4 (eBook)

Contents

List of Contributors

Athanasios Alegkakis
Laboratory of Toxicology, Medical School, University of Crete, Heraklion, Greece
Lifeplus S.A., Science & Technological Park of Crete, Vassilika Vouton, Heraklion, Greece

Evgenia Alexandrou
Dietitian-Nutritionist, Athens Euroclinic Hospital, D. Soutsou, Athens, Greece

Nicolina Anagnostatou
Department of Neonatology and Neonatal Intensive Care Unit, University Hospital of Heraklion, Heraklion, Greece

Michael Aschner
Department of Molecular Pharmacology, Albert Einstein College of Medicine, Bronx, New York, USA

Stella Baliou
Laboratory of Toxicology, Medical School, University of Crete, Heraklion, Greece
Lifeplus S.A., Science & Technological Park of Crete, Vassilika Vouton, Heraklion, Greece

Aikaterini Berdiaki
Laboratory of Histology-Embryology, School of Medicine, University of Crete, Heraklion, Greece

Félix Carvalho
Associate Laboratory i4HB—Institute for Health and Bioeconomy, Faculty of Pharmacy, University of Porto, Porto, Portugal
UCIBIO, REQUIMTE, Laboratory of Toxicology, Department of Biological Sciences, Faculty of Pharmacy, University of Porto, Porto, Portugal

Persefoni Fragkiadaki
Laboratory of Toxicology, Medical School, University of Crete, Heraklion, Greece
Lifeplus S.A., Science & Technological Park of Crete, Vassilika Vouton, Heraklion, Greece

Irene Fragkiadoulaki
Laboratory of Toxicology, Medical School, University of Crete, Heraklion, Greece
Lifeplus S.A., Science & Technological Park of Crete, Vassilika Vouton, Heraklion, Greece

Eleftheria Hatzidaki
Department of Neonatology and Neonatal Intensive Care Unit, University Hospital of Heraklion, Heraklion, Greece
School of Medicine, University of Crete, Heraklion, Greece

Petros Ioannou
School of Medicine, University of Crete, Heraklion, Greece

Fotios Kakridonis
25th Department of Orthopaedics, KAT Attica General Hospital, Athens, Greece

Mehtap Kara
Department of Pharmaceutical Toxicology, Faculty of Pharmacy, Istanbul University, Beyazıt, Istanbul, Turkey

Michael Koukakis
Laboratory of Toxicology, Medical School, University of Crete, Heraklion, Greece

Elisavet Kouvidi
Phenotypos Lab, Athens, Greece

Sabine Kruger-Krasagakis
Department of Dermatology & Venereology, General University Hospital of Heraklion, Faculty of Medicine, University of Crete, Greece

Petr Litvitsky
IM Sechenov First Moscow State Medical University, Sechenov University, Moscow, Russia

Lina Solange Matos
Associate Laboratory i4HB—Institute for Health and Bioeconomy, Faculty of Pharmacy, University of Porto, Porto, Portugal
UCIBIO, REQUIMTE, Laboratory of Toxicology, Department of Biological Sciences, Faculty of Pharmacy, University of Porto, Porto, Portugal

Dragana Nikitovic
Laboratory of Histology-Embryology, School of Medicine, University of Crete, Heraklion, Greece

Dimitra Nikolopoulou
Laboratory of Toxicology and Forensic Sciences, Medical School, University of Crete, Heraklion, Greece
Lifeplus S.A., Science & Technological Park of Crete, Vassilika Vouton, Heraklion, Crete, Greece

Taxiarchis Konstantinos Nikolouzakis
Department of Anatomy, Medical School, University of Crete, Crete, Greece

Eleni Ntoumou
School of Medicine, University of Thessaly, Viopolis, Larissa, Greece

Eren Ozcagli
Department of Pharmaceutical Toxicology, Faculty of Pharmacy, Istanbul University, Beyazıt, Istanbul, Turkey

Nikolaos Panagiotou
Lundbeck, 109 Kifisias Avenue & Sina, 151 24 Marousi, Athens, Greece
University of Glasgow, School of Molecular Biosciences, Glasgow, Scotland

George Pantazidis
PersonalWellness Health, Kalamaria, Greece

Monica Paoliello
Department of Molecular Pharmacology, Albert Einstein College of Medicine, Bronx, New York, USA

Emmanouel Papadakis
Onassis Cardiac Surgery Centre, Athens, Greece

Elisavet Renieri
Laboratory of Toxicology, Medical School, University of Crete, Heraklion, Greece
Lifeplus S.A., Science & Technological Park of Crete, Vassilika Vouton, Heraklion, Greece

Kleoniki Roka
Division of Pediatric Hematology Oncology, First Department of Pediatrics, National & Kapodistrian University of Athens," Aghia Sophia" Children's Hospital, Athens, Attiki, Greece

Abel Santamaria
Facultad de Ciencias, Universidad Nacional Autónoma de México, Mexico City, Mexico

Evangelia Sarandi
Metabolomic Medicine, Health Clinic for Autoimmune and Chronic Diseases, Athens, 10674, Greece
Laboratory of Toxicology and Forensic Sciences, Medical School, University of Crete, Voutes, Heraklion, Greece

Sergey Savko
Department of Medical Elementology, University Department, Peoples' Friendship University of Russia (RUDN University), Moscow, Russia

Çiğdem Sevim
Department of Medical Pharmacology, Faculty of Medicine, University of Kastamonu, Kastamonu, Turkey

Polytimi Sidiropoulou
1st Department of Dermatology-Venereology, Faculty of Medicine, "A. Sygros" Hospital, National and Kapodistrian University of Athens, Athens, Greece
Research Group of Clinical Pharmacology and Pharmacogenomics, Faculty of Pharmacy, School of Health Sciences, National and Kapodistrian University of Athens, Athens, Greece

Maria Sifaki
Skin Clinic, Heraklion, Crete, Greece

João Pedro Silva
Associate Laboratory i4HB—Institute for Health and Bioeconomy, Faculty of Pharmacy, University of Porto, Porto, Portugal
UCIBIO, REQUIMTE, Laboratory of Toxicology, Department of Biological Sciences, Faculty of Pharmacy, University of Porto, Porto, Portugal

Anatoly Skalny
IM Sechenov First Moscow State Medical University, Sechenov University, Moscow, Russia

Marios Spanakis
Department of Forensic Sciences and Toxicology, School of Medicine, University of Crete, Heraklion, Greece
Computational Bio-Medicine Laboratory, Institute of Computer Science, Foundation for Research and Technology—Hellas, Heraklion, Crete, Greece

Demetrios Spandidos
Laboratory of Clinical Virology, Medical School, University of Crete, Heraklion, Greece

Eftichia Stiakaki
Department of Pediatric Hematology-Oncology & Autologous Hematopoietic Stem Cell Transplantation Unit, University Hospital of Heraklion & Laboratory of Blood Diseases and Childhood Cancer Biology, School of Medicine, University of Crete, Voutes, Heraklion, Crete, Greece

Michael Stroumpakis
Historical Byzantine Musicology, Patriarchal University Ecclesiastical Academy of Crete, Greece

Andrey Svistunov
IM Sechenov First Moscow State Medical University, Sechenov University, Moscow, Russia

Lydia-Nefeli Thrapsanioti
Laboratory of Histology-Embryology, School of Medicine, University of Crete, Heraklion, Greece

Alexey Tinkov
Laboratory of Ecobiomonitoring and Quality Control, Yaroslavl State University, Yaroslavl, Russia

Konstantinos Tsarouhas
University Hospital of Larissa, Larissa, Greece

Aristidis Tsatsakis
Laboratory of Toxicology, Medical School, University of Crete, Heraklion, Greece
Lifeplus S.A., Science & Technological Park of Crete, Vassilika Vouton, Heraklion, Greece

John Tsiaoussis
Department of Anatomy, Medical School, University of Crete, Crete, Greece

Antonis Tsintarakis
Biomedical Applications Unit, Institute of Chemical Biology, National Hellenic Research Foundation, Athens, Greece

Christina Tsitsimpikou
General Chemical State Laboratory, Greece

Dimitris Tsoukalas
EINUMM, European Institute of Molecular Medicine, Rome, Italy
Metabolomic Medicine, Health Clinic for Autoimmune and Chronic Diseases, Athens, 10674, Greece

Manolis Tzatzarakis
Laboratory of Toxicology, Medical School, University of Crete, Heraklion, Greece

Elena Vakonaki
Laboratory of Toxicology, Medical School, University of Crete, Heraklion, Greece
Lifeplus S.A., Science & Technological Park of Crete, Vassilika Vouton, Heraklion, Greece

Maria Theodora Vitiadou
Laboratory of Toxicology, School of Medicine, University of Crete, Heraklion, Greece

Symeon Xenidis
Metabolomic Medicine, Health Clinic for Autoimmune and Chronic Diseases, Athens, 10674, Greece
Laboratory of Toxicology and Forensic Sciences, Medical School, University of Crete, Voutes, Heraklion, Greece

Konstantinos Xenos
Clinical Dietitian, Nutrigenetics Department, Athens Euroclinic Hospital, D. Soutsou, Athens, Greece

Esma Söylemez Yeşilçimen
Department of Pharmaceutical Toxicology, School of Pharmacy, University of Istanbul Medipol, Istanbul, Turkey

Ji-Chang Zhou
School of Public Health (Shenzhen), Sun Yat-sen University, Shenzhen, China

Evangelos Zoumpaneas
Founder, diatrofi.gr
Master Practitioner in Eating Disorders & Obesity, www.keadd.gr
CEO, Eating Disorders Education & Treatment Center, Nea Ionia, Athens, Greece

Vassilis Zoumpourlis
Biomedical Applications Unit, Institute of Chemical Biology, National Hellenic Research Foundation, Athens, Greece

About the Editor

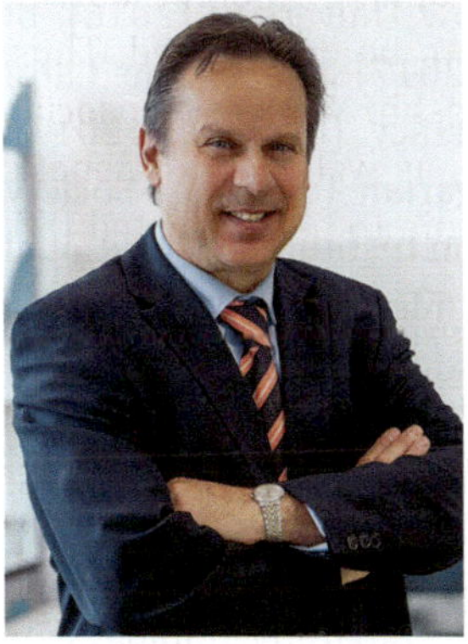

Professor and Academician Aristidis Tsatsakis,[1] an esteemed academic and researcher, holds the position of Director of the Department of Toxicology and Forensic Sciences[2] at the Medical School of the University of Crete, and the University Hospital of Heraklion. Additionally, he is the founder and chief scientific leader of the University of Crete spin-off company ToxPlus S.A.[3] and the startup LifePlus.[4]

Professor Tsatsakis has authored over 1300 publications (articles in journals, books, and abstract proceedings). Among these, more than 800 have been published in ISI journals and PubMed (715). Currently, his impact factor index stands at 109 (GS),[5] 90 (Scopus)[6] and 84 (Web of Science).[7] He has coordinated over 80 scientific research and technology projects as the Principal Investigator and has established worldwide collaborations, which include European, North American, and Asian teams well known for their excellence and innovation. He has additionally served as an

---

[1] Aristsatsakis (https://aristsatsakis.com/index.php)
[2] Laboratory of Toxicology (http://ctoxres.med.uoc.gr/index.php/en)
[3] ToxPlus (https://toxplus.gr/)
[4] LifePlus (https://life-plus.gr/)
[5] Google Scholar (https://scholar.google.gr/citations?sortby = pubdate&hl = en&user = hMJQ0nEAAAAJ&view_op= list_works)
[6] Scopus (https://www.scopus.com/authid/detail.uri?authorId = 35596169100)
[7] Web of Science (https://www.webofscience.com/wos/author/record/ H-2890-2013)

evaluator for many EU (HORIZON), UK (Public Health England, NHS, UK) and Asian research projects.

In 2012, he was elected President of the European Federation of European Societies of Toxicology (EUROTOX) and served in that position as President until 2016. He is a member of several Academies worldwide, including the Academy of Toxicological Sciences (FATS, USA), The World Academy of Sciences (WAS), the National Academy of Sciences of Russia (FMRAS) and the Academy of Europe (Academia Europaea). He is Emeritus Professor at the Federal Institute of Hygiene and Toxicology (Moscow, 2014), Doctor Honorary Causa of the Mendeleev Moscow University (2016), of the Far East Federal University (FEFU 2017) and of the Carol Davila University of Medicine and Pharmacy (Bucharest 2017). He was elected Honorary Member of Bulgarian Toxicology Society (2017), Honorary President of the European Institute of Nutritional Medicine (E.I.Nu.M.) (2018), Honorary Member of EUROTOX, Honorary Member of Slovak Society of Toxicology (SETOX) (2019) and most recently the Romanian Society of Toxicology (2023).

Professor Tsatsakis has an extensive career in the field of toxicology journal editing having served as both an Editor in Chief, Managing Editor, and Guest Editor for esteemed Elsevier Journals such as *Toxicology Reports*, *Food and Chemical Toxicology*, *Toxicology* and *Toxicology Letters*. More recently, he assumed the role of Editor-in-Chief for the newly established journal of European Publishing, *Public Health and Toxicology*.[8] His book *Toxicological Risk Assessment and Multi-System Health Impacts from Exposure* is currently the updated toxicology reference book for academics. He has also edited eminent books on risk assessment in agriculture and genetically modified organisms among others.[9] His upcoming book *Telomeres: Biomarkers of a Healthy Life and Successful Aging*, to be published by Jenny Stanford Publishing,[10] encompasses and discusses current knowledge on the role of telomeres as metabolic and genetic biomarkers.

---

[8] Public Health and Toxicology (https://www.publichealthtoxicology.com/)

[9] Toxicological Risk Assessment and Multi-System Health Impacts from Exposure (https://shop.elsevier.com/books/toxicological-risk-assessment-and-multi-system-health-impacts-from-exposure/tsatsakis/978-0-323-85215-9)

[10] Jenny Stanford Publishing (https://www.jennystanford.com/)

Professor Tsatsakis' primary research interests include biomonitoring and risk assessment of xenobiotic substances as well as linking chronic low-dose exposure to health problems and diseases. In 2015, he developed a novel risk analysis model, which incorporates multiple key factors such as the exposure to various environmental pollutants at low doses and their combinations with various everyday products as well as potential interactions of these pollutants with biological systems. This risk simulation model, known as "Real-Life Risk Simulation (RLRS)," examines these multifactorial systems on a long-term basis and since then, numerous related scientific studies have been conducted worldwide. The concept is based on the fact that in practice, the general population faces non-selective multichemical exposure from many different sources with long-term exposure to doses close to or below regulatory limits. There is a lack of such methodology from risk assessment practices and policies in the current worldwide regulatory framework.[11]

He has developed numerous exposure and effect biomarkers for various chemical substances, especially pesticides, pharmaceuticals, and others, revealing the mechanistic understanding of their mode of action and the adverse effects leading to clinical outcomes and chronic diseases (metabolic, autoimmune, cancer, etc.). Recent research has also highlighted telomeres as a genetic and metabolic phenotypic biomarker. Specifically, the percentage of "short telomeres" can indicate the onset of disease. As a biomarker, the percentage of short telomeres reflects genetic, environmental, and behavioral factors serving as an RLRS biomarker. The developed telomere measurement procedure realized by LifePlus is the most informative testing for clinical applications and phenotypic profiling and powerful biomarker of personalized medicine.

Professor Tsatsakis' long-term public engagement in promoting science for the safety of health and the environment has received repeated support and significant recognition from universities as well as national and international authorities. In 2020 and 2021,

[11]Wikipedia, A. Tsatsakis (https://en.wikipedia.org/wiki/Aristides_M._Tsatsakis)

he was recognized as a Highly Cited Researcher[12] by Clarivate Analytics—Web of Science in the field of Pharmacology and Toxicology of Biomedical Sciences earning a place on the list of researchers with the greatest global influence. Early in 2001, Dr Tsatsakis received the IRPC Gold Medal. In 2021, he was awarded the commemorative Medal "130 years of the Federal Scientific Center of Hygiene named after F.F. Erisman" and in 2022, the Academician Shitskova Medal of honors. In 2022, he was awarded the EUROTOX Merit Award 2022[13] by the European Federation of European Societies of Toxicology (EUROTOX) for his significant contributions to the field of Toxicology. Additionally, he was recently elected as a Member of the Academia Europaea[14] acknowledging his work and achievements in science.

His drive and mentality underscore the important role of academia in addressing societal issues. The concept of real-life risk simulation combines long-term exposures in relation to health issues and is an essential component and driving force for the application of theory to practice for safety evaluation in the 21st century.

Professor Tsatsakis is an eminent and pioneering scientist. The theme of Eurotox2025[15] is inspired by his personal attribution that "Toxicology addresses society's real life risks for sustainable health and well-being."[16]

---

[12] Highly Cited Researcher (https://recognition.webofscience.com/awards/highly-cited/2020/)
[13] EUROTOX Merit Award (https://www.eurotox.com/merit-award/)
[14] Academia Europaea (https://www.ae-info.org/ae/Member/Tsatsakis_Aristidis)
[15] EUROTOX2025 (https://www.eurotox2025.com/)
[16] BIONANOTOX (https://bionanotox.org/)

Preface

The subject of aging and its representative biomarkers have been under more active scrutiny recently with telomere length being the most indicative one. Aging is a multifaceted and complex process affected by genetics, epigenetics, lifestyle, nutrition, psychological, and socioeconomic factors starting even from the fetal stage of life.

Telomeres located at the distal ends of chromosomes preserve genetic information by sustaining chromosomes' structure shielding them from deconstruction, recombination, and fusion. Telomere length decreases as the cell divides. Once telomeres are reduced to a certain limit, cell mechanisms are activated leading to cellular senescence (aging) and apoptosis. According to numerous studies, the acceleration of this otherwise physiological process has been linked with age-related diseases and has been found to be induced by the factors mentioned previously. Hence, telomere length is a genetic and metabolic biomarker that reflects an individual's genotypic and phenotypic characteristics. Thus, we consider telomere length a valuable diagnostic tool for personalized health assessments and further treatment due to the ability to perform follow-up tests over time. Moreover, it fits well with our developed real-life risk simulation (RLRS) approach, which refers to the assessment of biological or clinical outcomes of chemical mixtures administered under a long-term, low-dose regimen, closer to real-life conditions.

Based on our research experience in telomeres in combination with systematic reviews and meta-analyses of several studies published lately led to the compilation of *Telomeres: Biomarkers of a Healthy Life and Successful Aging* with the aim to provide a comprehensive overview of the significance of various parameters on longevity and healthy aging. The book consists of five parts. Part I discusses the problems of an aging population globally, their impact on disease prevalence, and the associated economic implications, theories describing aging, biomarkers used, and reasons justifying why telomeres are the most suitable ones. A critical evaluation of the methodologies available for telomere length determination is presented in Part II. Lifestyle issues are the focus point of Part III. The way of life and complications during pregnancy as well as their impact on telomere length in in utero and post utero life are explained comprehensively. The importance of diet in the early days of life as well as of a balanced diet, the type and intensity of exercise, substance abuse, and exposure to toxic chemicals are the subjects scrutinized in association with telomere length. Part IV examines the link of telomere length to various diseases, such as aplastic anemia, osteoarthritis, autoimmune and cardiovascular diseases, male and female infertility, blood disorders and childhood cancer, and finally the effect of microbiota on telomere length. The final Part V analyzes the therapeutic approaches by specifying therapeutic targets at the site of telomere structures.

To our knowledge, this is the first attempt to describe the issue of aging in association with the telomeres in such a broad and extensive way, which makes this book an invaluable source of guidance and information to students, researchers new to the subject, scientists from various disciplines, and professionals, such as dieticians, nutritionists, doctors, toxicologists, just to name a few. Even the common reader will consider it a useful source of information about aging and the mechanisms describing it, and they might even extract some precious tips for everyday habits.

Aristidis Tsatsakis

Acknowledgments

It has been a joy to have "orchestrated" the creation of this book from being just a concept in my mind to the final product. However, I am indebted to my excellent editorial assistants Elli and Evi for their enthusiasm, organizational skills, patience, and a good sense of humor, which made the writing and compilation of the book a smooth and fun process.

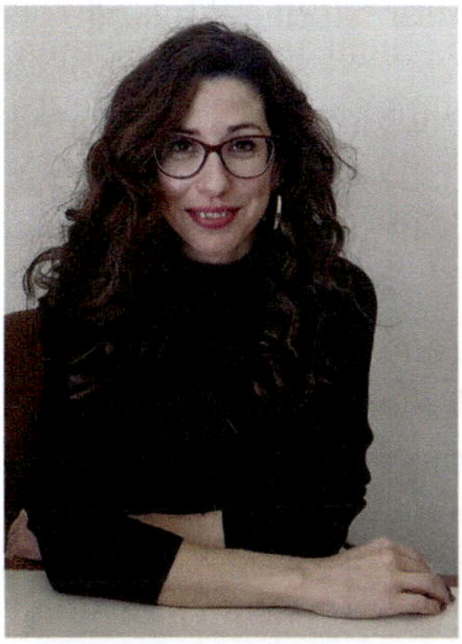

Elli (Elisavet Renieri) is a biologist (Department of Biology of the National and Kapodistrian University of Athens, Greece) and holds a PhD in toxicology related to human health risk assessment for cumulative exposure to chemicals, which took place in the Centre of Toxicology Science & Research (CTSAR), Faculty of Medicine of the University of Crete. She is currently a researcher at CTSAR for the development of risk assessment methods for human health from co-exposure to environmental pollutants and the development of methods for determining biological age by measuring the length of telomeric ends (Q-FISH) as well as the evaluation of telomeric length as a biomarker of the effect of exposure to exogenous chemical substances. She is also a postdoctoral researcher in the HERACLES Research Centre involved with the development of systemic biology models with the use of omics. She is a European Registered Toxicologist (ERT) and a member of the Hellenic Society of Toxicology.

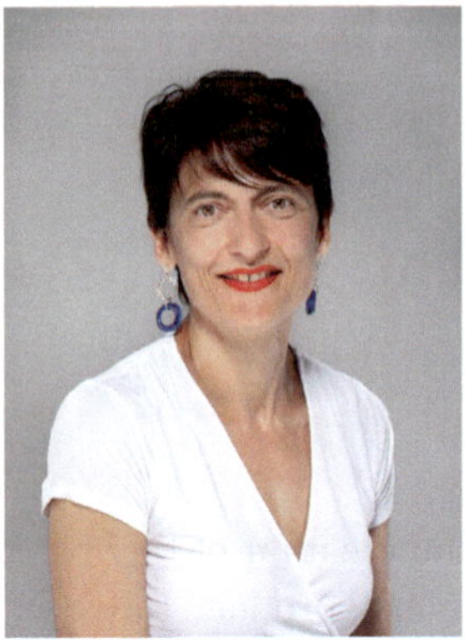

Evi (Paraskevi Kallinteri) is a pharmacist with an MSc and a PhD in the field of drug delivery (School of Pharmacy, University of Patras, Greece). She worked as a postdoctoral researcher on polymeric nanoparticles and their potential applications for the treatment of brain tumors at the University of Nottingham, UK. Then, she held a lecturing position in Pharmaceutics/Pharmaceutical Nanotechnology at the Medway School of Pharmacy, University of Kent, UK. Her research focused on the use of targeted arsonoliposomes for the treatment of leukemia and brain tumors. In 2010 she moved to Helsinki, Finland, and worked at the University of Helsinki as a teaching researcher. She is a Registered Pharmacist in Greece, the UK, and Finland. Currently, she has been working as a freelance translator, editor, and medical writer based in Finland.

I express my gratitude to all authors who have contributed their expertise and hard work to make the current edition for publication possible. I must emphasize that all authors are our close collaborators in various projects at the University of Crete and other universities worldwide as well as partners and colleagues in spinoff company ToxPlus and startup company LifePlus.

Special thanks to my parents from the island of Crete, who have been giving me inspiration to be creative and to follow their paradigm for a successful healthy aging.

Aristidis Tsatsakis

Endorsements

Ananya Nag
CEO, Aenaos Life

Delving into the mysteries of aging with *Telomeres: Biomarkers of a Healthy Life and Successful Aging*, by Prof. Aristidis Tsatsakis, has been an enlightening journey. This book, a treasure trove of knowledge, illuminates the significance of telomeres, those tiny guardians at the helm of our DNA, which play a crucial role far beyond merely marking the passage of time. They are the storytellers of our cellular legacy, intricately linked to our health and aging process.

As CEO of Aenaos Life, and having the privilege to collaborate with Prof. Aristidis Tsatsakis, I find this book aligns perfectly with both my personal experiences and our professional ethos. My life, shaped by the discipline of an athlete and challenged by personal health issues and genetic predispositions, has taught me the critical importance of understanding the cellular intricacies of aging. This insight has fuelled my passion for pioneering in the field of personalised medicine driven by the belief that healthcare must be as unique as the individuals it serves.

Prof. Tsatsakis' book masterfully demystifies the role of telomeres in dictating the pace of our biological clock through a narrative that is not only scientifically rich but also deeply personal. Each chapter unfolds the intricate dance of telomere replication, a process pivotal to our understanding of aging and the potential onset of senescence.

This work resonates with Aenaos Life Plus' mission to redefine preventive and regenerative healthcare. It mirrors our commitment to crafting wellness plans that honour the individuality of each person. The emphasis on lifestyle choices as sculptors of our telomere health reinforces our belief in the power of nutrition, physical activity, and mental well-being in preserving our vitality.

Our efforts at Aenaos Life to harness advanced technology and health analytics for exploring telomere length are a testament to the potential that understanding telomere dynamics holds for enriching our lives. This book champions the idea that a deep dive into our cellular makeup can chart a path to a future where aging is not merely slowed but is experienced with a richness that enhances every moment of our lives.

Telomeres: Biomarkers of a Healthy Life and Successful Aging takes us on a compelling journey from the very beginnings of our existence emphasising the impact of early life on our health trajectory. It invites us to embrace our biological uniqueness and to see wellness through the lens of personalization and proactive care.

I am proud to endorse this landmark publication, which not only highlights Prof. Tsatsakis' dedication to unveiling the mysteries of longevity but also serves as a beacon for Aenaos Life and everyone committed to navigating the future of health with wisdom, innovation, and care.

Let's join hands on this transformative journey to reshape the healthcare landscape, championing a future where personalised, celebrated health is the cornerstone of our lives.

In health and discovery,

Ananya Nag

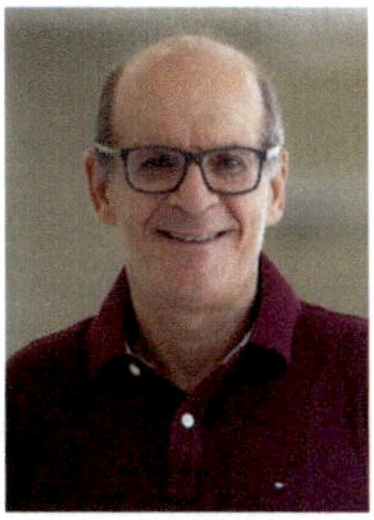

Michael Aschner
Department of Molecular Pharmacology
Albert Einstein College of Medicine
Forchheimer 209
1300 Morris Park Avenue
Bronx, NY 10461

Professor Tsatsakis has compiled an extended array of chapters, succinctly describing the latest developments in telomere research. The book is a multidisciplinary scientific endeavor, addressing methods in telomere length determination, impact of lifestyle and environmental factors on telomere length and their link to various diseases as well as therapeutic approaches to treat or prevent telomere length attrition.

The book assembled a series of chapters that advance the latest developments and scientific breakthroughs in this fast-paced research area. The first part discusses the mechanisms of aging and the health and socioeconomic problems arising due to a globally growing aging population as well as biomarkers used (telomeres included) to measure an individual's biological age. In the second part, a comprehensive analysis of all methods available to determine telomere length is presented. In the third part, several chapters highlight the significance of lifestyle and environmental parameters on telomere length and consequently biological age and healthy living. In the fourth part, the focus is directed at various diseases linked to telomere length attrition or anomalies in the telomeric topology. Therapeutic approaches for the prevention of telomere length change or correction of anomalies in the telomere locality are described. The book's primary goals were to provide the reader with information on mechanistic events of telomere length change leading to illness or comorbidities whether genetically or environmentally linked (or both).

Overall, the book provides state-of-the-art information and deepens the understanding of telomere importance in healthy life and aging written by internationally recognized experts in their own field. It provides a timely update on the latest research outcomes and scientific breakthroughs in the field of telomeres, and it should be of interest to students, researchers, experts in various disciplines and the general reader.

Michael D. Coleman, PhD, DSc
Professor of Toxicology
School of Pharmacy
Aston University
Birmingham B4 7ET, UK

Yesterday I saw an item on social media, when a lady exclaimed something to the effect of *'why am I working out so hard, when I am going to die eventually anyway!'* Indeed, not only is this subject area a matter of life and death for us all, but there is also conflict over what we want from our efforts to stave off aging and what we can realistically achieve with our particular genetic heritage. Publications in this area are usually the preserve of various lifestyle gurus from a variety of medical or psychology-based backgrounds, whose assertions are sometimes somewhat vaguely founded and essentially tell their audience what they want to hear.

However, the discipline of toxicology has quietly made vast strides in pursuit of our understanding of how our biological systems withstand attrition and aging. Much of this has been achieved through the study of the telomere, which has emerged as a precise and sensitive indicator of cell damage and ultimate cellular fate. Professor Tsatsakis' book has in a comprehensive and energetic way spotlighted these advances in our understanding of these cellular 'Swords of Damocles' and how telomeres can be our remorseless 'sell by date' for our fragile existences.

This book unsparingly lays out the challenges of worldwide aging and its growing and possibly insurmountable health and economic challenges. A powerful boost to the credibility of the book is its rigorous examination of the validity of the methods of telomere impact assessment, which facilitates understanding of what has been determined of the impact of our lifestyles on our telomere processes and also the effects of some major disease states. Critically, this publication also examines how our formative years govern our health and life expectancies and this is of particular importance to rapidly developing economies, where deprivation in the first few years of life will have disproportionate health and thus economic impact over the final years of those same populations. Finally, some promising drug targets in the telomere process are reviewed which provide some exciting possibilities, which may in the future claw back some of the now irreversible environmental, disease and lifestyle-mediated telomere attrition.

The book has a potentially wide readership and its accessibility, scope and timeliness bring not only the efforts of Professor Tsatsakis and his team to the fore in curating its themes, but also the growing effectiveness of toxicologically based scientific approaches in advancing our knowledge of the fabric of our health and vitality and how we can preserve those essentials as long as we humanly can.

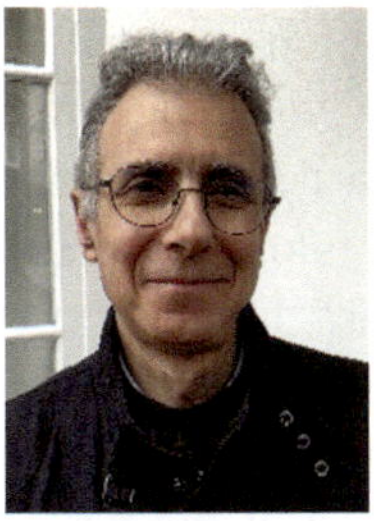

Prof. Michael Antoniou
Professor of Molecular Genetics and Toxicology
Head, Gene Expression and Therapy Group
King's College London
Faculty of Life Sciences & Medicine
Department of Medical and Molecular Genetics
Guy's Hospital, London SE1 9RT, UK

Telomere length is now a recognized and highly researched marker of aging. Thus, the theme of this book—*Telomeres: Biomarkers of a Healthy Life and Successful Aging*—is very topical and timely. Professor Aristidis Tsatsakis, a world-renowned expert in the field of chemical toxicology, has collated a comprehensive range of chapters, succinctly describing the latest developments in telomere and aging research. Among the many strengths of the book is that it is scientifically multidisciplinary in scope, addressing methods in telomere length determination, impact of lifestyle and environmental factors on telomere length, and the link of telomere length to various diseases as well as therapeutic approaches to treat or prevent telomere length attrition. Overall, the book's goal is to provide the reader with information on mechanistic events of telomere length change leading to illness or comorbidities whether either genetically or environmentally linked, or both.

The importance of the topic of telomere length in connection with aging is established from the outset with Chapter 1, which lays an excellent foundation. The book then logically progresses through a series of chapters that present and advance the latest developments and scientific breakthroughs in this rapidly advancing area of research. The first part of the book discusses the mechanisms of aging and the health and socioeconomic problems that have arisen due to a globally growing aging population as well as biomarkers used (including telomeres) to measure an individual's biological age. In the second part of the book, a comprehensive analysis of all methods available to determine telomere length is presented. In the third part, several chapters highlight the significance of lifestyle and environmental factors that impact telomere length and consequently biological age and a healthy life. Finally, the fourth part of the book is directed at discussing various diseases linked to telomere length attrition or anomalies in telomeric topology. The inclusion of therapeutic approaches for the prevention of telomere length change or correction of anomalies in telomere locality adds a much-needed practical dimension to the basic science presented and thus finishes on a theme with significant public health implications.

In summary, the book provides state-of-the-art information and deepens understanding of the importance of telomere integrity in maintaining healthy life and aging. The book is written by internationally recognized experts in their fields and provides a timely update on the latest research outcomes and scientific breakthroughs in telomere biology and disease/aging linkage. The comprehensive nature of the book makes it an excellent reference in telomere biology in general and constitutes a must-read for not only students, researchers, and experts in aging but also those in other disciplines as well as the general reader.

Mohammad Abdollahi, PharmD, PhD, FIAS
Professor, Tehran University of Medical Sciences
Editor-in-Chief, DARU Journal of Pharmaceutical Sciences
Country NGOs Correspondent to SAICM, UN
Council Member, Islamic World Academy of Sciences
Clarivate Highly Cited Researcher
Former Council Member, Committee on Publication Ethics (COPE)
Former Scientific Advisory Board Member, Organisation for the Prohibition of Chemical Weapons (OPCW)
Former Toxicology Advisor to the WHO

Dear Readers,

It is my distinct pleasure to bring to your attention the remarkable book *Telomeres: Biomarkers of a Healthy Life and Successful Aging*, edited by the esteemed Professor Aristidis Tsatsakis, director of the Department of Toxicology and Forensic Sciences at the University of Crete. He is one of the most highly cited researchers in the world and a former head of EUROTOX. This toxicologist's motivational manner makes him shed light on the science of toxicology. In this book, the prestigious authors and the prestigious editor help us understand the vital role of telomeres in human diseases and longevity.

This book comprehensively explores telomeres' role as a biomarker of aging and associated diseases in a five-part structure, ensuring a thorough understanding of the subject matter. Telomeres are the protective caps at the ends of chromosomes that shorten with each cell division and are associated with aging and age-related diseases. However, lifestyle choices that promote good health, such as a balanced diet, regular exercise, and avoiding harmful substances, can influence telomere length, making it an attractive area for research. Interestingly, the pursuit of good health and longevity is commendable in Islamic teachings as long as it is used for piety and good deeds. The Prophet Muhammad once said, "The best of people are those who live longest and excel in their deeds," highlighting the value placed on a long and virtuous life.

Climate change is a global problem that has far-reaching toxicological consequences. The impact of environmental toxicants on the human body is alarming. Epigenetics is an area of research that has gained significant attention in recent years. Environmental toxicants have been found to impact epigenetic processes, leading to various health problems. The impact of toxicants on telomeres, the protective caps at the end of chromosomes, is particularly concerning. This book provides critical insights into the complex interplay between environmental toxicants, epigenetics, and telomeres. The knowledge gained from this book will contribute to developing effective strategies to mitigate the impact of climate change and environmental toxicants on human health.

We must work together to develop innovative solutions to protect our environment and safeguard our health. This book is a starting point for anyone interested in understanding the impact of environmental toxicants on human biology and health. I highly recommend this book to anyone interested in understanding the complex relationship between our genetic blueprint and environment. This book offers a timely and critical exploration of telomeres and is sure to be of great value to all who seek to promote good health, longevity, and toxicants' role.

Sincerely,
Mohammad Abdollahi, PharmD, PhD, FIAS

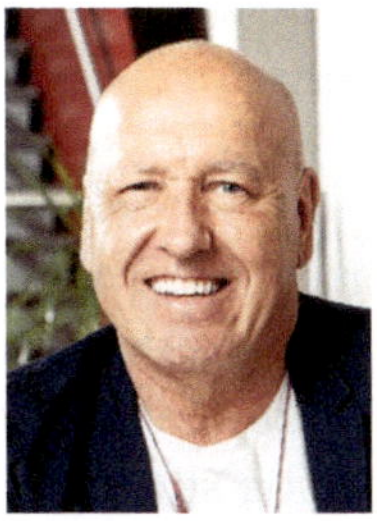

Thomas Hartung, MD
Environmental Health and Engineering (Primary)
Molecular Microbiology and Immunology (Joint)
Whiting School of Engineering (Joint)
Johns Hopkins Bloomberg School of Public Health
615 N. Wolfe Street, Room W7035
Baltimore Maryland 21205
USA

Brief Introduction

This enlightening book embarks on a detailed exploration of telomeres, the essential protective caps at the ends of chromosomes, unraveling their crucial role in the processes of aging and disease. It meticulously explains the function of telomeres in safeguarding genetic material and the consequences of their deterioration on cellular health. Through its pages, readers are invited to understand the intricate biological underpinnings of aging, providing a comprehensive look at how the stability and integrity of telomeres are central to maintaining genomic stability and preventing the onset of age-related diseases.

Unique Contributions

This text distinguishes itself with an extensive and insightful analysis that seamlessly connects fundamental biological understanding with the prospects of therapeutic intervention. It presents an unprecedented perspective on the realm of telomere research, shedding light on the latest strategies aimed at addressing telomere-associated diseases and promoting longevity. By bridging the gap between basic science and clinical application, the book introduces a groundbreaking approach to exploring the potential of telomere science in enhancing health span and offers a holistic view of the current landscape of research and therapy development.

Critical Analysis and Insights

The book delves deep into the dynamics of telomeres and their significant impact on health from the earliest stages of life through to old age. Providing a meticulous review of the latest research findings and the development of emerging therapeutic strategies, it emphasizes the critical role that telomere maintenance plays in the fight against age-related conditions. The analysis is rich with new perspectives, offering readers a comprehensive understanding of how telomere length and function influence overall health and longevity, and acknowledging the immense potential that lies in targeting these structures for therapeutic benefit.

Practical Implications

The implications of the book's findings are profound, offering new pathways for the medical community to explore in the quest to mitigate the effects of aging. It highlights the potential of telomere-focused research to pave the way for innovative treatments that could fundamentally alter our approach to preventing and managing age-related diseases. This work underscores the transformative power of telomere science, suggesting that it holds the key to unlocking novel therapeutic avenues that could significantly impact our approach to health and disease management in the aging population.

Target Audience

Designed with a broad audience in mind, this book is an invaluable resource for a diverse range of readers, from researchers and clinicians deeply entrenched in the study of genetics and aging, to those with a keen interest in the broader implications of telomere science for preventive medicine. It serves as an essential guide for anyone eager to dive into the complexities of how telomeres affect health and disease, offering insights that are both profound and accessible to those looking to deepen their understanding of this cutting-edge area of science.

Final Recommendation

For those deeply engrossed in the pursuit of knowledge on aging and telomere science, this book emerges as an essential read. Its contributions to advancing our comprehension of the complex biological mechanisms associated with aging are unrivaled, making it a cornerstone text for anyone looking to stay abreast of the latest developments in the field. The book not only educates but also inspires, encouraging further exploration and research into the promising horizons of telomere science and its potential to revolutionize our understanding of health and longevity.

Personal Endorsement

From a personal standpoint, this book has been a revelation, significantly enriching my understanding and approach to research in the field of aging and disease. Its in-depth analysis and groundbreaking insights have provided me with a new lens through which to view the intricate dance between genetics and the aging process, enhancing both my academic pursuits and professional practice. This text stands as a beacon of knowledge, guiding and inspiring those of us dedicated to exploring the frontiers of medicine and the science of longevity.

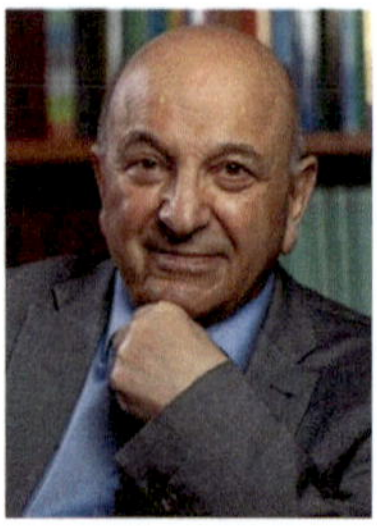

Victor A. Tutelyan, DSci, Professor
Full Member of the Russian Academy of Sciences
WHO Food Safety Expert
Member of Joint FAO/WHO Expert Committee on Food Additives
International Life Sciences Institute (ILSI) Board Member

Modern progressive scientific advancements have impacted all aspects of human life, even the most sacred such as birth and death. The discovery of telomeres has provided humanity with unprecedented opportunities to both predict and to control the life expectancy. The book systematizes and details all current knowledge on the aging mechanisms and solutions for their deceleration. These issues concern everyone. Therefore, this edition can be recommended to the widest range of readers.

PART I

AGING

Chapter 1

Aging

Nikolaos Panagiotou
Lundbeck, 109 Kifisias Avenue & Sina, 151 24 Marousi, Athens, Greece
University of Glasgow, School of Molecular Biosciences, Glasgow, Scotland
nipn@lundbeck.com

1.1 Introduction

Aging—A growing problem. A major issue that modern society must face is that of population aging. Population aging refers to the process through which elderly individuals constitute an increasing fraction of the overall population [1]. Specifically, population aging can be defined as an increase in the proportion of people within a population over a particular age, often 65 years of chronological age [2]. An increase in the median population age has also been employed for the purpose of studying the trends of population aging and predicting future projections [3].

1.2 Classical Demographic Transition Model

An ongoing demographic transition is the underlying cause of population aging. At the bottom of the demographic transition lies

Telomeres: Biomarkers of a Healthy Life and Successful Aging
Edited by Aristidis Tsatsakis

ISBN 978-981-5129-49-6 (Hardcover), 978-1-003-56809-4 (eBook)
www.jennystanford.com

a major shift from high birth and death rates to low birth and death rates. This transition is responsible for causing a demographic change over a period of time that leads to population aging. Consequently, reduced fertility rates and longer life expectancy are recorded at any age stratum [4].

In addition to the demographic transition, the epidemiological transition is responsible for the lower death rates and longer life expectancy [5, 6]. The epidemiological transition is defined by a move from deaths that were predominantly caused by infectious diseases to deaths which are caused by chronic diseases during old age [5]. Reductions in the number of deaths caused by infectious diseases, which disproportionately affect younger age groups, have occurred largely as a consequence of advances in public health. These include improved sanitation, health education, and better nutrition during childhood, as well as improvements in health-care, such as the development and availability of antibiotics and vaccinations (Centers for Disease Control and Prevention [298]). This has resulted in people living longer and consequently older individuals survive long enough to develop multiple age-associated disorders. Furthermore, improvements in healthcare, in addition to preventive pharmacological interventions, have allowed the older members of society to live significantly longer with chronic diseases and the comorbidities that are associated with them.

Collectively, the demographic transition along with the epidemi-ological transition constitutes the classical, or also termed Western, demographic transition model, which explains population aging [7].

1.3 Population Aging in Numbers

In agreement with the classical demographic transition model, currently, there is a rapidly growing number of aged individuals in the global population. This is also predicted to continue following an upward trajectory in the future [8]. Though over the past sixty years, there has only been a slight increase from 8% to 10% in the number of people aged 60 years and older, this group is expected to constitute 22% of the total global population in the next 30 years. This is representative of an elevation from 800 million elderly people to 2 billion people over the age of 60 by 2050 [9]. The number of people above the age of 80 is also projected to grow significantly, from 69 million recorded in 2000 to over 379 million by 2050. The proportion of this population, aged 80 years and over, is currently estimated to constitute approximately 1% of the total world population. This percentage has been predicted to increase by almost four-fold, reaching and surpassing an estimated 4.1% by 2050 [10]. Additionally, global population projections suggest that the median age of the world's population will increase accordingly, from 27 to 36 years of age by 2050 [303]. Furthermore, it is predicted that within the next few years, people aged 65 and older will outnumber children below the age of 5, for the first time in human history [11].

During the past three decades, life expectancy at 60 years of age has also increased in high- and middle-income countries, on account of novel biomedical interventions, coverage, and effectiveness of healthcare as well as due to reductions in exposure of populations to environmental, biological, and behavioral risk factors such as tobacco [12]. Noteworthy, while the average life expectancy has increased significantly, maximal longevity (i.e., maximal chronological age achieved by individuals) has shown little or modest evidence of increasing [13]. However, the Office for National Statistics has suggested that the number of centenarians in the United Kingdom (UK) has increased over five-fold since 1965 (Fig. 1.1) and it is expected to continue to show an elevating trend in the coming years [2]. Interestingly, the female centenarian population appears to grow at a much faster pace than the male population [2]. Moreover, it is anticipated that the global centenarian population may continue to live longer than it has ever been recorded before. Consequently, it is a possibility that maximal longevity may also demonstrate a significant rise in the near future [5].

Over the same period, fertility rates have shown a dramatic decline in the more developed regions of the world and this negative trend is expected to continue over the next 30 years. On average, women have fewer children and they become mothers at a later age than in the past due to continuing education as well as challenges associated with following a career [14]. Indeed, as observed in the Danish population, the total fertility rate has decreased from

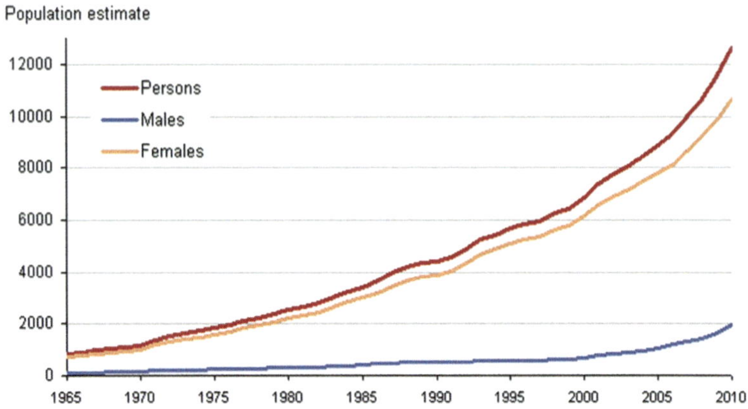

Figure 1.1 UK population aged 100 years and over. Total number of centenarians, males, and females in the UK from 1965 to 2010 (adapted from Office for National Statistics, 2012 [2]).

4.1 to 1.8 children per woman over the last century [15]. These observations suggest that, in the more developed countries and in agreement with the demographic transition model, fertility rates will continue to decrease dramatically to very low levels, while longevity is increasing. With respect to aging in low- and middle-income countries, the World Health Organization study on global aging and adult health aims to address this gap in reliable data and scientific knowledge [16, 17]. Indeed, this study has already begun to gradually increase our knowledge and understanding of the complex evolution of health and well-being and their determinants in the older members of society [16, 18, 19].

1.4 Impact of Population Aging on Disease Prevalence and the Associated Economic Implications

An increase in life expectancy and the aforementioned decrease in birth rates are currently transforming the shape of the age pyramid in the European Union (EU), as well as in other middle- and high-income populations across the globe. Additionally, they also raise the median age. In the past, the EU age pyramid comprised a wide base and narrow apex. However, due to population aging accompanied by a low birth rate, the traditional age pyramid has been replaced with a narrow base and blunt apex (Fig. 1.2) [304]. Over the next thirty years, the total number of individuals aged 65 or over is predicted to double in size. As a proportion of the working-age population, which is aged between 15 and 64 years, it will rise from one elderly individual for every four workers to one elderly individual for every two workers [304]. Therefore, it is estimated that people who are active in the labor force will unavoidably have to face an increasing tax burden and higher social contributions, as a means of supporting their elder members of society. Alternatively, older citizens may be required to either accept lower levels of financial, medical, and social support or a higher pension age. Additionally, the demographic data from the EU have depicted a narrowly based and blunt apex age pyramid for the year 2010, while future projections have estimated the EU-aged population increasing with the 2010 diamond shape becoming skinnier and heavier at the top by 2060 (Fig. 1.2) [304].

These projections highlight the major changes that are expected to happen in the next four decades, transforming the age profile

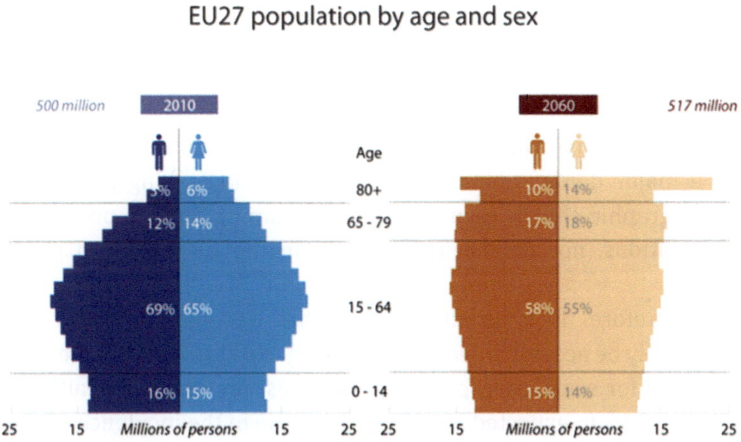

Figure 1.2 EU population demographic data and future projections. Percentage of individuals who lived in the EU in 2010, grouped by sex and age stratum, and future estimates for the year 2060 (adapted from the European Parliamentary Research Service, 2013).

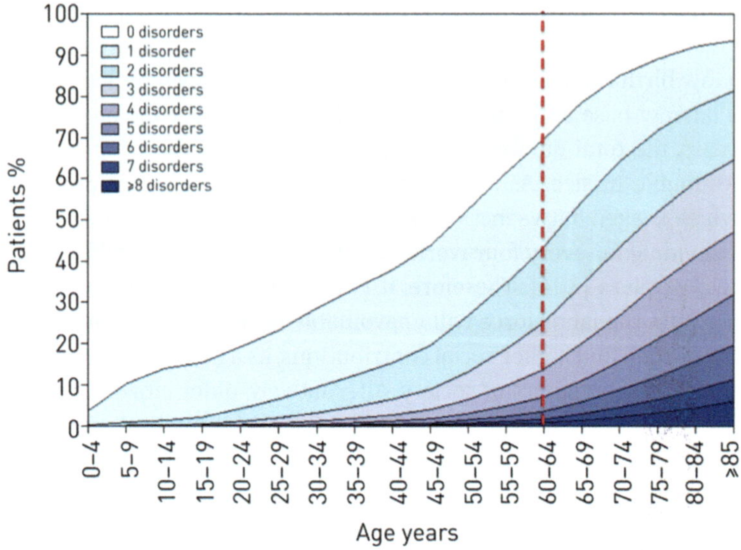

Figure 1.3 Number of age-related disorders that appear with age. The number of chronic comorbidities experienced by an individual elevates with age and is significantly larger in individuals who are older than 65 years of age (adapted from Divo et al., 2014 [21]).

of the EU dramatically. Life expectancy and median age are both expected to increase significantly, while the labor force in the member states is predicted to decrease [304]. The population data and future projections that have been discussed above are indicative of a major demographic shift that is currently taking place. This demographic shift is responsible for reshaping the composition of populations, not only in the UK and in the EU but on a global scale.

Therefore, it is predicted that this demographic shift will inevitably be accompanied by a shrinking workforce and an elevated demand for social care, pensions, and most importantly healthcare [20], due to an expected significant increase in the incidence of age-associated morbidities (Fig. 1.3) [21, 22]. Indeed, age is the primary risk factor for the prevalent diseases of developed countries that impact morbidity and mortality, including cancer, cardiovascular disease, chronic kidney disease, neurodegeneration, osteoarthritis,

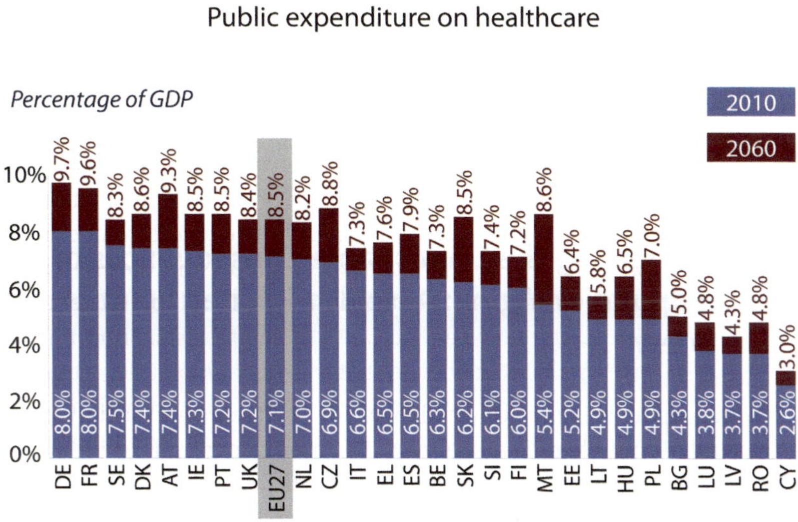

Figure 1.4 Public expenditure on healthcare and future estimates in the EU. Healthcare-associated costs in the EU in 2010 and future estimates for the year 2060 (adapted from European Parliamentary Research Service, 2013).

osteoporosis, type 2 diabetes, and many other major non-communicable diseases (i.e., not caused by infectious agents) that are tightly associated with aging [23, 24].

Consequently, this rise in cases of age-related disorders will financially burden healthcare and social security systems around the world. The global economic burden of healthcare is estimated at 35 trillion euros over the next two decades [25]. Additionally, the estimated economic impact of socioeconomic inequalities in health alone is 1 trillion euros per year, or 9.5% of the Gross Domestic Product accounting for 15% of the costs of social security systems and 20% of the costs of healthcare systems in the EU [26]. Hence, the implications of population aging are expected to heavily affect pensions, social expenditure, and healthcare systems (Fig. 1.4), not only in the EU but across the globe [304].

Moreover, it is worth highlighting that the association between health spending and health gains needs to be better measured and accounted for (National Research Council Panel2010) [305] as substantial differences have been observed in the health and functional status of older people in many developing countries as well as marked differences have been recorded in the health status within the UK and other developed countries [27]. This means that increasing expenditure on healthcare is not necessarily associated with increased health gains for the aged population.

1.5 Mitigating the Undesirable Consequences of Population Aging: A Health-Related Point of View

Overall, aging brings novel challenges for healthcare and society in general. Hence, there is a vital need to improve our understanding of the mechanisms underpinning aging [28]. This will allow the development of novel therapeutic strategies which can mitigate the undesirable effects of age-related morbidities and thus tackle the complications that are tightly associated with population aging.

The upshot will be an improvement in health span, which is defined by more years of healthy living and a reduction in age-associated comorbidities (Fig. 1.5) [29]. To address population aging, through the improvement of the health and well-being of elderly individuals, health promotion, disease prevention, and tissue regeneration interventions hold the promise of keeping older members of a society in good health and for significantly longer as they age [30, 31]. In this way, it is estimated that the public expenditure, associated with social care and healthcare, would decrease considerably.

1.6 What is Aging?

In order to address aging and to fully appreciate its impact on health status, disease susceptibility, progression, and outcome, it is essential to define it. This might seem like a simple task, as far as chronological age might be concerned, where chronological age corresponds to the total number of years that have elapsed since birth. However, aging is a complex process, and it is important

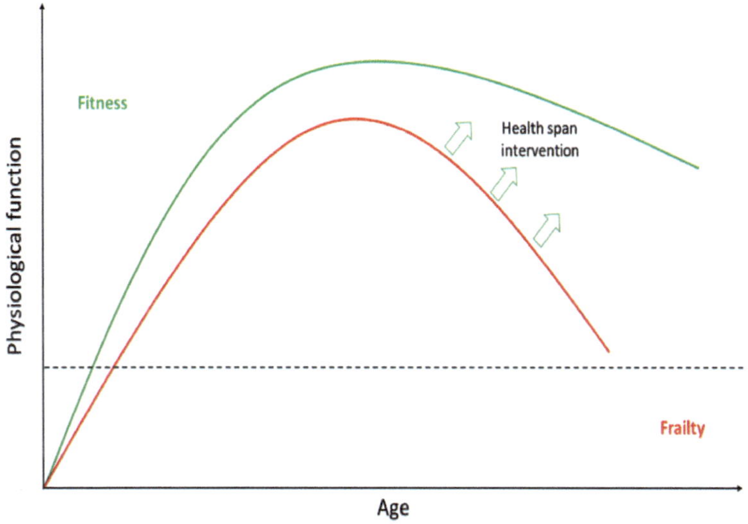

Figure 1.5 Schematic representation of two different trajectories of aging. The green line indicates a good trajectory for healthy aging. On the other hand, the red line indicates a poorer aging trajectory, associated with a steeper decline in age-related physiological functional capacity. Loss of functional capacity results in fitness decline, frailty, and a greater risk of mortality. Improving the human health span would require interventions that can push the poorer trajectory of aging up and to the right, providing more years of good health and vitality (adapted from Panagiotou et al., 2018 [29]).

that biological age (i.e., miles on a biological clock), which is defined by physiological functional capacity, must be taken into consideration.

For instance, two elderly individuals of the same chronological age can have significantly different biological ages and correspondingly very different physiological capabilities. Therefore, in this paradigm, one individual might be in better health than the other, who might be more biologically aged and thus of poorer health. This difference in biological age could be the outcome of the complex interplay between genetics, epigenetics, lifestyle, nutrition, psychology, socioeconomic factors, and other aspects of their exposomes (i.e., the measure of all the exposures of an individual over the life course that are related to health) [29, 32].

Therefore, it needs to be highlighted that, in contrast to chronological aging, biological aging is plastic and therefore it can be either accelerated or decelerated; for instance, by genetic, nutritional, or pharmacological interventions [33–35]. Chronological age is thus not the optimal method for determining the health status of an individual in late life. Hence, a definition for aging that encompasses biological aging would be more suitable.

1.6.1 Classical Definitions

Several definitions of aging have been proposed. Hence, it is important to discuss some of the initial classical definitions and observe how these evolved over the course of time.

In 1959, Strehler et al. described the process of aging by four main features [36]:

1) Aging is destructive and compromises functionality.
2) Aging is progressive and irreversible.
3) Aging is intrinsic and thus determined by internal rather than external factors.
4) Aging is universal and thus all living organisms are affected by it. Also, all individuals of the same species display a largely uniform pattern of aging.

However, these proposed features do not entirely reflect all aging characteristics and differ from our current understanding of aging. For instance, as discussed previously, evidence has been generated to support the thesis that aging is also determined by external factors, which can accelerate or delay biological aging, and not solely by internal elements.

In 1964, aging was termed by Comfort as the intrinsic, inevitable, and irreversible age-related process that leads to loss of viability and an increase in vulnerability [37]. Similarly, this definition also failed to incorporate the important role of environmental factors and how they can influence the aging process.

More than twenty years later, in 1991, in his book on the evolution of aging, Rose described the aging process as a persistent decline in the fitness of an organism due to degeneration of the internal physiology [38].

Almost after a decade, in 1999, aging was described by Partridge and Mangel as a progressive and gradual decline in capacity to function, associated with a gradual deterioration of physical function that comes with an increase in an individual's chronological age [39].

Although outdated in some of their views, all the above-mentioned classical definitions agreed upon the fact that aging is associated with a functional decline, which leads to multiple pathological consequences for the organism, and affects every individual, organ, and tissue.

As an inevitable outcome of the aging process, virtually all physiological functions lose efficiency. For instance, the effects of the aging processes may include:

- Appearance changes include a gradual loss of height, muscle, and bone mass as well as decreased elasticity in the skin.
- Deteriorations in sensory functioning, such as reductions in visual acuity and hearing capacity.
- Cognition problems like memory and cognitive impairment.
- Reduced capacity to maintain homeostasis.
- Deterioration of the force and elasticity of skeletal muscle.
- Increased susceptibility to stress, such as external temperature, infections, hyperglycemia, and trauma.
- Psychological changes such as frequent fluctuations in mood.

It has been discussed that aging phenotypes, such as the above, although genetically complex [40], overlap across species [35]. Indeed, some of the most common aging phenotypes in humans; for instance, decreased innate immunity, reduced memory, decreased cardiac function, changes in skin morphology, and abnormal sleep patterns, have also been observed in laboratory models, including mice (*Mus musculus*), worms (*Caenorhabditis elegans*) and flies (*Drosophila melanogaster*) [35]. Hence, some of the aging phenotypes appear to be conserved across species.

1.6.2 Modern Definitions

Currently, one of the most commonly accepted definitions for aging states that aging is a process defined by the accumulation of changes in an organism over time [41]. These changes can be genetic, epigenetic, environmental, and psychological in nature and are responsible for the transformation of an individual organism over the course of time. What this definition successfully takes into account that other modern definitions fail to incorporate, is that the aging process begins from the time of conception and not only later in life.

Specifically, the aging process is at its most rapid during the embryonic development period, where it results in organismal gain of functional capacity, through cell division, differentiation, and apoptosis. Additionally, this process promotes organismal growth and development early in life [42], so that the organism can achieve sexual maturity and successfully reproduce [41]. However, as life progresses, the aging process becomes deleterious; for instance, through the accumulation of cellular senescence, and is associated with loss of physiological capability which leads to disease and finally mortality [43]. Thus, it has been proposed that aging acts according to the antagonistic pleiotropy model, promoting growth and development early in life for the purpose of sexual reproduction, but driving senescence and loss of physiological capability later in life [26, 41, 42, 44].

Aging can be defined by the loss of functional capacity as time progresses either at the organismal or cellular level. It also needs to be highlighted that aging is not a passive process [45], but one actively regulated by distinct molecular pathways layered below a loss of functional physiological capacity which is experienced later in life and correlated with frailty and increased likelihood of death. The underpinning mechanisms are considered to be evolutionarily conserved across taxa [43, 46, 47] and have been reflected in nine distinct hallmarks [43]. These comprise genomic instability, telomere shortening, epigenetic alterations, loss of proteostasis, deregulated nutrient sensing, mitochondrial dysfunction, senescence, stem cell exhaustion, and altered intercellular communication [43]. More recently, a decade after the first publication of the hallmarks of aging, three more hallmarks have been recognized, including dysbiosis, chronic inflammation, and disabled macroautophagy [33]. In mammals, other features may also be present [69].

These features mirror the acquisition of allostatic load[a], which reflects the wear and tear on the organism [48], and eventual allostatic overload [49], correlated with dysregulated physiological function that comes with aging [50–52]. Consequently, they reflect the accumulation of cell and tissue damage, the loss of repair capacity, and an increased probability of neo-oncogenesis due to dysregulated cell proliferation [53–55].

Furthermore, it is important to recognize that not all individuals age at the same rate or in the same way [56]. In addition, individual organ systems, cells, organelles, and molecules, within an individual, may also age at significantly different rates [26]. In order to explain the inter- and intra-individual variation observed during aging, we need to further understand how extrinsic factors; for instance, environmental, physical, psychological, and socioeconomic factors, interplay with intrinsic elements, such as genetics and epigenetics. These factors may act synergistically, independently, or cumulatively. How they do so is still the focus of ongoing research. Recent studies focusing on the epigenetics of human aging and how epigenetic changes can significantly impact the way we age [57–61] have provided novel insight into a series of epigenetic modifications that influence the functional decline that is associated with organismal aging [62–66].

For instance, a Glasgow-based cohort, which included individuals of extreme socio-economic differences, lower socio-economic status, and poorer diet, has been tightly linked with accelerated biological aging and predisposition to early onset of disease, as indicated by telomere length measurements [67]. Specifically, age-related telomere attrition that occurred at a faster rate was significantly associated with low relative income, housing tenure, and poor diet. This study has also suggested potential links with elevated levels of Interleukin 6 (IL-6) in the circulation, which is a predictor of cardiovascular disease and diabetes with biological aging. Specifically, telomere length was demonstrated to be positively associated with low-density lipoprotein (LDL) and total cholesterol levels but inversely correlated to circulating IL-6 [67]. Elevated

[a]allostatic load: the cumulative wear and tear of the body that results from chronic exposure to various stressors and adjustments the body makes to maintain health.

IL-6 levels strongly support the hypothesis that the increased disease prevalence in these communities of higher deprivation status may be the outcome of underlying chronic inflammation [67]. Nevertheless, these observations require further study to discover potential mechanistic links. In other words, exactly how these changes are influenced by extrinsic factors among different individuals and different organ systems has yet to be determined. Thus, age-related morbidities and their relationship with psychosocial, economic, nutritional, and lifestyle factors as well as with genetic and epigenetic determinants of aging, remain to be elucidated [58, 68].

In this respect, the study of animals and how they mitigate some of the loss of physiological function, common to aging and diseases of aging in humans, may be of benefit. Interestingly, almost all the diseases that affect humans have an equivalent in the animal kingdom [69]. Hence, the success of such an approach depends on the study of biomimicry, as opposed to simply comparative biology. For instance, studying the long-lived naked mole rats (*Heterocephalus glaber*) and how they are protected from oxidative stress and cancer could assist in the development of strategies that prevent or slow down premature aging [301, 302]. Additionally, the study of rough eye rockfish (*Sebastes aleutianus*) and bowhead whale (*Balaena mysticetus*), which both have documented lifespans that surpass 200 years, could potentially enhance our understanding of autonomous and non-autonomous cellular senescence during aging [69], a process which undoubtedly plays a protagonist role in the age-related deterioration of physiological function within an organism.

1.7 Theories of Aging

Despite advances in molecular biology and genetics, the mechanisms that regulate aging and control lifespan remain unidentified [70]. There are numerous theories which have been proposed in order to explain the process of aging. However, none of them appears to be fully satisfactory [71]. Specifically, more than 300 of these theories of aging exist [72], although they are not necessarily mutually exclusive. In general, the theories can be grouped into three main mechanisms:

1) **Evolutionary mechanisms**: Aging is part of life's programming because the old need to remove themselves to make room for the next fertile generation, thus sustaining evolutionary turnover.
2) **Network mechanisms**: Multiple aging mechanisms work in parallel, and aging is the outcome of the interactions between cells, organs, and systems.
3) **Causative mechanisms**: Aging can be explained at the cellular level. For instance, the accumulation of cellular waste products might be responsible for causing cellular senescence, which is a cell state that is obtained by cells that cease to divide resulting in an impairment of function.

Moreover, modern biological theories of aging in humans can also be grouped into two main categories:

1) **Programmed theories**: These suggest that aging processes follow a biological timetable, perhaps a continuation of the one that regulates childhood growth and development as described above. This regulation would depend on changes in gene expression that affect the systems responsible for maintenance, repair, and defense responses.
2) **Damage or error theories**: These theories emphasize that environmental assaults on living organisms act as the cause of aging. These can induce cumulative damage at various levels and thus drive organismal aging.

1.7.1 Programmed Theories of Aging

The programmed theories of aging can be further divided into at least three sub-categories:

1) **Programmed longevity**: Aging is the result of successively switching on and off specific genes, with senescence being defined as the time when age-associated deficits are manifested. This topic is covered in depth by Davidovic et al., including the

role of genetic instability in aging and the dynamics of the aging process [71].

2) **Endocrine theory**: Biological clocks act through hormones to control the pace of aging within an individual. Recent studies have confirmed that aging is hormonally regulated and that the evolutionarily conserved insulin/insulin-like growth factor 1 (IGF-1) signaling (IIS) pathway plays a key role in the hormonal regulation of aging through collagen remodeling [73]. More extensive coverage of the potential mechanism underlying IIS and the aging process has been discussed by van Heemst [74].
3) **Immunological theory**: The immune system is programmed to decline over time. This leads to an increased vulnerability to infectious disease and thus aging and mortality. It is well documented that the effectiveness of the immune system peaks at puberty and then gradually declines with advances in age. For instance, as an individual grows older, antibodies lose their effectiveness and fewer new diseases can be combated effectively by the body. Consequently, this causes cellular stress and eventually death [75]. Indeed, dysregulated immune response has been linked to cardiovascular disease, inflammation, Alzheimer's disease, and cancer. Although direct causal relationships have not been established for all these detrimental outcomes, the immune system has been implicated [76].

1.7.2 Damage or Error Theories of Aging

Evolutionary considerations suggest that aging is not caused by active gene programming, but it is the outcome of evolved limitations in somatic maintenance, which ultimately leads to a build-up of damage [77]. Similarly, to the programmed theories, the damage or error theories of aging can also be divided further, into five sub-categories. These include:

1) **Wear and tear theory**: The wear and tear theory of aging was first introduced by August Weisman in 1882 [78]. Cells and tissues comprise vital parts that wear out over time resulting in aging. Parts of the body eventually wear out from repeated use

losing physiological capacity for function, and then becoming deleterious for the organism.

2) **Rate of living theory**: This theory, which was described initially by Raymond Pearl, states that the greater an organism's rate of oxygen basal metabolism, the shorter its lifespan [79]. The rate of living theory of aging, while helpful, has not been completely adequate in explaining the maximum lifespan [80, 81]. Hence, Rollo later proposed a modified version, highlighting the antagonism of growth, which is mediated by the target of rapamycin (TOR), and stress resistance, which is activated by the forkhead transcription factors (FOXOs) [82].
3) **Cross-linking theory**: The cross-linking theory of aging has been proposed by Johan Bjorksten [83]. According to this theory, an accumulation of cross-linked proteins damages cells and tissues within an organism slowing down bodily processes and thus resulting in aging. Indeed, it has been demonstrated that cross-linking reactions are involved in age-related changes in a number of proteins [84].
4) **Free radical theory**: The free radical theory of aging is one of the most prominent causative mechanism theories. This theory was first introduced in 1954 by Gerschman [85] and was later developed by Harman [86]. This theory proposes that an accumulation of free radicals derived from oxygen is responsible for the decline in biological functions associated with aging. Free radicals, which have also been termed reactive oxygen species (ROS), are primarily generated within cells by the mitochondrial respiratory chain, mainly due to the leakage of electrons. The body possesses natural antioxidants, in the form of enzymes, which assist in controlling the dangerous accumulation of these free radicals. Nevertheless, over time the antioxidant systems are unable to counteract the generated ROS including superoxide anion (O_2^-), hydrogen peroxide (H_2O_2), and peroxynitrite ($OONO^-$) [87]. These free radicals capture electrons from another molecule, which in turn becomes unstable and reacts with further molecules. As an outcome, oxidative damage occurs to lipids, DNA, and proteins within the cells, and therefore tissue damage is caused. This process has been termed as oxidative stress.

Experimental evidence in animal models supports this theory. Specifically, enhanced oxidative damage by ROS has been shown to result in lifespan shortening [88, 89], while antioxidants have been shown to extend the lifespan in flies [90]. In addition, transgenic mice that overexpress human catalase, which is responsible for removing H_2O_2, have been demonstrated to have their median and maximum lifespans significantly extended [91].

However, recent experiments in mice and worms have suggested that increased levels of ROS correlate with normal and sometimes extended lifespan, while the harmful effects of ROS were described to be the result of compromised signaling rather than direct oxidative damage occurring in sensitive targets [92]. Hence, the precise relationship between ROS-induced damage, mitochondrial damage, and aging remains to be elucidated. Nevertheless, it has been suggested that ROS signaling is probably the most important pathway responsible for the development of cell senescence and organismal aging and thus ROS signaling might be a strong candidate to be investigated in order to further develop the free radical theory of aging [93].

5) **Somatic DNA damage theory**: DNA damage occurs constantly in cells of all living organisms. While a large degree of DNA damage is repaired, some damage accumulates over time as the DNA repair mechanisms fail to repair it correctly. Evidence has been generated to suggest that DNA damage accumulation is occurring in non-dividing cells of mammals [94]. Genetic mutations occur and accumulate with increasing age, causing cells to deteriorate and malfunction. In addition, damage to mitochondrial DNA might lead to mitochondrial dysfunction, which could consequently result in vascular aging and contribute to the increased risk of cardiovascular diseases in the elderly [95]. Furthermore, it has been suggested that somatic mutagenesis in satellite cells, which are stem cells residing in muscle, has been associated with aging. Specifically, an increased incidence of mutations in exons and promoters targeting genes that are involved in satellite cell activity and muscle function could serve as a driving force for the age-related decline of skeletal muscle function [96]. Therefore, damage

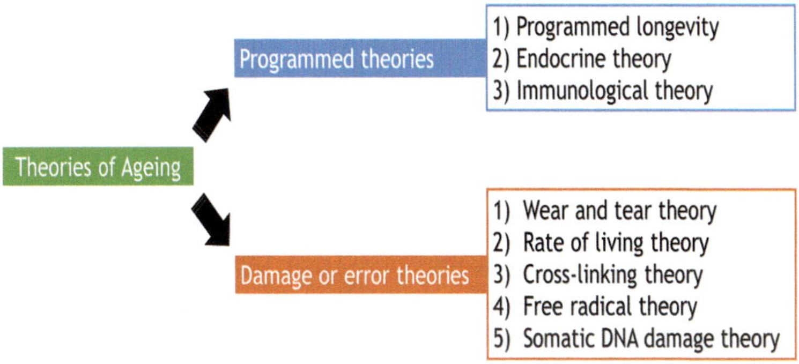

Figure 1.6 Theories of aging. Programmed theories and damage or error theories of aging and their sub-categories.

to the genetic integrity of the cells may be responsible for accelerating aging.

Overall, multiple theories of aging have been proposed (Fig. 1.6), while many interact with each other. Although currently there is no consensus on this issue, it has become evident that multiple factors and their interplay play an important role in driving the aging process. Hence, this further supports the fact that aging is a complex process, which is affected by the synergistic, independent, and cumulative action of many intrinsic and extrinsic factors. These elements can modify the trajectory of aging of an individual, either towards a good trajectory of healthy aging or towards a poorer trajectory of aging that is associated with frailty and a greater risk of mortality. Therefore, being able to account for states of healthy aging and frailty, would be beneficial when studying the impact of therapeutic interventions on human health span.

1.8 Healthy Aging

It has been discussed that the prevalence of chronic diseases and self-reported ill health shows an increase with chronological age [97]. This means that gains in healthy life expectancy (i.e., health span) are significantly less in comparison to the increase in total life expectancy. Consequently, a decline in the proportion of life spent in states of favorable health has also been recorded more recently [98].

Moreover, the proportion of people who report that they have a limiting and chronic disease is significantly higher in the elderly members of the population. Indeed, 37% of individuals between 65 and 74 years of age and 48% of individuals over the age of 75 have reported that they suffer from such an illness [98]. It has also been reported by the Scottish Health Survey that 13% of people over the age of 70 have a chronic illness and disability in comparison to an incidence of 2% in individuals between 30 and 39 years of age [99]. Furthermore, it has been indicated that elderly individuals were more likely to report poor health that directly impacts their daily life activities. For instance, 27% of men over the age of 75 reported that ill health was responsible for restricting them and limiting their ability to perform moderate activities in comparison to an incidence of 6% in men between 18 and 24 years of age [99]. Nevertheless, a significant number of the elderly were reported to still consider themselves to be in good health, even if they have a chronic disease that has a direct effect on their daily lives [98].

Age is considered to be the primary risk factor for chronic diseases, which can significantly limit the health status of an individual later in life, during aging [24]. Hence, it is of vital importance to better understand the biological processes that drive aging and how these affect the aging trajectory, both at an individual and population level. Healthy or normative (i.e., with good health) aging can be defined as optimizing the opportunities for good health, in order to allow older people to continue being active members of society and also enjoy an independent life of high quality [306].

There are primarily three components that need to be fulfilled for healthy aging:

1) Low probability of disease.
2) High cognitive and physical functional capacity.
3) Active engagement in life activities.

It has been recognized that a life course approach to healthy aging is necessary. Both internal (i.e., physical) and external (i.e., social) factors, which together comprise the exposome, have specifically been found to play important roles in altering the trajectory of aging [100]. Throughout the life course, critical periods, such as early life experiences, along with the accumulation of exposures and chain of risk, which refers to the sequence of linked exposures (i.e., the exposome), appear to impact the aging process. Accumulation of both observational and experimental evidence increasingly supports the thesis that a relationship exists between growth and development in early life and health later in life [101] in agreement with the antagonistic pleiotropy model. Therefore, this allows us to intervene in order to extend the health span, either through nutrition, exercise, and lifestyle routes or with the development of biomedical therapeutic strategies.

1.9 Frailty

Frailty has been defined as a syndrome of decreased reserve and resistance to stressors, which is responsible for causing vulnerability to adverse outcomes, such as physiological functional capacity decline, procedural complications, and prolonged periods of recovery as well as disability and mortality. It has also been proposed that frailty is characterized by an age-associated biological vulnerability to stressful stimuli and decreased physiological reserves [102]. In addition, it has been suggested that it may be more suitable to define frailty as clusters of vulnerabilities, weaknesses, instabilities, and limitations with shared root causes [103, 104].

Many of the definitions of frailty share commonality with the definitions of aging. There also appears to be significant variation in the frailty status of individuals who share the same chronological age, similar to biological age. More precisely, frailty, which is associated with impairment in cognitive and physical functional capacity and results in loss of resilience and reserve, may be driven by biological aging. Therefore, measurements of frailty have been implemented as a clinically important tool for assessing biological age.

Specifically, more than twenty clinical tools have been developed and employed in order to measure frailty status in patients [105]. Nevertheless, consensus has yet to be reached on which frailty tools are the most appropriate to use. Therefore, significant variability has been evidenced among studies. For instance, it has been reported that from 125 elderly individuals, frailty prevalence was found to range from 33% to 88% owing to the criteria that were used [106]. The majority of the tools emphasize one or more of the five core domains that describe the frailty phenotype. These include slowness, weakness, low physical activity, exhaustion, and unintentional weight loss. For instance, the Fried scale [107] incorporates slowness, weakness, low physical activity, exhaustion, and shrinking. It is required that at least three of the previous criteria must be satisfied for a diagnosis of frailty. It has also been proposed that frailty is not synonymous with comorbidity or disability. Instead, comorbidity is an etiologic risk factor for the manifestation of frailty, while disability is the outcome [107]. Currently, the Fried Scale is the most cited tool for measuring frailty and is a valuable predictor of mortality and disability risk, as it has been demonstrated in large cohorts of community-dwelling elderly individuals and patients suffering from cardiovascular disease [107]. In addition to the Fried Scale, the Short Physical Performance Battery (SPPB) includes scoring for slowness, weakness, and balance [108]. These are measured by a series of physical performance tests, gait speed, chair rises, and tandem balance. Furthermore, cognition and mood may also need to be considered as additional domains instead of simply modulating factors that play a role in the frailty-disability transition.

Contrary to the above-mentioned multi-domain frailty scales, it has been supported that five-meter gait velocity and handgrip strength could be utilized as single-item measures of frailty [109]. Indeed, the gait speed test is of significantly high inter-rater reliability [110]. This test has additionally been indicated to be sensitive to changes in mobility, while meaningful improvements in gait speed were also predictive of positive outcomes in frail elderly patients at a population level [111], although not necessarily at an individual patient level [112]. Variations, between three and ten meters, have been reported for the distance that was selected to measure gait speed. Nevertheless, the walking distance has appeared to be insignificant in measured velocity [113].

While the Fried scale, the SPPB, and single-item measures are employed to reflect the clinical phenotype of frailty, an alternative approach has been suggested to reflect the accumulation of deficits [114]. Deficits encompass a range of up to seventy different symptoms, signs, comorbidities, disabilities, and frailty traits, which are all counted and summed. For instance, the Frailty index has been developed to estimate the relative fitness and frailty. Specifically, this was based on twenty deficits [115]. The Frailty index can also be employed to assess aging status and mortality risk, with higher scores being linked to elevated risk of adverse outcomes. Moreover, the Frailty index better reflects physical than chronological age [115]. Nevertheless, the clinical phenotype approach has been favored by the International Academy on Nutrition and Aging Frailty Task Force, as comorbidities and disabilities have been suggested to be disentangled from frailty [116].

Disability, which is defined as difficulty or dependency in carrying out activities of daily living, is often used interchangeably with frailty. Nevertheless, disability is more accurately considered as an adverse outcome that is linked to frailty. Therefore, although certain tools may be effective at assessing frailty, other approaches may be required to study specific and potentially treatable domains. Hence, it is worth considering the use of alternative tools, which are based on challenging versions of the pre-existing scales with altered endpoints depending on the individual or the population that is under investigation. Furthermore, the heterogeneity that is evident in the patient groups is also indicative of the fact that the use of fixed endpoints may not be suitable to accurately assess the frailty status. One of the first studies to employ three different frailty tools with the aim to prospectively assess frailty and evaluate mortality risk in elderly patients suffering from cardiovascular diseases has demonstrated that there was significant variation in the prevalence of frailty and this observation was dependent upon which tool was selected [117].

Overall, being able to measure healthy aging and frailty is of significant clinical importance. However, inter-individual variation combined with a large number of tests available makes their assessment and interpretation a highly challenging task. Hence, more accurate tests and biological markers that are capable of correctly predicting an individual's health status during old age are required.

1.10 Biological Aging and Biomarkers of Aging

Aging is highly heterogeneous and as a result, determining healthy aging and frailty is a very desirable but challenging task, especially among individuals who share the same chronological age. Although increased chronological age is associated with diminished capability for physiological function and frailty, the degree of complex inter-individual variation in health and functional status is substantial and remains incompletely understood.

In contrast to chronological aging, which is easily defined and measured, biological aging involves variable structural and functional changes that occur at the cellular, tissue, and organ level. This ultimately affects the overall performance of the organism [118]. Biological age is widely accepted to vary between individuals of the same chronological age and to increase susceptibility to ill health and disease. Biological aging has also been described as a steady decrease in the physiological capability of an organism to meet its demands, which occurs with increased chronological age [119]. Biological aging is also thought to be the outcome of failure of intracellular and immune system repair mechanisms with resultant cellular damage [120]. The lack of a universal definition of biological age makes consistent measurement, reporting, and comparison of scientific data considerably difficult.

Research investigations typically use lifespan and survival rates when reporting on biomedical interventions with associated age-related benefits. However, these studies fail to reflect upon health span benefits. In other words, it is essential that research studies display the impact of intervention on health status, age-related disability, frailty, and age-associated onset of disease, both in model systems and in older populations [121]. Finally, it is also of major importance to be able to account for the inter-individual differences in aging, which are attributed to psychosocial and lifestyle confounders. Hence, more informative markers of biological age, which are defined as biomarkers of aging, are essential to determining health status in old age, both at organismal and cellular levels.

Biological age, which has also been regarded as miles on the clock [67], and in comparison, to chronological age appears to be a better reflection of inter-individual variation in the rate of growth and aging, given the heterogeneity of both lifespan and health span. There have been numerous studies which have used physical health as well as various biomarkers to assess biological age [122, 206] with particular interest in models which can be readily applied to the clinic [205]. Biomarkers of aging may include biochemical assays, gene expression assays, and physiological characteristic measurements, which can then indicate the presence or severity of an existing disease or physiological deterioration; for instance, lens opacity or psychological condition. The aim for successful biomarkers of aging would be to better predict organismal physiological functional capacity than chronological age by correlating more closely with the biological age of an individual. In particular, these biomarkers of aging are intended to identify individuals who are at greater risk of exhibiting age-associated pathology or developing it at a younger chronological age.

In 1988, Baker and Sprott suggested the following criteria to be fulfilled by potential biomarkers of biological aging [207]:

1) The rate of change of the biomarker must, at least in mathematical terms, reflect some measurable parameter which can be predicted at a later chronological age.
2) The biomarker should reflect some basic biological process of aging and certainly not a predisposition toward a disease state or some error in the metabolism.
3) The biomarker should have high reproducibility in cross-species comparisons of functional or physiological age versus chronological age, particularly within the same classes and certainly within the same families of species.
4) The biomarker should change independently with chronological age and reflect physiological age and functional capacity.
5) Assessment of the biomarker should be non-lethal in animal systems and should cause minimal trauma in humans, allowing for repeated measurements.
6) The biomarker should be reproducible and measurable during a relatively short time interval compared to the lifespan of the animal.

Subsequently, in 2004, a simpler set of criteria for biomarkers of aging was recommended by Butler et al. [208]:

1) The biomarker should predict the outcome of a wide range of age-sensitive tests in multiple physiological and behavioral domains in an age-coherent way and do so, better than chronological age.
2) It should predict remaining longevity at an age and do so for most of the specific illnesses that afflict the species under study.
3) Its measurement should not alter life expectancy or the outcome of subsequent tests or other age-sensitive tests.

The second criterion suggests that biomarkers of aging will also be biomarkers of age-related diseases rather than merely measures of degenerative changes. This is contentious because aging is thought to be a distinct process with specific pathways [26].

The American Federation for Aging Research has also proposed that a biomarker of aging should fulfill certain criteria, which were reviewed by Johnson in 2006 [209]:

1) The biomarker must be a good predictor of the rate of aging. In other words, it should tell exactly where a person is in their total lifespan and how many miles on the clock they have left. It must certainly be a better predictor of lifespan than chronological age.
2) It should monitor an underlying process of aging, and not the effects of disease.
3) It is also suggested that the biomarker can be tested repeatedly, without harming the individual. For instance, a blood test or an imaging technique would be required.
4) It needs to be measurable in humans as well as in laboratory animals. It must be indicative of a process that acts both in humans and laboratory animals such as mice, so that it can be tested on animal models before being tested on humans.

Nevertheless, even if a candidate biomarker of aging could be validated in model organisms, it remains unclear whether it would apply equally well in humans. Although several candidates have been examined, biomarkers capable of fulfilling the above-mentioned criteria are generally either lacking or proven insufficient [150, 210].

1.10.1 Physiological Biomarkers

Physiological biomarkers of aging comprise perceived age, body mass index, grip strength, systolic blood pressure, lipid concentrations, cognitive function, and lens opacity [206, 211, 212]. Furthermore, geriatric assessments [213] and measurements of frailty [100, 214] have also been proposed as complex aging biomarkers.

Biological markers that are capable of measuring inflammation, oxidative stress, protein glycation, cellular senescence, and hormonal deregulation have also been investigated for their potential as better predictors of biological age [212].

1.10.2 Inflammatory Biomarkers

The immune response in humans is a defense mechanism that can protect and respond to hazardous environmental exposures; for instance, infectious agents. The immune system does this in two ways; via an innate (or natural) response and an acquired (or adaptive) response [215]. The innate immunity includes a cellular response; for instance, macrophages and T-cells that secrete IL-6 [216], and a non-cellular response, comprising of C-reactive protein (CRP) and complementary cascade components [217]. Therefore, IL-6 and CRP are peripheral blood markers of inflammation.

IL-6 and CRP are non-specific. Nevertheless, abnormal levels have been suggested to indicate clinical or subclinical levels of chronic inflammation [218], which plays a key role in the aging process. Moreover, senescent cells, which are subject to inherent growth arrest and accumulate in tissues with age, have also been identified to secrete pro-inflammatory cytokines; for instance, interleukins [120]. Indeed, individuals with elevated levels of IL-6 have been demonstrated to have a significantly greater risk of developing disabilities of mobility, restraining them from activities of daily living over a four-year period [214] ostensibly due to elevated levels of underlying senescence. CRP has also been demonstrated to be an independent risk factor. Specifically, it has been linked to a two-fold risk of mortality in a cohort of higher-functioning elderly patients [219]. Although increased levels of both IL-6 and CRP were linked to higher concurrent risk of functional impairment, final levels of each biomarker appeared to be more important in determining the risk of subsequent events of cardiovascular disease and mortality than change over time [220]. Additionally, individuals from the 1958 British birth cohort with a high CRP score had a greater mortality risk in comparison to those with lower CRP scores [221]. The LIFEPATH project now aims to further understand the socioeconomic differences in health and some primary evidence has suggested that CRP is a very strong candidate for accurately predicting the lifespan [222].

1.10.3 Biomarkers of Oxidative Stress

In agreement with the free radical theory of aging [86], a number of ROS can be produced as a result of oxidative stress. These molecules are continuously being formed in cells and play key roles in a number of signaling pathways and the immune response [187]. ROS are removed from the cells by numerous antioxidant defense mechanisms. Oxidative stress is the imbalance between oxidative metabolism and antioxidant defenses. Throughout the lifespan, the accumulation of cellular damage that is caused by ROS has been proposed as an important factor that drives the aging process. Indeed, mitochondria from shorter-lived species have been indicated to produce higher amounts of ROS than mitochondria from longer-lived species [189–191].

Thus, several potential biomarkers of oxidative stress have been proposed. For instance, 8-hydroxydeoxyguanosine (8-OHdG) is produced when guanine, one of the four DNA nucleosides, is damaged by oxidative damage [192]. This molecule is excreted in urine and has been shown to increase with smoking [193]. Additionally, its levels have been indicated to be inversely associated with lifespan [194]. Moreover, senescent cells have also been associated with high levels of intracellular ROS and oxidative damage accumulation [122]. Shortening of the telomeres, which cap the DNA at the end of chromosomes, has been considered one of the primary causes of cellular replicative senescence and this process has been indicated to increase by oxidative stress [123].

Furthermore, the amino acid homocysteine, which is derived from dietary methionine, is thought to both increase the production of ROS and the ability of cells to protect themselves from ROS-induced damage [124]. Restriction of methionine consumption has been associated with increased lifespan [125]. Specifically, ample evidence exists to support the thesis that aging can be slowed down in rodents and monkeys, and their lifespan extended, either by caloric restriction or by diets which are low in methionine [126–130]. Mimetics of calorie restriction such as resveratrol, have also resulted in an increase in mitochondria density which might explain the prolonged lifespan [131, 132]. Thus, decreased mitochondrial density and higher ROS levels have been linked to shorter lifespans.

1.10.4 Advanced Glycation End Products (AGEs)

AGEs are proteins and lipids that are non-enzymatically glycated and that oxidize when in contact with sugars. AGEs can be either produced in cells or absorbed through diet. The formation of AGEs is also the outcome of complex ROS-dependent reactions that occur within cells [133]. Interestingly, cell activation by these AGEs leads to the generation of significantly more ROS resulting in oxidative damage. Accumulation of the AGE carboxy-methyl lysine (CML) has been linked to chronological age and age-related diseases; for instance, cataracts [134]. CML has also been indicated to be associated with diabetes disease progression and with an increased risk of developing retinopathy, nephrology, and cardiac disease [135].

1.10.5 Damage-Associated Molecular Pattern Molecules (DAMPs)

Cells which are dead, dying, or injured because of stress, release and expose on their cell surface certain endogenous molecules which are termed DAMPs. The DAMPs act as an alarm and warn the immune system to respond to tissue damage and promote repair [136, 137]. It has been indicated that DAMPs, including high mobility group box 1 (HMGB1), histones, S100, and heat shock proteins, play a significant intracellular and extracellular role that is location-dependent [138]. These molecules provide the platform for molecular interactions that have been tightly linked to common hallmarks of aging and cancer, comprising genomic instability, epigenetic alteration, aberrant telomeres, reprogrammed metabolism, impaired degradation, and impaired immune-inflammatory response [43, 138, 139].

Specifically, DAMPs can sense and mediate stress through cell surface receptors, intracellular recognition receptors, or following endocytic uptake. Additionally, circulating levels of DAMPs have been indicated to increase with aging and disease [140–142]. Thus, the DAMP hypothesis complements other theories that explain the features of aging, and therefore, DAMPs have the potential to be developed into useful diagnostic biomarkers, risk predictors, and theragnostics (i.e., treatment strategies that combine therapeutics with diagnostics) of clinical value. Hence, DAMPs represent ideal biomarkers of aging and may also provide a target for interventions to be developed in the field of aging and age-associated diseases [138].

1.10.6 Cellular Senescence

Cellular senescence was first described in 1961 when Hayflick noted that cell proliferation in the cell culture of human fibroblasts gradually declined over time [143]. Eventually, all cells in the culture lost the ability to divide, although they stayed viable and metabolically active for a long time afterward. They did so in a state of growth arrest described as cellular senescence. It has been proposed that this process resembles the aging process that occurs within systems and organisms.

Cellular senescence in primary somatic cells was demonstrated to be accompanied by attrition of the telomeres [144], which are the nucleoprotein complexes that cap and protect the ends of chromosomes. The DNA component of telomeres has been found to shorten as a function of replication in most human somatic cells [145]. Therefore, telomere length is a good indicator of a cell's replicative age, also termed cellular age. Accelerated telomere attrition has also been shown to be a feature of many pathologies, including cancer, vascular dementia, diabetes, and cardiovascular disease [146, 147].

Cellular senescence is also accompanied by the expression, or appearance of, markers, such as cyclin-dependent kinase inhibitor 2A (CDKN2A), cyclin-dependent kinase inhibitor 1A (CDKN1A), and senescence-associated β-galactosidase (SA β-gal). P16Ink4a, which is encoded by CDKN2A, appears to act as a tumor suppressor protein and maintains cells in a state of growth arrest during the establishment and maintenance of cellular senescence [148–150]. p21Cip1 (also called p21Waf1), which is the cognate protein of CDKN1A, is a p53-dependent cyclin-dependent kinase inhibitor that functions to regulate cell-cycle progression at the S phase [151–154]. SA β-gal activity, measured at pH 6.0, has also been suggested to be a reliable indicator of the switch mechanism used by cells to enter the senescent phenotype [155–157].

Primarily CDKN2A has been associated with senescence in cellular, animal, and human studies. Specifically, increasing levels of CDKN2A transcriptional expression (i.e., CDKN2A mRNA levels) have been found to be associated with increasing chronological age, both in solid organs and peripheral blood leucocytes [158, 159]. CDKN2A has also proven more effective in predicting physiological functional capacity [159–161] and its levels of expression have also been reported to positively associate with levels of pro-inflammatory cytokines such as IL-6 [158]. It has also been suggested that CDKN2A can better fulfill Baker and Sprott's criteria than other proposed biomarkers of aging including telomere length [162].

It has also been discussed that all these markers operate within the functional framework of the mitochondrion, telomere, and ribosome (MTR) trinity of aging [163, 164]. This suggests that aging is associated with interactions between cellular damage responses and any associated fuel utilization and energy production mechanisms. Thus, the level of damage accrued, and the level of energy expenditure required to facilitate repair dictate whether a cell will live (functioning or senescent) or die (apoptosis) [164, 165]. Consequently, the number of cells that die or become senescent correlates directly with organ functional capability and biological age.

Telomere length and expression levels of CDKN2A, CDKN1A, and SA β-gal will be discussed in more detail below for their role in aging and their predictive value of biological age.

1.10.7 Telomere Length

Telomere length has been proposed as a biomarker of aging repeatedly [166]. Given its association with chronological age and its role in cellular senescence, telomeres have been thought to be of importance in assessing cellular aging. This is due to telomeres shortening in primary cells with successive rounds of cellular proliferation and increasing chronological age. Therefore, measuring their attrition, which results as part of the end replication problem, allows their length to represent cellular aging [167, 168].

Telomeres are specialized nucleo-protein complexes, which cap the ends of eukaryotic chromosomes. The basic telomere structure consists of telomeric DNA and a series of bound proteins, which are vital for both the regulation of the telomere length and the functioning of the telomere [167]. Telomeres safeguard chromosomal integrity during cellular division by preventing DNA degradation at the chromosome terminus, due to the DNA polymerase complex being incapable of replicating to the end of the chromosomes. Without telomeres, this would result in significant loss of vital genetic information which is essential to sustain cellular activity. Through this process, the telomeres also act as an anti-oncogenic mechanism [169].

Telomere shortening occurs in almost all mitotic tissues, including peripheral blood leucocytes [158]. However, telomere attrition can be counteracted by the action of the enzyme telomerase, which is a reverse transcriptase that adds DNA repeats in the telomere region [167]. Telomerase is normally inactive in primary somatic cells but is functional in germ cells, stem cells, and lymphocyte subsets. Consequently, only germ cells, stem cells and activated leucocytes maintain their telomere length through the action of telomerase [169]. It has been reported that the action of telomerase can be employed to bypass cellular senescence in human cells [125]. Indeed, mice engineered to lack telomerase age prematurely, and this acceleration of aging can be reversed by reactivating the telomerase [170]. However, recently, it has been suggested that telomerase may also accelerate the telomere-associated aging process, through the paradoxical action of telomerase reverse transcriptase (TERT) and the gene that encodes telomerase [171]. Hence, the exact link between TERT, telomerase, and aging remains to be elucidated.

Gradual loss of telomeric DNA in dividing cells can result in cellular senescence due to the telomere length reaching a critical point. Cook and Smith were the first to link telomeres to the aging process as well as suggested a framework to explain the telomere attrition process and the Hayflick limit [172]. Thus, telomere shortening due to the end replication problem has also been suggested as a potential mechanism for a biological clock to determine cellular activity [173]. Indeed, it has been demonstrated that telomere length could be employed as a mitotic clock to study human hematopoietic stem cells [174]. However, the exact relationship between aging and telomere length has yet to be fully understood.

Telomere length fulfills several, but not all, of the criteria for a biomarker of aging. Although it decreases progressively with chronological age, considerable variability exists between individuals. Additionally, it only registers the life cycle of proliferative cells [175]. Hence, there is much debate as to whether it is a useful biomarker of aging [176].

Telomere length has been shown to be the longest at birth while shortening rapidly until 5 years of age and then remaining stable until early adulthood followed by a more gradual reduction thereafter [177]. This observation suggests that early life factors may constitute important determinants of adult telomere length. While high telomerase activity is likely in the rapidly dividing fetal cells, little is known about telomere length changes in utero. Evidence has suggested that antenatal stress and impaired intrauterine growth could be implicated in the acceleration of telomere attrition. Thus, shortened telomeres being present at birth may then result in shorter telomeres during adulthood [178]. A link has also been demonstrated to exist between dysfunctional growth during early life and the onset of disease in late life. The Barker Hypothesis has suggested that events leading to limited growth, while in utero may program the fetus for increased risk of adult cardiovascular disease among other conditions resulting in premature death [179]. It has been reported that adverse intrauterine conditions, such as those caused while mothers experience severe stress during pregnancy, are associated with shorter telomeres in cells of different tissues [180]. Therefore, stress during pregnancy has been associated with shorter telomere lengths in adult life. This restricted growth has been indicated to increase ROS and oxidative stress [181]. Therefore, a single measurement of telomere length could be representative of the combined effects of both telomere length at birth and the subsequent rate of attrition influenced by multiple factors. This observation agrees with the life-course approach to aging [101].

It has additionally been observed that telomere attrition is accelerated by disease. Hence, at a given chronological age, the average leucocyte telomere length in diseased individuals has been reported to be shorter than non-diseased individuals of the same chronological age [182, 183]. This has been suggested to arise as a result of elevated levels of oxidative stress increasing with pathology, superimposed on top of the end replication problem [184]. Another study has shown that those individuals over the age of 60 who had shorter telomeres also had poorer survival rates. This has been attributed to a higher mortality rate resulting from heart disease and infectious disease [185]. These results support the hypothesis that telomere attrition in humans contributes to mortality in a number of age-related diseases. However, only a small number of studies have examined the relationship between telomere attrition and age-related physiological functional decline. Data derived from these studies have been suggested to be equivocal, while also lacking statistical power [186].

It has been shown that shortened telomere length is associated with increased mortality risk [185]. Nevertheless, others have failed to show an analogous association [187]. Numerous other studies have also established the inverse relationship between telomere length and chronological aging [177, 194–196]. In the meanwhile, a systematic review has demonstrated that the association between telomere length, investigated in peripheral blood leucocytes, and age was a consistent observation in the literature [197]. This has been proposed to be the outcome of methodological issues and multiple confounders affecting epidemiological studies [150, 176]. Methodological issues have also beset the use of telomere length in inter-individual and inter-laboratory comparisons in epidemiological studies [183].

Moreover, human aging is heterogeneous and model systems investigating it have failed to fully account for the contribution of the exposome, including socio-economic, psychosocial, lifestyle, and nutritional factors [67, 198]. Therefore, telomere length has been proven to be a weak biomarker of aging and thus appears better employed as a composite biomarker [199].

1.10.8 CDKN2A/p16Ink4a, CDKN1A/p21Cip1, and SA *β*-gal

More robust biomarkers of aging are starting to emerge. The CDKN2A gene transcript is one such promising candidate. CDKN2A is cognate for the p16Ink4a tumor suppressor protein and acts as a cell cycle stop signal [148, 149]. Consequently, CDKN2A is a key effector of cellular senescence and the more CDKN2A is expressed by cells, tissues, or organs, the more biologically aged these are and the less functional capacity they are capable of exhibiting [26, 200].

Indeed, naturally occurring p16Ink4a-positive senescent cells shorten healthy lifespan in mice, while their clearance delays age-associated pathologies, as demonstrated in a mouse model of progeria caused by BubR1 insufficiency [201, 202]. Furthermore, late-life clearance of p16Ink4a-positive senescent cells can attenuate the progression of already established age-related disorders [202, 203]. Another study has also elegantly demonstrated that transplanting relatively small numbers of senescent cells into young mice is sufficient to cause persistent physical dysfunction as well as to spread cellular senescence to other host tissues. Transplantation of even fewer senescent cells had the same effect in older recipient animals and was accompanied by reduced survival indicating the potency of senescent cells to shorten both the health span and the lifespan [204]. The adverse effects have been demonstrated to be averted when a senolytic[b] cocktail, consisting of dasatinib plus quercetin, was employed. This caused selective elimination of senescent cells, decreased the amount of naturally occurring senescent cells, and their secretion of frailty-related pro-inflammatory cytokines was minimized in explants of human adipose tissue. Moreover, intermittent oral administration of senolytics, to both senescent cell–transplanted young mice and naturally aged mice, alleviated the physical dysfunction, and increased post-treatment survival rates by 36%, while also reducing mortality risk to 65% [204].

These findings have provided proof-of-concept evidence that senescent cells can cause physical dysfunction, generate age-related phenotypes, and decrease survival, while senolytic agents, which are capable of safely removing senescent cells, can enhance both the health span and the lifespan. This is also well supported by a series of studies which have demonstrated that organ function correlates more strongly with CDKN2A levels of expression than with chronological age and telomere length [159–161, 231].

In addition, it has also been suggested that the CDKN2A levels of expression elevate with disease-associated stress [205, 223, 224]. Cellular senescence thus provides a link between premature aging and inflammation, which is a key component of autoimmune and other chronic pathologies [26]. Indeed, senescent cells, which highly express CDKN2A, have been indicated to up-regulate pro-inflammatory cytokines as part of the senescence-associated secretory phenotype (SASP) which has been defined by the increased secretion of various secretory molecules including inflammatory cytokines, chemokines, growth factors, and extracellular vesicles, contributing to tumor suppression, wound healing, embryonic development but also tumorigenesis promotion [225, 226]. It is worth highlighting that non-autonomous cellular senescence processes may also be responsible for spreading the effects of a stressor systemically, thus contributing to the generation of allostatic load [49]. This is often reflected through a systemic increase in the expression of the CDKN2 locus despite a stressor being present in a single

[b]senolytic: a substance that selectively eliminates senescent cells in the body and promotes health span and longevity.

tissue or organ. For instance, incidents of infection with the chronic hepatitis C virus are associated with higher mortality rates due to disease-induced non-cell-autonomous senescence and the associated accelerated biological aging underlined by CDKN2 locus upregulation [227]. The infected individuals experience increased levels of cellular senescence, which coincides with chronic inflammation and oxidative stress. Likewise, patients infected with the human immunodeficiency virus (HIV) also display accelerated biological aging [223]. This is consistent with data suggesting that the expression of biomarkers, which are associated with senescence, elevates with infection [228]. Non-cell-autonomous senescence and paracrine[c] mediators of biological aging may thus provide a novel field for the study of systemic sclerosis, where relevant data remain sparse [229, 230].

Furthermore, a recent study has elegantly provided evidence that allografts are biologically older, centering on the CDKN2 and CDKN1 locus, producing less successful outcomes in renal transplantation and poorer post-transplant performance. Specifically, the CDKN2A and p16Ink4a expression levels were demonstrated to correlate strongly with delayed graft function occurrence and long-term allograft function post-transplantation [231]. The authors have suggested that underlying the associated reduced functional and repair capacity of the biologically aged renal allografts is allostatic overload caused by a significantly greater degree of allostatic load that has accumulated over time [231].

CDKN1A is another biomarker that has been discussed for its use as a biomarker of cellular aging and senescence, due to its role in cell cycle control [151–154]. Specifically, CDKN1A has been demonstrated to be upregulated in renal senescence [161]. Moreover, CDKN1A and p21Cip1 expression has been indicated to increase in a mouse model of Fuchs' endothelial corneal dystrophy, which is also associated with accelerated senescence [232]. In addition, another study has demonstrated that p21Cip1 was responsible for promoting the senescence of lens epithelial cells and cataract formation in BubR1 progeroid mice [233]. It is also worth

[c]paracrine: a mode of cell signaling where cells release signaling molecules (such as hormones or growth factors) into the extracellular fluid to affect nearby cells.

noting that the levels of CDKN1A expression have been shown to display significant positive correlations with the expression levels of CDKN2A [159, 234]. Therefore, CDKN1A is an important indicator of cellular senescence and aging.

SA β-gal activity has also been considered a valuable biomarker of replicative senescence that comes with aging and has become one of the most used biomarkers of cellular aging [53, 155, 235, 300]. For instance, it has been observed that the irreversibly growth-arrested normal somatic cells, due to extensive population doublings in culture, are defined by SA β-gal activity detectable at pH 6.0 [155] and increased expression levels of p53, p21Cip1, and p16Ink4a [236]. It has also been shown that during human fibroblast cultures, SA β-gal activity was low during the exponential growth phase with a defined significant increase in activity when the growth speed of the culture decreased as a high passage number was reached. This increase in SA β-gal activity was also a better predictor for the onset of the decreased growth speed than the chronological lifespan of the culture, which was expressed in population doublings [237]. SA β-gal activity, along with CDKN2A and p16Ink4a expression levels, have also been demonstrated to detect the accumulation of cellular senescence in rats, during the development, growth, and aging of the kidney despite the absence of telomere shortening [238]. SA β-gal has also been indicated to increase with stress. Specifically, its activity has been demonstrated to reversibly increase in quiescent cells induced by either serum starvation or confluence, while stress induced by H_2O_2 caused an irreversible increase [239].

However, it needs to be highlighted that not all cells that undergo replicative senescence express SA β-gal. For instance, it has been indicated that fibroblasts, derived from patients with autosomal recessive G(M1)-gangliosidosis, which expresses defective lysosomal β-gal, were not capable of expressing SA β-gal at late passages even though these cells underwent replicative senescence [240]. Furthermore, SA-β-gal activity alone is not sufficient on its own to allow conclusions to be drawn with confidence that cells are senescent, as positive staining can also occur in other biological contexts, such as in non-proliferating premalignant cells, in human and murine pancreatic intraepithelial neoplasia [241, 242].

Consequently, these observations suggest that SA β-gal is not essential for cellular senescence to be established and thus confounding factors may pose certain limitations to its use as a biomarker of aging.

In an attempt to overcome limitations, recent studies have demonstrated that conventional SA β-gal staining assays, combined with the use of additional biomarkers, such as p16Ink4a, Ki67, BrdU, and HMGB1, allow for the successful identification and quantification of senescent cells in tumors, fibrotic tissues and normal tissues of young and aged mice [243].

1.10.9 Fetuin-A

Fetuin-A is a serum protein that is secreted by the liver. It has multiple diverse effects throughout the body, and it has been demonstrated to inhibit vascular calcification, and it may be capable of controlling inflammatory processes [244, 245]. In addition, it has also been suggested to induce insulin resistance in muscle and fat and has been linked to clinical and sub-clinical type 2 diabetes and cardiovascular disease [246]. Moreover, it has also been linked to a reduced risk of cognitive function impairment and was found to be of low levels in Alzheimer's disease patients [247].

It has also been suggested that decreased fetuin-A accompanied by telomere attrition can be an indicator of accelerated biological aging [248]. Indeed, telomere attrition associated with inflammation and low fetuin-A levels have been associated with the accelerated aging phenotype and the increased mortality risk observed in chronic kidney disease patients who undergo hemodialysis [58, 249].

1.10.10 Phosphate

Control of phosphate metabolism also appears crucial in regulating aging. It has been demonstrated that mice that are mutant or deficient in Klotho, which is an anti-aging factor that regulates the metabolism of phosphate, exhibit a premature aging phenotype that is accompanied by shorter lifespan, osteoporosis, arteriosclerosis and chronic kidney disease-associated mineral and bone disorder [47, 250]. The transmembrane form of Klotho functions as a co-receptor for fibroblast growth factor-23 (FGF23) and together these are responsible for regulating phosphate as well as calcium and vitamin D metabolism [251]. Specifically, excess phosphate is excreted into urine and this process is mediated by FGF23 acting on a bone-kidney endocrine axis. FGF23 also reduces the level of vitamin D in the serum in order to suppress intestinal phosphate absorption [252]. However, during chronic kidney disease, a decreased Klotho expression is experienced from the early stages of the disease, and this continues to decline further with disease progression causing FGF-23 resistance. Thus, phosphate cannot be efficiently removed, and the associated hyperphosphatemia drives the premature aging phenotype [253]. Specifically, the increased phosphate levels in the uremic serum exert their cytotoxic effect by forming insoluble nanoparticles with calcium and fetuin-A termed calciprotein particles. The serum phosphate and calciprotein particles, which are highly bioactive ligands, have been identified as capable of inducing osteogenic transformation of vascular smooth muscle cells, cell death of vascular endothelial cells, and renal tubular epithelial cells, while also significantly increasing the risk of mortality among people with chronic kidney disease [254, 255]. Hence, phosphate has been regarded as a pro-aging factor in mammals [256]. Recently, it has also been shown that the ectonucleotide pyrophosphatase/phosphodiesterase 1 (Enpp1) is essential for Klotho expression under phosphate overload. Hence, Enpp1 has also been suggested to regulate aging via Klotho expression [257].

1.10.11 Sirtuins

Sirtuins are a family of proteins whose function has been linked to cellular metabolism in a number of tissues, such as the liver, muscle, adipose tissue, heart, and endothelium. It has been indicated that sirtuins do not only play a role as energy status sensors but also protect cells from metabolic stresses. Additionally, sirtuins have been implicated in preserving genomic stability. An association with aging has been suggested through the observation that sirtuins coordinate a range of cellular responses that have frequently been observed to be dysregulated with aging [178, 258, 259]. For instance, Sirtuin 2 has been indicated to play a key role in the repair of DNA and has also been found to regulate genes that their expression alters during aging in yeast [259]. Overexpression of Sirtuin 6 in transgenic mice has also allowed for an increased lifespan of 15% in males [178]. Sirtuin 1 has also been indicated to behave in humans similarly to yeast Sirtuin 2 by regulating the biogenesis of mitochondria [219].

1.10.12 DNA Methylation and Epigenetic Clocks

Epigenetics can be defined as the study of heritable changes in gene expression that are not the result of DNA sequence changes. It was first suggested that between the genotype and phenotype, and connecting them to each other, lies a whole complex of developmental processes, called the epigenotype [260]. Epigenetic changes; for instance, DNA methylation (DNAm), appear to regulate gene expression by switching genes on and off. Epigenetic silencing is responsible for turning genes off contributing to differential gene expression. Silencing might also partly explain why genetic twins are not phenotypically identical. In addition, epigenetics plays an essential role in the inactivation of the X-chromosome in female mammals, which is required so that female mammals do not express twice the number of X-chromosome genes [261]. Thus, there is evidence of regulation of gene expression via epigenetic changes.

Within cells, there are three systems that can interact with each other and are responsible for silencing gene expression:

1) **DNA methylation**: A chemical process which adds methyl groups to DNA.
2) **Histone modifications**: Histones are proteins which can influence how chromatin is arranged, which in turn can determine whether the associated chromosomal DNA will be transcribed or not.
3) **RNA interference (RNAi) silencing**: RNAi molecules can also negatively affect gene expression.

DNA methylation involves the addition of a methyl group to the DNA nucleosides cytosine and adenine. The pattern of DNA methylation regulates the binding of proteins to target sites in the DNA. Thus, DNA methylation can generate changes in chromatin organization and ultimately gene expression. For instance, methylation at gene promoter regions can silence gene expression. Research investigating saliva samples from 34 pairs of identical male twins between the ages of 21 and 55 indicated that 88 sites exist on the DNA where DNA methylation strongly correlated with chronological age [262]. The levels of global DNA methylation have also been demonstrated to correlate with frailty status in middle and advanced-age individuals, but not with chronological age [263]. A follow-up study has also revealed that deterioration in frailty status was linked with significantly reduced global DNA methylation levels [263]. A potential role for age-related changes in the methylation status of CpG islands (i.e., short stretches of DNA in which the CG sequence frequency is higher than other regions) in the development of frailty has also been demonstrated [264].

Moreover, DNA methylation age has been proposed as a measure of the cumulative effect of an epigenetic maintenance system. Specifically, this novel epigenetic clock can be used to address a host of questions in developmental biology, cell differentiation, tissue homeostasis, cancer, and aging research [265]. In accordance with the epigenetic clock, DNA methylation age is close to 0 for embryonic and induced pluripotent stem cells, it correlates well with cell passage number at the cellular level, it gives rise to a highly heritable measure of age acceleration, and it is also applicable to chimpanzee tissues [57]. Recently, six types of potential biological age estimators, comprising epigenetic clocks, telomere length, transcriptomic-based, proteomic-based, and metabolomic-based estimators and composite biomarkers, have been cross-compared. The outcome of the study has indicated that the epigenetic clock is the most promising molecular estimator of biological age [266], while for age estimation DNA methylation is the most promising age-predictive biomarker [267]. Epigenetic age estimators are sets of CpGs (i.e., CpG dinucleotides) that coupled with a mathematical algorithm can estimate the age of a DNA source, including cells, tissues, and organs. The estimated age, also referred to as epigenetic age or more precisely as DNAm age, is not only a reflection of chronological age but also of the biological age of the DNA source [265]. Interestingly, although senescent cells can also exhibit methylation changes and these have been recorded in some specific CpGs, these changes are in general different from age-related CpGs [268]. Hence, it has been suggested that cellular senescence and epigenetic aging are distinct phenomena [269]. Further evidence to support this hypothesis has been generated by studies which have demonstrated that irradiation-induced senescent cells do not exhibit epigenetic aging [57, 269], while immortalized cells, which do not undergo replicative senescence, continue to exhibit epigenetic aging [269, 270]. What cellular senescence and methylation aging can become entwined remains to be elucidated.

Recently, a novel epigenetic biomarker of phenotypic aging, termed DNAm PhenoAge, strongly outperformed the first generation of DNAm age estimators for predicting a variety of aging outcomes, including all-cause mortality, cancer, health span, physical functioning, and disease [271]. An increase in the epigenetic age has also been associated with increased activation of pro-inflammatory and interferon pathways as well as decreased activation of the transcriptional and translational machinery, DNA damage response, and mitochondrial signatures [271]. Therefore, both DNAm age and DNAm PhenoAge have been established as epigenetic biomarkers of aging that are better suited for satisfying the formerly elusive properties of molecular biomarkers of aging [265].

1.10.13 Non-Coding RNAs

Finally, recent evidence has suggested that non-coding RNAs are key determinants of biological aging processes. Specifically, microRNAs (miRNAs) can be valuable as potential circulatory biomarkers of aging. They may also provide a mechanism which mediates the spread of allostatic load across the body over time, ultimately reflecting the immunological health and physiological status of tissues and organs within an individual [49]. The interplay between extracellular vesicle microRNAs and aging processes remains relatively unexplored, although circulating microRNAs have been linked to the regulation of a range of physiological and pathological processes and offer insight into mechanistic determinants of health span.

Although there is a plethora of evidence for potential biomarkers of aging, it has been advocated that no single or simple combination of biomarkers is likely to deliver a clinically valuable estimate of biological age [272, 273]. This suggestion adopts the thesis that biological aging results from the deterioration of multiple systems and no single biological or genetic cause of aging exists. From this hypothesis, we are led to conclude that a panel of biomarkers that reflect the functional capacity of an array of key systems within an individual may be required to evaluate biological age. Additionally, the complexity that underlines the aging process means that the search for candidate biomarkers will probably continue assuming that biological clocks indeed exist. It is also worth noting that biomarkers may undergo changes over different critical points in life. In other words, biomarkers of aging that are of predictive value early in life may not be as predictive later in life and vice versa. Therefore, instead of selecting a single panel of biomarkers to be examined periodically over the life course, it may be more sensible to assess a large variety of biomarkers treating each one as a separate tool of different predictive value, depending on the time point in life at which it is examined.

Finally, despite advances in geroscience, which have allowed us to better understand and predict how we age, there is still a pressing need to better understand the mechanisms that drive aging throughout the life course and not just in the latter half of life.

1.11 Telomeres' Associations with Diseases

Chronic kidney disease, which is a debilitating and life-shortening disease whose prevalence is increasing globally, is a long-term condition that is characterized by a gradual loss of kidney function. Usually, other conditions that put a strain on the kidneys are responsible for the development of chronic kidney disease. In addition, it can often be the result of a combination of problems including hypertension, diabetes, elevated levels of cholesterol, and kidney infections, among many others [274, 275, 299].

Clinicians use a scale to define the severity of chronic kidney disease. This relies on the estimation of glomerular filtration rate and albuminuria [276–279]. According to this method, stage 1 chronic kidney disease patients demonstrate normal to high glomerular filtration rates, while stage 4 is associated with severely decreased glomerular filtration rates, and stage 5 corresponds to kidney failure [276].

Chronic kidney disease has also been defined as an independent risk factor for cardiovascular disease, cognitive dysfunction, hospitalization, and all-cause mortality. Interestingly, the risk of developing cardiovascular disease and all-cause mortality has been reported higher than the risk for progression to end-stage renal disease in older patients [280–282]. At the other end of the spectrum, when chronic kidney disease occurs at a much younger age and progresses to end-stage renal disease, the risk of cardiovascular mortality increases exponentially [280, 283]. Hence, this suggested that chronic kidney disease could be a clinical model of premature aging [58, 284].

Premature aging is a common feature of chronic kidney disease and other chronic diseases; for instance, heart failure, chronic obstructive pulmonary disease, HIV infection, and rheumatoid arthritis [58, 26]. Progressive accumulation of deleterious changes over time, impairment of physiologic functions, and increased risk of disease and mortality are tightly associated with premature aging [284]. Indeed, clinical, and pathophysiological evidence suggest that premature aging is involved in the pathogenesis of systemic complications of many chronic organ diseases, which result in analogous phenotypes including premature vascular aging, osteoporosis, and muscle wasting [59]. Hence, improving the understanding of fundamental aging processes may be important in comprehending the complications associated with organ diseases such as chronic kidney disease.

Chronic kidney disease is responsible for promoting cellular senescence, and thus a premature aging phenotype, through toxic alterations in the internal milieu. Several mechanisms are accountable for these changes including DNA and mitochondria damage, increased reactive oxygen species generation, persistent inflammation, stem cell exhaustion, decreased klotho expression, telomere attrition, and altered nutrient sensing [68, 284]. Indeed, all nine hallmarks of aging [43] were found relevant for the pathogenesis of premature aging processes in chronic kidney disease [59]. Accelerated aging has also been associated with elevated levels of serum phosphate [285], which is increased in the uremic serum of chronic kidney disease patients. In addition, it has been indicated that, besides a sedentary lifestyle, psychosocial and socioeconomic factors, four major mechanisms underlie the premature aging phenotype that is caused by the manifestation of chronic kidney disease [58]:

1. An increase in allostatic load.
2. Activation of the stress resistance response.
3. Activation of age-promoting mechanisms.
4. Impairment of anti-aging pathways.

Apoptosis, cellular senescence, and osteogenic transformation have also been reported as key mediators of the progeric phenotype [286–291]. Nevertheless, to appropriately test these factors in model organisms has proven challenging. Therefore, the progeric vascular phenotype has been investigated directly in man. Several studies have associated single nucleotide polymorphisms on chromosome 9p21, close to the CDKN2A and CDKN2B genes, with risk for cardiovascular disease in the general population [292–296]. As the CDKN2A and CDKN2B protein derivatives are functionally involved in maintaining cells in a state of growth arrest, and cellular senescence increases with age, expression of CDKN2A increases as a function of increasing cellular stress and organismal aging [200, 297]. Indeed, CDKN2A gene expression appears to be superior to telomere length as a biomarker of biological age [160–162, 199]. Thus, elevated CDKN2A expression correlates with increased biological aging as well as increased frequency of a frailty phenotype [223].

1.12 Telomeres' Role in Aging

Either at the organismal or cellular level, aging can be defined by loss of functional capacity over time [43]. It also needs to be highlighted that aging is not a passive process [45], but one actively regulated by distinct molecular pathways layered below a loss of functional physiological capability and correlated with frailty and increased likelihood of death [26, 107]. The underpinning mechanisms are considered to be evolutionarily conserved across taxa [46, 47] and have been reflected in twelve distinct hallmarks [33]. These comprise telomere shortening, genomic instability, epigenetic alterations, loss of proteostasis, deregulated nutrient sensing, mitochondrial dysfunction, cellular senescence, stem cell exhaustion, altered intercellular communication, dysbiosis, chronic inflammation, and disabled macroautophagy [43].

As far as the telomere's role in aging is concerned, telomere attrition has been identified as a key mechanism of aging. Specifically, replicative DNA polymerases are unable to completely copy the telomeric DNA and with time, after several rounds of cell division, telomeres undergo substantial shortening. This shortening then induces DNA damage and genomic instability at the end of chromosomes throughout life and finally leads to either apoptosis or cell senescence, hence contributing to aging and age-related diseases [33]. The speed of telomere shortening can then be associated with either accelerated or decelerated aging phenotypes, health span, and longevity.

References

1. Nations, U. (2013). *World Population Aging 2013*. New York: United Nations.
2. Gavrilov, L. A., & Heuveline, P. (2003). Aging of population. In P. Demeny & G. McNicoll (Eds.), *The Encyclopedia of Population* (pp. 32–37). Macmillan, New York.
3. Statistics, O. f. N. (2012). *Population Ageing in the United Kingdom, its Constituent Countries and the European Union*. London: Office for National Statistics.
4. Tulchinsky, T. H., & Varavikova, E. A. (2009). *The New Public Health*. 2nd ed. Burlington, MA: Elsevier academic press.
5. Fontana, L. (2009). Modulating human aging and age-associated diseases, *Biochimica et Biophysica Acta*, **1790**, pp. 1133–1138. https://doi.org/10.1016/j.bbagen.2009.02.002

6. Government, S. (2008). *Equally Well: Report of the Ministerial Task Force on Inequalities*. Scottish Government: Edinburgh.
7. Caldwell, J. C., Caldwell, B. K., Caldwell, P., McDonald, P. F., & Schindlmayr, T. (2006). *Demographic Transition Theory*. https://doi.org/10.1007/978-1-4020–4498-4
8. Kinsella, K. G. (2005). Future longevity-demographic concerns and consequences, *J Am Geriatr Soc*, **53**, pp. S299–303. https://doi.org/10.1111/j.1532-5415.2005.53494.x
9. Bloom, D. E., Chatterji, S., Kowal, P., Lloyd-Sherlock, P., McKee, M., Rechel, B., *et al.* (2015). Macroeconomic implications of population ageing and selected policy responses, *Lancet*, **385**, pp. 649–657. https://doi.org/10.1016/s0140-6736(14)61464-1
10. Nations, U. (2002). *World Population Ageing: 1950–2050*. New York: United Nations Publications.
11. Suzman, R., Beard, J. R., Boerma, T., & Chatterji, S. (2015). Health in an ageing world-what do we know? *Lancet*, **385**, pp. 484–486. https://doi.org/10.1016/s0140-6736(14)61597-x
12. Mathers, C. D., Stevens, G. A., Boerma, T., White, R. A., & Tobias, M. I. (2015). Causes of international increases in older age life expectancy, *Lancet*, **385**, pp. 540–548. https://doi.org/10.1016/s0140-6736(14)60569-9
13. Carnes, B. A., Olshansky, S. J., & Hayflick, L. (2013). Can human biology allow most of us to become centenarians? *J Gerontol A Biol Sci Med Sci*, **68**, pp. 136–142. https://doi.org/10.1093/gerona/gls142
14. Cohen, J. E. (2003). Human population: the next half century, *Science*, **302**, pp. 1172–1175. https://doi.org/10.1126/science.1088665
15. Blomberg Jensen, M., Priskorn, L., Jensen, T. K., Juul, A., & Skakkebaek, N. E. (2015). Temporal trends in fertility rates: a nationwide registry-based study from 1901 to 2014, *PLoS One*, **10**, e0143722. https://doi.org/10.1371/journal.pone.0143722
16. Kowal, P., Chatterji, S., Naidoo, N., Biritwum, R., Fan, W., Lopez Ridaura, R., *et al.* (2012). Data resource profile: the World Health Organization Study on global AGEing and adult health (SAGE), *Int J Epidemiol*, **41**, pp. 1639–1649. https://doi.org/10.1093/ije/dys210
17. Suzman, R. (2010). Guest Editorial: The INDEPTH WHO-SAGE multicentre study on ageing, health and well-being among people aged 50 years and over in eight countries in Africa and Asia. *Global Health Action*, **3**, 10.3402/gha.v3403i3400.5480. https://doi.org/10.3402/gha.v3i0.5480

18. Kowal, P., Kahn, K., Ng, N., Naidoo, N., Abdullah, S., Bawah, A., *et al.* (2010). Ageing and adult health status in eight lower-income countries: the INDEPTH WHO-SAGE collaboration, *Glob Health Action*, **3**. https://doi.org/10.3402/gha.v3i0.5302
19. Ng, N., Kowal, P., Kahn, K., Naidoo, N., Abdullah, S., Bawah, A., *et al.* (2010). Health inequalities among older men and women in Africa and Asia: evidence from eight health and demographic surveillance system sites in the INDEPTH WHO-SAGE Study, *Glob Health Action*, **3**, pp. 96–107. https://doi.org/10.3402/gha.v3i0.5420
20. Beard, J. R., & Bloom, D. E. (2015). Towards a comprehensive public health response to population ageing, *Lancet*, **385**, pp. 658–661. https://doi.org/10.1016/s0140-6736(14)61461-6
21. Divo, M. J., Martinez, C. H., & Mannino, D. M. (2014). Ageing and the epidemiology of multimorbidity, *Eur Respir J*, **44**, pp. 1055–1068. https://doi.org/10.1183/09031936.00059814
22. Gems, D. (2015). The aging-disease false dichotomy: understanding senescence as pathology. *Frontiers in Genetics*, **6**, pp. 212. https://doi.org/10.3389/fgene.2015.00212
23. Ding, D., Lawson, K. D., Kolbe-Alexander, T. L., Finkelstein, E. A., Katzmarzyk, P. T., van Mechelen, W., *et al.* (2016). The economic burden of physical inactivity: a global analysis of major non-communicable diseases, *Lancet*, **388**, pp. 1311–1324. https://doi.org/10.1016/s0140-6736(16)30383-x
24. Niccoli, T., & Partridge, L. (2012). Ageing as a risk factor for disease, *Current Biology*, **22**, pp. R741–R752. https://doi.org/https://doi.org/10.1016/j.cub.2012.07.024
25. Bloom, D. E., Cafiero, E.T., Jané-Llopis, E., Abrahams-Gessel, S., Bloom, L.R., Fathima, S., *et al.* (2011). The global economic burden of non-communicable diseases, *Geneva: World Economic Forum*, pp. 1–48.
26. Shiels, P. G., & Ritzau-Reid, K. (2015). Biological ageing, inflammation and nutrition: how might they impact on systemic sclerosis? *Current Aging Science*, **8**, pp. 123–130.
27. Lloyd-Sherlock, P., McKee, M., Ebrahim, S., Gorman, M., Greengross, S., Prince, M., *et al.* (2012). Population ageing and health, *The Lancet*, **379**, pp. 1295–1296. https://doi.org/10.1016/S0140-6736(12)60519-4
28. Kirkwood, T. B. (2008a). A systematic look at an old problem, *Nature*, **451**, pp. 644–647. https://doi.org/10.1038/451644a

29. Panagiotou, N., Neytchev, O., Selman, C., & Shiels, P. (2018). Extracellular vesicles, ageing, and therapeutic interventions, *Cells*, **7**, pp. 110. http://www.mdpi.com/2073-4409/7/8/110
30. Chatterji, S., Byles, J., Cutler, D., Seeman, T., & Verdes, E. (2015). Health, functioning, and disability in older adults-present status and future implications, *Lancet*, **385**, pp. 563–575. https://doi.org/10.1016/s0140-6736(14)61462-8
31. Prince, M. J., Wu, F., Guo, Y., Gutierrez Robledo, L. M., O'Donnell, M., Sullivan, R., *et al.* (2015). The burden of disease in older people and implications for health policy and practice, *Lancet*, **385**, pp. 549–562. https://doi.org/10.1016/s0140-6736(14)61347-7
32. Panagiotou, N., McGuinness, D., Jaminon, A. M. G., Mees, B., Selman, C., Schurgers, L., *et al.* (2023). Microvesicle-mediated tissue regeneration mitigates the effects of cellular ageing, *Cells*, **12**, pp. 1707. https://www.mdpi.com/2073-4409/12/13/1707
33. López-Otín, C., Blasco, M. A., Partridge, L., Serrano, M., & Kroemer, G. (2023). Hallmarks of aging: an expanding universe, *Cell*, **186**, pp. 243–278. https://doi.org/10.1016/j.cell.2022.11.001
34. Panagiotou, N., Wayne Davies, R., Selman, C., & Shiels, P. G. (2016). Microvesicles as vehicles for tissue regeneration: changing of the guards, *Current Pathobiology Reports*, **4**, pp. 181–187. https://doi.org/10.1007/s40139-016-0115-5
35. Vijg, J., & Campisi, J. (2008). Puzzles, promises and a cure for ageing [Review], *Nature*, **454**, pp. 1065–1071. https://doi.org/10.1038/nature07216
36. Strehler, B. L., Mark, D. D., Mildvan, A. S., & Gee, M. V. (1959). Rate and magnitude of age pigment accumulation in the human myocardium [Article], *Journals of Gerontology*, **14**, pp. 430–439. https://doi.org/10.1093/geronj/14.4.430
37. Comfort, A. (1964). *Ageing: The Biology of Senescence*. Holt, Rinehart and Winston, Inc., New York. <Go to ISI>://BCI:BCI19654600002339
38. Rose, M. R. (1991). *Evolutionary Biology of Ageing*. <Go to ISI>://BCI:BCI199141102512
39. Partridge, L., & Mangel, M. (1999). Messages from mortality: the evolution of death rates in the old, *Trends Ecol Evol.*, **14**, pp. 438–442.
40. Kirkwood, T. B. (2008b). Understanding ageing from an evolutionary perspective, *Journal of Internal Medicine*, **263**, pp. 117–127. https://doi.org/doi:10.1111/j.1365-2796.2007.01901.x

41. Bowen, R. L., & Atwood, C. S. (2004). Living and dying for sex: a theory of aging based on the modulation of cell cycle signaling by reproductive hormones, *Gerontology*, **50**, pp. 265–290. https://doi.org/10.1159/000079125
42. de Magalhaes, J. P. (2012). Programmatic features of aging originating in development: aging mechanisms beyond molecular damage? *Faseb j*, **26**, pp. 4821–4826. https://doi.org/10.1096/fj.12-210872
43. Lopez-Otin, C., Blasco, M. A., Partridge, L., Serrano, M., & Kroemer, G. (2013). The hallmarks of aging [Review], *Cell*, **153**, pp. 1194–1217. https://doi.org/10.1016/j.cell.2013.05.039
44. Williams, G. C. (1957). Pleiotropy, natural selection, and the evolution of senescence, *Evolution*, **11**, pp. 398–411. https://doi.org/10.2307/2406060
45. Kirkwood, T. B. L., & Austad, S. N. (2000). Why do we age? [Review], *Nature*, **408**, pp. 233–238. https://doi.org/10.1038/35041682
46. Kenyon, C. J. (2010). The genetics of ageing, *Nature*, **464**, pp. 504–512. https://doi.org/10.1038/nature08980
47. Xu, Y., & Sun, Z. (2015). Molecular basis of Klotho: from gene to function in aging, *Endocr Rev*, **36**, pp. 174–193. https://doi.org/10.1210/er.2013-1079
48. Seeman, T. E., McEwen, B. S., Rowe, J. W., & Singer, B. H. (2001). Allostatic load as a marker of cumulative biological risk: MacArthur studies of successful aging, *Proc Natl Acad Sci USA*, **98**, pp. 4770–4775. https://doi.org/10.1073/pnas.081072698
49. Shiels, P. G., Stenvinkel, P., Kooman, J. P., & McGuinness, D. (2017). Circulating markers of ageing and allostatic load: a slow train coming, *Practical Laboratory Medicine*, **7**, pp. 49–54. https://doi.org/10.1016/j.plabm.2016.04.002
50. Adams, P. D. (2009). Healing and hurting: molecular mechanisms, functions, and pathologies of cellular senescence [Review], *Molecular Cell*, **36**, pp. 2–14. https://doi.org/10.1016/j.molcel.2009.09.021
51. Campisi, J. (2005). Senescent cells, tumor suppression, and organismal aging: good citizens, bad neighbors [Review], *Cell*, **120**, pp. 513–522. https://doi.org/10.1016/j.cell.2005.02.003
52. Collado, M., Blasco, M. A., & Serrano, M. (2007). Cellular senescence in cancer and aging [Review], *Cell*, **130**, pp. 223–233. https://doi.org/10.1016/j.cell.2007.07.003
53. Campisi, J. (2013). Aging, cellular senescence, and cancer. *Annual Review of Physiology*, **75**, pp. 685–705. https://doi.org/10.1146/annurev-physiol-030212-183653

54. Hodzic, M., Naaldijk, Y., & Stolzing, A. (2013). Regulating aging in adult stem cells with microRNA [Article], *Zeitschrift Fur Gerontologie Und Geriatrie*, **46**, pp. 629–634. https://doi.org/10.1007/s00391-013-0531-7
55. Reya, T., Morrison, S. J., Clarke, M. F., & Weissman, I. L. (2001). Stem cells, cancer, and cancer stem cells [Review], *Nature*, **414**, pp. 105–111. https://doi.org/10.1038/35102167
56. Fulop, T., Larbi, A., Witkowski, J. M., McElhaney, J., Loeb, M., Mitnitski, A., *et al.* (2010). Aging, frailty and age-related diseases [Article], *Biogerontology*, **11**, pp. 547–563. https://doi.org/10.1007/s10522-010-9287-2
57. Horvath, S. (2013). DNA methylation age of human tissues and cell types, *Genome Biol*, **14**, pp. R115. https://doi.org/10.1186/gb-2013-14-10-r115
58. Kooman, J. P., Kotanko, P., Schols, A., Shiels, P. G., & Stenvinkel, P. (2014). Chronic kidney disease and premature ageing [Article], *Nature Reviews Nephrology*, **10**, pp. 732–742. https://doi.org/10.1038/nrneph.2014.185
59. Kooman, J. P., Shiels, P. G., & Stenvinkel, P. (2015). Premature aging in chronic kidney disease and chronic obstructive pulmonary disease: similarities and differences, *Curr Opin Clin Nutr Metab Care*, **18**, pp. 528–534. https://doi.org/10.1097/mco.0000000000000218
60. McGuinness, D., McGlynn, L. M., Johnson, P. C., MacIntyre, A., Batty, G. D., Burns, H., *et al.* (2012). Socio-economic status is associated with epigenetic differences in the pSoBid cohort, *Int J Epidemiol*, **41**, pp. 151–160. https://doi.org/10.1093/ije/dyr215
61. Stenvinkel, P., Kooman, J. P., & Shiels, P. G. (2016). Nutrients and ageing: what can we learn about ageing interactions from animal biology? *Curr Opin Clin Nutr Metab Care*, **19**, pp. 19–25. https://doi.org/10.1097/mco.0000000000000234
62. Cole, J. J., Robertson, N. A., Rather, M. I., Thomson, J. P., McBryan, T., Sproul, D., *et al.* (2017). Diverse interventions that extend mouse lifespan suppress shared age-associated epigenetic changes at critical gene regulatory regions [Article], *Genome Biol*, **58**, pp. 16. https://doi.org/10.1186/s13059-017-1185-3
63. Jin, S. L., Zhang, Y., Chen, Z. H., Qian, D. W., Qine, Y. J., Yongjie, Q., *et al.* (2015). Epigenetic changes of the Klotho gene in age-related cataracts [Article], *European Review for Medical and Pharmacological Sciences*, **19**, pp. 2544–2551. <Go to ISI>://WOS:000358790400005

64. Lardenoije, R., van den Hove, D. L. A., Havermans, M., Van Casteren, A., Le, K. X., Palmour, R., *et al.* (2018). Age-related epigenetic changes in hippocampal subregions of four animal models of Alzheimer's disease [Article], *Molecular and Cellular Neuroscience*, **86**, pp. 1–15. https://doi.org/10.1016/j.mcn.2017.11.002

65. Przybilla, J., Rohlf, T., Loeffler, M., & Galle, J. (2014). Understanding epigenetic changes in aging stem cells: a computational model approach [Article], *Aging Cell*, **13**, pp. 320–328. https://doi.org/10.1111/acel.12177

66. Qian, Y., Tu, J. J., Tang, N. L. S., Kong, G. W. S., Chung, J. P. W., Chan, W. Y., *et al.* (2015). Dynamic changes of DNA epigenetic marks in mouse oocytes during natural and accelerated aging [Article], *International Journal of Biochemistry & Cell Biology*, **67**, pp. 121–127. https://doi.org/10.1016/j.biocel.2015.05.005

67. Shiels, P. G., McGlynn, L. M., MacIntyre, A., Johnson, P. C., Batty, G. D., Burns, H., *et al.* (2011). Accelerated telomere attrition is associated with relative household income, diet and inflammation in the pSoBid cohort, *PLoS One*, **6**, pp. e22521. https://doi.org/10.1371/journal.pone.0022521

68. Shiels, P. G., McGuinness, D., Eriksson, M., Kooman, J. P., & Stenvinkel, P. (2017). The role of epigenetics in renal ageing, *Nat Rev Nephrol*, **13**, pp. 471–482. https://doi.org/10.1038/nrneph.2017.78

69. Stenvinkel, P., Painer, J., Kuro, O. M., Lanaspa, M., Arnold, W., Ruf, T., *et al.* (2018). Novel treatment strategies for chronic kidney disease: insights from the animal kingdom, *Nat Rev Nephrol*, **14**, pp. 265–284. https://doi.org/10.1038/nrneph.2017.169

70. Jin, K. (2010). Modern biological theories of aging, *Aging and Disease*, **1**, pp. 72–74. http://www.ncbi.nlm.nih.gov/pmc/articles/PMC2995895/

71. Davidovic, M., Sevo, G., Svorcan, P., Milosevic, D. P., Despotovic, N., & Erceg, P. (2010). Old age as a privilege of the "selfish ones," *Aging Dis*, **1**, pp. 139–146.

72. Vina, J., Borras, C., & Miquel, J. (2007). Theories of ageing, *IUBMB Life*, **59**, pp. 249–254. https://doi.org/10.1080/15216540601178067

73. Ewald, C. Y., Landis, J. N., Abate, J. P., Murphy, C. T., & Blackwell, T. K. (2014). Dauer-independent insulin/IGF-1-signalling implicates collagen remodelling in longevity, *Nature*, **519**, pp. 97. https://doi.org/10.1038/nature14021

74. van Heemst, D. (2010). Insulin, IGF-1 and longevity, *Aging Dis*, **1**, pp. 147–157.

75. Cornelius, E. (1972). Increased incidence of lymphomas in thymectomized mice-evidence for an immunological theory of aging, *Experientia*, **28**, pp. 459.
76. Rozemuller, A. J., van Gool, W. A., & Eikelenboom, P. (2005). The neuroinflammatory response in plaques and amyloid angiopathy in Alzheimer's disease: therapeutic implications, *Curr Drug Targets CNS Neurol Disord*, **4**, pp. 223–233.
77. Kirkwood, T. B. L. (2005). Understanding the odd science of aging [Review], *Cell*, **120**, pp. 437–447. https://doi.org/10.1016/j.cell.2005.01.027
78. Kirkwood, T. B., & Cremer, T. (1982). Cytogerontology since 1881: a reappraisal of August Weismann and a review of modern progress, *Hum Genet*, **60**, pp. 101–121.
79. Pearl, R. (1928). *The Rate of Living*, University of London Press, London.
80. Brys, K., Vanfleteren, J. R., & Braeckman, B. P. (2007). Testing the rate-of-living/oxidative damage theory of aging in the nematode model Caenorhabditis elegans, *Exp Gerontol*, **42**, pp. 845–851. https://doi.org/10.1016/j.exger.2007.02.004
81. Hulbert, A. J., Pamplona, R., Buffenstein, R., & Buttemer, W. A. (2007). Life and death: metabolic rate, membrane composition, and life span of animals, *Physiol Rev*, **87**, pp. 1175–1213. https://doi.org/10.1152/physrev.00047.2006
82. Rollo, C. D. (2010). Aging and the Mammalian regulatory triumvirate, *Aging Dis*, **1**, pp. 105–138.
83. Bjorksten, J. (1968). The crosslinkage theory of aging, *J Am Geriatr Soc*, **16**(4), pp. 408–427. https://doi.org/doi:10.1111/j.1532-5415.1968.tb02821.x
84. Bjorksten, J., & Tenhu, H. (1990). The crosslinking theory of aging—added evidence, *Exp Gerontol*, **25**, pp. 91–95. https://doi.org/https://doi.org/10.1016/ 0531-5565(90)90039-5
85. Gerschman, R., Gilbert, D. L., Nye, S. W., Dwyer, P., & Fenn, W. O. (1954). Oxygen poisoning and X-irradiation: a mechanism in common, *Science*, **119**, pp. 623–626. https://doi.org/10.1126/science.119.3097.623
86. Harman, D. (1956). Aging: a theory based on free radical and radiation chemistry, *J Gerontol*, **11**, pp. 298–300.
87. Finkel, T., & Holbrook, N. J. (2000). Oxidants, oxidative stress and the biology of ageing, *Nature*, **408**, pp. 239–247. https://doi.org/10.1038/35041687

88. Arking, R., Burde, V., Graves, K., Hari, R., Feldman, E., Zeevi, A., Soliman, S., Saraiya, A., Buck, S., Vettraino, J., & Sathrasala, K. (2000). Identical longevity phenotypes are characterized by different patterns of gene expression and oxidative damage, *Exp Gerontol*, **35**, pp. 353–373.
89. Yanase, S., Yasuda, K., & Ishii, N. (2002). Adaptive responses to oxidative damage in three mutants of Caenorhabditis elegans (age-1, mev-1 and daf-16) that affect life span, *Mech Ageing Dev*, **123**, pp. 1579–1587.
90. Magwere, T., West, M., Riyahi, K., Murphy, M. P., Smith, R. A., & Partridge, L. (2006). The effects of exogenous antioxidants on lifespan and oxidative stress resistance in Drosophila melanogaster, *Mech Ageing Dev*, **127**, pp. 356–370. https://doi.org/10.1016/j.mad.2005.12.009
91. Schriner, S. E., Linford, N. J., Martin, G. M., Treuting, P., Ogburn, C. E., Emond, M., *et al.* (2005). Extension of murine life span by overexpression of catalase targeted to mitochondria, *Science*, **308**, pp. 1909. http://science.sciencemag.org/content/308/5730/1909.abstract
92. Liochev, S. I. (2013). Reactive oxygen species and the free radical theory of aging, *Free Radic Biol Med*, **60**, pp. 1–4. https://doi.org/10.1016/j.freeradbiomed.2013.02.011
93. Afanas'ev, I. (2010). Signaling and damaging functions of free radicals in aging-free radical theory, hormesis, and TOR, *Aging Dis*, **1**, pp. 75–88.
94. Iyama, T., & Wilson, D. M. (2013). DNA repair mechanisms in dividing and non-dividing cells, *DNA Repair*, **12**, pp. 620–636. https://doi.org/https://doi.org/10.1016/j.dnarep.2013.04.015
95. Mikhed, Y., Daiber, A., & Steven, S. (2015). Mitochondrial oxidative stress, mitochondrial DNA damage and their role in age-related vascular dysfunction, *International Journal of Molecular Sciences*, **16**, pp. 15918–15953. https://doi.org/10.3390/ijms160715918
96. Franco, I., Johansson, A., Olsson, K., Vrtačnik, P., Lundin, P., Helgadottir, H. T., *et al.* (2018). Somatic mutagenesis in satellite cells associates with human skeletal muscle aging, *Nature Communications*, **9**, pp. 800. https://doi.org/10.1038/s41467-018-03244-6
97. Brubaker, T. H., & Powers, E. A. (1976). The stereotype of "old": a review and alternative approach, *J Gerontol*, **31**, pp. 441–447.
98. Government, S. (2007). *All Our Futures: Planning for a Scotland with an Ageing Population: 3,* The Evidence Base. Scottish Government: Edinburgh.
99. Executive, S. (2005). *Scottish Health Survey 2003: Summary of key findings*. Edinburgh: Scottish Executive the Stationery Office: Edinburgh.

100. Kuh, D. (2007). A life course approach to healthy aging, frailty, and capability, *J Gerontol A Biol Sci Med Sci*, **62**, pp. 717–721.

101. Ben-Shlomo, Y., & Kuh, D. (2002). A life course approach to chronic disease epidemiology: conceptual models, empirical challenges and interdisciplinary perspectives, *Int J Epidemiol*, **31**, pp. 285–293.

102. Mohler, M. J., Fain, M. J., Wertheimer, A. M., Najafi, B., & Nikolich-Zugich, J. (2014). The Frailty syndrome: clinical measurements and basic underpinnings in humans and animals, *Exp Gerontol*, **54**, pp. 6–13. https://doi.org/10.1016/j.exger.2014.01.024

103. Bergman, H., Ferrucci, L., Guralnik, J., Hogan, D. B., Hummel, S., Karunananthan, S., *et al.* (2007). Frailty: an emerging research and clinical paradigm-issues and controversies, *J Gerontol A Biol Sci Med Sci*, **62**, pp. 731–737.

104. Walston, J., Hadley, E. C., Ferrucci, L., Guralnik, J. M., Newman, A. B., Studenski, S. A., *et al.* (2006). Research agenda for frailty in older adults: toward a better understanding of physiology and etiology: summary from the American Geriatrics Society/National Institute on Aging Research Conference on Frailty in Older Adults, *J Am Geriatr Soc*, **54**, pp. 991–1001. https://doi.org/10.1111/j.1532-5415.2006.00745.x

105. Afilalo, J., Alexander, K. P., Mack, M. J., Maurer, M. S., Green, P., Allen, L. A., *et al.* (2014). Frailty assessment in the cardiovascular care of older adults, *J Am Coll Cardiol*, **63**, pp. 747–762. https://doi.org/10.1016/j.jacc.2013.09.070

106. van Iersel, M. B., & Rikkert, M. G. (2006). Frailty criteria give heterogeneous results when applied in clinical practice, *J Am Geriatr Soc*, **54**, pp. 728–729. https://doi.org/10.1111/j.1532-5415.2006.00668_14.x

107. Fried, L. P., Tangen, C. M., Walston, J., Newman, A. B., Hirsch, C., Gottdiener, J., *et al.* (2001). Frailty in older adults: evidence for a phenotype, *J Gerontol A Biol Sci Med Sci*, **56**, pp. M146–156.

108. Guralnik, J. M., Simonsick, E. M., Ferrucci, L., Glynn, R. J., Berkman, L. F., Blazer, D. G., *et al.* (1994). A short physical performance battery assessing lower extremity function: association with self-reported disability and prediction of mortality and nursing home admission, *J Gerontol*, **49**, pp. M85–94.

109. Gary, R. (2012). Evaluation of frailty in older adults with cardiovascular disease: incorporating physical performance measures, *J Cardiovasc Nurs*, **27**, pp. 120–131. https://doi.org/10.1097/JCN.0b013e318239f4a4

110. Munoz-Mendoza, C. L., Cabanero-Martinez, M. J., Millan-Calenti, J. C., Cabrero-Garcia, J., Lopez-Sanchez, R., & Maseda-Rodriguez, A. (2011). Reliability of 4-m and 6-m walking speed tests in elderly people with cognitive impairment, *Arch Gerontol Geriatr*, **52**, pp. e67–70. https://doi.org/ 10.1016/j.archger.2010.06.020

111. van Iersel, M. B., Munneke, M., Esselink, R. A., Benraad, C. E., & Olde Rikkert, M. G. (2008). Gait velocity and the Timed-Up-and-Go test were sensitive to changes in mobility in frail elderly patients, *J Clin Epidemiol*, **61**, pp. 186–191. https://doi.org/ 10.1016/j.jclinepi.2007.04.016

112. Hardy, S. E., Perera, S., Roumani, Y. F., Chandler, J. M., & Studenski, S. A. (2007). Improvement in usual gait speed predicts better survival in older adults, *J Am Geriatr Soc*, **55**, pp. 1727–1734. https://doi.org/10.1111/j.1532-5415.2007.01413.x

113. Graham, J. E., Ostir, G. V., Kuo, Y. F., Fisher, S. R., & Ottenbacher, K. J. (2008). Relationship between test methodology and mean velocity in timed walk tests: a review, *Arch Phys Med Rehabil*, **89**, pp. 865–872. https://doi.org/10.1016/j.apmr.2007.11.029

114. Rockwood, K., Song, X., MacKnight, C., Bergman, H., Hogan, D. B., McDowell, I., *et al.* (2005). A global clinical measure of fitness and frailty in elderly people, *Cmaj*, **173**, pp. 489–495. https://doi.org/10.1503/cmaj.050051

115. Mitnitski, A. B., Song, X., & Rockwood, K. (2004). The estimation of relative fitness and frailty in community-dwelling older adults using self-report data, *J Gerontol A Biol Sci Med Sci*, **59**, pp. M627–632.

116. Abellan van Kan, G., Rolland, Y., Bergman, H., Morley, J. E., Kritchevsky, S. B., & Vellas, B. (2008). The I.A.N.A Task Force on frailty assessment of older people in clinical practice, *J Nutr Health Aging*, **12**, pp. 29–37.

117. Purser, J. L., Kuchibhatla, M. N., Fillenbaum, G. G., Harding, T., Peterson, E. D., & Alexander, K. P. (2006). Identifying frailty in hospitalized older adults with significant coronary artery disease, *J Am Geriatr Soc*, **54**, pp. 1674–1681. https://doi.org/10.1111/j.1532-5415.2006.00914.x

118. Fedarko, N. S. (2011). The biology of aging and frailty [Article], *Clinics in Geriatric Medicine*, **27**, pp. 27–37. https://doi.org/ 10.1016/j.cger.2010.08.006

119. Adams, J. M., & White, M. (2004). Biological ageing: a fundamental, biological link between socio-economic status and health? *Eur J Public Health*, **14**, pp. 331–334.

120. Fulop, T., Fortin, C., Lesur, O., Dupuis, G., Kotb, J. R., Lord, J. M., *et al.* (2012). The innate immune system and aging: what is the contribution to immunosenescence? *Open Longevity Science,* **6**, pp. 121–132.
121. Kirkland, J. L., & Peterson, C. (2009). Health span, translation, and new outcomes for animal studies of aging, *J Gerontol A Biol Sci Med Sci*, **64**, pp. 209–212. https://doi.org/10.1093/gerona/gln063
122. Martin-Ruiz, C., Jagger, C., Kingston, A., Collerton, J., Catt, M., Davies, K., *et al.* (2011). Assessment of a large panel of candidate biomarkers of ageing in the Newcastle 85+ study, *Mech Ageing Dev*, **132**, pp. 496–502. https://doi.org/10.1016/j.mad.2011.08.001
123. Kawanishi, S., & Oikawa, S. (2004). Mechanism of telomere shortening by oxidative stress, *Ann N Y Acad Sci*, **1019**, pp. 278–284. https://doi.org/10.1196/annals.1297.047
124. Gomez, J., Sanchez-Roman, I., Gomez, A., Sanchez, C., Suarez, H., Lopez-Torres, M., *et al.* (2011). Methionine and homocysteine modulate the rate of ROS generation of isolated mitochondria in vitro, *J Bioenerg Biomembr*, **43**, pp. 377–386. https://doi.org/10.1007/s10863-011-9368-1
125. Bodnar, A. G., Ouellette, M., Frolkis, M., Holt, S. E., Chiu, C. P., Morin, G. B., *et al.* (1998). Extension of life-span by introduction of telomerase into normal human cells, *Science*, **279**, pp. 349–352. http://science.sciencemag.org/content/sci/279/5349/349.full.pdf
126. Mattison, J. A., Colman, R. J., Beasley, T. M., Allison, D. B., Kemnitz, J. W., Roth, G. S., *et al.* (2017). Caloric restriction improves health and survival of rhesus monkeys [Article], *Nature Communications*, **8**, pp. 14063. https://doi.org/10.1038/ncomms14063
127. Orentreich, N., Matias, J. R., DeFelice, A., & Zimmerman, J. A. (1993). Low methionine ingestion by rats extends life span, *J Nutr*, **123**, pp. 269–274. https://doi.org/10.1093/jn/123.2.269
128. Sun, L., Sadighi Akha, A. A., Miller, R. A., & Harper, J. M. (2009). Life-span extension in mice by preweaning food restriction and by methionine restriction in middle age, *The Journals of Gerontology Series A: Biological Sciences and Medical Sciences*, **64A**, pp. 711–722. https://doi.org/10.1093/gerona/glp051
129. Weindruch, R., Walford, R. L., Fligiel, S., & Guthrie, D. (1986). The retardation of aging in mice by dietary restriction: longevity, cancer, immunity and lifetime energy intake, *J Nutr*, **116**, pp. 641–654. https://doi.org/10.1093/jn/116.4.641
130. Zimmerman, J. A., Malloy, V., Krajcik, R., & Orentreich, N. (2003). Nutritional control of aging, *Exp Gerontol*, **38**, pp. 47–52.

131. Baur, J. A., Pearson, K. J., Price, N. L., Jamieson, H. A., Lerin, C., Kalra, A., *et al.* (2006). Resveratrol improves health and survival of mice on a high-calorie diet, *Nature*, **444**, pp. 337–342. https://doi.org/10.1038/nature05354

132. F., P. J., Thomas, v. Z., & B.L., K. T. (2007). Mitochondria and ageing: winning and losing in the numbers game, *BioEssays*, **29**, pp. 908–917. https://doi.org/doi:10.1002/bies.20634

133. Uribarri, J., del Castillo, M. D., de la Maza, M. P., Filip, R., Gugliucci, A., Luevano-Contreras, C., *et al.* (2015). Dietary advanced glycation end products and their role in health and disease, *Adv Nutr*, **6**, pp. 461–473. https://doi.org/10.3945/an.115.008433

134. Franke, S., Dawczynski, J., Strobel, J., Niwa, T., Stahl, P., & Stein, G. (2003). Increased levels of advanced glycation end products in human cataractous lenses, *J Cataract Refract Surg*, **29**, pp. 998–1004.

135. Schmidt, A. M., Yan, S. D., Wautier, J. L., & Stern, D. (1999). Activation of receptor for advanced glycation end products: a mechanism for chronic vascular dysfunction in diabetic vasculopathy and atherosclerosis, *Circ Res*, **84**, pp. 489–497.

136. Matzinger, P. (2002). The danger model: a renewed sense of self [10.1126/science.1071059], *Science*, **296**, pp. 301. http://science.sciencemag.org/content/296/5566/301.abstract

137. Matzinger, P. (2007). Friendly and dangerous signals: is the tissue in control? *Nat Immunol*, **8**, pp. 11. https://doi.org/10.1038/ni0107-11

138. Huang, J., Xie, Y., Sun, X., Zeh, H. J., III, Kang, R., Lotze, M. T., *et al.* (2015). DAMPs, ageing, and cancer: The 'DAMP Hypothesis', *Ageing Res Rev*, **24**(Pt A), pp. 3–16. https://doi.org/10.1016/j.arr.2014.10.004

139. Hanahan, D., & Weinberg, R. A. (2000). The hallmarks of cancer, *Cell*, **100**, pp. 57–70.

140. Kang, R., Zhang, Q., Hou, W., Yan, Z., Chen, R., Bonaroti, J., *et al.* (2014). Intracellular Hmgb1 inhibits inflammatory nucleosome release and limits acute pancreatitis in mice, *Gastroenterology*, **146**, pp. 1097–1107. https://doi.org/10.1053/j.gastro.2013.12.015

141. Tang, D., Kang, R., Zeh, H. J., & Lotze, M. T. (2010). High-mobility group box 1, oxidative stress, and disease, *Antioxidants & Redox Signaling*, **14**, pp. 1315–1335. https://doi.org/10.1089/ars.2010.3356

142. Zhang, Q., Kang, R., Zeh, I. I. I. H. J., Lotze, M. T., & Tang, D. (2013). DAMPs and autophagy, *Autophagy*, **9**, pp. 451–458. https://doi.org/10.4161/auto.23691

143. Hayflick, L., & Moorhead, P. S. (1961). The serial cultivation of human diploid cell strains, *Experimental Cell Research*, **25**, pp. 585–621. https://doi.org/https://doi.org/10.1016/0014-4827(61)90192-6

144. Bernadotte, A., Mikhelson, V. M., & Spivak, I. M. (2016). Markers of cellular senescence: telomere shortening as a marker of cellular senescence, *Aging (Albany NY)*, **8**, pp. 3–11. http://www.ncbi.nlm.nih.gov/pmc/articles/PMC4761709/

145. Moyzis, R. K., Buckingham, J. M., Cram, L. S., Dani, M., Deaven, L. L., Jones, M. D., *et al.* (1988). A highly conserved repetitive DNA sequence, (TTAGGG)n, present at the telomeres of human chromosomes, *Proc Natl Acad Sci U S A*, **85**, pp. 6622–6626.

146. Blasco, M. A. (2005). Telomeres and human disease: ageing, cancer and beyond. *Nat Rev Genet*, **6**, pp. 611–622. https://doi.org/10.1038/nrg1656

147. Rizvi, S., Raza, S. T., & Mahdi, F. (2014). Telomere length variations in aging and age-related diseases, *Curr Aging Sci*, **7**, pp. 161–167.

148. Roussel, M. F. (1999). The INK4 family of cell cycle inhibitors in cancer [Original Paper], *Oncogene*, **18**, pp. 5311. https://doi.org/10.1038/sj.onc.1202998

149. Serrano, M., Hannon, G. J., & Beach, D. (1993). A new regulatory motif in cell-cycle control causing specific inhibition of cyclin D/CDK4, *Nature*, **366**, pp. 704–707. https://doi.org/10.1038/366704a0

150. Shiels, P. G. (2012). CDKN2A might be better than telomere length in determining individual health status, *Bmj*, **344**, pp. e1415. https://doi.org/10.1136/bmj.e1415

151. El-Deiry, W. S., Tokino, T., Velculescu, V. E., Levy, D. B., Parsons, R., Trent, J. M., *et al.* (1993). WAF1, a potential mediator of p53 tumor suppression, *Cell*, **75**, pp. 817–825.

152. Harper, J. W., Adami, G. R., Wei, N., Keyomarsi, K., & Elledge, S. J. (1993). The p21 Cdk-interacting protein Cip1 is a potent inhibitor of G1 cyclin-dependent kinases, *Cell*, **75**, pp. 805–816.

153. Harper, J. W., & Elledge, S. J. (1996). Cdk inhibitors in development and cancer, *Curr Opin Genet Dev*, **6**, pp. 56–64.

154. Xiong, Y., Hannon, G. J., Zhang, H., Casso, D., Kobayashi, R., & Beach, D. (1993). p21 is a universal inhibitor of cyclin kinases, *Nature*, **366**, pp. 701. https://doi.org/10.1038/366701a0

155. Dimri, G. P., Lee, X., Basile, G., Acosta, M., Scott, G., Roskelley, C., *et al.* (1995). A biomarker that identifies senescent human cells in culture

and in aging skin in vivo, *Proc Natl Acad Sci USA*, **92**, pp. 9363–9367. http://www.ncbi.nlm.nih.gov/pmc/articles/PMC40985/

156. Hall, B. M., Balan, V., Gleiberman, A. S., Strom, E., Krasnov, P., Virtuoso, L. P., *et al.* (2016). Aging of mice is associated with p16(Ink4a)- and beta-galactosidase-positive macrophage accumulation that can be induced in young mice by senescent cells, *Aging (Albany NY)*, **8**, pp. 1294–1315. https://doi.org/10.18632/aging.100991
157. Ravelojaona, V., Robert, A. M., & Robert, L. (2009). Expression of senescence-associated beta-galactosidase (SA-beta-Gal) by human skin fibroblasts, effect of advanced glycation end-products and fucose or rhamnose-rich polysaccharides, *Arch Gerontol Geriatr*, **48**, pp. 151–154. https://doi.org/10.1016/j.archger.2007.12.004
158. Liu, Y., Sanoff, H. K., Cho, H., Burd, C. E., Torrice, C., Ibrahim, J. G., *et al.* (2009). Expression of p16(INK4a) in peripheral blood T-cells is a biomarker of human aging, *Aging Cell*, **8**, pp. 439–448. https://doi.org/10.1111/j.1474-9726.2009.00489.x
159. McGlynn, L. M., Stevenson, K., Lamb, K., Zino, S., Brown, M., Prina, A., *et al.* (2009). Cellular senescence in pretransplant renal biopsies predicts postoperative organ function, *Aging Cell*, **8**, pp. 45–51. https://doi.org/10.1111/j.1474-9726.2008.00447.x
160. Gingell-Littlejohn, M., McGuinness, D., McGlynn, L. M., Kingsmore, D., Stevenson, K. S., Koppelstaetter, C., *et al.* (2013). Pre-transplant CDKN2A expression in kidney biopsies predicts renal function and is a future component of donor scoring criteria, *PLoS One*, **8**, pp. e68133. https://doi.org/10.1371/journal.pone.0068133
161. Koppelstaetter, C., Schratzberger, G., Perco, P., Hofer, J., Mark, W., Ollinger, R., *et al.* (2008). Markers of cellular senescence in zero-hour biopsies predict outcome in renal transplantation, *Aging Cell*, **7**, pp. 491–497. https://doi.org/10.1111/j.1474-9726.2008.00398.x
162. Shiels, P. G. (2010). Improving precision in investigating aging: why telomeres can cause problems, *The Journals of Gerontology: Series A*, **65A**, pp. 789–791. https://doi.org/10.1093/gerona/glq095
163. Maguire, D., Neytchev, O., Talwar, D., McMillan, D., & Shiels, P. G. (2018). Telomere homeostasis: interplay with magnesium, *International Journal of Molecular Sciences*, **19**, pp. 157. https://doi.org/10.3390/ijms19010157
164. Shiels, P. G., & Davies, R. W. (2004). Ageing and the death of neurones. In *Molecular Biology of the Neuron*. Oxford University Press. https://doi.org/10.1093/acprof:oso/9780198509981.003.0016

165. Lamb, K. J., & Shiels, P. G. (2009). Telomeres, ageing and oxidation, *SEB Exp Biol Ser*, **62**, pp. 117–137.

166. von Zglinicki, T., & Martin-Ruiz, C. M. (2005). Telomeres as biomarkers for ageing and age-related diseases, *Curr Mol Med*, **5**, pp. 197–203.

167. Chan, S. R. W. L., & Blackburn, E. H. (2004). Telomeres and telomerase, *Philosophical Transactions of the Royal Society B: Biological Sciences*, **359**, pp. 109–121. http://www.ncbi.nlm.nih.gov/pmc/articles/PMC1693310/

168. Levy, M. Z., Allsopp, R. C., Futcher, A. B., Greider, C. W., & Harley, C. B. (1992). Telomere end-replication problem and cell aging, *Journal of Molecular Biology*, **225**, pp. 951–960. https://doi.org/https://doi.org/10.1016/0022-2836(92)90096-3

169. Shammas, M. A. (2011). Telomeres, lifestyle, cancer, and aging, *Curr Opin Clin Nutr Metab Care*, **14**, pp. 28–34. https://doi.org/10.1097/MCO.0b013e32834121b1

170. Jaskelioff, M., Muller, F. L., Paik, J.-H., Thomas, E., Jiang, S., Adams, A. C., *et al.* (2010). Telomerase reactivation reverses tissue degeneration in aged telomerase-deficient mice, *Nature*, **469**, pp. 102. https://doi.org/10.1038/nature09603

171. Mendelsohn, A. R., & Larrick, J. W. (2018). Telomerase may paradoxically accelerate aging of the DNA methylome, *Rejuvenation Res*, **21**, pp. 168–172. https://doi.org/10.1089/rej.2018.2073

172. Cooke, H. J., & Smith, B. A. (1986). Variability at the telomeres of the human X/Y pseudoautosomal region, *Cold Spring Harb Symp Quant Biol*, **51**(1), pp. 213–219.

173. Olovnikov, A. M. (1996). Telomeres, telomerase, and aging: origin of the theory, *Exp Gerontol*, **31**, pp. 443–448.

174. Vaziri, H., Dragowska, W., Allsopp, R. C., Thomas, T. E., Harley, C. B., & Lansdorp, P. M. (1994). Evidence for a mitotic clock in human hematopoietic stem cells: loss of telomeric DNA with age, *Proc Natl Acad Sci U S A*, **91**, pp. 9857–9860. http://www.ncbi.nlm.nih.gov/pmc/articles/PMC44916/

175. Hunt, S. C., Chen, W., Gardner, J. P., Kimura, M., Srinivasan, S. R., Eckfeldt, J. H., *et al.* (2008). Leukocyte telomeres are longer in African Americans than in whites: the national heart, lung, and blood institute family heart study and the Bogalusa heart study, *Aging Cell*, **7**, pp. 451–458. https://doi.org/10.1111/j.1474-9726.2008.00397.x

176. von Zglinicki, T. (2012). Will your telomeres tell your future? *Bmj*, **344**, pp. e1727. https://doi.org/10.1136/bmj.e1727

177. Frenck, R. W., Jr., Blackburn, E. H., & Shannon, K. M. (1998). The rate of telomere sequence loss in human leukocytes varies with age, *Proc Natl Acad Sci U S A*, **95**, pp. 5607–5610.

178. Chen, J., Zhou, Y., Mueller-Steiner, S., Chen, L. F., Kwon, H., Yi, S., *et al.* (2005). SIRT1 protects against microglia-dependent amyloid-beta toxicity through inhibiting NF-kappaB signaling, *J Biol Chem*, **280**, pp. 40364–40374. https://doi.org/10.1074/jbc.M509329200

179. Barker, D. J. (2012). Sir Richard Doll Lecture: Developmental origins of chronic disease, *Public Health*, **126**, pp. 185–189. https://doi.org/10.1016/j.puhe.2011.11.014

180. Entringer, S., Epel, E. S., Kumsta, R., Lin, J., Hellhammer, D. H., Blackburn, E. H., *et al.* (2011). Stress exposure in intrauterine life is associated with shorter telomere length in young adulthood, *Proc Natl Acad Sci U S A*, **108**, pp. E513–518. https://doi.org/10.1073/pnas.1107759108

181. Tchirkov, A., & Lansdorp, P. M. (2003). Role of oxidative stress in telomere shortening in cultured fibroblasts from normal individuals and patients with ataxia–telangiectasia, *Human Molecular Genetics*, **12**, pp. 227–232. https://doi.org/10.1093/hmg/ddg023

182. Gardner, M., Bann, D., Wiley, L., Cooper, R., Hardy, R., Nitsch, D., *et al.* (2014). Gender and telomere length: systematic review and meta-analysis, *Exp Gerontol*, **51**, pp. 15–27. https://doi.org/10.1016/j.exger.2013.12.004

183. Martin-Ruiz, C. M., Baird, D., Roger, L., Boukamp, P., Krunic, D., Cawthon, R., *et al.* (2015). Reproducibility of telomere length assessment: an international collaborative study, *Int J Epidemiol*, **44**, pp. 1673–1683. https://doi.org/10.1093/ije/dyu191

184. Hjelmborg, J. B., Dalgard, C., Moller, S., Steenstrup, T., Kimura, M., Christensen, K., *et al.* (2015). The heritability of leucocyte telomere length dynamics, *J Med Genet*, **52**, pp. 297–302. https://doi.org/10.1136/jmedgenet-2014-102736

185. Cawthon, R. M., Smith, K. R., O'Brien, E., Sivatchenko, A., & Kerber, R. A. (2003). Association between telomere length in blood and mortality in people aged 60 years or older, *Lancet*, **361**, pp. 393–395. https://doi.org/10.1016/s0140-6736(03)12384-7

186. Mather, K. A., Jorm, A. F., Parslow, R. A., & Christensen, H. (2011). Is telomere length a biomarker of aging? A review, *J Gerontol A Biol Sci Med Sci*, **66**, pp. 202–213. https://doi.org/10.1093/gerona/glq180

187. Droge, W. (2002). Free radicals in the physiological control of cell function, *Physiol Rev*, **82**, pp. 47–95. https://doi.org/10.1152/physrev.00018.2001

188. Barja, G. (2002). Rate of generation of oxidative stress-related damage and animal longevity, *Free Radic Biol Med*, **33**, pp. 1167–1172.

189. Barja, G., Cadenas, S., Rojas, C., Perez-Campo, R., & Lopez-Torres, M. (1994). Low mitochondrial free radical production per unit O2 consumption can explain the simultaneous presence of high longevity and high aerobic metabolic rate in birds, *Free Radic Res*, **21**, pp. 317–327.

190. Sohal, R. S., Svensson, I., Sohal, B. H., & Brunk, U. T. (1989). Superoxide anion radical production in different animal species, *Mech Ageing Dev*, **49**, pp. 129–135. https://doi.org/https://doi.org/10.1016/0047-6374(89)90096-1

191. Loft, S., Vistisen, K., Ewertz, M., Tjonneland, A., Overvad, K., & Poulsen, H. E. (1992). Oxidative DNA damage estimated by 8-hydroxydeoxyguanosine excretion in humans: influence of smoking, gender and body mass index, *Carcinogenesis*, **13**, pp. 2241–2247.

192. Adelman, R., Saul, R. L., & Ames, B. N. (1988). Oxidative damage to DNA: relation to species metabolic rate and life span, *Proc Natl Acad Sci U S A*, **85**, pp. 2706–2708.

193. Miller, R. A., Buehner, G., Chang, Y., Harper, J. M., Sigler, R., & Smith-Wheelock, M. (2005). Methionine-deficient diet extends mouse lifespan, slows immune and lens aging, alters glucose, T4, IGF-I and insulin levels, and increases hepatocyte MIF levels and stress resistance, *Aging Cell*, **4**, pp. 119–125. https://doi.org/10.1111/j.1474-9726.2005.00152.x

194. Chen, W., Kimura, M., Kim, S., Cao, X., Srinivasan, S. R., Berenson, G. S., *et al.* (2011). Longitudinal versus cross-sectional evaluations of leukocyte telomere length dynamics: age-dependent telomere shortening is the rule, *J Gerontol A Biol Sci Med Sci*, **66**, pp. 312–319. https://doi.org/10.1093/gerona/glq223

195. Ren, F., Li, C., Xi, H., Wen, Y., & Huang, K. (2009). Estimation of human age according to telomere shortening in peripheral blood leukocytes of Tibetan, *Am J Forensic Med Pathol*, **30**, pp. 252–255. https://doi.org/10.1097/PAF.0b013e318187df8e

196. Tsuji, A., Ishiko, A., Takasaki, T., & Ikeda, N. (2002). Estimating age of humans based on telomere shortening, *Forensic Sci Int*, **126**, pp. 197–199.

197. Muezzinler, A., Zaineddin, A. K., & Brenner, H. (2013). A systematic review of leukocyte telomere length and age in adults, *Ageing Res Rev*, **12**, pp. 509–519. ttps://doi.org/10.1016/j.arr.2013.01.003

198. Robertson, T., Batty, G. D., Der, G., Green, M. J., McGlynn, L. M., McIntyre, A., *et al.* (2012). Is telomere length socially patterned? Evidence from the West of Scotland Twenty-07 Study, *PLoS One*, **7**, pp. e41805. https://doi.org/10.1371/journal.pone.0041805

199. Der, G., Batty, G. D., Benzeval, M., Deary, I. J., Green, M. J., McGlynn, L., *et al.* (2012). Is telomere length a biomarker for aging: cross-sectional evidence from the west of Scotland? *PLoS One*, **7**, pp. e45166. https://doi.org/10.1371/journal.pone.0045166

200. Krishnamurthy, J., Torrice, C., Ramsey, M. R., Kovalev, G. I., Al-Regaiey, K., Su, L., *et al.* (2004). Ink4a/Arf expression is a biomarker of aging, *J Clin Invest*, **114**(9), pp. 1299–1307. https://doi.org/10.1172/jci22475

201. Baker, D. J., Jeganathan, K. B., Cameron, J. D., Thompson, M., Juneja, S., Kopecka, A., *et al.* (2004). BubR1 insufficiency causes early onset of aging-associated phenotypes and infertility in mice, *Nat Genet*, **36**, pp. 744–749. https://doi.org/10.1038/ng1382

202. Baker, D. J., Wijshake, T., Tchkonia, T., LeBrasseur, N. K., Childs, B. G., van de Sluis, B., *et al.* (2011). Clearance of p16Ink4a-positive senescent cells delays ageing-associated disorders, *Nature*, **479**, pp. 232–236. https://doi.org/10.1038/nature10600

203. Baker, D. J., Childs, B. G., Durik, M., Wijers, M. E., Sieben, C. J., Zhong, J., *et al.* (2016). Naturally occurring p16(Ink4a)-positive cells shorten healthy lifespan [Article], *Nature*, **530**, pp. 184–189. https://doi.org/10.1038/nature16932

204. Xu, M., Pirtskhalava, T., Farr, J. N., Weigand, B. M., Palmer, A. K., Weivoda, M. M., *et al.* (2018). Senolytics improve physical function and increase lifespan in old age, *Nature Medicine*, **24**, pp. 1246–1256. https://doi.org/10.1038/s41591-018-0092-9

205. Pathai, S., Gilbert, C. E., Lawn, S. D., Weiss, H. A., Peto, T., Cook, C., *et al.* (2013). Assessment of candidate ocular biomarkers of ageing in a South African adult population: relationship with chronological age and systemic biomarkers, *Mech Ageing Dev*, **134**, pp. 338–345. https://doi.org/10.1016/j.mad.2013.05.002

206. Moreno-Villanueva, M., & Burkle, A. (2011). MARK-AGE: European study to establish biomarkers of human ageing [Meeting Abstract], *Exp Gerontol*, **46**, pp. 212–212. https://doi.org/10.1016/j.exger.2010.11.025

207. Baker, G. T., 3rd, & Sprott, R. L. (1988). Biomarkers of aging, *Exp Gerontol*, **23**, pp. 223–239.

208. Butler, R. N., Sprott, R., Warner, H., Bland, J., Feuers, R., Forster, M., *et al.* (2004). Biomarkers of aging: from primitive organisms to humans, *J Gerontol A Biol Sci Med Sci*, **59**, pp. B560–567.

209. Johnson, T. E. (2006). Recent results: biomarkers of aging, *Exp Gerontol*, **41**, pp. 1243–1246. https://doi.org/10.1016/j.exger.2006.09.006

210. Martin-Ruiz, C., & von Zglinicki, T. (2013). *A Life-Course Approach to Biomarkers of Ageing*, Oxford University Press (in press).

211. Christensen, K., Thinggaard, M., McGue, M., Rexbye, H., Hjelmborg, J. V., Aviv, A., *et al.* (2009). Perceived age as clinically useful biomarker of ageing: cohort study, *Bmj*, **339**, pp. b5262.

212. Martin-Ruiz, C., & von Zglinicki, T. (2014). Biomarkers of healthy ageing: expectations and validation, *Proc Nutr Soc*, **73**, pp. 422–429. https://doi.org/10.1017/s0029665114000147

213. Kristjansson, S. R. (2011). The role of geriatric assessment and frailty measurements in predicting surgical risk and survival in elderly patients with colorectal cancer, *Doktoravhandling*, University of Oslo.

214. Ferrucci, L., Harris, T. B., Guralnik, J. M., Tracy, R. P., Corti, M. C., Cohen, H. J., *et al.* (1999). Serum IL-6 level and the development of disability in older persons, *J Am Geriatr Soc*, **47**, pp. 639–646.

215. Tomar, N., & De, R. K. (2014). A brief outline of the immune system, *Methods Mol Biol*, **1184**, pp. 3–12. https://doi.org/10.1007/978-1-4939-1115-8_1

216. Hunter, C. A., & Jones, S. A. (2015). IL-6 as a keystone cytokine in health and disease, *Nat Immunol*, **16**, pp. 448–457. https://doi.org/10.1038/ni.3153

217. Mortensen, R. F. (2001). C-reactive protein, inflammation, and innate immunity, *Immunol Res*, **24**, pp. 163–176. https://doi.org/10.1385/ir:24:2:163

218. Panichi, V., Migliori, M., De Pietro, S., Taccola, D., Bianchi, A. M., Norpoth, M., *et al.* (2000). C-reactive protein as a marker of chronic inflammation in uremic patients, *Blood Purif*, **18**, pp. 183–190. https://doi.org/10.1159/000014417

219. Harris, T. B., Ferrucci, L., Tracy, R. P., Corti, M. C., Wacholder, S., Ettinger, W. H., Jr., *et al.* (1999). Associations of elevated interleukin-6 and C-reactive protein levels with mortality in the elderly, *Am J Med*, **106**, pp. 506–512.

220. Jenny, N. S., French, B., Arnold, A. M., Strotmeyer, E. S., Cushman, M., Chaves, P. H. M., *et al.* (2012). Long-term assessment of inflammation and healthy aging in late life: the cardiovascular health study all stars, *The Journals of Gerontology Series A: Biological Sciences and Medical Sciences*, **67**, pp. 970–976. https://doi.org/10.1093/gerona/glr261

221. Castagné, R., Garès, V., Karimi, M., Chadeau-Hyam, M., Vineis, P., Delpierre, C., *et al.* (2018). Allostatic load and subsequent all-cause mortality: which biological markers drive the relationship? Findings from a UK birth cohort [journal article], *European Journal of Epidemiology*, **33**, pp. 441–458. https://doi.org/10.1007/s10654-018-0364-1

222. Vineis, P., Avendano-Pabon, M., Barros, H., Chadeau-Hyam, M., Costa, G., Dijmarescu, M., *et al.* (2017). The biology of inequalities in health: the LIFEPATH project, *Longitudinal and Life Course Studies*, **8**, pp. 417–439. https://doi.org/10.14301/llcs.v8i4.448

223. Pathai, S., Lawn, S. D., Gilbert, C. E., McGuinness, D., McGlynn, L., Weiss, H. A., *et al.* (2013). Accelerated biological ageing in HIV-infected individuals in South Africa: a case-control study, *Aids*, **27**, pp. 2375–2384. https://doi.org/10.1097/QAD.0b013e328363bf7f

224. Pathai, S., Shiels, P. G., Weiss, H. A., Gilbert, C. E., Peto, T., Bekker, L. G., *et al.* (2013). Ocular parameters of biological ageing in HIV-infected individuals in South Africa: relationship with chronological age and systemic biomarkers of ageing, *Mech Ageing Dev*, **134**, pp. 400–406. https://doi.org/10.1016/j.mad.2013.08.002

225. Coppe, J. P., Desprez, P. Y., Krtolica, A., & Campisi, J. (2010). The senescence-associated secretory phenotype: the dark side of tumor suppression, *Annu Rev Pathol*, **5**, pp. 99–118. https://doi.org/10.1146/annurev-pathol-121808-102144

226. Watanabe, S., Kawamoto, S., Ohtani, N., & Hara, E. (2017). Impact of senescence-associated secretory phenotype and its potential as a therapeutic target for senescence-associated diseases, *Cancer Science*, **108**, pp. 563–569. https://doi.org/10.1111/cas.13184

227. Robinson, M. W., McGuinness, D., Swann, R., Barclay, S., Mills, P. R., Patel, A. H., *et al.* (2013). Non cell autonomous upregulation of CDKN2 transcription linked to progression of chronic hepatitis C disease, *Aging Cell*, **12**, pp. 1141–1143. https://doi.org/10.1111/acel.12125

228. Deeks, S. G. (2011). HIV: How to escape treatment, *Nature*, **477**, pp. 36–37. https://doi.org/10.1038/477036a

229. Broen, J. C., Coenen, M. J., & Radstake, T. R. (2012). Genetics of systemic sclerosis: an update, *Curr Rheumatol Rep*, **14**, pp. 11–21. https://doi.org/10.1007/s11926-011-0221-7

230. Dehbi, A. Z., Radstake, T. R., & Broen, J. C. (2013). Accelerated telomere shortening in rheumatic diseases: cause or consequence? *Expert Rev Clin Immunol*, **9**, pp. 1193–1204. https://doi.org/10.1586/1744666x.2013.850031

231. McGuinness, D., Mohammed, S., Monaghan, L., Wilson, P. A., Kingsmore, D. B., Shapter, O., *et al.* (2018). A molecular signature for delayed graft function, *Aging Cell*, **17**, pp. e12825. https://doi.org/10.1111/acel.12825

232. Matthaei, M., Meng, H., Meeker, A. K., Eberhart, C. G., & Jun, A. S. (2012). Endothelial Cdkn1a (p21) overexpression and accelerated senescence in a mouse model of Fuchs endothelial corneal dystrophy, *Investigative Ophthalmology & Visual Science*, **53**, pp. 6718–6727. https://doi.org/10.1167/iovs.12-9669

233. Baker, D. J., Weaver, R. L., & van Deursen, J. M. (2013). p21 both attenuates and drives senescence and aging in BubR1 progeroid mice, *Cell Rep*, **3**, pp. 1164–1174. https://doi.org/10.1016/j.celrep.2013.03.028

234. Jennings, P., Koppelstaetter, C., Aydin, S., Abberger, T., Wolf, A. M., Mayer, G., *et al.* (2007). Cyclosporine A induces senescence in renal tubular epithelial cells, *Am J Physiol Renal Physiol*, **293**, pp. F831–838. https://doi.org/10.1152/ajprenal.00005.2007

235. Munoz-Espin, D., & Serrano, M. (2014). Cellular senescence: from physiology to pathology, *Nat Rev Mol Cell Biol*, **15**, pp. 482–496. https://doi.org/10.1038/nrm3823

236. Dimri, G. P., Testori, A., Acosta, M., & Campisi, J. (1996). Replicative senescence, aging and growth-regulatory transcription factors, *Neurosignals*, **5**, pp. 154–162. https://www.karger.com/DOI/10.1159/000109185

237. Maier, A. B., Westendorp, R. G. J., & Van Heemst, D. (2007). Beta-galactosidase activity as a biomarker of replicative senescence during the course of human fibroblast cultures. In S. I. S. Rattan & S. Akman (Eds.), *Biogerontology: Mechanisms and Interventions*, **1100**, pp. 323–332. https://doi.org/10.1196/annals.1395.035

238. Melk, A., Kittikowit, W., Sandhu, I., Halloran, K. M., Grimm, P., Schmidt, B. M., *et al.* (2003). Cell senescence in rat kidneys in vivo increases with growth and age despite lack of telomere shortening, *Kidney Int*, **63**, pp. 2134–2143. https://doi.org/10.1046/j.1523-1755.2003.00032.x

239. Yang, N. C., & Hu, M. L. (2005). The limitations and validities of senescence associated-beta-galactosidase activity as an aging marker for human foreskin fibroblast Hs68 cells, *Exp Gerontol*, **40**, pp. 813–819. https://doi.org/10.1016/j.exger.2005.07.011
240. Lee, B. Y., Han, J. A., Im, J. S., Morrone, A., Johung, K., Goodwin, E. C., Kleijer, W. J., DiMaio, D., & Hwang, E. S. (2006). Senescence-associated beta-galactosidase is lysosomal beta-galactosidase. *Aging Cell*, **5**(2), pp. 187–195. https://doi.org/10.1111/j.1474-9726.2006.00199.x
241. Caldwell, M. E., DeNicola, G. M., Martins, C. P., Jacobetz, M. A., Maitra, A., Hruban, R. H., *et al.* (2012). Cellular features of senescence during the evolution of human and murine ductal pancreatic cancer, *Oncogene*, **31**, pp. 1599–1608. https://doi.org/10.1038/onc.2011.350
242. Kuilman, T., Michaloglou, C., Mooi, W. J., & Peeper, D. S. (2010). The essence of senescence, *Genes Dev*, **24**, pp. 2463–2479. https://doi.org/10.1101/gad.1971610
243. Biran, A., Zada, L., Abou Karam, P., Vadai, E., Roitman, L., Ovadya, Y., Porat, Z., & Krizhanovsky, V. (2017). Quantitative identification of senescent cells in aging and disease, *Aging Cell*, **16**, pp. 661–671. https://doi.org/10.1111/acel.12592
244. Schafer, C., Heiss, A., Schwarz, A., Westenfeld, R., Ketteler, M., Floege, J., *et al.* (2003). The serum protein alpha 2-Heremans-Schmid glycoprotein/fetuin-A is a systemically acting inhibitor of ectopic calcification, *J Clin Invest*, **112**, pp. 357–366. https://doi.org/10.1172/jci17202
245. Stefan, N., Hennige, A. M., Staiger, H., Machann, J., Schick, F., Krober, S. M., *et al.* (2006). Alpha2-Heremans-Schmid glycoprotein/fetuin-A is associated with insulin resistance and fat accumulation in the liver in humans, *Diabetes Care*, **29**, pp. 853–857.
246. Mori, K., Emoto, M., Yokoyama, H., Araki, T., Teramura, M., Koyama, H., *et al.* (2006). Association of serum fetuin-A with insulin resistance in type 2 diabetic and nondiabetic subjects, *Diabetes Care*, **29**, pp. 468–468. https://doi.org/10.2337/diacare.29.02.06.dc05-1484
247. Puchades, M., Hansson, S. F., Nilsson, C. L., Andreasen, N., Blennow, K., & Davidsson, P. (2003). Proteomic studies of potential cerebrospinal fluid protein markers for Alzheimer's disease, *Brain Res Mol Brain Res*, **118**, pp. 140–146.
248. Maxwell, F. (2013). The influence of biological ageing in the pathogenesis of colorectal cancer, MD thesis, University of Glasgow.

249. Carrero, J. J., Stenvinkel, P., Fellstrom, B., Qureshi, A. R., Lamb, K., Heimburger, O., *et al.* (2008). Telomere attrition is associated with inflammation, low fetuin-A levels and high mortality in prevalent haemodialysis patients, *J Intern Med*, **263**, pp. 302–312. https://doi.org/10.1111/j.1365-2796.2007.01890.x

250. Kuro-o, M., Matsumura, Y., Aizawa, H., Kawaguchi, H., Suga, T., Utsugi, T., *et al.* (1997). Mutation of the mouse klotho gene leads to a syndrome resembling ageing, *Nature*, **390**, pp. 45–51. https://doi.org/10.1038/36285

251. Kuro-o, M. (2009). Klotho and aging, *Biochim Biophys Acta*, **1790**, pp. 1049–1058. https://doi.org/10.1016/j.bbagen.2009.02.005

252. Kuro-o, M. (2010). A potential link between phosphate and aging—lessons from Klotho-deficient mice, *Mech Ageing Dev*, **131**, pp. 270–275. https://doi.org/10.1016/j.mad.2010.02.008

253. Kuro-o, M. (2011). Phosphate and Klotho [Review], *Kidney Int*, **79**, pp. S20–S23. https://doi.org/10.1038/ki.2011.26

254. Kestenbaum, B., Sampson, J. N., Rudser, K. D., Patterson, D. J., Seliger, S. L., Young, B., *et al.* (2005). Serum phosphate levels and mortality risk among people with chronic kidney disease, *J Am Soc Nephrol*, **16**, pp. 520–528. https://doi.org/10.1681/asn.2004070602

255. Kuro-o, M. (2013). Klotho, phosphate and FGF-23 in ageing and disturbed mineral metabolism, *Nat Rev Nephrol*, **9**, pp. 650–660. https://doi.org/10.1038/nrneph.2013.111

256. Kuro, O. M. (2018). Molecular mechanisms underlying accelerated aging by defects in the FGF23-Klotho system, *Int J Nephrol*, **2018**, pp. 9679841. https://doi.org/10.1155/2018/9679841

257. Watanabe, R., Fujita, N., Sato, Y., Kobayashi, T., Morita, M., Oike, T., *et al.* (2017). Enpp1 is an anti-aging factor that regulates Klotho under phosphate overload conditions, *Scientific Reports*, **7**, pp. 7786. https://doi.org/10.1038/s41598-017-07341-2

258. Kanfi, Y., Naiman, S., Amir, G., Peshti, V., Zinman, G., Nahum, L., *et al.* (2012). The sirtuin SIRT6 regulates lifespan in male mice, *Nature*, **483**, pp. 218–221. https://doi.org/10.1038/nature10815

259. McGuinness, D., McGuinness, D. H., McCaul, J. A., & Shiels, P. G. (2011). Sirtuins, bioageing, and cancer, *J Aging Res*, **2011**, pp. 235754. https://doi.org/10.4061/2011/235754

260. Waddington, C. H. (1942). Canalization of development and the inheritance of acquired characters [Article], *Nature*, **150**, pp. 563. https://doi.org/10.1038/150563a0

261. Egger, G., Liang, G., Aparicio, A., & Jones, P. A. (2004). Epigenetics in human disease and prospects for epigenetic therapy, *Nature*, **429**, pp. 457–463. https://doi.org/10.1038/nature02625

262. Bocklandt, S., Lin, W., Sehl, M. E., Sanchez, F. J., Sinsheimer, J. S., Horvath, S., *et al.* (2011). Epigenetic predictor of age, *PLoS One*, **6**, pp. e14821. https://doi.org/10.1371/journal.pone.0014821

263. Bellizzi, D., D'Aquila, P., Montesanto, A., Corsonello, A., Mari, V., Mazzei, B., *et al.* (2012). Global DNA methylation in old subjects is correlated with frailty, *Age*, **34**, pp. 169–179. https://doi.org/10.1007/s11357-011-9216-6

264. Collerton, J., Gautrey, H. E., van Otterdijk, S. D., Davies, K., Martin-Ruiz, C., von Zglinicki, T., *et al.* (2014). Acquisition of aberrant DNA methylation is associated with frailty in the very old: findings from the Newcastle 85+ Study, *Biogerontology*, **15**, pp. 317–328. https://doi.org/10.1007/s10522-014-9500-9

265. Horvath, S., & Raj, K. (2018). DNA methylation-based biomarkers and the epigenetic clock theory of ageing, *Nature Reviews Genetics*, **19**, pp. 371–384. https://doi.org/10.1038/s41576-018-0004-3

266. Jylhava, J., Pedersen, N. L., & Hagg, S. (2017). Biological age predictors, *EBioMedicine*, **21**, pp. 29–36. https://doi.org/10.1016/j.ebiom.2017.03.046

267. Lee, H. Y., Lee, S. D., & Shin, K. J. (2016). Forensic DNA methylation profiling from evidence material for investigative leads, *BMB Rep*, **49**, pp. 359–369.

268. Franzen, J., Zirkel, A., Blake, J., Rath, B., Benes, V., Papantonis, A., et al. (2017). Senescence-associated DNA methylation is stochastically acquired in subpopulations of mesenchymal stem cells, *Aging Cell*, **16**, pp. 183–191. https://doi.org/10.1111/acel.12544

269. Lowe, D., Horvath, S., & Raj, K. (2016). Epigenetic clock analyses of cellular senescence and ageing, *Oncotarget*, **7**, pp. 8524–8531. https://doi.org/10.18632/oncotarget.7383

270. Lu, A. T., Xue, L., Salfati, E. L., Chen, B. H., Ferrucci, L., Levy, D., *et al.* (2018). GWAS of epigenetic aging rates in blood reveals a critical role for TERT, *Nat Commun*, **9**, pp. 387. https://doi.org/10.1038/s41467-017-02697-5

271. Levine, M. E., Lu, A. T., Quach, A., Chen, B. H., Assimes, T. L., Bandinelli, S., *et al.* (2018). An epigenetic biomarker of aging for lifespan and health span, *Aging (Albany NY)*, **10**, pp. 573–591. https://doi.org/10.18632/aging.101414

272. Goffaux, J., Friesinger, G. C., Lambert, W., Shroyer, L. W., Moritz, T. E., McCarthy, M., Jr., *et al.* (2005). Biological age-a concept whose time has come: a preliminary study, *South Med J*, **98**, pp. 985–993. https://doi.org/10.1097/01.smj.0000182178.22607.47

273. Zhang, W. G., Zhu, S. Y., Bai, X. J., Zhao, D. L., Jian, S. M., Li, J., Li, Z. X., Fu, B., Cai, G. Y., Sun, X. F., & Chen, X. M. (2014). Select aging biomarkers based on telomere length and chronological age to build a biological age equation, *Age (Dordr)*, **36**, pp. 9639. https://doi.org/10.1007/s11357-014-9639-y

274. Krop, J. S., Coresh, J., Chambless, L. E., Shahar, E., Watson, R. L., Szklo, M., *et al.* (1999). A community-based study of explanatory factors for the excess risk for early renal function decline in blacks vs whites with diabetes: the atherosclerosis risk in communities study, *Arch Intern Med*, **159**, pp. 1777–1783.

275. Levey, A. S., de Jong, P. E., Coresh, J., El Nahas, M., Astor, B. C., Matsushita, K., *et al.* (2011). The definition, classification, and prognosis of chronic kidney disease: a KDIGO controversies conference report, *Kidney Int*, **80**, pp. 17–28. https://doi.org/10.1038/ki.2010.483

276. Drawz, P., & Rahman, M. (2015). Chronic kidney disease, *Ann Intern Med*, **162**, ITC1. https://doi.org/10.7326/AITC201506020

277. Fink, H. A., Ishani, A., Taylor, B. C., Greer, N. L., MacDonald, R., Rossini, D., *et al.* (2012). AHRQ comparative effectiveness reviews. In chronic kidney disease stages 1–3: screening, monitoring, and treatment, *Agency for Healthcare Research and Quality (US)*, Report No.: **11**(12)-EHC075-EF.

278. Levey, A. S., Stevens, L. A., Schmid, C. H., Zhang, Y. L., Castro, A. F., III, Feldman, H. I., *et al.* (2009). A new equation to estimate glomerular filtration rate, *Ann Intern Med*, **150**, pp. 604–612.

279. Matsushita, K., Mahmoodi, B. K., Woodward, M., Emberson, J. R., Jafar, T. H., Jee, S. H., *et al.* (2012). Comparison of risk prediction using the CKD-EPI equation and the MDRD study equation for estimated glomerular filtration rate, *Jama*, **307**, pp. 1941–1951. https://doi.org/10.1001/jama.2012.3954

280. Go, A. S., Chertow, G. M., & Fan, D. (2005). Chronic kidney disease and the risks of death, cardiovascular events, and hospitalization, *Journal of Vascular Surgery*, **41**, pp. 177. https://doi.org/10.1016/j.jvs.2004.10.020

281. Hallan, S. I., Matsushita, K., Sang, Y., Mahmoodi, B. K., Black, C., Ishani, A., *et al.* (2012). Age and association of kidney measures with

mortality and end-stage renal disease, *Jama*, **308**, pp. 2349–2360. https://doi.org/10.1001/jama.2012.16817

282. Rahman, M., Pressel, S., Davis, B. R., Nwachuku, C., Wright, J. T., Jr., Whelton, P. K., *et al.* (2006). Cardiovascular outcomes in high-risk hypertensive patients stratified by baseline glomerular filtration rate, *Ann Intern Med*, **144**, pp. 172–180.
283. Foley, R. N. (2010). Clinical epidemiology of cardiovascular disease in chronic kidney disease, *J Ren Care*, **36**, pp. 4–8. https://doi.org/10.1111/j.1755-6686.2010.00171.x
284. Stenvinkel, P., & Larsson, T. E. (2013). Chronic kidney disease: a clinical model of premature aging [Review], *American Journal of Kidney Diseases*, **62**, pp. 339–351. https://doi.org/10.1053/j.ajkd.2012.11.051
285. McClelland, R., Christensen, K., Mohammed, S., McGuinness, D., Cooney, J., Bakshi, A., *et al.* (2016). Accelerated ageing and renal dysfunction links lower socioeconomic status and dietary phosphate intake, *Aging (Albany NY)*, **8**, pp. 1135–1148. https://doi.org/10.18632/aging.100948
286. Byon, C. H., Javed, A., Dai, Q., Kappes, J. C., Clemens, T. L., Darley-Usmar, V. M., *et al.* (2008). Oxidative stress induces vascular calcification through modulation of the osteogenic transcription factor Runx2 by AKT signaling, *J Biol Chem*, **283**, pp. 15319–15327. https://doi.org/10.1074/jbc.M800021200
287. Hale, J. E., Fraser, J. D., & Price, P. A. (1988). The identification of matrix Gla protein in cartilage, *J Biol Chem*, **263**, pp. 5820–5824.
288. Luo, G., Ducy, P., McKee, M. D., Pinero, G. J., Loyer, E., Behringer, R. R., *et al.* (1997). Spontaneous calcification of arteries and cartilage in mice lacking matrix GLA protein, *Nature*, **386**, pp. 78–81. https://doi.org/10.1038/386078a0
289. Shanahan, C. M., Crouthamel, M. H., Kapustin, A., & Giachelli, C. M. (2011). Arterial calcification in chronic kidney disease: key roles for calcium and phosphate, *Circ Res*, **109**, pp. 697–711. https://doi.org/10.1161/circresaha.110.234914
290. Shroff, R. C., McNair, R., Figg, N., Skepper, J. N., Schurgers, L., Gupta, A., *et al.* (2008). Dialysis accelerates medial vascular calcification in part by triggering smooth muscle cell apoptosis, *Circulation*, **118**, pp. 1748–1757. https://doi.org/10.1161/circulationaha.108.783738
291. Speer, M. Y., Li, X., Hiremath, P. G., & Giachelli, C. M. (2010). Runx2/Cbfa1, but not loss of myocardin, is required for smooth

muscle cell lineage reprogramming toward osteochondrogenesis, *J Cell Biochem*, **110**, pp. 935–947. https://doi.org/10.1002/jcb.22607

292. Adams, J. N., Raffield, L. M., Freedman, B. I., Langefeld, C. D., Ng, M. C., Carr, J. J., *et al.* (2014). Analysis of common and coding variants with cardiovascular disease in the diabetes heart study, *Cardiovasc Diabetol*, **13**, pp. 77. https://doi.org/10.1186/1475-2840-13-77.
293. Ferguson, J. F., Matthews, G. J., Townsend, R. R., Raj, D. S., Kanetsky, P. A., Budoff, M., *et al.* (2013). Candidate gene association study of coronary artery calcification in chronic kidney disease: findings from the CRIC study (Chronic Renal Insufficiency Cohort), *J Am Coll Cardiol*, **62**, pp. 789–798. https://doi.org/10.1016/j.jacc.2013.01.103
294. Helgadottir, A., Thorleifsson, G., Manolescu, A., Gretarsdottir, S., Blondal, T., Jonasdottir, A., *et al.* (2007). A common variant on chromosome 9p21 affects the risk of myocardial infarction, *Science*, **316**, pp. 1491–1493. https://doi.org/10.1126/science.1142842
295. Larson, M. G., Atwood, L. D., Benjamin, E. J., Cupples, L. A., D'Agostino, R. B., Sr., Fox, C. S., *et al.* (2007). Framingham Heart Study 100K project: genome-wide associations for cardiovascular disease outcomes, *BMC Med Genet*, **8**, pp. S5. https://doi.org/10.1186/1471-2350-8-s1-s5
296. Lee, J. Y., Lee, B. S., Shin, D. J., Woo Park, K., Shin, Y. A., Joong Kim, K., *et al.* (2013). A genome-wide association study of a coronary artery disease risk variant, *J Hum Genet*, **58**, pp. 120–126. https://doi.org/10.1038/jhg.2012.124
297. Sun, L. Q., Lee, D. W., Zhang, Q., Xiao, W., Raabe, E. H., Meeker, A., *et al.* (2004). Growth retardation and premature aging phenotypes in mice with disruption of the SNF2-like gene, PASG, *Genes Dev*, **18**, pp. 1035–1046. https://doi.org/10.1101/gad.1176104
298. Fee, E. (1991). Save the babies: American public health reform and the prevention of infant mortality, 1850–1929, *Medical History*, **35**, pp. 374–375. http://www.ncbi.nlm.nih.gov/pmc/articles/PMC1036505/
299. Foundation, N. K. (2002). K/DOQI clinical practice guidelines for chronic kidney disease: evaluation, classification, and stratification, *Am J Kidney Dis*, **39**(2 Suppl 1), pp. S1–266.
300. Itahana, K., Campisi, J., & Dimri, G. P. (2007). Methods to detect biomarkers of cellular senescence: the senescence-associated beta-galactosidase assay, *Methods Mol Biol*, **371**, pp. 21–31.
301. Keane, M., Craig, T., Alföldi, J., Berlin, A. M., Johnson, J., Seluanov, A., *et al.* (2014). The naked mole rat genome resource: facilitating

analyses of cancer and longevity-related adaptations, *Bioinformatics*, **30**, pp. 3558–3560. https://doi.org/10.1093/bioinformatics/btu579

302. Tian, X., Azpurua, J., Hine, C., Vaidya, A., Myakishev-Rempel, M., Ablaeva, J., *et al.* (2013). High-molecular-mass hyaluronan mediates the cancer resistance of the naked mole rat, *Nature*, **499**, pp. 346. https://doi.org/10.1038/nature12234
303. UN Department of Economic and Social Affairs (2010). *World Population Prospects, The 2012 Revision*. New York: United Nations.
304. European Parliamentary Research Service (2013). *Ageing Population: Projections 2010–2060 for the EU27*.
305. National Research Council Panel to Advance a Research Program on the Design of National Health (2010). The National Academies Collection: Reports funded by National Institutes of Health, *Accounting for Health and Health Care: Approaches to Measuring the Sources and Costs of Their Improvement,* Washington (DC): National Academies Press (US).
306. The Swedish National Institute of Public Health (2007). Healthy ageing a challenge for Europe, *NRS Tryckeri AB: Huskvarna*

Part II

Telomere Length

Chapter 2

Telomere Length as a Marker of Biological Age

Stella Baliou,[a,b] Persefoni Fragkiadaki,[a,b] Elena Vakonaki,[a,b] Petros Ioannou,[c] Elisavet Renieri,[a,b] Manolis Tzatzarakis,[a] and Aristidis Tsatsakis[a,b]

[a]*Laboratory of Toxicology, Medical School, University of Crete, Heraklion, Greece*
[b]*Lifeplus S.A., Science & Technological Park of Crete, Vassilika Vouton, Heraklion, Greece*
[c]*School of Medicine, University of Crete, Heraklion, Greece*
tsatsaka@uoc.gr

2.1 Introduction

Aging is a process in which multiple organ systems are functionally dysregulated [1]. This gradual and progressive degenerative state is characterized by stem cell exhaustion, genomic instability, epigenetic reprogramming, telomere shortening, cellular senescence, dysregulated metabolism, loss of proteostasis, and aberrations in both intercellular communication and nutrient sensing [2], thereby contributing to limited healthy lifespan.

An individual's chronological age measures physical decline, whereas an individual's biological age measures functional decline

Telomeres: Biomarkers of a Healthy Life and Successful Aging
Edited by Aristidis Tsatsakis

ISBN 978-981-5129-49-6 (Hardcover), 978-1-003-56809-4 (eBook)
www.jennystanford.com

[3]. Indeed, the biological age of one individual is distinguished from the other, despite having the same chronological age [4, 5]. Biological age is an estimator of cell aging, monitoring the cellular DNA damage over time on an individual basis [6, 7]. As such, biological age can be considered a more critical and precise marker for the risk of age-associated disorders and eventual mortality than chronological age [8]. In most cases, biological age appears to be increased compared to chronological age forming age acceleration residual (AAR) [5]. Individuals with positive AAR have more attenuated functional capacity than their peers, conferring higher disease-risk. In contrast, individuals with a perfect balance between biological and chronological age should exhibit a zero value of AAR (Fig. 2.1) [5]. As a result, biomarkers of biological age are considered more reliable than those of chronological age, providing comprehensive insights into the disease risk and mortality [9]. Identifying biological age predictors is particularly important because they can serve as predictive tools for increased susceptibility to many age-related diseases [9].

Indeed, an individual's biological age is delayed from the chronological age, due to genetic predisposition, environmental and lifestyle factors (lack of sleep, sedentary behavior, smoking, unhealthy nutrition, stress), and estrogens [4, 5]. The unhealthy lifestyle of one individual has been associated with an increased biological age, while a healthy lifestyle seems beneficial through preventing cell aging [10].

On the one hand, the rejuvenating effect of calorie restriction on prolonging lifespan is attributed to the attenuation of the aging process through epigenetic alterations, such as DNA methylation (DNAm) and histone modifications (Fig. 2.1) [11, 12]. As shown in primates, the restricted dietary composition can reduce the susceptibility to age-related disorders by 40% [13]. It can exert a beneficial effect on the aging process by ameliorating liver function and preventing oxidative stress [13]. On the other hand, deficits in physical activity, unhealthy dietary composition, alcohol use, and smoking are accompanied by disturbances of normal metabolism, as evidenced by the accumulation of low-density lipoproteins, high levels of glucose, triglycerides, and high blood pressure [10]. In a molecular setting, the high consumption of

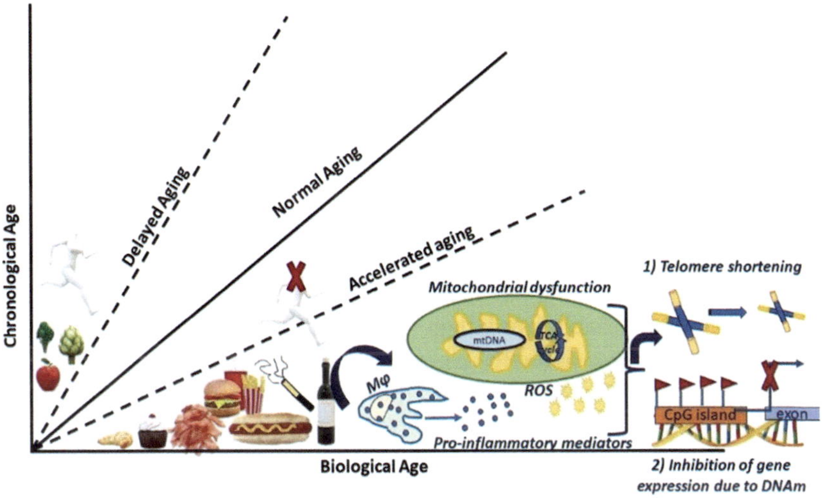

Figure 2.1 The rate of cell aging is mainly genetic-dependent but also affected by environmental inputs. An unhealthy lifestyle (smoking, not exercising, and excessive salt and fatty acids in diet) causes inflammation and oxidative stress that account for telomere shortening. In parallel, the increased methylation at CpG islands accounts for the silencing of gene expression at specific genes. Abbreviations: macrophage ($M\varphi$), mitochondrial DNA (mtDNA), telomere length combing assay (TCA), cytosine phosphate-guanine dinucleotides (CpG), and DNA methylation (DNAm).

saturated fat and the increased salt intake exert a pronounced effect on accelerating the biological age, through the induction of oxidative stress and inflammation with detrimental effects on telomere length (TL) [14]. A possible explanation for this positive correlation of TL with an unhealthy lifestyle is the increased secretion of oxidant, and pro-inflammatory mediators, which account for telomere shortening (Fig. 2.1) [15]. In vitro and in vivo setting, it has been proved that telomere shortening can be accelerated through an unhealthy diet-mediated oxidative stress and inflammatory effects [14, 16, 17]. Indeed, the accumulation of reactive oxygen species (ROS) that exceeds the cellular antioxidant defenses [18–20], can cause 8-oxo-7,8-dihydro-2′-deoxyguanine (8-oxoG) DNA lesions contributing to telomere shortening. The G-rich content of 5'TTAGGG3' telomeric repeats makes them sensitive to oxidative stress impairing telomere length and integrity [21]. In this manner, DNA replication is inhibited [21] and mitochondrial function and energy production are attenuated, thus generating a positive feedforward loop (Fig. 2.1) [21, 22]. Besides, the premature aging phenotypes have been observed in telomerase-deficient mice [23] and mice bearing mitochondrial dysfunction [24]. On the other hand, the durable inflammation has been illustrated to cause telomere shortening. Telomere shortening is one example of the triggers that can promote cell senescence [25]. Senescent cells are characterized by senescence-associated secretory phenotype (SASP) that creates an inflammatory microenvironment, which induces senescence in bystander cells. The SASP profile differs among cell types and is composed of pro-inflammatory mediators, such as tumor necrosis factor-a (TNFa), C-reactive protein (CRP), interleukin-6 (IL-6), growth factors [e.g., vascular endothelial growth factor (VEGF) and epidermal growth factor (EGF) and], chemokines and proteases such as matrix-metalloproteinases-1/3 (MMP-1/3) (Fig. 2.1) [26–29]. The SASP of senescent cells has been acknowledged to drive the pathogenesis of age-related diseases [30]. In contrast, exercise can strongly ameliorate muscle function by reprogramming DNA methylation (DNAm) and histone modifications, thus attenuating biological aging through contributing to telomere length maintenance or elongation (Fig. 2.1.) [31–35]. Likewise, a balanced diet seems to positively influence biological aging, preventing telomere shortening [10, 13].

2.2 Determination of Biological Age Predictors

The characterization of driving factors that cause a divergence between an individual's chronological and biological age, thus aiding in identifying new therapeutic interventions to halt the aging process. Importantly, this chapter provides an overview of the current knowledge about the methods of biological age determination, thus improving risk prediction for the onset of age-related diseases [36]. The common biomarkers are categorized into three types: (a) molecular and cellular (relied on DNA, RNA, etc.), (b) functional and structural (clinical parameters), and (c) composite biomarker predictors after the combination of omics data [37].

Such biomarkers of biological age determination are the following: estimating TL [38], patterns of DNAm [39], transcriptomic signatures [40], and proteomic profiles [41]. DNAm and TL have been documented to be highly efficient and precise biomarkers of the aging process [42]. However, the association between DNAm and TL and other clinical parameters seems low or non-significant [42–44]. Importantly, DNAm and TL are independently linked to chronological age and mortality [42].

Other age-associated epigenetic markers can be changes in the transcription of noncoding RNAs (ncRNAs), especially in miRNAs [45], post-translational modifications like those implicated in histones [46], and chromatin reprogramming [2]. Quantitative polymerase chain reaction (qPCR) and sequencing analysis have been used to detect changes in miRNA expression across tissues with high sensitivity, specificity, and stability [47]. Aging can also be determined by the microbe prevalence suggesting the microbiome as a biological age estimator and its targeting through therapeutic approaches [48, 49]. Besides, the potential involvement of gut microbiota in mediating such effects needs to be clarified through further research.

To leverage a transcriptome as a biological age predictor, nine cohorts have employed blood-based tests to elucidate the gene expression profiles of the elderly compared to the young. The gene expression levels of five transcripts were initially analyzed in the InCHIANTI cohort. The five-transcript model was also evaluated in two additional cohorts (Exeters with 95 samples and San Antonio Family Heart Study (SAFHS) with 1240 samples) together with the InCHIANTI cohort with 698 samples [50]. In another six independent cohorts, the expression levels of 1497 transcripts were examined in 7074 human blood samples of European ancestry populations [51] after adjusting the transcriptome to their age and lifestyle. The discrepancy between chronological age and biological age was attributed to different biological attributes of aging, like body mass index (BMI), glucose, cholesterol, and pressure [51]. As a result, the predicted biological age based on transcriptome differed from the chronological age from 4.84 to 11.21 years (mean = 7.8 years). Accordingly, two important transcriptomes emerged in the blood through Self-Organizing Maps ML (SOM-ML) analysis.

Recently, researchers used transcriptome to develop the binarized transcriptomic aging "BiT age" clock in C. elegans and human fibroblasts to provide accurately predicted biological age [52]. Notably, the transcriptome of the "BiT age" clock was composed of genes related to the immune and neural systems, which are crucial for the progression of aging [52].

In line with this, proteome derived from the plasma of patients has been used to predict age acceleration compared to their chronological age [53]. The "PROAge" clock was composed of 76 proteins implicated in aging. Similarly, proteome from the plasma of 491 patients has been leveraged to provide information about the susceptibility to age-related pathologies [54].

Apart from the proteome itself, several studies have illustrated that post-translational modifications of glycans in either human serum or plasma can be used to estimate biological age [55]. More insights into proteins' impact have come from studies that evaluated Immunoglobulin G (IgG) glycosylation (including glycans, such as FA2B, FA2G2, and FA2BG2) related to chronological age [56].

Growing evidence has also suggested metabolome is a major determinant factor behind the evaluation of biological age. Different measurement techniques, such as mass-spectrometry and proton nuclear magnetic resonance (H1 NMR), have been used for the identification of metabolites, thereby forming the Metabolic Age Score that is correlated to the clinical manifestations of patients irrespective of their age [57]. In other cases, the characterization of metabolites related to aging through ultra-high-performance liquid chromatography–mass spectrometry (UHPLC-MS) has enabled the identification of biological age relying on the overall snapshot of metabolic pathways [58, 59].

Furthermore, routine clinical tests have been used to estimate the overall lipid and glucose metabolism. The accurate assessment of biological age can also be accomplished through measurements of cholesterols [high-density lipoprotein (HDL) and low-density lipoprotein (LDL)] [60], glucose tests [oral glucose tolerance test (OGTT) and glycated hemoglobin (Hba1c)] [61], levels of pro-inflammatory mediators like [IL-15, IL-6, IL-1β, IL-8, and TNFα] [62], oxidative stress [2], and renal parameters like albumin, creatinine, ureal, and systolic blood pressure with maximal oxygen consumption [63], thus estimating overall physical health.

Since biological aging is a multiparametric and incredibly complicated process, there is not a single marker that can precisely estimate the biological age considering every facet of the aging process [64]. Using single-molecule biomarkers makes the biological age prediction very simplistic, so a more precise "blueprint" of aging can arise from omics data [65]. The high-throughput omics technologies compiled several omics data like metabolomics, transcriptomics, epigenomics, transcriptomics, and proteomics, enabling more accurate prediction of aging trajectories than single biomarkers. For example, the combination of omics data has enabled the quantification of biological age, therefore offering new perspectives regarding the precise estimation of developing age-related diseases [6, 43, 66–72].

To sum up, there is escalating interest in predicting biological age, focusing on both DNAm and TL, but metabolomics and a combination of omics data have been shown to provide convincing clues about the susceptibility for age-related diseases [6, 73–75].

2.3 DNA Methylation as a Biological Age Predictor

The overall content of methylation at cytosine phosphate-guanine dinucleotides (CpG) sites can indicate an accurate prediction of cell aging in humans [74]. Growing evidence has proved that DNAm is a crucial factor in regulating gene expression [76–82] since DNAm exerts a significant impact on the recruitment of transcription factors and mapping of related histone modifications, which themselves orchestrate the transcriptional landscape and regulate the gene expression, respectively [83–85]. For example, a meta-analysis has shown that hypermethylation at CpG islands (CGIs) occurs in many tissues and accounts for preventing the expression of many genes [86, 87].

Across the genome, 28 million CpG sites undergo DNAm, and they are clustered in CGIs, which are usually located at gene promoters at a 60–70% rate [88, 89]. However, CGIs within transcriptional start sites (TSSs) of active genes are generally hypomethylated [90]. With the advanced age, CGIs seem to be hypermethylated [91, 92] in both bivalent promoters [93] and Polycomb target genes [87, 94], thereby causing this epigenetic mode of silencing. Age-related hypomethylated regions are preferentially found in non-CGI promoters, enhancers, and late-replicating domains [95].

In the past two decades, DNAm has appeared to be a precise estimator to predict biological age. Bocklandt et al. reported the first clock based on methylation of 88 CpG sites to indicate age [96]. The "Hannum and Horvath" clocks were mainly acknowledged as robust calculators of chronological age. Still, they displayed variations in the calculation of chronological age (r_2 = 0.91 for the "Hannum" clock and r_2 = 0.96 for the "Horvath" clock) [65]. Then, other epigenetic clocks were leveraged to estimate biological age. The "Horvath" clock was considered the epigenetic clock that provided a rough calculation of age in a tissue and cell-specific manner based on 353 CpG sites derived from the Illumina 27 K array [97]. It should be noted that the mean difference was 3.2% per CpG in individuals up to 35 years old compared to those above 55 years old [5]. In parallel, the "Hannum clock" was created to predict the age in tissue and a cell-specific manner, using only 71 CpG sites derived from the Illumina 450 K array in whole blood samples [98]. In principle, the "Hannum and Horvath" clocks shared the capacity to predict all-cause mortality [74]. The "Horvath" clock is regarded as a multi-tissue clock because it is applied in various tissues [whole blood, peripheral blood mononuclear cells (PBMCs), brain, cerebellar samples, liver, saliva, buccal epithelium, colon, lung, adipose tissue, liver, and lungs] [97]. On the contrary, the "Hannum" clock appears after measurements in blood cell proportions [98]. Indeed, the "Horvath" clock can describe the whole aging process, whereas a tissue-specific clock like the "Hannum" clock provides insights into the susceptibility to age-dependent pathologies [99]. The results, as mentioned above, emerged given that the total sample size was composed of 800 individuals in the "Horvath" clock, and 656 participants were enrolled in the "Hannum" clock [97, 98].

In line with this, a mitotic-like biological DNAm "epiTOC" clock was created after mapping 385 CpGs at the promoters of Polycomb target genes, which were unmethylated at the fetal stage [100]. In 2017, Zhang et al. developed a clock that showed the risk for all-cause mortality to a greater extent than that derived from the "Horvath and Hannum" clocks, relying on 10 CpG sites [101]. Accordingly, Youn et al. developed a mitotic-like "MiAge" clock, relying on 268 CpGs across the genome, which showed enhanced DNAm with each cell division [102]. Even though the "MiAge" clock originated from studies in the field of cancer, the "MiAge" clock can be leveraged as a biomarker relative to aging [102].

In addition to those above first-generation epigenetic clocks, second-generation epigenetic clocks (PhenoAge, GrimAge, and ScAge) have emerged, due to their capacity to assess the risk of age-specific diseases [9, 103, 104]. The second-generation epigenetic clocks enable the identification of underlying differences behind the risk of age-related diseases in a personalized manner [10, 113, 114]. The main characteristic of second-generation epigenetic clocks lies in their ability to precisely predict the biological age on an individual basis based on their specific biological attribute (DNAm) [9, 103, 104]. In particular, the "PnenoAge clock" served as a predictive biomarker of biological age after incorporating the analysis of DNAm with other 42 clinical covariates derived from 9926 participants recruited at the National Health and Nutrition Examination Survey (NHANES) [105]. The biological age was determined in that analysis after adjusting DNAm to different clinical parameters like white blood cell (WBC), CRP, and creatine. Compared to first-generation clocks that predicted mortality [106], the "PhenoAge clock" provided deep insight into predicting all-cause mortality from 10 to 20 years and evaluating the risk of age-related comorbidities even adjusting to their chronological age [107]. In that context, Levine et al. developed a "DNAmPhenoAge" epigenetic clock that exerted high predictive value for mortality and risk of unhealthy outcomes after the incorporation of DNAm at 513 CpG sites with nine markers of tissue function and immune function adjusting to chronological age [103]. Increased "DNAmPhenoAge" clock was related to the stimulation of pro-inflammatory and interferon pathways as well as the downregulation of transcriptional/translational machinery, DNA damage response (DDR), and mitochondrial pathways, proposing the importance of signaling pathways in aging [103]. In that manner, Levine et al. developed a multi-estimator of biological age and confirmed the results through a meta-analysis of five large populations. The meta-analysis results illustrated that an acceleration in the "DNAm PhenoAge" clock for one year was related to an increased risk for all-cause mortality by 4.5% [103]. Based on the above, the "DNAmPhenoAge" clock seems superior to previous ones in providing insight into survival and health outcomes [103].

The "GrimAge" clock was used to calculate biological age and all-cause mortality after combining the analysis of DNAm levels of 88 proteins in plasma and the packs of cigarettes for years [9, 108]. The "GrimAge" clock is considered a sensitive epigenetic clock for providing information regarding susceptibility for different clinical phenotypes [9]. Notably, it has been substantiated that "GrimAge" clock outweighed other epigenetic clocks, such as "Horvath", "Hannum", and "DNAmPhenoAge" epigenetic clocks in providing all-cause mortality risk [9].

To sum up, second-generation clocks, such as the "PhenoAge and GrimAge", predict morbidity and mortality with high accuracy at a greater extent as compared to the first-generation clocks [9, 103]. Indeed, the "PnenoAge and GrimAge" clocks provide an accurate quantitative estimate of biological age and the onset of aging-related diseases [103, 108]. Based on methylation levels at a single-cell level, the "ScAge" clock is used as an epigenetic clock to separate young from aged cells in heterogeneous tissues since aging differs among cell types within a tissue [109].

2.4 Telomere Length as a Biological Age Predictor

Initially, Harley et al. were the pioneers who demonstrated that telomere shortening occurred with each cell division [110]. Leucocyte telomere length (LTL) has been widely substantiated as a very strong biomarker of aging [111], but inconsistency among studies has underestimated its use [38, 112, 113]. There is also considerable research regarding the use of TL as a significant contributor to age-related disorders [114, 115]. To support the causal role of telomere shortening in aging, cells with short telomeres exhibit cellular senescence and death due to the induction of DDR [116].

Senescence does not necessarily show cell aging, but telomere attrition is undoubtedly implicated in both aging and senescence [117].

Within the last few years, the TL has been addressed through several approaches (Table 2.1) [118, 119]. Terminal restriction fragment (TRF) analysis was reported as the "gold standard" technique for relative quantification of TL and substrate for the following techniques [120]. The TRF method was the first one that revealed TL's inverse relationship with aging [110]. The principle behind TRF analysis is based on three steps: DNA digestion with different combinations of restriction enzymes that do not have recognition sites, then agarose gel electrophoresis of DNA, and, finally, visualization through Southern blot [120]. In the TRF technique, the quantification of average TL is accomplished after labeling the telomere smear with a radioactive telomere probe adjusting to the known intensity and size of the DNA ladder since repetitive telomere sequences remain intact [120–122]. However, a smear of variable lengths of telomeres is visualized through Southern blot analysis, but the telomeres of the shortest length cannot be visualized [120–122]. Accordingly, many shortcomings have limited the use of TRF analysis, such as the difficulties in the extraction of genomic DNA due to possible DNA degradation, the high quantity of genomic DNA, lack of information about single and short telomeres, not application to epidemiological studies and polymorphisms in telomeres complicating TL measurement [123]. Then, researchers proceeded to the relative quantification of average TL through qPCR [124, 125]. In this procedure, TL is measured after dividing the amplified fluorescence intensity signal of telomere repeat copy numbers by that of autosomal single copy gene (T/S ratio) using a standard curve [126]. In this manner, a relative measure of average TL is provided in the population of cells of every tissue examined [124, 125]. Indeed, TL measurements arise through a linear regression equation. It is important to note that qPCR has the advantage of being applied to large-scale studies in a high-throughput manner using only 50 ng as a starting genetic material and being of high quality, not amenable to DNA degradation [123, 127]. Even though qPCR has received considerable attention as a recommended method for

Table 2.1 Telomere length determination methods

Method	Principle	Starting material	Application	Property	Reference
TRF	Relative quantification of average TL through digestion of genomic DNA with restriction enzymes, leaving intact the telomeres	Approx. 1–3 μg DNA	Not applied to large populations	Gold standard for TL measurement, time-consuming, laborious, not recognition of short telomeres	[123]
qPCR	Relative quantification of average TL	Approx. 20–50 ng DNA	Population-based studies	Rapid, laborious, not recognition of short telomeres	[124–128]
Metaphase FISH	Quantification of absolute TL in individual chromosomes at single cells in metaphase	Metaphase chromosomes	Not applied to large populations	Low detection limit, laborious, time-consuming, low throughput	[129-132]
Interphase Q-FISH	Quantification of TL in single cells at interphase	Interphase nuclei	Not applied to large populations	Labor-intensive	[133]
Flow-FISH	Relative quantification of average TL	Interphase nuclei	Clinical diagnostic tool, not suited for large studies	Evaluation of mean telomere content in single cells, tedious	[134]
HT Q-FISH	Relative quantification of average TL	Interphase nuclei	Applied to large populations	Very accurate, no detection of telomere free ends and telomere clusters at interphase, no measurement of TL in individual chromosomes	[135]

PRINS	Relative quantification of average TL	Interphase or metaphase nuclei	Not applied to large populations	Faster alternative to FISH	[119]
PHAST	Telomere relative measurement as short as 100 bp	DNA	A small number of cells	Measurement of telomeres shorter than 15 kb	[138, 139]
STELA	Absolute abundance of shortest telomeres in a chromosome-specific manner	DNA	A small subset of single chromosomes	Measurement of chromosome-specific TL, absolutely low throughput, laborious, no recognition of telomere-free ends	[140, 141]
Universal STELA	Absolute quantification of shortest telomeres	DNA	Not applied to large populations	Laborious, low-throughput, no detection of TL over 8 kb	[142]
TeSLA	Measurement of telomeres less than 1 kb up to 18 kbs in all chromosomes	Less than 1 μg DNA	Applied to many studies, diagnostic tools for disease development	Precise, sensitive, unbiased, laborious, low- throughput, without detection of ITSs	[143]
TCA	Measurement of absolute TL (range from less than 1 kb up to 80 kbs)	DNA	Applied to large populations	High-throughput, information about TL distribution	[144]
STAR	Measurement of absolute TL (range from 0.2 kb up to 320 kbs)	DNA less than 1 ng	Applied to large populations	High-throughput, information about TL distribution	[145]

providing a relatively average TL in large-scale epidemiological studies, there are inconsistencies in results due to different DNA extraction methods, post-extraction processes from various tissue types, and storage conditions [120, 128, 129]. The inter-assay variability through qPCR has been calculated to range from 2.27% to 28% [130]. The significant addressed limitations of qPCR are the precise detection of very short telomeres and accurate telomere length measured in kilobases (kbs) [131]. The major shortcoming of qPCR is its inability to provide information concerning the TL differences between cells and chromosomes in every individual [111]. Some other modifications of qPCR [monochrome multiplex quantitative PCR (MMqPCR) and absolute telomere length (aTL) qPCR] have been introduced to address some challenges of qPCR. The MMqPCR can have telomeric and reference signals in the same tube, avoiding the variation between tubes [119, 125] and the aTL qPCR can provide an absolute quantification of TL [119, 126]. Then, quantitative fluorescence in situ hybridization (Q-FISH) has been proposed to quantify critically short repeated telomeric sequences, which are very important in chromatin stability and cell viability [121, 132]. The metaphase Q-FISH method has been proven more reliable and precise for mapping telomere ends at individual chromosomes than other techniques, providing the median TL of an individual's TL distribution [133] and absolute TL in each chromosome at a single-cell level [121, 132]. The metaphase Q-FISH method is a valuable approach to recognizing "telomere-free" ends, the ends of chromosomes without detectable telomeres' sequences. In addition, the metaphase q-FISH method measures the telomere length on each chromosome of every individual, avoiding to provide measures regarding the interstitial telomeric repeat (ITR) regions, studied as interstitial telomeric sequences (ITSs), that comprise repetitive telomeric sequences detected within intrachromosomal regions. Researchers have shown that differences in TL were attributed more to inter-individual variations than intra-individual variations [134]. In addition to the above, it has been substantiated that TL represents an individual's signature from birth, which displays a progressive shortening with each cell division. The telomere attrition is potentiated with advanced age [135].

Besides, other types of FISH comprise the interphase FISH, which measures telomeres at cells in interphase [136], and Flow-FISH, in which FISH was combined with fluorescence-activated cell sorting (FACS) technology measuring mainly median TL of an individual's TL distribution in single suspended lymphocytes [137]. However, the limitations of Flow-FISH have focused on studying cells in suspension and additionally, the peptide nucleic acid (PNA) probe could bind to random cytoplasmic artifacts [123]. Commercial modification of interphase Q-FISH, named high-throughput Q-FISH (HT Q-FISH) [138], is an automated procedure that is often used in large-scale studies on fixed lymphocytes at interphase providing a relative quantification of average TL [138]. Studies have proven that HT Q-FISH is as powerful and accurate as conventional Q-FISH for average telomere length measurement. For that reason, all the versions of FISH have been proven meaningful, enabling the visualization of shortest telomeres in single cells.

Besides, the primed in situ (PRINS) approach has been developed as a faster alternative to the FISH method at metaphase or interphase cells, in which telomeres are amplified through the use of fluorescent-tagged nucleotides [119]. The results of the PRINS method are like those of the FISH method, but they differ in their principle [119].

Similarly, another technique named peptide nucleic acid hybridization and analysis of single telomere (PHAST) has been shown to leverage fluorescent intensity to provide relative quantification of TL after the hybridization of DNA with fluorescently labeled probe [141]. The unique property of this method is the quantification of telomeres as short as 100 bp up to 15 kb [142]. Then, the single telomere length analysis (STELA) was created relying on principles of PCR and Southern blot analysis [143]. The critical characteristic of this method is the accurate measurement of telomere length with limited starting DNA material [144]. However, the STELA technique can be performed in a few chromosomes due to a lack of primers designed for all chromosome ends [143]. To overcome the hurdle above, Universal STELA emerged and reported a strong association of telomeres at short length with cellular senescence [145]. The Universal STELA can recognize any critically short telomere in chromosomes [123].

In addition, telomere shortest length (TeSLA) method was introduced, shedding light on average TL in the following range (less than 1 kb up to 18 kbs) in all chromosomes [137, 146]. The TeSLA method is considered superior to other methods because it can precisely estimate the mean TL in a sample [137, 146].

Like the PHAST method, the telomere length combing assay (TCA) method measures TL at absolute values (below 1 kb up to 80 kbs) [147]. The principle behind this method is based on stretching DNA fibers on the slide and hybridizing DNA with PNA probes, enabling the evaluation of TL in a high-throughput manner [147]. Besides, the TCA method provides insights into the distribution of TL in cell populations at a single-cell level [147]. In the single telomere absolute-length rapid (STAR) method, DNA digestion occurs. Then DNA is mixed with primers for the qPCR chip providing information about absolute TL (varying from 0.2 kb to 320 kb) [142, 148]. Indeed, the STAR method was devised to tackle the hurdle of standardization developed through qPCR [142, 148]. The STAR method has attracted much attention, owing to its high throughput use and its application in many samples rapidly with limited starting DNA material [142, 148].

The evaluation of aging rate can offer significant information about mortality and disease risk. Initially, Cawthon et al. used 143 individuals aged 60–97 years and showed that telomere shortening can be a predictive marker for all-cause mortality [124]. Then, many epidemiological studies provided convincing clues about the critical involvement of telomere shortening in escalating mortality risk [73, 149–151]. For example, the results of the Swedish Twin Registry study illustrated that individuals with the shortest leukocyte TL (LTL) had susceptibility for mortality at a greater extent by 44% folds than those bearing long telomeres [152]. Accordingly, a systematic review showed that participants with short telomeres had higher all-cause mortality than others with long ones, implying the inverse relationship of telomere length with mortality [153]. As a result, many epidemiological studies have highlighted the importance of telomere shortening in predicting mortality, the inter-individual variabilities among participants of studies [73, 149–153]. However, different assays for TL measurement are considered to complicate the precise estimation of mortality risk.

From the epidemiological side, all TL techniques have proved to be accurate with a small range (31–64 base pairs per year) after evaluation of TL derived from 154 healthy individuals of different age groups (from newborn to 81 years) [154]. Accordingly, Ye et al. have performed a recent meta-analysis of 414 studies of 743,019 individuals aged 0–112 years [155], examining the effect of TL using different TL methods during the lifespan of participants [155]. The results of the systematic review showed the gradual telomere shortening in a non-linear manner, with an average decrease of 23 base pairs for a year using cross-sectional data and a mean decline of 38 base pairs for a year using longitudinal data [155].

Epidemiological studies have also shown a positive association between TL and severe health complications [156, 157]. After evaluating results derived from a meta-analysis of 23,379 cases, there was a link between TL and cancer risk with different hazard ratios depending on the cancer type [158]. In another systematic review of 8400 events, TL was reported as an essential determinant for coronary heart disease [159].

Compared to other biological age estimators, TL has emerged to be very important in determining biological age in a sex-dependent manner. In particular, a meta-analysis composed of 36,230 individuals [160] and another study comprising 105,539 participants [161] has shown that women have an extended lifespan compared to men as determined by their longer telomeres. Those conclusions about biological age were in line with those derived from DNAm.

2.5 Metaphase Quantitative Fluorescence in situ Hybridization in Peripheral Blood Cells

This Q-FISH on cells at metaphase can quantify critically short repeated telomeric sequences, essential in chromatin stability and cell viability [121, 132]. It is generally known that tissues exhibit a distinct age-related rate of telomere shortening, but most focus is given to studying TL in leukocytes [134, 162]. In humans, white blood is usually used as a source for evaluating TL since it provides a general framework about the heterogeneous cell composition of blood and the average of different doubling times of involved different cells [163, 164]. It has been reported that a strong association of germ-line mutated genes involved in telomere maintenance with syndromes linked to short telomeres [165]. Based on this, it has been highlighted that telomere shortening triggers the onset and the progression of age-related diseases. Indeed, there is a growing number of studies that have linked short leukocyte telomere length with the pathology of many diseases like Covid-19 infection [166, 167], autoimmune diseases [168, 169], cardiovascular diseases [170], metabolic syndrome and diabetes [171, 172], and neoplasms [173, 174]. Critical short telomeres are implicated in various types of cancer since critical short telomeres function as flags for induction of non-homologous end joining (NHEJ) signaling pathway, thus leading to end-to-end fusions of chromosomes and aberrant recombination [116, 175]. Accordingly, genome-wide association studies (GWASs) have underlined the causal role of TL in many diseases, using 62,271 individuals [176]. On the other hand, several studies have also shown that highly long telomeres are associated with an increased risk for cancers including melanomas and pulmonary cancers. Still, the mechanism in which TL is implicated in cancer is unknown [177, 178]. Telomere length also seems to be a reliable biomarker for female and male infertility [184]. Many studies have revealed the role of telomere length as a predictive biomarker in osteoporosis and osteoarthritis patients [180, 185]. Additionally, it has been shown that there is an association between nutraceutical supplements with longer telomere length and with common mental disorders [179–185].

From a molecular perspective, the metaphase Q-FISH quantifies the TL distribution in each chromosome in either fresh or frozen cells or paraffin-embedded tissue, providing precise evidence about absolute TL in each chromosome at a single-cell level [121, 132]. In this manner, the median of the whole TL in each cell and the shortest TL in each cell are provided through metaphase Q-FISH, thereby developing a general snapshot of the average TL in all cells. Furthermore, the percentage of the critically short and long telomeres and the presence or absence of the fused chromosomes is only supplied through metaphase Q-FISH [123]. Metaphase Q-FISH is superior to other techniques because it can evaluate an average chromosome instability due to identification of "telomere-free ends" [133, 186]. Rearrangements between chromosomes usually occur in chromosomes with "telomere-free" ends. Such chromosome replacements include chromosome fusions or chromosomal structures named rings [123]. In addition to the above, this technique can be used in multiple aspects and several cell types, even rare ones [187, 188]. However, metaphase Q-FISH cannot be applied to senescent cells (mitotically inactive) and low-proliferated cells [128]. TL is usually examined in blood and is not used in the following organs: heart, muscle, and central nervous system. This is because it is a tissue-specific marker that complicates the whole snapshot of the aging process [189]. Other drawbacks of metaphase Q-FISH that hinder its application in extensive epidemiological studies are the high cost, the technical expertise, extensive work, and the proper equipment [123].

The starting material for metaphase Q-FISH is blood, which needs to be cultured with a medium, and then the cells are arrested at the metaphase stage. The basic steps of the procedure are the following: (a) fixation and permeabilization of the samples, (b) denaturation of the DNA sequence, (c) hybridization with a fluorescent probe for telomeric repeats [136], and another for chromosome, such as 4,6-diamidino-2-phenylindole dihydrochloride (DAPI), (d) washing to remove unbound probes, and (e) visualization of telomeres in the individual chromosome in each sample by using fluorescence microscopy with specific software for telomere ends measurement (Fig. 2.2). Then, the fluorescence intensities are converted into telomere length values (measured in kbs).

The primary principle behind this method is the hybridization of the fluorophore-conjugated probe with denatured nuclear DNA at metaphase chromosomes [190]. Importantly, formamide is usually used to cause a decline in the melting point of denaturation [190]. The probe can hybridize to complementary DNA sequence at a 100% rate, owing to its unique structure and non-charged sequence giving rise to very stable duplexes [190]. The hybridization procedure is affected by the number of C-G bonds and hybridization temperature [190]. The following washing steps are required to remove

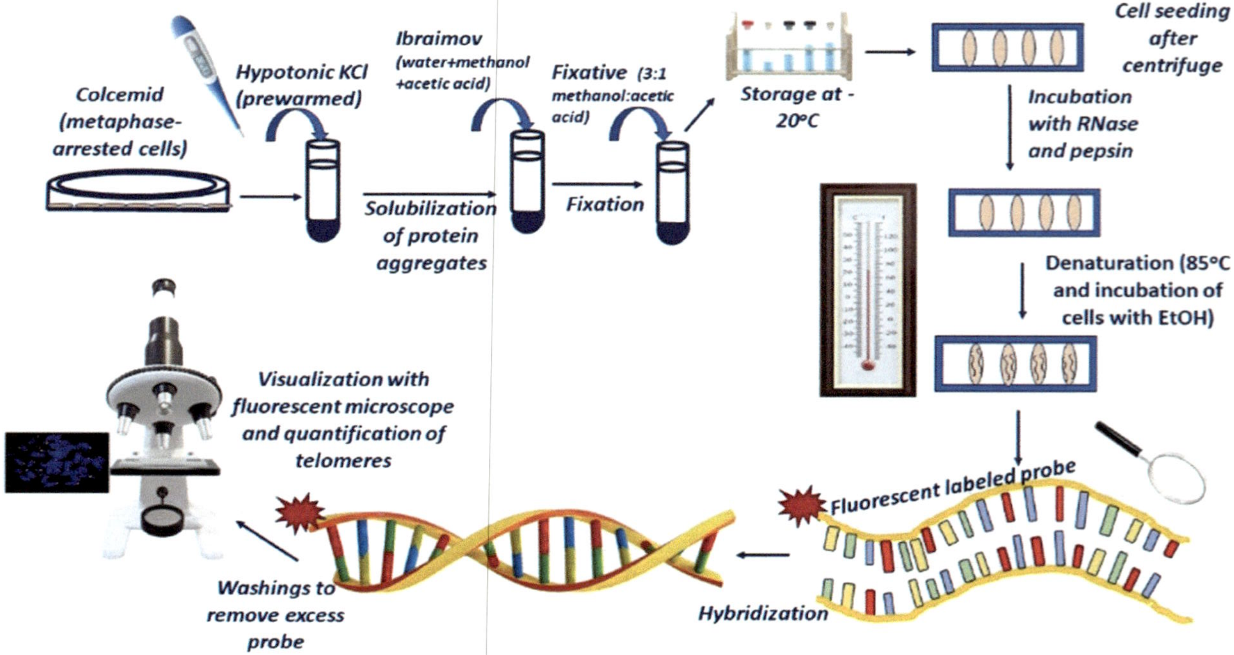

Figure 2.2 The steps of the metaphase Q-FISH method.

non-specific DNA molecules, which can increase the background in a fluorescence microscope [190]. Then, data are analyzed using a functional semi-automated worksheet called BIOTEL ver. 2.4, providing a precise TL statistic [183, 191]. The principle of BIOTEL ver. 2.4 is based on using short and long telomere ends of an individual's chromosomes to estimate the biological age through the rate of telomere shortening.

Following Biotel, statistical analysis and the personalized questionnaire of an examinee can function as complementary. In this manner, personalized consultation for wellness and longevity can be provided for every individual. A flow chart is presented below (Fig. 2.3).

2.6 Overview of Aging Markers

These findings shed light on the large spectrum of biomarkers of aging available, each with its benefits and side effects. Through an overview of all aging markers, there is evidence concerning a partial overlap among them at the epidemiological and genetic levels [192]. Epidemiological evidence has supported the significant equivalence of diverse aging markers as part of the aging network [193]. In this direction, Gialluisi et al. have provided convincing evidence that all the aging markers based on either TL or DNAm exert a similar effect on mortality [192]. Indeed, further epidemiological studies have evaluated the association across different biological age markers and have supported that the approaches complement each other, as they are used for assessing the different aspects of the multidimensional aging process [64, 194–196]. For example, in a single longitudinal cohort, researchers have reported a partial overlap among nine different biological aging methods including TL and DNAm [197]. In another longitudinal study, authors compared genomics, proteomics, metabolomics, and clinical variables of 3558 individuals after deep phenotyping, suggesting the precise calculation of biological age can be through quantification of proteins associated with detoxification, metabolism, and inflammation [66].

Even though various markers have been used to predict biological age, they mainly provide a suboptimal estimation of biological

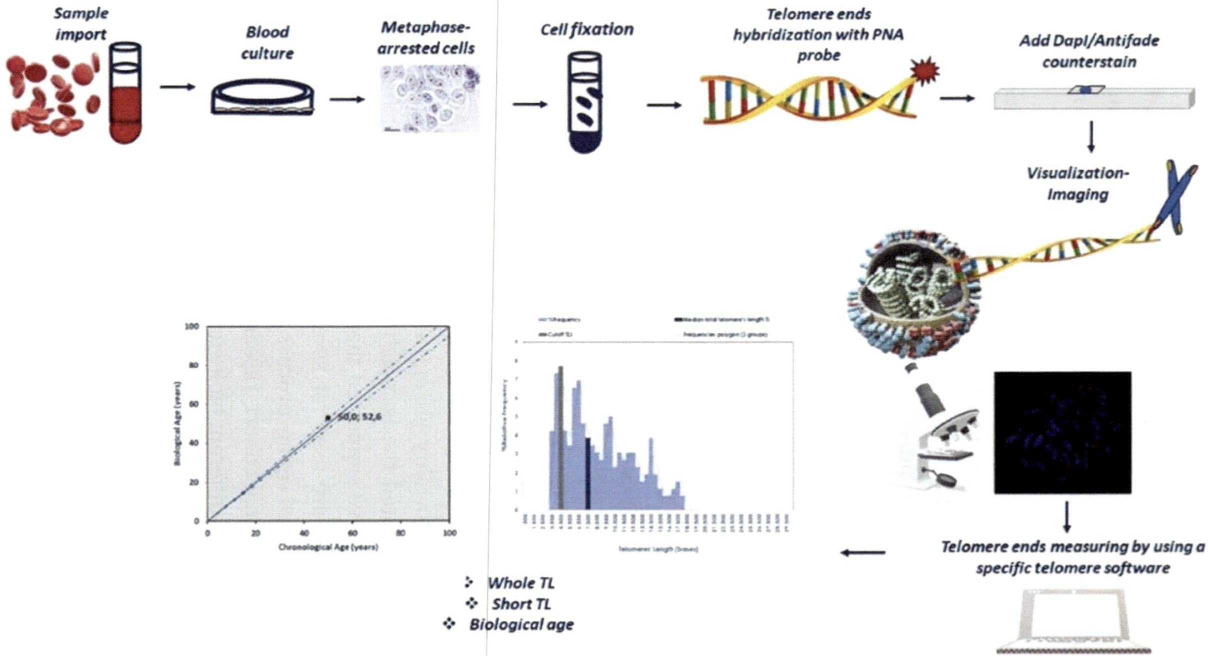

Figure 2.3 The flow chart of metaphase Q-FISH. Fluorescence intensity values are measured on blood cells. Statistical analysis provides data about telomere length distribution and an individual's biological age.

age. Indeed, there is no consensus to infer biological age as a single quantitative value, probably due to the complicated nature of aging and differences among individuals [198]. As a result, identifying sensitive and specific biomarkers that can precisely assess the onset of aging is very important for alleviating the onset or retarding the progression of aging and its related disorders through therapeutics. Therapeutic interventions are directed toward reversing the epigenetic framework or restoring telomere maintenance [36, 198, 199]. To sum up, the biological age estimators and especially telomere length can be regarded as markers monitoring the onset and the progression of age-related diseases.

Abbreviations

4,6-Diamidino-2-phenylindole dihydrochloride (DAPI)
8-Oxo-7,8-dihydro-2′-deoxyguanine (8-oxoG)
Absolute telomere length (aTL)
Age acceleration residual (AAR)
Body mass index (BMI)
CpG islands (CGIs)
C-reactive protein (CRP)
Cytosine phosphate-guanine dinucleotides (CpG)
DNA damage response (DDR)
DNA methylation (DNAm)
Epidermal growth factor (EGF)
Fluorescence-activated cell sorting (FACS)
Genome-wide association studies (GWASs)
Glycated hemoglobin (Hba1c)
High-density lipoprotein (HDL)
High-throughput Q-FISH (HT Q-FISH)
Immunoglobulin G (IgG)
Interleukin-6 (IL-6)
Interstitial telomeric sequences (ITSs)
Leucocyte telomere length (LTL)
Low-density lipoprotein (LDL)
Matrix-metalloproteinases-1/3 (MMP-1/3)
Monochrome multiplex quantitative PCR (MMqPCR)

National Health and Nutrition Examination Survey (NHANES)
Noncoding RNAs (ncRNAs)
Non-homologous end joining (NHEJ)
Oral glucose tolerance test (OGTT)
Peptide nucleic acid (PNA)
Peptide nucleic acid hybridization and analysis of single telomere (PHAST)
Peripheral blood mononuclear cells (PBMCs)
Primed In Situ (PRINS)
Proton nuclear magnetic resonance (H1 NMR)
Quantitative fluorescence in situ hybridization (Q-FISH)
Quantitative polymerase chain reaction (qPCR)
Reactive oxygen species (ROS)
San Antonio Family Heart Study (SAFHS)
Self-Organizing Maps ML (SOM-ML)
Senescence-associated secretory phenotype (SASP)
Single telomere absolute-length rapid (STAR)
Single telomere length analysis (STELA)
Telomere length (TL)
Telomere length combing assay (TCA)
Telomere shortest length assay (TeSLA)
Terminal restriction fragment (TRF)
Transcriptional start sites (TSSs)
Tumor necrosis factor-a (TNFa)
Ultra-high-performance liquid chromatography–mass spectrometry (UHPLC-MS)
Vascular endothelial growth factor (VEGF)
White blood cell (WBC)

References

1. Kirkwood, T. B. L. (2005). Understanding the odd science of aging, *Cell*, **120**, pp. 437–447.
2. López-Otín, C., Blasco, M. A., Partridge, L., Serrano, M. and Kroemer, G. (2013). The hallmarks of aging, *Cell*, **153**, pp. 1194–1217.

3. Ashapkin, V. V., Kutueva, L. I. and Vanyushin, B. F. (2019). Epigenetic clock: just a convenient marker or an active driver of aging? *Adv. Exp. Med. Biol.*, **1178**, pp. 175–206.
4. Nwanaji-Enwerem, J. C., Weisskopf, M. G. and Baccarelli, A. A. (2018). Multi-tissue DNA methylation age: molecular relationships and perspectives for advancing biomarker utility, *Ageing Res. Rev.*, **45**, pp. 15–23.
5. Field, A. E., Robertson, N. A., Wang, T., Havas, A., Ideker, T. and Adams, P. D. (2018). DNA Methylation clocks in aging: categories, causes, and consequences, *Mol. Cell*, **71**, pp. 882–895.
6. Levine, M. E. (2013). Modeling the rate of senescence: can estimated biological age predict mortality more accurately than chronological age?, *J. Gerontol. A. Biol. Sci. Med. Sci.*, **68**, pp. 667–674.
7. Jia, L., Zhang, W., Jia, R. Zhang, H. and Chen, X. (2016). Construction formula of biological age using the principal component analysis, *BioMed Res. Int.*, **2016**, pp. 1–8.
8. Jackson, S. H. D., Weale, M. R. and Weale, R. A. (2003). Biological age-what is it and can it be measured? *Arch. Gerontol. Geriatr.*, **36**, pp. 103–115.
9. McCrory, C., Fiorito, G., Hernandez B., Polidoro S., O'Halloran A.M., Hever A., *et* al. (2021). GrimAge outperforms other epigenetic clocks in the prediction of age-related clinical phenotypes and all-cause mortality, *J Gerontol A Biol Sci Med Sci.*,**76**, pp. 741–749.
10. Strasser B. (2013). Physical activity in obesity and metabolic syndrome, *Ann. N. Y. Acad. Sci.*, **1281**, pp. 141–159.
11. Cohen, H. Y., Miller, C., Bitterman, K.J., Wall, N.R., Hekking, B., Kessler B., *et al.* (2004). Calorie restriction promotes mammalian cell survival by inducing the SIRT1 deacetylase, *Science*, **305**, pp. 390–392.
12. Hahn, O., Grönke S., Stubbs, T.M., Ficz, G., Hendrich, O., Krueger, F., *et al.* (2017). Dietary restriction protects from age-associated DNA methylation and induces epigenetic reprogramming of lipid metabolism, *Genome Biol.*, **18**, pp. 56.
13. Redman, L. M., Smith, S. R., Burton, J. H., Martin, C. K., Il'yasova, D. and Ravussin, E. (2018). Metabolic slowing and reduced oxidative damage with sustained caloric restriction support the rate of living and oxidative damage theories of aging, *Cell Metab.*, **27**, pp. 805–815.e4.
14. Navarro-Ibarra, M. J., Hernández, J. and Caire-Juvera, G. (2019). Diet, physical activity and telomere length in adults, *Nutr. Hosp.*, **36**, pp. 1403–1417.

15. Castro, A. M., Macedo-de la Concha, L. E. and Pantoja-Meléndez, C. A. (2017). Low-grade inflammation and its relation to obesity and chronic degenerative diseases, *Rev. Médica Hosp. Gen. México*, **80**, pp. 101–105.
16. Ahmed, W. and Lingner, J. (2018). Impact of oxidative stress on telomere biology, *Differ. Res. Biol. Divers.*, **99**, pp. 21–27.
17. Barnes, R. P., Fouquerel, E. and Opresko, P. L. (2019). The impact of oxidative DNA damage and stress on telomere homeostasis, *Mech. Ageing Dev.*, **177**, pp. 37–45.
18. Hegde, M. L., Mantha, A. K., Hazra, T. K., Bhakat, K. K., Mitra, S. and Szczesny, B. (2012). Oxidative genome damage and its repair: implications in aging and neurodegenerative diseases, *Mech. Ageing Dev.*, **133**, pp. 157–168.
19. Malinin, N. L., West, X. Z. and Byzova, T. V. (2011). Oxidation as "the stress of life", *Aging*, **3**, pp. 906–910.
20. Reuter, S., Gupta, S. C., Chaturvedi, M. M. and Aggarwal, B. B. (2010). Oxidative stress, inflammation, and cancer: how are they linked? *Free Radic. Biol. Med.*, **49**, pp. 1603–1616.
21. Von Zglinicki, T. (2002). Oxidative stress shortens telomeres, *Trends Biochem. Sci.*, **27**, pp. 339–344.
22. Fouquerel, E., Barnes, R. P., Uttam, S., Watkins, S. C., Bruchez, M. P. and Opresko, P. L. (2019). Targeted and persistent 8-oxoguanine base damage at telomeres promotes telomere loss and crisis, *Mol. Cell*, **75**, pp. 117–130.
23. Sahin, E., Colla, S., Liesa, M., Moslehi, J., Müller, F.L., Guo M, *et al.* (2011). Telomere dysfunction induces metabolic and mitochondrial compromise, *Nature*, **470**, pp. 359–365.
24. Trifunovic, A., Wredenberg, A., Falkenberg, M., Spelbrink, J.N., Rovio, A.T., Bruder, C.E., *et al.* (2004). Premature ageing in mice expressing defective mitochondrial DNA polymerase, *Nature*, **429**, pp. 417–423.
25. Di Micco, R., Krizhanovsky, V. Baker, D., and d'Adda di Fagagna, F. (2021). Cellular senescence in ageing: from mechanisms to therapeutic opportunities, *Nat. Rev. Mol. Cell Biol.*, **22**, pp. 75–95.
26. Squassina, A., Pisanu, C. and Vanni, R. (2019). Mood disorders, accelerated aging, and inflammation: is the link hidden in telomeres? *Cells*, **8**, pp. 52.
27. Chen, R., Zhang, K., Chen, H., Zhao, X., Wang, J., Li, L., *et al.* (2015). Telomerase deficiency causes alveolar stem cell senescence-associated low-grade inflammation in lungs, *J. Biol. Chem.*, **290**, pp. 30813–30829.

28. Coppé, J.P., Desprez, P.Y., Krtolica, A. and Campisi, J. (2010). The senescence-associated secretory phenotype: the dark side of tumor suppression, *Annu. Rev. Pathol.*, **5**, pp. 99–118.

29. Basisty, N., Kale, A., Jeon, O.H., Kuehnemann, C., Payne, T., Rao, C., *et al.* (2020). A proteomic atlas of senescence-associated secretomes for aging biomarker development, *PLoS Biol.*, **18**, pp. e3000599.

30. Tominaga, K. (2015). The emerging role of senescent cells in tissue homeostasis and pathophysiology, *Pathobiol. Aging Age Relat. Dis.*, **5**, pp. 27743.

31. Barrès, R., Yan, J., Egan, B., Treebak, J.T., Rasmussen, M., Fritz, T., *et al.* (2012). Acute exercise remodels promoter methylation in human skeletal muscle, *Cell Metab.*, **15**, pp. 405–411.

32. Nitert, M. D., Dayeh T, Volkov P, Elgzyri T, Hall E, Nilsson E, *et al.* (2012). Impact of exercise intervention on DNA methylation in skeletal muscle from first-degree relatives of patients with type 2 diabetes, *Diabetes*, **61**, pp. 3322–3332.

33. Egan, B., Carson, B.P., Garcia-Roves, P.M., Chibalin, A.V., Sarsfield, F.M., Barron, N., *et al.* (2010). Exercise intensity-dependent regulation of peroxisome proliferator-activated receptor γ coactivator-1α mRNA abundance is associated with differential activation of upstream signalling kinases in human skeletal muscle: exercise intensity and PGC-1α regulation, *J. Physiol.*, **588**, pp. 1779–1790.

34. Ruple, B. A., Godwin, J.S., Mesquita, P.H.C., Osburn, S.C., Vann, C.G., Lamb, D.A., *et al.* (2021). Resistance training rejuvenates the mitochondrial methylome in aged human skeletal muscle, *FASEB J.*, **35**, pp. e21864.

35. Rubenstein, A.B., Hinkley, J.M., Nair, V.D., Nudelman, G., Standley, R.A., Yi, F., *et al.* (2022). Skeletal muscle transcriptome response to a bout of endurance exercise in physically active and sedentary older adults, *Am. J. Physiol. Endocrinol. Metab.*, **322**, pp. E260–E277.

36. Kennedy, B. K., Berger, S.L., Brunet, A., Campisi, J., Cuervo, A.M., Epel, E.S., *et al.* (2014). Geroscience: linking aging to chronic disease, *Cell*, **159**, pp. 709–713.

37. Ferrucci, L., Levine, M. E., Kuo, P.-L. and Simonsick, E. M. (2018). Time and the metrics of aging, *Circ. Res.*, **123**, pp. 740–744.

38. Lulkiewicz, M., Bajsert, J., Kopczynski, P., Barczak, W. and Rubis, B. (2020). Telomere length: how the length makes a difference, *Mol. Biol. Rep.*, **47**, pp. 7181–7188.

39. Horvath, S. and Raj, K. (2018). DNA methylation-based biomarkers and the epigenetic clock theory of ageing, *Nat. Rev. Genet.*, **19**, pp. 371–384.

40. Stegeman, R. and Weake, V. M. (2017). Transcriptional signatures of aging, *J. Mol. Biol.*, **429**, pp. 2427–2437.
41. Lehallier, B., Gate, D., Schaum, N., Nanasi, T., Lee, S.E., Yousef, H., *et al.* (2019). Undulating changes in human plasma proteome profiles across the lifespan, *Nat. Med.*, **25**, pp. 1843–1850.
42. Marioni, R. E., Harris, S.E., Shah, S., McRae, A.F., von Zglinicki, T., Martin-Ruiz, C., *et al.* (2016). The epigenetic clock and telomere length are independently associated with chronological age and mortality, *Int. J. Epidemiol.*, **45**, pp. 424–432.
43. Belsky, D.W., Moffitt, T.E., Cohen, A.A., Corcoran, D.L., Levine, M.E., Prinz, J.A., *et al.* (2017). Eleven telomere, epigenetic clock, and biomarker-composite quantifications of biological aging: do they measure the same thing?, *Am. J. Epidemiol.*, **187**, pp. 1220–1230.
44. Breitling, L. P., Saum, K.-U., Perna, L., Schöttker, B., Holleczek, B. and Brenner, H. (2016). Frailty is associated with the epigenetic clock but not with telomere length in a German cohort, *Clin. Epigenetics*, **8**, pp. 21.
45. Noren Hooten, N., Abdelmohsen, K., Gorospe, M., Ejiogu, N., Zonderman, A. B. and Evans, M. K. (2010). MicroRNA expression patterns reveal differential expression of target genes with age, *PLoS ONE*, **5**, pp. e10724.
46. Han, S. and Brunet, A. (2012). Histone methylation makes its mark on longevity, *Trends Cell Biol.*, **22**, pp. 42–49.
47. Cortez, M. A., and Calin, G. A. (2009). MicroRNA identification in plasma and serum: a new tool to diagnose and monitor diseases, *Expert Opin. Biol. Ther.*, **9**, pp. 703–711.
48. Galkin, F., Mamoshina, P., Aliper, A., Putin, E., Moskalev, V., Gladyshev, V.N. *et al.* (2020). Human gut microbiome aging clock based on taxonomic profiling and deep learning, *iScience*, **23**, pp. 101199.
49. Wilmanski, T., Diener, C., Rappaport, N., Patwardhan, S., Wiedrick, J., Lapidus, J., *et al.* (2021). Gut microbiome pattern reflects healthy ageing and predicts survival in humans, *Nat. Metab.*, **3**, pp. 274–286.
50. Holly, A.C., Melzer, D., Pilling, L.C., Henley, W., Hernandez, D.G., Singleton, A.B., *et al.* (2013). Towards a gene expression biomarker set for human biological age, *Aging Cell*, **12**, pp. 324–326.
51. Peters, M.J., Joehanes, R., Pilling, L.C., Schurmann, C, Conneely, KN, Powell, J, *et al.* (2015). The transcriptional landscape of age in human peripheral blood, *Nat. Commun.*, **6**, pp. 8570.

52. Meyer, D. H. and Schumacher, B. (2021). BiT age: A transcriptome-based aging clock near the theoretical limit of accuracy, *Aging Cell*, **20**, pp. e13320.

53. Tanaka, T., Basisty, N., Fantoni, G., Candia, J., Moore, A.Z., Biancotto, A., *et al.* (2020). Plasma proteomic biomarker signature of age predicts health and life span, *eLife*, **9**, pp. e61073.

54. Lehallier, B., Shokhirev, M. N., Wyss-Coray, T. and Johnson, A. A. (2020). Data mining of human plasma proteins generates a multitude of highly predictive aging clocks that reflect different aspects of aging, *Aging Cell*, **19**, pp. e13256.

55. Knežević, A., Gornik, O., Polasek, O., Pucic, M., Redzic, I., Novokmet, M., *et al.* (2010). Effects of aging, body mass index, plasma lipid profiles, and smoking on human plasma N-glycans, *Glycobiology*, **20**, pp. 959–969.

56. Ruhaak, L.R., Uh, H.W., Beekman, M., Koeleman, C.A., Hokke, C. H., Westendorp, R.G., *et al.* (2010). Decreased levels of bisecting glcnac glycoforms of IgG are associated with human longevity, *PLoS ONE*, **5**, pp. e12566.

57. Ishikawa, M., Maekawa, K., Saito, K., Senoo, Y., Urata, M., Murayama, M., *et al.* (2014). Plasma and serum lipidomics of healthy white adults shows characteristic profiles by subjects' gender and age, *PLoS ONE*, **9**, pp. e91806.

58. Johnson, L. C., Parker, K., Aguirre, B. F., Nemkov, T. G., D'Alessandro, A., Johnson S. A., *et al.* (2019). The plasma metabolome as a predictor of biological aging in humans, *GeroScience*, **41**, pp. 895–906.

59. Robinson, O., Chadeau Hyam, M., Karaman, I., Climaco Pinto, R., Ala-Korpela, M., Handakas, E., *et al.* (2020). Determinants of accelerated metabolomic and epigenetic aging in a UK cohort, *Aging Cell*, **19**, pp. e13149.

60. Niedernhofer, L. J., Kirkland, J. L. and Ladiges, W. (2017). Molecular pathology endpoints useful for aging studies, *Ageing Res. Rev.*, **35**, pp. 241–249.

61. Dubowitz, N., Xue, W., Long, Q., Ownby, J.G., Olson, D.E., Barb, D., *et al.* (2014). Aging is associated with increased HbA1c levels, independently of glucose levels and insulin resistance, and also with decreased HbA1c diagnostic specificity, *Diabet. Med. J. Br. Diabet. Assoc.*, **31**, pp. 927–935.

62. Khan, S. S., Singer, B. D. and Vaughan, D. E. (2017). Molecular and physiological manifestations and measurement of aging in humans, *Aging Cell*, **16**, pp. 624–633.

63. Jee, H., Jeon, B.H., Kim, Y.H., Kim, H.K., Choe, J., Park, J. and Jin, Y. (2012). Development and application of biological age prediction models with physical fitness and physiological components in Korean adults, *Gerontology*, **58**, pp. 344–353.
64. Vetter, V. M., Kalies, C. H., Sommerer, Y., Spira, D., Drewelies, J., Regitz-Zagrosek, V., *et al.* (2022). Relationship between 5 epigenetic clocks, telomere length, and functional capacity assessed in older adults: cross-sectional and longitudinal analyses, *J. Gerontol. Ser. A*, **77**, pp. 1724–1733.
65. Jylhävä, J., Pedersen, N. L. and Hägg, S. (2017). Biological age predictors, *EBioMedicine*, **21**, pp. 29–36.
66. Earls, J.C., Rappaport, N., Heath, L., Wilmanski, T., Magis, A.T., Schork, N.J., *et al.* (2019). Multi-omic biological age estimation and its correlation with wellness and disease phenotypes: a longitudinal study of 3,558 individuals, *J. Gerontol. Ser. A*, **74**, pp. S52–S60.
67. Rutledge, J. Oh, H. and Wyss-Coray, T. (2022). Measuring biological age using omics data, *Nat. Rev. Genet.*, **23**, pp. 715–727.
68. Ahadi, S., Zhou, W., Schüssler-Fiorenza Rose, S.M., Sailani, M.R., Contrepois, K., Avina, M., Ashland, M., Brunet, A. and Snyder, M. (2020). Personal aging markers and ageotypes revealed by deep longitudinal profiling, *Nat. Med.*, **26**, pp. 83–90.
69. Zierer, J., Pallister, T., Tsai, P.C., Krumsiek, J., Bell, J.T., Lauc, G., Spector, T.D., Menni, C. and Kastenmüller, G. (2016). Exploring the molecular basis of age-related disease comorbidities using a multi-omics graphical model, *Sci. Rep.*, **6**, pp. 37646.
70. Delude, C. M. (2015). Deep phenotyping: the details of disease, *Nature*, **527**, pp. S14–S15.
71. Belsky, D.W., Caspi, A., Houts, R., Cohen, H.J., Corcoran, D.L., Danese, A., *et al.* (2015). Quantification of biological aging in young adults, *Proc. Natl. Acad. Sci. U. S. A.*, **112**, pp. E4104–4110.
72. Sebastiani, P., Thyagarajan, B., Sun, F., Schupf, N., Newman, A.B., Montano, *et al.* (2017). Biomarker signatures of aging, *Aging Cell*, **16**, pp. 329–338.
73. Rode, L., Nordestgaard, B. G. and Bojesen, S. E. (2015). Peripheral blood leukocyte telomere length and mortality among 64 637 individuals from the general population, *JNCI J. Natl. Cancer Inst.*, **107**, pp. 1–8.
74. Chen, B.H., Marioni, R.E., Colicino, E., Peters, M.J., Ward-Caviness, C.K., Tsai, P.C., *et al.* (2016). DNA methylation-based measures of biological age: meta-analysis predicting time to death, *Aging*, **8**, pp. 1844–1865.

75. Hertel, J., Friedrich, N., Wittfeld, K., Pietzner, M., Budde, K., Van der Auwera, S., *et al.* (2016). Measuring biological age via metabonomics: the metabolic age score, *J. Proteome Res.*, **15**, pp. 400–410.

76. Gregory, D. J., Zhang, Y., Kobzik, L. and Fedulov, A. V. (2013). Specific transcriptional enhancement of inducible nitric oxide synthase by targeted promoter demethylation, *Epigenetics*, **8**, pp. 1205–1212.

77. Saunderson, E. A., Stepper, P., Gomm, J. J., Hoa, L., Morgan, A., Allen, M. D., *et al.* (2017). Hit-and-run epigenetic editing prevents senescence entry in primary breast cells from healthy donors, *Nat. Commun.*, **8**, pp. 1450.

78. Davies, M. N., Volta, M., Pidsley, R., Lunnon, K., Dixit, A, Lovestone, S., *et al.* (2012). Functional annotation of the human brain methylome identifies tissue-specific epigenetic variation across brain and blood, *Genome Biol.*, **13**, pp. R43.

79. Laurent, L., Wong, E., Li G., Huynh, T., Tsirigos, A., Ong, C.T., *et al.* (2010). Dynamic changes in the human methylome during differentiation, *Genome Res.*, **20**, pp. 320–331.

80. Irizarry, R. A., Ladd-Acosta, C., Wen B., Wu, Z., Montano, C., Onyango, P., *et al.* (2009). The human colon cancer methylome shows similar hypo- and hypermethylation at conserved tissue-specific CpG island shores, *Nat. Genet.*, **41**, pp. 178–186.

81. Deaton, A. M. and Bird, A. (2011). CpG islands and the regulation of transcription, *Genes Dev.*, **25**, pp. 1010–1022.

82. Nagae, G., Isagawa, T., Shiraki, N., Fujita, T., Yamamoto, S., Tsutsumi, S., *et al.* (2011). Tissue-specific demethylation in CpG-poor promoters during cellular differentiation, *Hum. Mol. Genet.*, **20**, pp. 2710–2721.

83. Yin, Y., Morgunova, E., Jolma A., Kaasinen, E., Sahu, B., Khund-Sayeed, S., *et al.* (2017). Impact of cytosine methylation on DNA binding specificities of human transcription factors, *Science*, **356**, pp. eaaj2239.

84. Reddington, J. P., Perricone, S. M., Nestor, C. E., Reichmann, J., Youngson, N. A., Suzuki, M., *et al.* (2013). Redistribution of H3K27me3 upon DNA hypomethylation results in de-repression of Polycomb target genes, *Genome Biol.*, **14**, pp. R25.

85. Rose, N. R. and Klose, R. J. (2014). Understanding the relationship between DNA methylation and histone lysine methylation, *Biochim. Biophys. Acta*, **1839**, pp. 1362–1372.

86. Lu, A. T., Fei, Z., Haghani, Robeck, T. R., Zoller, J. A., Li, C. Z., *et al.* (2022). Universal DNA methylation age across mammalian tissues, *bioRxiv*, pp. 2021.

87. Slieker, R. C., van Iterson, M., Luijk R., Beekman, M., Zhernakova, D. V., Moed, M. H., *et al.* (2016). Age-related accrual of methylomic variability is linked to fundamental ageing mechanisms, *Genome Biol.*, **17**, pp. 191.
88. Schübeler, D. (2015). Function and information content of DNA methylation, *Nature*, **517**, pp. 321–326.
89. Jones, P. A. (2012). Functions of DNA methylation: islands, start sites, gene bodies and beyond, *Nat. Rev. Genet.*, **13**, pp. 484–492.
90. Suzuki M. M. and Bird, A. (2008). DNA methylation landscapes: provocative insights from epigenomics, *Nat. Rev. Genet.*, **9**, pp. 465–476.
91. Maegawa, S., Lu, Y., Tahara, T., Lee, J.T., Madzo, J., Liang, S., *et al.* (2017). Caloric restriction delays age-related methylation drift, *Nat. Commun.*, **8**, pp. 539.
92. Heyn, H., Li N., Ferreira, H. J., Moran, S., Pisano, D. G., Gomez, A., *et al.* (2012). Distinct DNA methylomes of newborns and centenarians, *Proc. Natl. Acad. Sci. U. S. A.*, **109**, pp. 10522–10527.
93. Rakyan, V. K., Down T. A., Maslau, S., Andrew, T., Yang, T. P., Beyan, H., *et al.* (2010). Human aging-associated DNA hypermethylation occurs preferentially at bivalent chromatin domains, *Genome Res.*, **20**, pp. 434–439.
94. Beerman, I., Bock, C., Garrison, B. S., Smith, Z. D., Gu, H., Meissner, A. *et al.* (2013). Proliferation-dependent alterations of the DNA methylation landscape underlie hematopoietic stem cell aging, *Cell Stem Cell*, **12**, pp. 413–425.
95. Zhou, W., Dinh H. Q., Ramjan, Z., Weisenberger, D. J., Nicolet, C. M., Shen, H., *et al.* (2018). DNA methylation loss in late-replicating domains is linked to mitotic cell division, *Nat. Genet.*, **50**, pp. 591–602.
96. Bocklandt, S., Lin, W., Sehl, M. E., Sánchez, F. J., Sinsheimer, J. S., Horvath, S. *et al.* (2011). Epigenetic predictor of age, *PLoS ONE*, **6**, pp. e14821.
97. Horvath, S. (2013). DNA methylation age of human tissues and cell types, *Genome Biol.*, **14**, pp. R115.
98. Hannum, G., Guinney, J., Zhao, L., Zhang, L., Hughes, G., Sadda, S., *et al.* (2013). Genome-wide methylation profiles reveal quantitative views of human aging rates, *Mol. Cell*, **49**, pp. 359–367.
99. Bell, C. G, Lowe, R., Adams, P. D., Baccarelli, A. A., Beck, S., Bell, J. T., *et al.* (2019). DNA methylation aging clocks: challenges and recommendations, *Genome Biol.*, **20**, pp. 249.

100. Yang, Z., Wong, A., Kuh, D., Paul, D. S., Rakyan, V. K., Leslie, R. D., *et al.* (2016). Correlation of an epigenetic mitotic clock with cancer risk, *Genome Biol.*, **17**, pp. 205

101. Zhang, Y., Wilson, R., Heiss, J., Breitling, L. P., Saum, K. U., Schöttker, B., *et al.* (2017). DNA methylation signatures in peripheral blood strongly predict all-cause mortality, *Nat. Commun.*, **8**, pp. 14617.

102. Youn A. and Wang, S. (2018). The MiAge Calculator: a DNA methylation-based mitotic age calculator of human tissue types, *Epigenetics*, **13**, pp. 192–206.

103. Levine, M. E., Lu, A. T., Quach, A., Chen, B. H., Assimes, T. L., Bandinelli, S, *et al.* (2018). An epigenetic biomarker of aging for lifespan and healthspan, *Aging*, **10**, pp. 573–591.

104. Trapp, A., Kerepesi, C. and Gladyshev, V. N. (2021). Profiling epigenetic age in single cells, Nat. *Aging*, **1**, pp. 1189–1201.

105. Burt, V. L. and Harris, T. (1994). The third national health and nutrition examination survey: contributing data on aging and health, *The Gerontologist*, **34**, pp. 486–490.

106. Marioni, R. E., Shah, S., McRae, A. F., Chen, B. H., Colicino E, Harris S. E., *et al.* (2015). DNA methylation age of blood predicts all-cause mortality in later life, *Genome Biol.*, **16**, pp. 25.

107. Zhang, Q., Vallerga, C. L., Walker, R. M., Lin T., Henders A. K., Montgomery G. W., *et al.* (2019). Improved precision of epigenetic clock estimates across tissues and its implication for biological ageing, *Genome Med.*, **11**, pp. 54.

108. Lu, A. T., Quach, A., Wilson, J. G., Reiner, A. P., Aviv, A., Raj, K., *et al.* (2019). DNA methylation GrimAge strongly predicts lifespan and healthspan, *Aging*, **11**, pp. 303–327.

109. Rattan, S. I. S. (2018). Biogerontology: research status, challenges and opportunities, *Acta Bio Medica Atenei Parm.*, **89**, pp. 291–301.

110. Harley, C. B., Futcher, A. B. and Greider, C. W. (1990). Telomeres shorten during ageing of human fibroblasts, *Nature*, **345**, pp. 458–460.

111. Vaiserman, A. and Krasnienkov, D. (2021). Telomere length as a marker of biological age: state-of-the-art, open issues, and future perspectives, *Front. Genet.*, **11**, pp. 630186.

112. Deng, Y., Chan, S. S. and Chang, S. (2008). Telomere dysfunction and tumour suppression: the senescence connection, *Nat. Rev. Cancer*, **8**, pp. 450–458.

113. Bernardes de Jesus, B., Vera, E., Schneeberger, K., Tejera, A.M., Ayuso, E., Bosch, F. *et al.* (2012). Telomerase gene therapy in adult and old mice

delays aging and increases longevity without increasing cancer, *EMBO Mol. Med.*, **4**, pp. 691–704.

114. McHugh, D. and Gil, J. (2018). Senescence and aging: causes, consequences, and therapeutic avenues, *J. Cell Biol.*, **217**, pp. 65–77.
115. Fasching, C. L. (2018). Telomere length measurement as a clinical biomarker of aging and disease, *Crit. Rev. Clin. Lab. Sci.*, **55**, pp. 443–465.
116. Blasco, M. A. (2005). Telomeres and human disease: ageing, cancer and beyond, *Nat. Rev. Genet.*, **6**, pp. 611–622.
117. Daniali, L., Benetos, A., Susser, E., Kark, J. D., Labat, C., Kimura, M., *et al.* (2013). Telomeres shorten at equivalent rates in somatic tissues of adults, *Nat. Commun.*, **4**, pp. 1597.
118. Martin-Ruiz, C. M., Baird, D., Roger L, Boukamp, P., Krunic, D., Cawthon, R., *et al.* (2015). Reproducibility of telomere length assessment: an international collaborative study, *Int. J. Epidemiol.*, **44**, pp. 1673–1683.
119. Sarandi, E., Georgaki, S., Renieri, E., Fragkiadaki, P., Tsatsakis, A. and Tsoukalas, D. (2022). *Telomeres and Telomerase, in Reference Module in Biomedical Sciences*, Elsevier.
120. Kimura, M., Stone, R.C., Hunt, S.C., Skurnick, J., Lu, X., Cao, X., *et al.* (2010). Measurement of telomere length by the Southern blot analysis of terminal restriction fragment lengths, *Nat. Protoc.*, **5**, pp. 1596–1607.
121. Lansdorp, P. (1996). Heterogeneity in telomere length of human chromosomes, *Hum. Mol. Genet.*, **5**, pp. 685–691.
122. Mender I. and Shay, J. (2015). Telomere restriction fragment (TRF) analysis, *BIO-Protoc.*, **5**, pp. e1658
123. Montpetit, A.J., Alhareeri, A.A., Montpetit, M., Starkweather, A.R., Elmore, L.W., Filler, K., *et al.* (2014). Telomere length: a review of methods for measurement, *Nurs. Res.*, **63**, pp. 289–299.
124. Cawthon, R. M., Smith, K. R., O'Brien, E., Sivatchenko, A. and Kerber, R. A. (2003). Association between telomere length in blood and mortality in people aged 60 years or older, *The Lancet*, **361**, pp. 393–395.
125. Cawthon, R. M. (2009). Telomere length measurement by a novel monochrome multiplex quantitative PCR method, *Nucleic Acids Res.*, **37**, pp. e21–e21.
126. O'Callaghan, N. J. and Fenech, M. (2011). A quantitative PCR method for measuring absolute telomere length, *Biol. Proced. Online*, **13**, pp. 3.

127. Aubert, G., Hills, M. and Lansdorp, P. M. (2012). Telomere length measurement—caveats and a critical assessment of the available technologies and tools, *Mutat. Res. Mol. Mech. Mutagen.*, **730**, pp. 59–67.

128. Wynford-Thomas, D. and Kipling, D. (1997). Cancer and the knockout mouse, *Nature*, **389**, pp. 551–552.

129. Raschenberger, J., Lamina, C., Haun, M., Kollerits, B., Coassin, S., Boes, E., *et al.* (2016). Influence of DNA extraction methods on relative telomere length measurements and its impact on epidemiological studies, *Sci. Rep.*, **6**, pp. 25398.

130. Willeit, P., Willeit, J., Brandstätter, A., Ehrlenbach, S., Mayr, A., Gasperi, A., *et al.* (2010). Cellular aging reflected by leukocyte telomere length predicts advanced atherosclerosis and cardiovascular disease risk, *Arterioscler. Thromb. Vasc. Biol.*, **30**, pp. 1649–1656.

131. Gutierrez-Rodrigues, F., Santana-Lemos, B. A., Scheucher, P. S., Alves-Paiva, R. M. and Calado, R. T. (2014). Direct comparison of flow-FISH and qPCR as diagnostic tests for telomere length measurement in humans, *PloS One*, **9**, pp. e113747.

132. Hemann, M. T., Strong, M. A., Hao, L. Y. and Greider, C. W. (2001). The shortest telomere, not average telomere length, is critical for cell viability and chromosome stability, *Cell*, **107**, pp. 67–77.

133. Vera, E. and Blasco, M. A. (2012). Beyond average: potential for measurement of short telomeres, *Aging*, **4**, pp. 379–392.

134. Toupance, S., Villemonais, D., Germain, D., Gegout-Petit, A., Albuisson, E. and Benetos, A. (2019). The individual's signature of telomere length distribution, *Sci. Rep.*, **9**, pp. 685.

135. Gorenjak, V., Petrelis, A. M., Stathopoulou, M. G. and Visvikis-Siest, S. (2020). Telomere length determinants in childhood, *Clin. Chem. Lab. Med.*, **58**, pp. 162–177.

136. Canela, A., Vera, E., Klatt, P. and Blasco, M. A. (2007). High-throughput telomere length quantification by FISH and its application to human population studies, *Proc. Natl. Acad. Sci.*, **104**, pp. 5300–5305.

137. Rufer, N., Dragowska, W., Thornbury, G., Roosnek, E. and Lansdorp, P. M. (1998). Telomere length dynamics in human lymphocyte subpopulations measured by flow cytometry, *Nat. Biotechnol.*, **16**, pp. 743–747.

138. Baerlocher, G. M., Vulto, I., de Jong, G. and Lansdorp, P. M. (2006). Flow cytometry and FISH to measure the average length of telomeres (flow FISH), *Nat. Protoc.*, **1**, pp. 2365–2376.

139. Flores, I., Canela, A., Vera, E., Tejera, A., Cotsarelis, G. and Blasco, M. A. (2008). The longest telomeres: a general signature of adult stem cell compartments, *Genes Dev.*, **22**, pp. 654–667.

140. Meyne, J., Baker, R.J., Hobart, H.H., Hsu, T.C., Ryder, O.A., Ward, O.G., *et al.* (1990). Distribution of non-telomeric sites of the (TTAGGG)n telomeric sequence in vertebrate chromosomes, *Chromosoma*, **99**, pp. 3–10.

141. Beh, C. W., Zhang, Y., Zheng, Y.-L., Sun, B. and Wang, T.-H. (2018). Fluorescence spectroscopic detection and measurement of single telomere molecules, *Nucleic Acids Res.*, **46**, pp. e117–e117.

142. Luo, Y., Viswanathan, R., Hande, M. P., Loh, A. H. P. and Cheow, L. F. (2020). Massively parallel single-molecule telomere length measurement with digital real-time PCR, *Sci. Adv.*, **6**, pp. eabb7944.

143. Baird, D. M., Rowson, J., Wynford-Thomas, D. and Kipling, D. (2003). Extensive allelic variation and ultrashort telomeres in senescent human cells, *Nat. Genet.*, **33**, pp. 203–207.

144. Abdallah, P., Luciano, P., Runge, K.W., Lisby, M., Géli, V., Gilson, E., *et al.* (2009). A two-step model for senescence triggered by a single critically short telomere, *Nat. Cell Biol.*, **11**, pp. 988–993.

145. Alter, B. P., Rosenberg, P. S., Giri, N., Baerlocher, G. M., Lansdorp, P. M. and Savage, S. A. (2012). Telomere length is associated with disease severity and declines with age in dyskeratosis congenita, *Haematologica*, **97**, pp. 353–359.

146. Bendix, L., Horn, P. B., Jensen, U. B., Rubelj, I. and Kolvraa, S. (2010). The load of short telomeres, estimated by a new method, Universal STELA, correlates with number of senescent cells, *Aging Cell*, **9**, pp. 383–397.

147. Lai, T. P., Zhang, N., Noh, J., Mender, I., Tedone, E., Huang, E., *et al.* (2017). A method for measuring the distribution of the shortest telomeres in cells and tissues, *Nat. Commun.*, **8**, pp. 1356.

148. Lin, J., Smith, D. L., Esteves, K. and Drury, S. (2019). Telomere length measurement by qPCR – summary of critical factors and recommendations for assay design, *Psychoneuroendocrinology*, **99**, pp. 271–278.

149. Needham, B. L., Rehkopf, D., Adler, N., Gregorich, S., Lin, J., Blackburn, E. H. *et al.* (2015). Leukocyte telomere length and mortality in the National Health and Nutrition Examination Survey, 1999–2002, *Epidemiol. Camb. Mass*, **26**, pp. 528–535.

150. Deelen, J., Beekman, M., Codd, V., Trompet, S., Broer, L, Hägg, S., *et al.* (2014). Leukocyte telomere length associates with prospective

mortality independent of immune-related parameters and known genetic markers, *Int. J. Epidemiol.*, **43**, pp. 878–886.

151. Bakaysa, S. L., Mucci, L. A., Slagboom, P. E., Boomsma, D. I., McClearn, G. E., Johansson B., *et al.* (2007). Telomere length predicts survival independent of genetic influences, *Aging Cell*, **6**, pp. 769–774.

152. Wang, Q., Zhan, Y., Pedersen, N. L., Fang, F. and Hägg, S. (2018). Telomere length and all-cause mortality: a meta-analysis, *Ageing Res. Rev.*, **48**, pp. 11–20.

153. Mons, U., Müezzinler, A., Schöttker, B., Dieffenbach, A.K., Butterbach, K., Schick, M., *et al.* (2017). Leukocyte telomere length and all-cause, cardiovascular disease, and cancer mortality: results from individual-participant-data meta-analysis of 2 large prospective cohort studies, *Am. J. Epidemiol.*, **185**, pp. 1317–1326.

154. Behrens, A., Sibilia, M. and Wagner, E. F. (1999). Amino-terminal phosphorylation of c-Jun regulates stress-induced apoptosis and cellular proliferation, *Nat. Genet.*, **21**, pp. 326–329.

155. Ye, Q., Apsley, A. T., Etzel, L., Hastings, W. J., Kozlosky, J. T., Walker, C., *et al.* (2023). Telomere length and chronological age across the human lifespan: a systematic review and meta-analysis of 414 study samples including 743,019 individuals, *Ageing Res. Rev.*, **90**, pp. 102031.

156. De Meyer, T., Nawrot, T., Bekaert, S., De Buyzere, M. L., Rietzschel, E. R., and Andrés, V. (2018). Telomere length as cardiovascular aging biomarker: JACC review topic of the week, *J. Am. Coll. Cardiol.*, **72**, pp. 805–813.

157. Aviv, A. and Shay, J. W. (2018). Reflections on telomere dynamics and ageing-related diseases in humans, *Philos. Trans. R. Soc. Lond. B. Biol. Sci.*, **373**, pp. 20160436.

158. Zhu, X., Han, W., Xue, W., Zou, Y., Xie, C., Du, J. *et al.* (2016). The association between telomere length and cancer risk in population studies, *Sci. Rep.*, **6**, pp. 22243.

159. Haycock, P. C., Heydon, E. E., Kaptoge, S., Butterworth, A. S., Thompson, A. and Willeit, P. (2014). Leucocyte telomere length and risk of cardiovascular disease: systematic review and meta-analysis, *BMJ*, **349**, pp. g4227.

160. Gardner, M., Bann, D., Wiley, L., Cooper, R., Hardy, R., Nitsch, D., *et al.* (2014). Gender and telomere length: systematic review and meta-analysis, *Exp. Gerontol.*, **51**, pp. 15–27.

161. Lapham, K., Kvale, M. N., Lin, J., Connell, S., Croen, L. A., Dispensa, B. P., *et al.* (2015). Automated assay of telomere length measurement and

informatics for 100,000 subjects in the genetic epidemiology research on adult health and aging (GERA) cohort, *Genetics*, **200**, pp. 1061–1072.

162. Demanelis, K., Jasmine, F, Chen, L.S., Chernoff, M., Tong L., Delgado D., *et al.* (2020). Determinants of telomere length across human tissues, *Science*, **369**, pp. eaaz6876.
163. Ouyang, Q., Baerlocher, G., Vulto, I. and Lansdorp, P. M. (2007). Telomere length in human natural killer cell subsets, *Ann. N. Y. Acad. Sci.*, **1106**, pp. 240–252.
164. Lin, J. and Epel, E. (2022). Stress and telomere shortening: insights from cellular mechanisms, *Ageing Res. Rev.*, **73**, pp. 101507.
165. Grill, S. and Nandakumar, J. (2021). Molecular mechanisms of telomere biology disorders, *J. Biol. Chem.*, **296**, pp. 100064.
166. Noppert, G. A., Feinstein, L., Dowd, J. B., Stebbins, R. C., Zang, E., Needham, B. L., *et al.* (2020). Pathogen burden and leukocyte telomere length in the United States, *Immun. Ageing A*, **17**, pp. 36.
167. Froidure, A., Mahieu, M., Hoton, D., Laterre, P. F., Yombi, J. C., Koenig, S., *et al.* (2020). Short telomeres increase the risk of severe COVID-19, *Aging*, **12**, pp. 19911–19922.
168. Habib, R., Ocklenburg, S., Hoffjan, S., Haghikia, A., Epplen, J. T. and Arning, L. (2020). Association between shorter leukocyte telomeres and multiple sclerosis, *J. Neuroimmunol.*, **341**, pp. 577187.
169. Zeng, Z., Zhang, W., Qian, Y., Huang, H., Wu, D.J.H., He, Z., *et al.* (2020). Association of telomere length with risk of rheumatoid arthritis: a meta-analysis and Mendelian randomization, *Rheumatol. Oxf. Engl.*, **59**, pp. 940–947.
170. Yeh, J.-K. and Wang, C.-Y. (2016). Telomeres and telomerase in cardiovascular diseases, *Genes*, **7**, pp. 58.
171. Cheng, F., Carroll, L., Joglekar, M. V., Januszewski, A. S., Wong, K. K., Hardikar, A. A., *et al.* (2021). Diabetes, metabolic disease, and telomere length, *Lancet Diabetes Endocrinol.*, **9**, pp. 117–126.
172. Jenkins, A. J., Syreeni, A., Mutter, S., Januszewski, A. S. and Groop, P.-H. (2022). Telomeres in clinical diabetes research: moving towards precision medicine in diabetes care? *Diabetes Res. Clin. Pract.*, **194**, pp. 110178.
173. Chen, B., Yan, Y., Wang, H., and Xu, J. Association between genetically determined telomere length and health-related outcomes: a systematic review and meta-analysis of Mendelian randomization studies, *Aging Cell*, **22**, pp. e13874, Jul. 2023, doi: 10.1111/acel.13874.

174. Tsatsakis, A., Oikonomopoulou, T., Nikolouzakis, T.K., Vakonaki E., Tzatzarakis, M., Flamourakis, M., *et al.* (2023). Role of telomere length in human carcinogenesis (review), *Int J Oncol.*, **63**, pp. 78.

175. Kong, C. M., Lee, X. W. and Wang, X. (2013). Telomere shortening in human diseases, *FEBS J.*, **280**, pp. 3180–3193.

176. Allaire, P., He, J., Mayer, J., Moat, L., Gerstenberger, P., Wilhorn, R., *et al.* (2023). Genetic and clinical determinants of telomere length, *HGG Adv.*, **4**, pp. 100201.

177. Gong, Y., Stock, A. J. and Liu, Y. (2020). The enigma of excessively long telomeres in cancer: lessons learned from rare human POT1 variants, *Curr. Opin. Genet. Dev.*, **60**, pp. 48–55.

178. Rode, L., Nordestgaard, B. G. and Bojesen, S. E. (2016). Long telomeres and cancer risk among 95 568 individuals from the general population, *Int. J. Epidemiol.*, **45**, pp. 1634–1643, Oct. 2016, doi: 10.1093/ije/dyw179.

179. Fragkiadaki, P., Tsoukalas, D., Fragkiadoulaki, I., Psycharakis, C., Nikitovic, D., Spandidos, D.A. *et al.* (2016). Telomerase activity in pregnancy complications (review), *Mol. Med. Rep.*, **14**, pp. 16–21.

180. Fragkiadaki, P., Nikitovic, D., Kalliantasi, K., Sarandi, E., Thanasoula, M., Stivaktakis, P.D., *et al.* (2019). Telomere length and telomerase activity in osteoporosis and osteoarthritis (review), *Exp. Ther. Med.*, **19**, pp. 1626–1632.

181. Nikolouzakis, T.K., Vassilopoulou, L., Fragkiadaki, P., Mariolis Sapsakos, T., Papadakis, G.Z., Spandidos, D.A., *et al.* (2018). Improving diagnosis, prognosis and prediction by using biomarkers in CRC patient (review), *Oncol. Rep.*, **39**, pp. 2455–2472.

182. Vakonaki, E., Tsiminikaki, K., Plaitis S., Fragkiadaki, P., Tsoukalas, Katsikantami, I., *et al.* (2018). Common mental disorders and association with telomere length, *Biomed. Rep.*, **8**, pp. 111–116.

183. Tsoukalas, D., Fragkiadaki, P., Docea, A.O., Alegakis, A.K., Sarandi, E., Vakonaki, E., *et al.* (2019). Association of nutraceutical supplements with longer telomere length, *Int. J. Mol. Med.*, **44**, pp. 218–226.

184. Vasilopoulos, E., Fragkiadaki, P., Kalliora, C., Fragou, D., Docea, A.O., Vakonaki, E., *et al.* (2019). The association of female and male infertility with telomere length (review), *Int. J. Mol. Med.*, **44**, pp. 375–389

185. Kakridonis, F., Pneumatikos, S.G., Vakonaki, E., Berdiaki, A., Tzatzarakis, M.N., Fragkiadaki, P., *et al.* (2023). Telomere length as a predictive biomarker in osteoporosis (review), *Biomed Rep.*, **19**, pp. 87.

186. Aubert, G. and Lansdorp, P. M. (2008). Telomeres and aging, *Physiol. Rev.*, **88**, pp. 557–579.

187. Artandi, S. E., Chang, S., Lee, S. L., Alson, S., Gottlieb, G. J., Chin, L. *et al.* (2000). Telomere dysfunction promotes non-reciprocal translocations and epithelial cancers in mice, *Nature*, **406**, pp. 641–645.

188. Goldman, F. D., Aubert, G., Klingelhutz, A. J., Hills, M., Cooper, S. R., Hamilton, W. S., *et al.* (2008). Characterization of primitive hematopoietic cells from patients with dyskeratosis congenita, *Blood*, **111**, pp. 4523–4531.

189. Mensà, E., Latini, S., Ramini, D., Storci, G., Bonafè, M. and Olivieri, F. (2019). The telomere world and aging: Analytical challenges and future perspectives, *Ageing Res. Rev.*, **50**, pp. 27–42.

190. Frickmann, H., Zautner, A. E., Moter, A., Kikhney, J., Hagen, R. M., Stender, H. *et al.* (2017). Fluorescence in situ hybridization (FISH) in the microbiological diagnostic routine laboratory: a review, *Crit. Rev. Microbiol.*, **43**, pp. 263–293.

191. Tsatsakis, A., Tsoukalas, D., Fragkiadaki, P., Vakonaki, E., Tzatzarakis, M., Sarandi, E., *et al.* (2019). Developing BIOTEL: a semi-automated spreadsheet for estimating telomere length and biological age, *Front. Genet.*, **10**, pp. 84.

192. Gialluisi, A., Santoro, A., Tirozzi, A., Cerletti, C., Donati, M.B., de Gaetano, G., *et al.* (2021). Epidemiological and genetic overlap among biological aging clocks: new challenges in biogerontology, *Ageing Res. Rev.*, **72**, pp. 101502.

193. Whitwell, H.J., Bacalini, M.G., Blyuss, O., Chen, S., Garagnani, P., Gordleeva S.Y., *et al.* (2020). The human body as a super network: digital methods to analyze the propagation of aging, *Front. Aging Neurosci.*, **12**, pp. 136.

194. Fiorito, G., Caini, S., Palli, D., Bendinelli, B., Saieva, C., Ermini, I., *et al.* (2021). DNA methylation-based biomarkers of aging were slowed down in a two-year diet and physical activity intervention trial: the DAMA study, *Aging Cell*, **20**, pp. e13439.

195. McCrory, C., Fiorito, G., McLoughlin, S., Polidoro, S., Cheallaigh, C. N., Bourke, N., *et al.* (2020). Epigenetic clocks and allostatic load reveal potential sex-specific drivers of biological aging, *J. Gerontol. A. Biol. Sci. Med. Sci.*, **75**, pp. 495–503.

196. Vetter, V. M., Meyer, A., Karbasiyan, M., Steinhagen-Thiessen, E., Hopfenmüller, W. and Demuth, I. (2019). Epigenetic clock and relative telomere length represent largely different aspects of aging in the

berlin aging study II (BASE-II), *J. Gerontol. A. Biol. Sci. Med. Sci.*, **74**, pp. 27–32.

197. Li, X., Ploner, A., Wang, Y., Magnusson, P. K., Reynolds, C., Finkel, D., *et al.* (2020). Longitudinal trajectories, correlations, and mortality associations of nine biological ages across 20-years follow-up, *eLife*, **9**, pp. e51507.
198. Mitnitski, A., Collerton, J., Martin-Ruiz, C., Jagger, C., von Zglinicki, T., Rockwood, K. *et al.* (2015). Age-related frailty and its association with biological markers of ageing, *BMC Med.*, **13**, pp. 161.
199. Nelke, C., Schroeter, C. B., Pawlitzki, M., Meuth, S. G. and Ruck, T. (2022). Cellular senescence in neuroinflammatory disease: new therapies for old cells? *Trends Mol. Med.*, **28**, pp. 850–863.

Chapter 3

Computational Tools for Telomere Length Measurement

Irene Fragkiadoulaki,[a,b] Athanasios Alegkakis,[a,b] Elisavet Renieri,[a,b] and Aristidis Tsatsakis[a,b]

[a] *Laboratory of Toxicology, Medical School, University of Crete, Heraklion, Greece*
[b] *Lifeplus S.A., Science & Technological Park of Crete, Vassilika Vouton, Heraklion, Greece*
eirinimbg@hotmail.gr

3.1 Introduction

Telomeres, the protective sequences of nucleotides found at the ends of linear chromosomes, play a crucial role in safeguarding genomic stability and contributing to overall cellular well-being. These specialized structures, composed of repetitive DNA sequences and associated proteins, act as caps that shield chromosomes from degradation preserving the integrity of genetic information. Over the past decades, telomeric length has been linked to a biological clock offering insights into human aging [1, 2]. Moreover, it has emerged as a valuable individual marker and, when combined with other biological metrics, serves as a reliable predictor of life

Telomeres: Biomarkers of a Healthy Life and Successful Aging
Edited by Aristidis Tsatsakis

ISBN 978-981-5129-49-6 (Hardcover), 978-1-003-56809-4 (eBook)
www.jennystanford.com

expectancy. Numerous studies have linked telomeric length to the presence of various diseases including gene mutations [3] and the severity of conditions, such as aplastic anemia [4].

Therefore, the assessment of telomere length emerges as a crucial metric in delving into the complexities of various biological phenomena. It acts as a key to unraveling the intricacies of cellular dynamics providing valuable insights into the factors influencing lifespan, aging patterns, and potential connections to a range of pathologies. The significance of these measurements underscores the need for procedures and software capable of robustly estimating telomeric length ensuring validated and accurate results. Given the diverse techniques available for telomere length estimation, including PCR, Q-FISH, and TRF [5, 6], multiple approaches have been developed to address this need.

This chapter embarks on an exploration of the diverse computational techniques that have become integral to telomere length measurement. Ranging from sophisticated fluorescence microscopy image analysis tools to high-throughput methodologies leveraging next-generation sequencing (NGS) technologies, these computational tools reflect the dynamic and evolving nature of telomere research.

3.2 Computational Tools Used in Fluorescence in situ Hybridization

Fluorescence in situ hybridization (FISH) image analysis stands as a foundational pillar in the accurate assessment of telomere length offering researchers a window into the intricate world of chromosomal dynamics. A variety of computational tools are available for telomere length estimation using FISH. The most important are described in this paragraph.

TeloView is a software tool designed for telomere length analysis providing detailed visualization and data statistical analysis. Even though specific details about TeloView may vary based on its version and updates, there are some general features. TeloView is dedicated to the analysis of telomere lengths. It facilitates the measurement and characterization of telomeres within biological samples (blood, urine, saliva, etc.). The software offers detailed visualization tools allowing researchers to observe and analyze telomeric structures within fluorescence microscopy images or other relevant data sources, such as Microarray Data, ChIP-Seq Data, RNA-Seq Data, Clinical Data, etc. [7]. Visual representation is crucial for understanding the distribution and patterns of telomere lengths. TeloView offers the ability of statistical analysis so quantitative insights into telomere dynamics can be achieved. Such quantitative insights are the generation of summary statistics, identification of correlations, or telomere lengths comparison across different conditions or sample groups. Like many image analysis tools, TeloView typically provides a user-friendly interface making it accessible to researchers with diverse backgrounds and levels of expertise. An intuitive interface enhances the usability of the software. TeloView can be applied in various research settings including studies related to cellular aging, cancer research, and investigations into the impact of telomere dynamics on biological processes.

ImageJ is an open-source platform for image analysis, and FIJI is a distribution of ImageJ that extends its functionality with additional plugins and features. Developed by the National Institutes of Health (NIH), ImageJ/FIJI is widely used in the scientific community for various biological image analysis tasks including the analysis of FISH images [8]. It provides an extensive set of tools and plugins making it a versatile and customizable solution for researchers in the field of microscopy and bioimage analysis. ImageJ and FIJI are freely available and open source allowing for widespread adoption and community contributions. Users can enhance the capabilities of ImageJ/FIJI by installing a variety of plugins and extensions. This extensibility makes it suitable for a wide range of image analysis applications. Specific plugins within ImageJ/FIJI are designed for telomere length analysis using FISH data. These plugins often provide tools for measuring fluorescence intensity, quantifying signals, and analyzing the distribution of telomere lengths in a population of cells [7]. ImageJ/FIJI supports the analysis of various types of microscopy images, making it suitable for researchers working with diverse imaging techniques. ImageJ/FIJI's user-friendly interface, combined with its powerful analysis capabilities and community support, makes it a valuable tool for researchers involved in telomere length analysis using FISH data.

BIOTEL, a spreadsheet software developed by a research team in Greece, estimates telomeric length from Q-FISH fluorescence data and generates individual and population measurements [9]. Positioned as a practical tool for laboratory and clinical research, BIOTEL employs a structured set of worksheets encompassing various inputs, parameters, and procedures. Input data includes demographic information such as age, sex, presence of chronic diseases, and personal habits, along with raw fluorescence data exported from Q-FISH measurements. The software incorporates parameters linked to experiment dates and cell line characteristics. Procedures within BIOTEL encompass tasks for cleaning and transforming fluorescence data into telomeric length estimating specific statistics like telomeric short ranges and medians and providing a rough estimation of biological age (Fig. 3.1). Program outputs comprise individual characteristics, age and sex-based population statistics, and graphical representations such as telomeric distribution plots, biological and chronological age plots, and individual positions within age population distributions. BIOTEL has been referenced in a series of articles focused on telomere length estimations [10, 11].

The advantages of BIOTEL can be summarized as: (a) it is an easy-to-use software -mainly the spreadsheet view option, (b) it is based on entries made by the researcher and can produce both individual profiles and population statistics, and (c) the researcher can develop new techniques on estimation/presentation on fluorescence/telomeric data. The disadvantages of BIOTEL can be summarized as: (a) there is no detailed user manual and (b) it is focused on Q-FISH techniques.

As telomere biology continues to unravel its complexities, the significance of fluorescence microscopy image analysis, coupled with advanced computational tools, becomes increasingly evident. These tools not only provide accurate measurements but also pave the way for deeper insights into the role of telomeres in cellular health, aging, and diseases positioning them as invaluable assets in the researcher's toolkit.

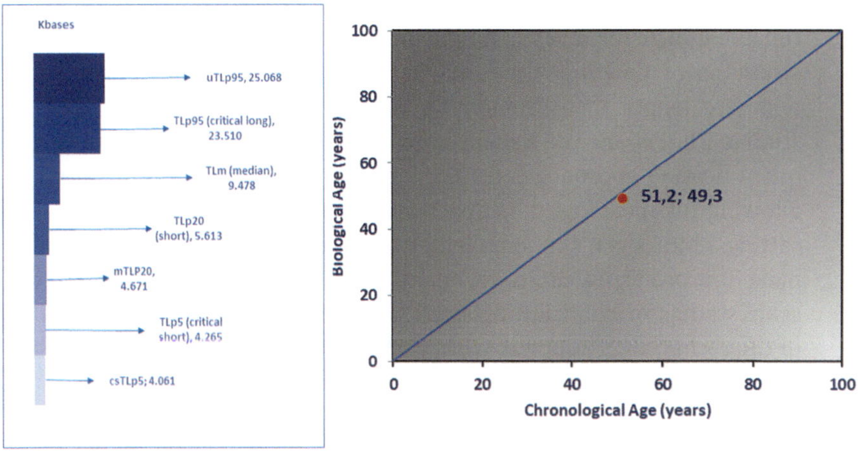

Figure 3.1 Representation of telomere length distribution (left) and chronological vs. biological age (plot) using BIOTEL software based on Q-FISH fluorescence data.

3.3 Computational Tools Used in Quantitative Polymerase Chain Reaction

In the realm of telomere length measurement, quantitative polymerase chain reaction (qPCR) approaches have emerged as powerful and widely employed methods supported by robust computational methodologies.

Cawthon's method, introduced in 2002, stands as a cornerstone in qPCR-based telomere length measurement and has become a benchmark for researchers in the field [12]. This method offers a robust and standardized framework for estimating telomere length by leveraging the principles of relative quantification. The fundamental premise of Cawthon's method is based on the determination of the ratio of telomere repeats copy number to single-copy gene copy number within a given sample. This ratio is then normalized against a reference sample facilitating the establishment of a relative measurement of telomere length. The use of a single-copy gene as a reference helps account for variations in DNA input, amplification efficiency, and other factors that may influence the qPCR assay. The result is a quantifiable and comparable measure of telomere length across samples providing researchers with a reliable metric for investigating telomere dynamics. One of the key strengths of Cawthon's method lies in its ability to standardize telomere length measurements across different laboratories and studies. The reliance on a single-copy gene reference and the relative quantification approach contribute to the reproducibility of results allowing for meaningful comparisons across diverse experimental settings. Moreover, the simplicity and accessibility of the method make it a preferred choice for many researchers conducting large-scale studies or clinical investigations. The use of widely available qPCR technology, coupled with a straightforward computational analysis, enhances the method's applicability and scalability.

Qbase+ stands as an indispensable and comprehensive software tool tailored for the intricate analysis of qPCR data with a specialized focus on telomere length analysis [13]. Developed by Biogazelle, qBase+ addresses the complexities of qPCR experiments and streamlines the process of deriving accurate and reliable measurements of telomere lengths. One of the primary strengths of qBase+ lies in its ability to calculate relative telomere lengths. This is achieved by comparing the cycle threshold (Ct) values of telomere repeats with those of carefully selected reference genes [14]. The utilization of reference genes helps account for variability in the sample input and other experimental factors contributing to the normalization of telomere length data. The software provides a user-friendly interface that facilitates efficient data input and manipulation making it accessible to researchers with varying levels of expertise. Qbase+ offers a range of normalization options, allowing researchers to account for variations in sample quality and quantity, as well as other potential sources of bias [15]. This normalization step is crucial for obtaining accurate and biologically relevant telomere length measurements. To enhance the robustness of telomere length measurements, qBase+ incorporates statistical analysis tools. These tools enable researchers to assess the significance of observed differences in telomere lengths among experimental conditions, providing a deeper understanding of the biological implications of the data. The software has been widely adopted in telomere research, where accurate measurement of telomere length is essential for understanding cellular aging, disease processes, and the impact of various interventions. Researchers appreciate the versatility and reliability of qBase+ in handling qPCR data specific to telomere length analysis.

The qPCR package, an essential component of the R programming language, stands out as a flexible and powerful tool designed for the in-depth analysis of qPCR data. Its versatility makes it particularly well-suited for the nuanced examination of relative telomere length offering researchers a robust set of functionalities to obtain valuable insights from their experiments [16]. The most important capability of qPCR is the analysis of relative telomere length. Leveraging established methods, the package facilitates the comparison of telomere repeat abundance with that of carefully selected reference genes. This approach is crucial in order to normalize telomere length data taking into account sample variations as well as other potential sources of experimental variability. QPCR provides researchers with the flexibility to adapt their analyses to specific experimental designs. The package accommodates various qPCR assay configurations making it suitable for a wide range of experimental setups and conditions. Being an open-source tool within the R programming environment, qPCR allows users to customize analyses and workflows according to their specific research needs. This adaptability is invaluable for tailoring the software to the intricacies of telomere length studies. R's open-source nature enables seamless integration with other bioinformatics tools and statistical packages. The combination of qPCR's flexibility and R's extensive capabilities makes it a valuable tool in the toolkit of researchers investigating telomere length dynamics and associated phenomena using qPCR methodologies.

LinRegPCR stands as a specialized tool meticulously designed to assess polymerase chain reaction (PCR) amplification efficiency directly from raw data. Developed to enhance the accuracy of quantification in qPCR experiments, LinRegPCR is particularly valuable in the context of telomere length measurements [17]. This tool offers a unique perspective by considering and calculating the amplification efficiency, a critical parameter for accurate quantification in qPCR analyses. In the realm of telomere research, where precise measurements are paramount, LinRegPCR plays a pivotal role in refining the analysis process. By evaluating and incorporating the PCR amplification efficiency, LinRegPCR contributes to more accurate and reliable quantification of telomere length from qPCR data. The tool addresses the inherent variability in amplification across samples and reactions, offering a more nuanced understanding of telomere dynamics within experimental datasets [18]. LinRegPCR excels in determining the amplification efficiency of PCR reactions. This information is crucial for correcting biases and variations in the amplification process ultimately leading to more accurate and reproducible results. Moreover, LinRegPCR operates directly on raw data allowing for a detailed examination of the kinetics of the PCR reaction. This approach provides a more granular view of the amplification process enabling researchers to identify and correct potential sources of variability. By considering and accounting for amplification efficiency, LinRegPCR significantly improves the accuracy of quantification in qPCR experiments. This is particularly beneficial in telomere length measurements, where precision is essential for understanding cellular aging and related processes. LinRegPCR's emphasis on amplification efficiency assessment makes it an invaluable tool for researchers striving to achieve high precision in telomere length measurements and other qPCR-based analyses.

TeloTool is recognized for its proficiency in analyzing telomere length from qPCR data analysis. This versatility positions TeloTool as a comprehensive software solution, catering to the diverse needs of researchers engaged in telomere length measurement across various experimental techniques. In the context of qPCR, TeloTool emerges as a valuable resource by facilitating the processing and analysis of raw qPCR data [19]. This includes essential steps such as signal detection, background correction, and the derivation of telomere length results. The software's user-friendly interface streamlines these complex analytical processes, allowing researchers to navigate and interpret qPCR data effectively. TeloTool is equipped to handle raw qPCR data efficiently. It assists researchers in organizing and preprocessing their qPCR datasets, laying the groundwork for subsequent analyses. The software excels in detecting signals relevant to telomere repeats within qPCR data. This step is crucial for accurately identifying and quantifying telomere-specific signals against the background noise ensuring the precision of subsequent measurements. Also, TeloTool incorporates sophisticated algorithms for background correction. This feature is vital in minimizing the impact of non-specific fluorescence and noise refining the accuracy of telomere length measurements derived from qPCR experiments. Finally, one of TeloTool's notable strengths lies in its adaptability across multiple telomere length measurement techniques. Researchers can seamlessly transition between TRF and qPCR data analyses within the same software platform streamlining their workflow and promoting consistency in their analyses. TeloTool's adaptability to multiple telomere length measurement techniques makes it as an asset for researchers seeking a unified and user-friendly platform for their telomere studies, whether employing TRF or qPCR methodologies.

3.4 Computational Tools Used in Southern Blot Analysis

Terminal restriction fragment (TRF) analysis is a traditional method for measuring telomere length. Several computational tools are used in conjunction with TRF experiments to analyze the resulting data and estimate telomere length accurately. Here are some commonly used computational tools for TRF analysis.

TeloTool stands out as a versatile and comprehensive software tool designed to analyze telomere length, seamlessly accommodating data from qPCR and TRF analyses, as well. TeloTool has been extended to cater to the unique requirements of TRF experiments. This adaptability makes TeloTool a valuable resource for researchers engaged in telomere length studies across different experimental methodologies. In the context of TRF analysis, TeloTool plays a crucial role in streamlining data processing and enhancing the accuracy of telomere length quantification [19]. TeloTool aids researchers in efficiently processing TRF data. It handles the intricacies of digitized gel images allowing for the extraction of essential information required for subsequent analyses. The software incorporates algorithms for background correction, a critical step in minimizing non-specific signals and noise inherent in TRF experiments. This correction ensures that telomere length measurements are more precise and reflective of the true biological signal. In addition, TeloTool excels in quantifying telomere lengths from TRF data. Researchers obtain reliable and reproducible measurements through automation of the detection and analysis of terminal restriction fragments. TeloTool's adaptability is a notable strength. Researchers can seamlessly transition between PCR and TRF analyses within the same software platform. This versatility not only simplifies workflow management but also ensures consistency in data analysis and interpretation. TeloTool's double applicability in qPCR and TRF analyses makes it a valuable tool for researchers seeking a unified platform for telomere length studies regardless of the specific experimental techniques employed. Its user-friendly interface and robust analytical features contribute to the precision and efficiency of telomere length quantification in diverse research contexts.

Telometric stands as a dedicated software package meticulously crafted for the analysis of telomere length specifically tailored for TRF data. TRF analysis involves resolving DNA fragments on agarose gels, and Telometric streamlines this process by providing essential functions for precise quantification [20]. Telometric includes functions for the automated identification and delineation of lanes on agarose gels. This is a crucial initial step, as it enables the software to isolate individual lanes corresponding to different samples facilitating focused analysis for each. The software is equipped with tools for generating intensity profiles from the resolved DNA fragments. These profiles serve as a representation of the signal intensity along the length of the gel lanes providing a visual representation of telomeric DNA fragments. Telometric incorporates algorithms for calculating telomere lengths based on the intensity profiles generated. This step involves quantifying the size of the telomeric DNA fragments within each lane ultimately providing researchers with accurate and reproducible telomere length measurements. Telometric is particularly designed for quantifying TRF lengths from agarose gels, a common medium for separating DNA fragments based on size. The software's specialization in handling agarose gel data makes it a valuable tool for researchers employing this traditional approach in telomere length analysis. Its automation of lane finding, intensity profile generation, and telomere length calculation collectively contribute to the efficiency and accuracy of telomere analysis in agarose gel electrophoresis.

The WALTER toolset addresses the need for a user-friendly and robust tool for the reproducible evaluation of TRF data. It allows the analysis of TRF scans with non-unimodal distributions of telomere signals overcoming limitations of existing tools [21]. WALTER uses an innovative approach by automatically setting a threshold to interpret a specific part of the telomere-specific signal reducing user bias. This approach enables the analysis of TRF scans with technical defects or high signal intensity, which might be challenging for other tools. A key advantage of WALTER is demonstrated in cases where TeloTool overestimated telomere lengths, particularly when TeloTool indicated low fit quality. WALTER provides in-house statistical evaluation of data allowing for comparisons between control and case groups or among all groups [22]. The toolset offers transparency and reproducibility in the analysis, presenting input gel images and final log files. While WALTER offers versatility and advantages in certain scenarios, the authors emphasize the importance of following best practices and carefully reading the user manual to avoid potential biases. Overall, WALTER addresses the challenges in TRF data analysis and provides a valuable tool for researchers seeking precise and reproducible evaluation of telomere lengths.

3.5 Computational Tools Used in Next-Generation Sequencing Analysis

Next-generation sequencing (NGS) has become an increasingly powerful tool for telomere length measurement providing a high-throughput and genome-wide perspective. Here are some computational tools commonly used for telomere length analysis with NGS data.

TelSeq is a sophisticated bioinformatics tool tailored for the precise analysis of telomere length using NGS data. With a focus on efficiency and accuracy, TelSeq has gained widespread popularity for its ability to handle large-scale sequencing datasets making it an invaluable resource for researchers studying telomeres across various organisms and conditions [23]. TelSeq harnesses the power of whole genome sequencing data allowing researchers to leverage comprehensive genomic information for accurate telomere length estimation. By utilizing the entire genome, TelSeq provides a more holistic view of telomere dynamics. TelSeq employs a read-counting strategy to estimate telomere lengths. Specifically, it counts the number of sequencing reads that align to telomeric repeats providing a quantitative measure of telomere abundance. This approach is robust and enables the analysis of telomeres on a genome-wide scale [24]. Known for its accuracy, TelSeq ensures reliable telomere length estimates. This is crucial for studies where precise measurements are essential, such as investigations into the impact of telomere length on various biological processes, diseases, and aging. TelSeq is designed to handle large-scale sequencing datasets efficiently [25]. Its computational efficiency makes it suitable for processing extensive genomic data generated by modern NGS technologies facilitating high-throughput analysis. TelSeq proves its significance in telomere research through its application of whole-genome sequencing data, utilization of a read-counting approach, and prioritization of accuracy. Its widespread adoption speaks to its reliability and efficiency in handling the complexities of NGS datasets for telomere length analysis.

Qmotif, an advanced R package, is developed for in-depth analysis of telomere length using NGS data. It utilizes a k-mer-based approach designed for precise quantification of telomere repeats within sequencing reads. Particularly adept at handling short-read data, Qmotif is advantageous for telomere length studies with NGS platforms [26]. The k-mer-based strategy allows for a nuanced and accurate assessment of telomere lengths, robustly capturing the repetitive nature of telomeric DNA sequences. Tailored for short-read data from various NGS platforms, Qmotif considers the characteristics of short-read sequencing technologies ensuring reliable telomere length measurements [27]. Integrated as an R package, Qmotif seamlessly merges with the R environment, offering users flexibility for additional statistical analyses and visualizations. This integration boosts the overall analytical capabilities of researchers working with telomere length data. Qmotif's design specifically targets telomeric sequences within the complex genomic landscape, heightening its sensitivity and specificity in detecting and quantifying telomere repeats [28]. Its focus on k-mer-based quantification and compatibility with short-read NGS data highlights its efficacy in the detailed analysis of telomere length. The integration with the R environment empowers researchers to conduct comprehensive analyses and extract meaningful insights from datasets related to telomeres.

Computel is a crucial tool in the field of NGS offering a specialized solution for accurately estimating telomere length. The repetitive nature of telomeres poses challenges in analysis, but Computel effectively addresses these issues providing a robust and accurate method for estimating telomere length from high-throughput NGS data [29]. Computel aligns short reads to a specialized index crafted to ensure exclusive mapping of telomeric reads which leads to enhanced accuracy of telomere length estimation. The software demonstrates robust performance in short-read lengths, fold coverage, and insert sizes. This versatility ensures consistent and reliable results under varying experimental conditions, such as different sample types, sequencing platforms, library preparation methods, sequencing protocols, quality of sequencing data, and different research objectives. Computel excels in scenarios with sequencing errors, providing accurate results even when common types of sequencing errors are present in the data. The software is designed to handle such challenges and mitigate the impact of errors on the accuracy of telomere length measurements. Another important feature is Computel's ability to minimize misclassification of reads originating from interspersed telomeric repeats (interstitial telomeric repeats) in other chromosomal regions. This enhances the tool's accuracy in distinguishing true telomeric reads. Computel outperforms TelSeq in scenarios with a variation of short-read lengths offering consistent performance. Its threshold-free approach contributes to improved accuracy, especially in diverse experimental settings. The "threshold-free approach" mentioned in this context indicates that Computel does not rely on a predetermined threshold for certain parameters, as opposed to methods that involve setting fixed thresholds for specific criteria. In the context of telomere length estimation, thresholds might be used for criteria such as the number of telomeric repeats in a sequencing read. With parameters easily adjustable through a single configuration file, Computel ensures user-friendliness. This accessibility is particularly beneficial for researchers with basic programming skills. Computel acknowledges limitations such as the inability to handle variable telomeric patterns and aims to address these in future versions. The software may have challenges when dealing with diverse or non-standard patterns of telomeric DNA because telomeric patterns can vary among organisms or even within a species. Consideration for implementation with alternative short-read alignment programs is also on the agenda for enhancing versatility. Its strengths in accurate alignment, robust performance, and user-friendly configuration contribute to its significance in advancing research related to telomeres, cellular dynamics, and their implications in health and disease.

Telomerecat emerges as a powerful bioinformatics tool designed to unravel the mysteries of telomere length using whole-genome sequencing data. Telomeres are investigated with precision through Telomerecat's sophisticated mapping and clustering strategies because the software can identify telomeric repeats, even in regions rich in telomeric sequences, through whole genome analysis [30]. Therefore, Telomerecat provides higher accuracy in telomere length distribution determination. Leveraging advanced clustering strategies, Telomerecat groups mapped reads enabling a comprehensive and nuanced understanding of telomere length distributions. Telomerecat proves invaluable in diverse biological investigations shedding light on aging processes, disease mechanisms, and cellular function. Overall, Telomerecat stands as a sophisticated bioinformatics ally empowering researchers to decode the intricate language of telomere length through whole-genome sequencing data. Its precision in mapping, clustering strategies, and comprehensive insights contribute to advancing our understanding of telomere biology and its implications in health and disease.

TelomereHunter emerges as a cutting-edge bioinformatics tool meticulously crafted for the analysis of telomere lengths from NGS data [31]. Deploying a sophisticated machine learning approach, TelomereHunter stands at the forefront of telomere research because it is engineered to handle challenging datasets characterized by low coverage and high noise. This approach ensures a high degree of accuracy in telomere length estimation. Designed to confront challenges posed by datasets with low coverage and high noise, TelomereHunter exhibits robust performance making it a reliable companion for researchers dealing with diverse experimental conditions, such as differences in biological samples, variability in sequencing platforms, fluctuations in sequencing depth, noise, and error handling, etc. TelomereHunter's core strength lies in its ability to provide accurate and reliable telomere length estimates, a critical metric for understanding cellular processes and health. Researchers benefit from TelomereHunter's versatility allowing them to seamlessly integrate telomere length analysis into a wide array of genomic studies. For example, researchers can use TelomereHunter across a wide array of genomic investigations, such as those focused on gene expression, epigenetics, or disease-associated studies. TelomereHunter emerges as a formidable asset in the realm of telomere research seamlessly merging bioinformatics prowess with machine learning sophistication. Its ability to navigate through complex NGS datasets, identify telomeric signals, and provide accurate length estimates makes it a valuable tool for researchers unraveling the mysteries of genomic telomeres.

3.6 Conclusion

Computational tools, from the foundational fluorescence microscopy image analysis tools like TeloTool to the high-throughput capabilities of NGS technologies, have become indispensable allies in studying the telomeric ends of DNA with higher accuracy and precision (Table 3.1).

The evolution of telomere research, marked by the transition from traditional Southern blot analyses to sophisticated, high-throughput methodologies, reflects the dynamic nature of the field. The precision and efficiency afforded by computational tools have not only enhanced our understanding of telomere dynamics but have also paved the way for groundbreaking discoveries. Notably, the work of Deng et al. exemplifies the power of these tools, showcasing their ability to extract meaningful insights from

Table 3.1 An overview of computational tools used in telomere length measurement, along with the methodologies they are typically employed with

Computational tool	Description	Methodology
TeloView	Software for telomere length analysis, offering detailed visualization and statistical analysis of the data	FISH
ImageJ/FIJI	An open-source platform for image analysis, including specific plugins for telomere length analysis from FISH images	FISH
BIOTEL	A spreadsheet software tailored for telomeric length estimation from Q-FISH fluorescence, providing individual and population measurements, demographic data, and statistics	Q-FISH
Qbase+	Software for qPCR data analysis, including telomere length measurements and relative expression analysis	qPCR
LinRegPCR	A method and software tool for real-time PCR analysis, commonly used for quantifying telomere length using qPCR data	qPCR
TeloTool	An open-source software facilitating data preprocessing, visualization, statistical analysis, and interpretation	PCR and TRF analysis
Telometric	A software package for the automated analysis of telomere length, offering precise measurements and statistical analysis	TRF analysis
Walter	An automated telomere analysis tool facilitating efficient and accurate quantification of telomere length and interpretation of telomere length data	TRF analysis
TelSeq	Utilizes whole-genome sequencing data and read-counting approach for accurate telomere length estimation, particularly adept at handling short-read data	NGS

Qmotif	An R package employing a k-mer-based approach for quantifying telomere repeats within sequencing reads, designed for short-read data analysis	NGS
Computel	Open-source software for estimating telomere length from high-throughput NGS data, addressing challenges like repetitive sequences, and providing accurate estimations	NGS
Telomerecat	A bioinformatics tool for telomere length estimation using whole genome sequencing data, employing a mapping and clustering strategy for accurate length distribution analysis	NGS
TelomereHunter	A bioinformatics tool employing a machine learning approach to identify telomere signals in NGS data, offering accurate length estimates even under challenging conditions	NGS

large-scale genomic data, ultimately contributing to our understanding of subtelomere chromatin organization [32].

As we stand at the intersection of technology and telomere biology, the impact of computational tools extends far beyond mere measurements. These tools facilitate nuanced analyses, uncover variations in telomere length distributions, and offer a genome-wide perspective that was once unimaginable. The dynamic landscape of telomere research continues to be shaped by the ongoing refinement of computational algorithms, the integration of multi-omics approaches, and the pursuit of standardized methodologies.

Looking forward, the challenges that lie ahead include further refining computational methodologies addressing data interpretation complexities and harmonizing high-throughput protocols. The future of telomere research holds promise for more sophisticated tools, deeper insights into telomere dynamics across diverse contexts, and a holistic understanding of telomere biology within the broader cellular and molecular landscape.

In this book chapter, we have described the variety and efficacy of computational tools available for telomere length determination, telomere length distribution, method accuracy and precision, method challenges, etc. From the microscopic intricacies of fluorescence image analysis to the genome-wide perspectives offered by high-throughput technologies, these tools not only serve as instruments of measurement but also as catalysts for unlocking the secrets encoded in the protective caps of our chromosomes. The collaborative synergy between experimental techniques and computational methodologies will undoubtedly continue to shape the trajectory of telomere research offering new vistas for exploration and contributing to our understanding of fundamental biological processes and their implications for human health and longevity.

References

1. Fasching, C. L. (2018). Telomere length measurement as a clinical biomarker of aging and disease, *Crit. Rev. Clin. Lab. Sci.*, **55**, pp. 443–465.
2. Vaiserman, A., Krasnienkov, D. (2020). Telomere length as a marker of biological age: state-of-the-art, open issues, and future perspectives, *Front. Genet.*, **11**, pp. 630186.

3. Aubert, G., Lansdorp, P. M. (2008). Telomeres and aging, *Physiol. Rev.*, **88**, pp. 557–579.
4. Polychronopoulou, S., Koutroumba, P. (2004). Telomere length variation and telomerase activity expression in patients with congenital and acquired aplastic anemia, *Acta Haematol.*, **111**, pp. 125–131.
5. Montpetit, A. J., Alhareeri, A. A., Montpetit, M., Starkweather, A. R., Elmore, L. W., Filler, K. *et al.* (2014). Telomere length: a review of methods for measurement, *Nurs. Res.*, **63**, pp. 289–299.
6. Lai, M. C., Lombardo, M. V., Auyeung, B., Chakrabarti, B., Baron-Cohen, S. (2015). Sex/gender differences and autism: setting the scene for future research, *J. Am. Acad. Child Adolesc. Psychiatry*, **54**, pp. 11–24.
7. Adam, N., Degelman, E., Briggs, S., Wazen, R. M., Colarusso, P., Riabowol, K., *et al.* (2019). Telomere analysis using 3D fluorescence microscopy suggests mammalian telomere clustering in hTERT immortalized Hs68 fibroblasts, *Commun. Biol.*, **2**, pp. 451.
8. Schindelin, J., Arganda-Carreras, I., Frise, E., Kaynig, V., Longair, M., Pietzsch, T., *et al.* (2012). Fiji: an open-source platform for biological-image analysis, *Nat. Methods*, **9**, pp. 676–682.
9. Tsatsakis, A., Tsoukalas, D., Fragkiadaki, P., Vakonaki, E., Tzatzarakis, M., Sarandi, E., *et al.* (2019). Developing BIOTEL: a semi-automated spreadsheet for estimating telomere length and biological age, *Front. Genet.*, **10**, pp. 84.
10. Tsatsakis, A., Renieri, E., Tsoukalas, D., Buga, A. M., Sarandi, E., Vakonaki, E., *et al.* (2023). A novel nutraceutical formulation increases telomere length and activates telomerase activity in middle-aged rats, *Mol. Med. Rep.*, **28**, pp. 232.
11. Tsoukalas, D., Fragkiadaki, P., Docea, A. O., Alegakis, A. K., Sarandi, E., Vakonaki, E., *et al.* (2019). Association of nutraceutical supplements with longer telomere length, *Int. J. Mol. Med.*, **44**, pp. 218–226.
12. Cawthon, R. M. (2002). Telomere measurement by quantitative PCR, *Nucleic Acids Res.*, **30**, pp. e47.
13. Hellemans, J., Mortier, G., De Paepe, A., Speleman, F., Vandesompele, J. (2007). qBase relative quantification framework and software for management and automated analysis of real-time quantitative PCR data, *Genome Biol.*, **8**, pp. 19.
14. Martens, D. S., Plusquin, M., Gyselaers, W., De Vivo, I., Nawrot, T. S. (2016). Maternal pre-pregnancy body mass index and newborn telomere length, *BMC Med.*, **14**, pp. 148.
15. Prieto-Botella, D., Martens, D. S., Valera-Gran, D., Subiza-Perez, M., Tardon, A., Lozano, M., *et al.* (2023). Sedentary behaviour and

telomere length shortening during early childhood: evidence from the multicentre prospective INMA cohort study, *Int. J. Environ. Res. Public Health*, **20**, pp. 5134.

16. Ruijter, J. M., Ramakers, C., Hoogaars, W. M., Karlen, Y., Bakker, O., van den Hoff, M. J., *et al.* (2009). Amplification efficiency: linking baseline and bias in the analysis of quantitative PCR data, *Nucleic Acids Res.*, **37**, pp. 45.
17. Ramakers, C., Ruijter, J. M., Deprez, R. H., Moorman, A. F. (2003). Assumption-free analysis of quantitative real-time polymerase chain reaction (PCR) data, *Neurosci. Lett.*, **339**, pp. 62–66.
18. Hastings, W. J., Eisenberg, D. T. A., Shalev, I. (2021). Impact of amplification efficiency approaches on telomere length measurement via quantitative-polymerase chain reaction, *Front. Genet.*, **12**, pp. 728603.
19. Gohring, J., Fulcher, N., Jacak, J., Riha, K. (2014). TeloTool: a new tool for telomere length measurement from terminal restriction fragment analysis with improved probe intensity correction, *Nucleic Acids Res.*, **42**, pp. 21.
20. Grant, J. D., Broccoli, D., Muquit, M., Manion, F. J., Tisdall, J., Ochs, M. F. (2001). Telometric: a tool providing simplified, reproducible measurements of telomeric DNA from constant field agarose gels, *Biotechniques*, **3**, pp. 1314–1316, 1318.
21. Lycka, M., Peska, V., Demko, M., Spyroglou, I., Kilar, A., Fajkus, J., *et al.* (2021). WALTER: an easy way to online evaluate telomere lengths from terminal restriction fragment analysis, *BMC Bioinformatics*, **22**, pp. 145.
22. Kimura, M., Stone, R. C., Hunt, S. C., Skurnick, J., Lu, X., Cao, X., *et al.* (2010). Measurement of telomere length by the Southern blot analysis of terminal restriction fragment lengths, *Nat. Protoc.*, **5**, pp. 1596–1607.
23. Ding, Z., Mangino, M., Aviv, A., Spector, T., Durbin, R., Consortium UK. (2014). Estimating telomere length from whole genome sequence data, *Nucleic Acids Res.*, **42**, pp. 75.
24. Taub, M. A., Conomos, M. P., Keener, R., Iyer, K. R., Weinstock, J. S., Yanek, L. R., *et al.* (2022). Genetic determinants of telomere length from 109,122 ancestrally diverse whole-genome sequences in TOPMed, *Cell Genom.*, **2**, pp. 100084. doi: 10.1016/j.xgen.2021.100084. Epub 2022 Jan 13.
25. Al Khleifat, A., Iacoangeli, A., Jones, A. R., van Vugt, J., Moisse, M., Shatunov, A., *et al.* (2022). Telomere length analysis in amyotrophic lateral sclerosis using large-scale whole genome sequence data, *Front. Cell Neurosci.*, **16**, pp. 1050596.

26. Holmes, O., Nones, K., Tang, Y. H., Loffler, K. A., Lee, M., Patch, A. M., *et al.* (2022). Qmotif: determination of telomere content from whole-genome sequence data, *Bioinform. Adv.*, **2**, pp. vbac005. doi: 10.1093/bioadv/vbac005. eCollection 2022.

27. Lee, M., Napier, C. E., Yang, S. F., Arthur, J. W., Reddel, R. R., Pickett, H. A. (2017). Comparative analysis of whole genome sequencing-based telomere length measurement techniques, *Methods*, **114**, pp. 4–15.

28. Wang, C., Gu, Y., Zhou, J., Zang, J., Ling, X., Li, H., *et al.* (2022). Leukocyte telomere length in children born following blastocyst-stage embryo transfer, *Nat. Med.*, **28**, pp. 2646–2653.

29. Nersisyan, L., Arakelyan, A. (2015). Computel: computation of mean telomere length from whole-genome next-generation sequencing data, *PLoS One*, **10**, pp. 0125201.

30. Farmery, J. H. R., Smith, M. L., Diseases NB-R, Lynch, A. G. (2018). Telomerecat: a ploidy-agnostic method for estimating telomere length from whole genome sequencing data, *Sci. Rep.*, **8**, pp. 1300. doi: 10.1038/s41598-017-14403-y.

31. Feuerbach, L., Sieverling, L., Deeg, K. I., Ginsbach, P., Hutter, B., Buchhalter, I., *et al.* (2019). TelomereHunter - in silico estimation of telomere content and composition from cancer genomes, *BMC Bioinformatics*, **20**, pp. 272.

32. Deng, Z., Wang, Z., Strong, N., Plasschaert, R., Moczan, A., Chen, H. S., *et al.* (2012). A role for CTCF and cohesin in subtelomere chromatin organization, TERRA transcription, and telomere end protection, *Embo Journal*, **31**, pp. 4165–4178.

Part III

Lifestyle

Chapter 4

The Impact of the First 1000 Days of Human Life on Telomere Length

Maria Theodora Vitiadou,[a] Nicolina Anagnostatou,[b] Elena Vakonaki,[a,d] Aristidis Tsatsakis,[a,d] and Eleftheria Hatzidaki[b,c]

[a]*Laboratory of Toxicology, School of Medicine, University of Crete, Heraklion, Greece*
[b]*Department of Neonatology and Neonatal Intensive Care Unit, University Hospital of Heraklion, Heraklion, Greece*
[c]*School of Medicine, University of Crete, Heraklion, Greece*
[d]*Lifeplus S.A., Science & Technological Park of Crete, Vassilika Vouton, Heraklion, Greece*
elhatzidaki@gmail.com

4.1 Introduction

Telomeres, DNA-protein structures found at the ends of chromosomes, play a crucial role in health and longevity. It is already known that telomeres are at their maximum length at birth, and with each cell division, they shorten due to incomplete synthesis of DNA. After approximately 50–70 cell divisions, they reach a critically short length, called the Hayflick limit, which triggers cellular apoptosis [1].

Telomeres: Biomarkers of a Healthy Life and Successful Aging
Edited by Aristidis Tsatsakis

ISBN 978-981-5129-49-6 (Hardcover), 978-1-003-56809-4 (eBook)
www.jennystanford.com

Telomere length (TL) exhibits considerable variation among individuals of the same age, and this variability is also observed at birth. During critical cellular growth, differentiation, and maturation, the fetus's internal and external environments form interactions that lead to alterations in the structure and function of cells, tissues, and organs [1, 2]. These changes can have significant impacts on health and disease susceptibility throughout an individual's lifespan, either independently or in combination with subsequent developmental processes and environmental insults [3]. Consequently, it is highly likely that an individual's telomere length in later life is greatly influenced by their telomere length at birth and the subsequent attrition of telomeres during early life [4]. These ideas are known as Baker's hypothesis called the "Developmental Origin of Health and Disease" (DOHaD) theory, which states that the interaction between genes and the environment during conception, embryonic, fetal, and neonatal stages can affect the occurrence of lifestyle-related diseases [5]. Under this context, the TL at birth can also be viewed as a significant programmed biological marker that potentially shapes a portion of an individual's aging phenotype later in life.

The first 1000 days of human life, from conception to the second year of postnatal life, have been identified as an essential phase of rapid growth and development. During this time, maternal factors such as lifestyle, nutrition, stress levels, and various disorders and pregnancy complications, along with early postnatal environmental exposure, can ultimately impact the individual's health later in life by influencing the offspring's telomere length. Shorter fetal telomeres have been associated with an increased risk of cardiovascular disease, cancer, neurodegenerative disorders, and other chronic conditions. However, it is important to note that the relationship between TL and age-related diseases is complex and multifaced. While shorter telomeres often correlate with disease risk, this does not necessarily imply a direct cause-and-effect relationship. Instead, it influences an individual's susceptibility or propensity for diseases in later life by shaping responsiveness to subsequent conditions.

In this chapter, we will delve into the recent findings or current knowledge around fetal telomere programming in utero and subsequently during the first two years of an infant's life. At the same time, we will discuss the maternal influence that has been noted regarding these mechanisms, as well as the importance of telomeres in disease susceptibility over the lifespan.

4.2 Basic Principles of Telomere Programming during Fetal Development

4.2.1 Telomere Attrition during the Third Trimester of Pregnancy

The stable telomeric structure during fetal and neonatal development is likely determined during the final months of pregnancy, possibly due to changes in fetal metabolism as birth approaches [1, 6]. During this time, excessively long telomeres in embryonic stem cells are "trimmed back" to the correct length by specific proteins known as telomeric zinc-finger associated proteins (TZAPs) [7]. Following this step, telomere repair is restricted in most somatic cells, which means that the initial telomere length determines the cell's lifespan by influencing the rate at which it can divide before reaching the final telomere attrition and cell apoptosis. In addition, although all cells in an organism are derived from the zygote, differences in telomere lengths are observed over time and can be linked to a variety of factors, including DNA replication errors, exonuclease activity errors, deletion of t-loops by homologous recombination damage and damage induced by exposure to oxidative stress, stress hormones, inflammation, UV radiation, or toxic chemicals [8–11].

In order to further emphasize that fetal telomeres undergo different shaping dynamics compared to those of newborns, Holmes, and his colleagues compared the TL dynamics between fetuses at 23–26 weeks of gestation for a period of 8–12 weeks and preterm born neonates that had reached the same age while being nursed in a special care unit. Over this period, fetal leukocytes gained an average of 19 bp per week, while newborn leukocytes consistently lost an average of 231 bp per week during the same period [6]. These findings imply that the ways in which telomeres are kept at their optimal length during fetal development differ from those during post-natal life, which are mostly associated with age and potential health issues.

4.2.2 In utero Telomerase Activity

Another known mechanism that has been proven to contribute to determining TL is the rate of telomerase activity during fetal development. The telomerase enzyme is a major regulator of TL and comprises two main components: an RNA known as TERC or TER or TR and a catalytic protein domain called TERT. Typically, most adult somatic cells experience reduced or lack telomerase activity, but during fetal development, this pattern appears to be different. In 1996, Wright et al. discovered that while mature sperm and unfertilized eggs do not exhibit telomerase activity, they become rapidly activated and detectable as early as the blastocyst stage of embryonic development [12]. From 16 weeks of gestation on, telomerase activity is also observed in a diverse range of tissues. Previous research has indicated that telomerase is present in certain human tissues, such as the testis, ovary, and fetal adrenal glands [13–15]. Fetal lung, liver, and spleen cells also have active telomerase at least until the 21st gestational week [16]. On the contrary, during this period, the fetal brain shows either a weak presence or a complete absence of telomerase activity. Toward the third trimester of pregnancy, telomerase activity declines, but the limited research that has been done until today limits the ability to fully examine this decrease. After birth, telomerase activity was not found in tissues such as the liver, skin, lung, muscle, or adrenal tissue in neonates at 2 months of age [12]. The exact mechanisms through which telomerase exhibits telomere elongation and/or preservation are discussed in other parts of this book.

4.2.3 Oxidative Stress Is the Major Cause of Telomere Attrition during Fetal Development

Oxidative stress is considered to play a role in the development of various diseases. Reactive oxygen species (ROS) are molecules that contain at least one oxygen atom and can generate free radicals. Normally, ROS is involved in essential cell signaling pathways that are important for cellular function. However, an excessive amount of ROS can result in damage to cellular DNA, lipids, and proteins, leading to cellular dysfunction and potential disease development [17].

Oxidative damage primarily occurs when the body's antioxidant defenses are unable to fully neutralize reactive oxygen species (ROS) generated in the mitochondria. Telomeres are especially susceptible to oxidative damage, possibly due to the high content of guanine residues. The repair process for damage to telomeres differs from that in other parts of the genome. Oxidative lesions can disrupt shelterin proteins leading to dysfunction in telomeres [7]. At the same time, it can significantly speed up the process of telomere shortening by reducing the activity of telomerase and triggering either cellular senescence or apoptosis through the activation of the p53 pathway, which is involved in DNA damage response. Additionally, oxidative stress can cause the relocation of TERT from the nucleus to the cytoplasm and mitochondria resulting in a decrease in telomerase activity [1].

Some researchers suggest that the heightened cell-cycle arrest and cell death observed after continuous exposure to oxidative stress may be primarily caused by oxidative damage to the entire genome rather than being solely triggered by telomere shortening. However, it is important to note that under natural circumstances, the extent of unrepaired oxidative damage in the telomeres is likely related to the overall level of damage experienced throughout the entire genome [7].

4.3 In utero Life: Maternal Pregnancy Lifestyle and Its Influence on Fetal Telomeres

The field of fetal telomere biology has gained significant attention, due to its potential implications for long-term health outcomes in offspring. While the mechanisms regarding telomere dynamics during fetal development are complex and not fully understood yet, emerging evidence suggests that maternal determinants play a crucial role in shaping fetal telomeres. Maternal factors, including lifestyle, stress levels, nutrition habits, and certain obstetric complications, have been implicated in influencing the telomere length and function of the developing fetus. In this section, we explore the current knowledge on maternal determinants highlighting the potential implications for the fetus's health and telomere programming.

4.3.1 Active Lifestyle and Exercise during Pregnancy

Maintaining adequate levels of physical activity is essential for a healthy pregnancy. However, during pregnancy, physical activity often decreases due to various factors, including the physical and psychological changes experienced by the mother. Nowadays, there is a common and mistaken belief that resting is the safest approach for a healthy pregnancy without complications.

In 2017 and 2018, the American College of Obstetricians and Gynecologists (ACOG) and the U.S. Department of Health and Human Services, respectively, suggested that pregnant women should engage in regular physical activity, aiming for at least 150 minutes of moderate-intensity aerobic exercise per week. The recommended physical activity during pregnancy should be distributed across the week, and certain adjustments to exercise routines might be required due to normal anatomical and physiological changes in the mother's body [18]. Types of activity that are considered safe and beneficial for both the mother and the fetus are walking, stationary cycling, open-air and water aerobics, dancing, stretching, and resistance exercises using light weights or elastic bands [19].

4.3.1.1 Benefits of physical activity during pregnancy

Maternal exercise during pregnancy does not appear to have a direct impact on fetal telomere length. The only association that has been documented is that since exercise has been found to have antioxidant effects, it can positively influence telomere length by affecting the oxidation-inflammation pathway. However, it seems to indirectly benefit the mother's and fetus's health both during fetal development and postnatal life, especially when combined with a proper diet [20].

Engaging in low-intensity exercise during early pregnancy has been found to enhance umbilical blood flow, leading to improved placental circulation and better fetal cardiac adaptation to the surrounding environment [21]. It also appears to lower the risk of gestational diabetes by reducing maternal blood glucose levels without increasing the risk of hypoglycemia [22]. Additionally, it has been associated with a decreased risk of cesarean section [21] and a trend toward preventing pre-eclampsia [23]. Furthermore, maternal exercise seems to be linked to a lower likelihood of preterm birth [24]. It is important to note that while many studies demonstrate positive trends in preventing these negative pregnancy outcomes through physical activity, most of the time, the results are not statistically significant. Further research needs to be done incorporating better control of parallel maternal nutrition, the avoidance of unsupervised exercise, and a more diverse study group that does not include only healthy women [21].

4.3.2 Maternal Nutrition

A rich-in-nutrient maternal diet before and during pregnancy is associated with optimal fetal birth weight and improved fetal and postnatal health [25]. Over the years, many studies have been conducted in an attempt to check whether certain foods and macro- and/or micronutrients play a crucial role in the fetus's health and development including potential effects on telomere length.

4.3.2.1 The importance of proper maternal nutrition before and during pregnancy

A balanced diet before conception ensures that the preimplantation and early differentiation environments are prepared to support the initial development of the fetus and placenta [25]. After conception, it appears that the fertilized ovum and early blastocyst can detect and respond to the nutritional quality of the fallopian tube environment even before implantation occurs [25]. Throughout the first 10 weeks of pregnancy, the developing fetus seems to nourish solely from the fluid produced by the endometrial glands. Studies conducted on mice and other animals have shown that there is no access to the maternal bloodstream for the embryo until 10 weeks of gestation, and the fluid present in the fallopian tubes is similar to that found in the endometrial glands [26]. This finding is of great significance considering that all organ differentiation takes place within the first 11 weeks of gestation.

In 2004, Gluckman and Hanson formed a hypothesis according to which the fetus can "predict" the postnatal environment and adapt its development accordingly. Studies conducted on living organisms have shown that a shortage of specific micronutrients like folic acid and vitamin B12 can modify gene expression and elevate the probability of chronic ailments, emphasizing the significance of appropriate maternal nutrition during pregnancy [5]. A dietary pattern that includes protein-rich foods and whole grains is linked to a lower likelihood of preterm delivery. Adhering to a Mediterranean dietary pattern is associated with a reduced risk of maternal gestational diabetes and atopy in offspring. Conversely, unhealthy dietary patterns characterized by high consumption of refined grains, processed meat, and foods rich in saturated fat and sugar are connected to lower newborn birth weight and an increased risk of preterm birth [27]. It is important to emphasize that the overall dietary pattern and nutrient balance have a more significant impact on fetal telomeres than individual foods. Hence, it is generally recommended to follow a diverse and nutritious diet before and during pregnancy in order to promote normal fetal development [28].

4.3.2.2 Essential nutrients that affect fetal telomeres during pregnancy

Various micro- and macro-nutrients play crucial roles in DNA synthesis maintaining DNA stability and preserving fetal telomere integrity [27]. In a prospective cohort study involving 62 women, increased maternal fat consumption was linked to shorter telomere length as measured in umbilical cord blood in comparison to carbohydrate consumption, which didn't show any statistically significant association with fetal telomere length [29]. Daily maternal energy intake also appears to be positively correlated with fetal telomeres, although there was no association between protein, carbohydrate, or fat intake — regarding their percentage of total energy intake — and fetal telomere length [27]. Animal studies have shown that temporary caloric restriction can increase the number of mitochondria and enhance the function of the respiratory chain, leading to reduced ROS production, thus preventing telomere shortening. However, the specific associations between the proportions of dietary carbohydrates and fats with telomere length have not been thoroughly investigated [30].

On the contrary, the effects of certain micronutrients on telomeres have been studied in greater depth. These studies have provided more detailed insights into how micronutrients may influence telomere biology.

4.3.2.3 Folate

Folate is a B vitamin that is soluble in water. It occurs naturally in certain foods, can be found added to various food products, and can also be obtained through dietary supplements [31]. Folate plays a vital role in maintaining DNA integrity and DNA methylation, both of which have an impact on telomere length. Its significance has generally been established in relation to DNA synthesis, cell proliferation, and the development of the neural tube [32]. According to a 2015 study by Entringer et al., higher maternal folate concentrations during early pregnancy show a positive association with newborns' telomere length as measured from cord blood. The fetus seems to rely entirely on the maternal supply of folate, which occurs through a unidirectional process of folate transport from the mother to the fetus. Additionally, maternal folate intake during pregnancy has been linked to the methylation status and phenotypic outcomes of the offspring [32].

4.3.2.4 Folic acid

While folate refers to all naturally occurring forms of vitamin B9, folic acid is a specific synthetic vitamin B9 form that is often used as a supplement in pregnancy due to its better stability and absorbance [33, 34]. Folic acid plays a critical role in the synthesis of purines and thymine, which are essential components of DNA. More specifically, it is involved in the conversion of deoxyuridine monophosphate (dUMP) to deoxythymidine monophosphate (dTMP) through a process known as reductive methylation. When folic acid is deficient, the dUMP/dTMP ratio can become imbalanced resulting in an abnormal increase in dUMP levels. This imbalance can lead to the incorporation of excessive uracil instead of thymine during DNA replication resulting in DNA strand breakage. Studies have shown that such DNA damage can eventually lead to shorter telomeres and quicker cell apoptosis in offspring [35].

4.3.2.5 Vitamin D

Vitamin D, also known as calciferol, is a type of fat-soluble vitamin. It naturally occurs in a limited number of foods like fatty fish, egg yolks, and orange juice, and, as folate, it can also be obtained as a supplement [36, 37]. The body can produce vitamin D internally when the skin is exposed to UV rays from sunlight stimulating its synthesis. It is important to note that the fetus is unable to produce vitamin D, so it relies on the transfer of maternal vitamin D or its biologically active forms, such as 25-hydroxyvitamin D [25(OH)D] and 1,25-dihydroxyvitamin D [1,25(OH)D] through the placenta [37, 38].

Maintaining sufficient levels of vitamin D during pregnancy is crucial for the healthy development of the fetal skeleton, the formation of tooth enamel, and overall fetal growth and development [39]. Lower levels of cholecalciferol in cord blood are associated with increased inflammation, and cord blood vitamin D levels are influenced by maternal vitamin D status. Considering the mechanisms involving vitamin D and its role in reducing oxidative stress and inflammation, it seems that lower maternal vitamin D concentrations contribute to shorter telomeres in offspring [27, 40].

4.3.2.6 Caffeine intake

Caffeine is a stimulant found in various foods and beverages including tea, coffee, soft drinks, and chocolate, as well as over-the-counter medications [40]. The effects of caffeine on telomeres are thought to be mediated by the phosphoinositide 3-kinase-related protein kinases Tel1 and MEc1, which are known to regulate telomere length [40]. Interestingly, higher caffeine intake may have a protective effect on telomere length. In a study involving 57 multiracial mother–newborn pairs, it was found that higher caffeine intake, categorized as consuming more than 200mg, was associated with longer telomere length in cord blood [27].

However, it is important to note that the current recommendations from the World Health Organization (WHO) advise pregnant women to limit their total caffeine consumption to less than 300 mg per day. This limitation, though, derives from the fact that caffeine is probably associated with general pregnancy complications like pregnancy loss and low-birth-weight neonates, which are not directly related to fetal telomeres [41].

4.3.3 Maternal Obesity

Body mass index (BMI) is a widely used measurement for determining obesity. A BMI value above 25 kg/m^2 is typically regarded as an indicator of being overweight, while a BMI exceeding 30 kg/m^2 is indicative of obesity [42]. Prenatal care guidelines address the significance of ensuring appropriate maternal weight gain throughout gestation. For overweight women (BMI 25–29,9), their gestational weight gain should be in the range of 7–11 kg. Meanwhile, obese women (BMI >30) are advised to gain between 5 and 9 kg [43].

Maternal overweight and obesity are widely recognized as factors that increase the chances of complications during pregnancy [44]. Maternal body mass index (BMI) is linked to elevated levels of blood glucose in pregnant women as well as a greater likelihood of experiencing pregnancy complications including pre-eclampsia, gestational diabetes, hypertensive disorders, and cesarean delivery [45]. Excessive weight gain during pregnancy has been linked to adverse neonatal outcomes such as perinatal asphyxia, birth injuries, hypoglycemia, and delivering large-for-gestational-age infants [43].

4.3.3.1 Obesity effects on fetal telomeres

Apart from the consequences that maternal BMI has on pregnancy as a process, it has also been found to influence the fetus by affecting the length of its telomeres. Studies have suggested that higher maternal BMI, particularly in the overweight or obese range, may be associated with alterations in fetal telomere length. Paternal BMI showed no significant correlation with fetal TL [46]. Additionally, the exact mechanisms through which maternal low weight gain during pregnancy influences fetal TL are not fully comprehended yet. However, it is reasonable to consider that these effects may be attributed to increased and persistent inflammatory, and oxidative conditions during fetal development [46]. Pre-pregnancy BMI in an obese category is also associated with shorter placental and cord blood telomeres [45]. Additionally, childhood obesity, childhood asthma, and cardiovascular diseases have been linked to maternal obesity aligned with the Developmental Origin of Disease hypothesis [45].

4.3.4 Prenatal Smoking

Maternal smoking has been linked to various negative outcomes, including preterm birth, placental abruption, low birth weight, fetal growth restriction, and sudden infant death syndrome (SIDS). Despite the well-documented adverse effects of maternal smoking during pregnancy on offspring, it is concerning that, according to a survey in 2016, approximately one in 14 mothers in the USA reported smoking during pregnancy [47], while many more are still exposed as passive smokers in public places [48].

4.3.4.1 Effects of maternal smoking on fetal telomeres

Smoking during pregnancy is responsible for the transfer of harmful chemicals, such as nicotine and other toxins, into the maternal bloodstream, which can cross the placenta and reach the developing fetus. Various mechanisms have been suggested to connect tobacco exposure and the shortening of fetal TL, including oxidative stress and inflammation [49]. The reactive oxygen substances (ROS) tend to damage the rich in guanine telomeric DNA, among other parts of the genome, even before birth. Following Baker's hypothesis, prenatal exposure to substances and toxins found in tobacco can be linked to diseases associated with early telomere attrition later in life.

Fetal telomere shortening due to maternal smoking can be associated with abnormal lung development during both prenatal and postnatal stages, as well as lung disorders like idiopathic pulmonary fibrosis (IPF), COPD, emphysema, asthma, and lung cancer in adulthood [50]. Additionally, maternal tobacco smoking during pregnancy has also been associated with an increased risk of attention-deficit/hyperactivity disorder (ADHD) in children [47].

4.3.5 Maternal Stress

Maternal stress has been studied in relation to various aspects of fetal development and can affect long-term health issues negatively [51, 52]. It can exert several physiological effects on the body, including oxidative stress, inflammatory responses, as well as alterations in stress hormone levels that can affect the fetus during intrauterine life.

4.3.5.1 Regulation of the hypothalamic-pituitary-adrenal axis

The hypothalamic-pituitary-adrenal axis (HPA) is a neuroendocrine system that plays a crucial role in the body's response to stress [52]. When the brain detects stress, it activates the hypothalamus triggering the release of corticotropin-releasing hormone (CRH). CRH then stimulates the pituitary gland to secrete adrenocorticotropic hormone (ACTH) which enters the bloodstream and reaches the adrenal glands. The adrenal glands respond by producing and releasing cortisol, the primary stress hormone. Normally, cortisol helps the body adapt to stress by mobilizing energy and suppressing non-essential functions. Under normal conditions, once cortisol levels reach a certain point, a feedback mechanism reduces CRH and ACTH release maintaining cortisol balance. However, chronic stress can disrupt this axis leading to sustained high cortisol levels which can adversely affect various physiological systems (Fig. 4.1) [52].

Dysregulation of the HPA axis and elevated cortisol levels are thought to contribute to oxidative stress and inflammation, potentially resulting in telomere shortening. Studies have suggested

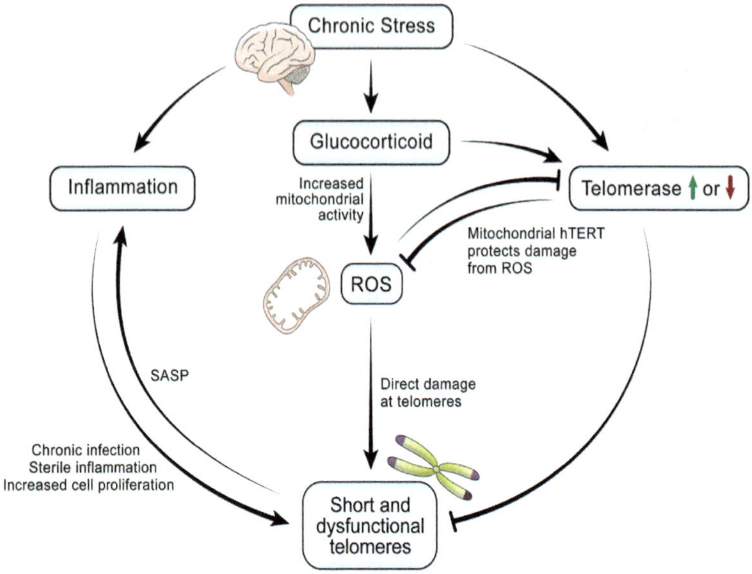

Figure 4.1 Republished from Lin & Epel., 2022, showing the main molecular and cellular pathways (oxidative stress, hormonal pathways, and inflammatory mediators) that connect stress with shorter telomeres [53].

a potential association between maternal stress and shorter fetal telomeres with cortisol playing a potential role. When a pregnant woman experiences stress, cortisol levels rise, and part of it can cross the placenta affecting the fetus [53]. The precise impact of cortisol on fetal telomere shortening is still not fully understood, although recent findings suggest that immune cells from individuals who display greater cortisol responses to stress may have a reduced capacity to induce telomerase activity [1].

4.3.5.2 Association of maternal stress with fetal telomere length

Maternal psychological stress, such as anxiety, depression, or perceived stress levels, has been linked to shorter telomeres in offspring. Prenatal stressors, including major life events or socio-environmental stress, have also been associated with fetal telomere length. The timing and duration of maternal stress during pregnancy may also be important, with long-term or chronic stress having potential effects on telomere length shortening [54].

Studies have found associations between maternal stress during pregnancy and shorter telomere length in newborns as measured in umbilical cord blood. Entringer et al. (2013) examined 27 mother–newborn pairs and discovered that pregnancy-related stress, assessed early in gestation, was linked to shorter TL in newborn cord blood [55]. Similarly, two other studies reported associations between higher maternal perceived stress and shorter TL in newborns. Another study involving 24 mother–newborn pairs revealed that newborns of mothers with higher reported levels of psychological stress had significantly shorter TL compared to newborns of mothers with lower stress levels [56]. Overall, throughout the course of our lives, we encounter different stressors that elicit physiological stress responses through established mechanisms. Yet, the precise mechanisms by which stress impacts our cells, accelerates cellular aging, and increases susceptibility to diseases are not fully understood [57].

4.4 Maternal Pregnancy Conditions and Complications: Their Role in Fetal Telomere Length Regulation

The development of the placenta, which is the distinctive organ responsible for exchanging nutrients and gases between the mother and fetus, is critical for ensuring a healthy pregnancy and fetal development. Initially formed from extraembryonic tissues, the placenta rapidly grows during the first weeks of pregnancy as trophoblasts undergo extensive proliferation and invasion [58, 59]. Throughout the course of pregnancy, the placenta performs various essential functions, including physiological adjustments to accommodate the mother's environment, immune tolerance, and provision of nourishment and support to the growing fetus [60]. As pregnancy continues, the placental cells start to age, and their lifespan is closely regulated to determine the duration of the pregnancy. Toward the end of gestation, intrinsic and extrinsic factors such as oxidative stress and DNA damage trigger the placental cells to enter a senescent apoptotic state [61].

Recent studies have indicated that various intrauterine factors that are associated with maternal health and potential pregnancy complications can be transferred to the fetus influencing its health condition and the telomere length in various cell types. These findings highlight the significance of prenatal and early life exposures in determining telomere length at birth, which can subsequently impact aging, disease susceptibility, and molecular longevity later in life [45].

4.4.1 Intrauterine Fetal Hypoxia

One of the most vital gases being transported via the placenta to the fetus is oxygen, which is essential for the growth and maturation of all organ systems. The fetal environment supports typical growth and development as it provides more oxygen than the developing fetus requires for oxidative processes [62]. If the oxygen supply to the fetus is reduced such as in cases of placental ischemia, the fetus initiates adaptive responses that can impact fetal metabolism and oxygen transport [63]. This condition, called intrauterine hypoxia, affects the mother, placenta, and fetus, and the nature and magnitude of these responses depend on the severity and duration of the oxygen deprivation. Kingdom and Kaufmann proposed a classification of hypoxic pregnancy conditions into three subtypes [62]:

1. Preplacental hypoxia, which involves both the mother and her fetus experiencing hypoxia (i.e., maternal cardiovascular diseases).
2. Uteroplacental hypoxia, in which the mother's oxygenation is normal, but there's impaired blood circulation in the uteroplacental region (i.e., pre-eclampsia).
3. Postplacental hypoxia, in which only the fetus faces hypoxic conditions.

Intrauterine hypoxia triggers the production of hypoxia-inducible factors, which respond to various changes in pregnancy, including low oxygen levels and the renin-angiotensin system,

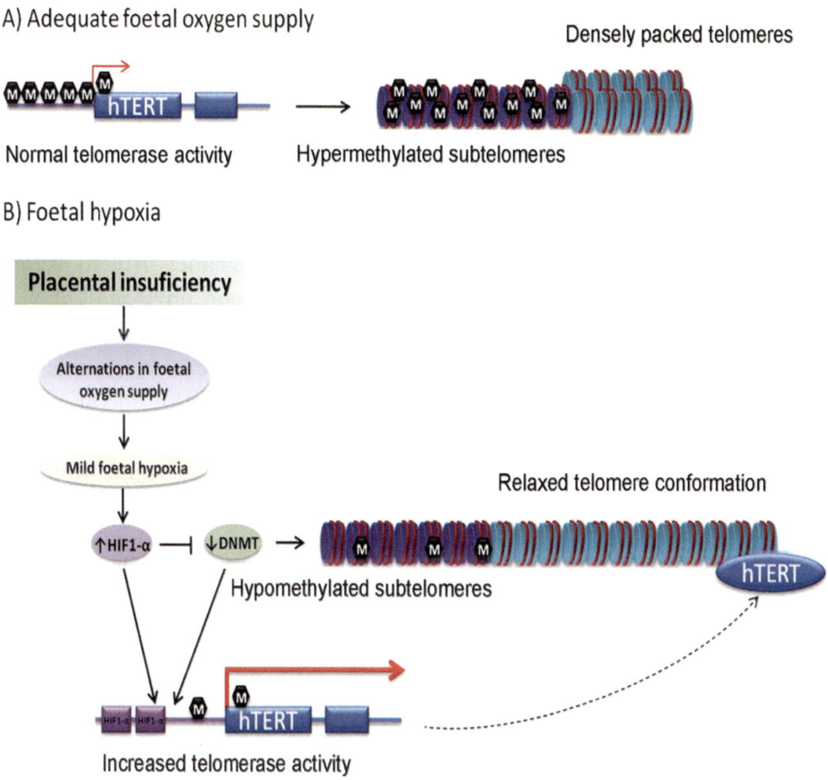

Figure 4.2 Republished from Ravlić et al., 2018, showing the conformation of fetal telomeres, in both normal and insufficient oxygen supply conditions [67].

cytokines, and growth factors, all of which regulate placental function. Telomere length varies with different levels of hypoxia, and mild hypoxia has been shown to increase telomerase activity and elongate telomeres [64, 65]. Figure 4.2 illustrates a possible molecular pathway that underlines the telomeric changes observed in a low-oxygen environment. During pregnancy and under hypoxic conditions, the downregulation of DNMT1 (as described in paragraph 4.4.1.1) results in looser telomeres, that seem longer even if they have the same bp. This modification though, makes telomeres more prone to increased shortage later in life so during adulthood they tend to have shorter telomere length.

4.4.1.1 Mechanisms of telomere length regulation in a hypoxic environment

Hypoxia-inducible factor-1 (HIF-1) is a protein transcription factor composed of two subunits (HIF-1a and HIF-1b) that have a crucial function in the organism's reaction to reduced levels of oxygen. HIF-1α is sensitive to oxygen levels and quickly degrades and remains inactive under normal oxygen conditions, while HIF-1β is constantly active [64]. In the early stages of pregnancy, HIF-1α is extensively expressed in the placenta's low-oxygen environment, where it plays a critical function in the development and function of the placenta. Later in pregnancy and in the case of a hypoxic environment, the expression of the HIF-1α transcription factor is elevated, which in turn enhances telomerase expression by binding to the hTERT promoter and, thus, boosting its activity. The duration of hypoxia exposure has been found to correlate with changes in the levels of HIF-1α, telomerase, and telomere length. Simultaneously, HIF-1α reduces the expression of DNA methyltransferases (DNMT1), especially DNMT1, which is involved in maintaining DNA methylation patterns. This DNMT1 downregulation leads to decreased methylation of subtelomeric DNA and the regulatory region of hTERT. These changes can result in elongated telomeres but also decreased stability, increasing the likelihood of accelerated shortening during adulthood [66].

4.4.2 Intrauterine Growth Restriction (IUGR)

Intrauterine growth restriction (IUGR) is characterized by the fetus exhibiting a rate of growth that is lower than expected based on the growth potential specific to the infant's race and gender [67]. IUGR primarily derives from inadequate placental function but can also stem from various factors such as infections, chromosomal or genetic anomalies, congenital malformations, or maternal smoking. The pathophysiology of this condition is not fully known but typically emerges from trophoblast invasion deficiencies, leading to irregular blood flow within the intervillous space [68].

Research has indicated that IUGR may contribute to shorter telomeres in affected fetuses. The underlying mechanisms behind this association are not fully understood, but it is believed that IUGR-related factors such as reduced nutrient supply, placental insufficiency, and increased oxidative stress may play a role in telomere shortening [61, 68].

4.4.3 Gestational Diabetes Mellitus and Its Impact on Fetal Telomeres

Gestational diabetes mellitus (GDM) is a prevalent medical complication that frequently occurs during pregnancy and is characterized by high blood sugar levels due to insulin resistance [69]. In a normal pregnancy, insulin resistance (IR) gradually develops starting in mid-pregnancy and progressing further in the third trimester. Hormones and adipokines released by the placenta, such as TNF-α, human placental lactogen, and human placental growth hormone, are potential factors contributing to IR during pregnancy. Additionally, elevated levels of estrogen, progesterone, and cortisol disrupt the balance between glucose and insulin. To counterbalance the IR experienced during pregnancy, the pancreas increases insulin secretion. GDM can occur when the pancreas fails to secrete sufficient insulin to cope with the metabolic demands of insulin resistance [70]. Factors such as maternal obesity, reduced physical exercise, and rising caloric intake contribute to this state of impaired glucose tolerance during pregnancy [71–73].

4.4.3.1 GDM and fetal telomere shortening

GDM can lead to the production of excessive free radicals and impaired mechanisms to eliminate them indicating the involvement of oxidative stress in its pathophysiology [61]. Several studies have observed fetal telomere shortening from pregnancies complicated by GDM [74, 75]. Biron-Shental et al. conducted a study in 2015, where they compared placental biopsies obtained from 16 pregnant women in the third trimester diagnosed with poorly controlled gestational diabetes with placental biopsies from 16 healthy pregnancies serving as the control group. Trophoblasts derived from diabetic mothers exhibited a significantly higher occurrence of shortened telomeres in comparison to the control group. The researchers concluded that uncontrolled hyperglycemia leads to telomere attrition triggering trophoblast senescence and potentially increasing fetal morbidity [61, 75]. Studies also demonstrate a higher proportion of cells with short telomeres, with oxidative stress due to GDM triggering the upregulation and translocation of hTERT from the nuclei to mitochondria [76]. Since TERT is a catalytic subunit of telomerase responsible for TL maintenance, its absence from the nucleus further enhances the connection between TL shortening and hyperglycemia.

4.4.3.2 Contradictory evidence regarding GDM and fetal telomere length

It is worth noticing that, even though the majority of studies show a negative correlation between GDM and fetal TL, conflicting results have also been reported. Some studies found similar [77, 78] or longer telomeres in these newborns compared to those from mothers without GDM [79]. This discrepancy may be attributed to variations in oxidative stress levels among fetuses born to mothers with GDM and pre-eclampsia. While oxidative stress was consistently enhanced in fetuses of diabetic women, the findings regarding oxidative stress in pre-eclamptic pregnancies have been inconsistent with reports of increased, unchanged, or even decreased oxidative status. Nevertheless, these differences in oxidative stress status between pre-eclampsia and GDM could be one of the factors contributing to the varying telomere lengths observed [80]. Additionally, variations in study populations, glycemic control, and telomere length measurement methods may also contribute to the different findings [61].

4.4.4 Infection during Pregnancy and Inflammatory Activation

Regarding how the telomere system is influenced during a maternal infection, activation of the maternal and/or fetal immune response, characterized by increased expression of pro-inflammatory cytokines due to various adverse conditions during pregnancy, might potentially affect fetal telomere length [81].

4.4.4.1 Viral and bacterial infections

Viral or bacterial infections are frequently observed in pregnant women, and studies indicate that such infections can affect fetal telomeres [82]. Human herpesvirus 6 (HHV-6) can integrate itself into specific sites in the human genome through homologous recombination between telomeric regions of human chromosomes and HHV-6 sequences. HHV-6 infections occur in approximately 1% of neonates and can be transmitted through two main modalities. In about 86% of cases, the virus becomes integrated into either maternal or paternal chromosomes and can, thus, be transmitted to the fetus. In the rest of the cases, transmission through the transplacental route has been observed [83]. Chromosomally integrated HHV-6 has been associated with cellular malfunctions, including telomere abnormalities and impaired chromosome stability affecting both the mother and the fetus.

Additionally, bacterial infections are believed to have a negative impact on telomere length through the activation of mechanisms such as oxidative stress and inflammatory responses. Tung et al. have demonstrated that group B streptococcus infection was linked to shorter telomere length in cord blood [82].

4.4.4.2 The role of TNF-a and NF-κB inflammatory factors in telomere shortening

In adults, having high levels of pro-inflammatory substances like tumor necrosis factor α (TNF-α) and interleukin 6 (IL-6) has been associated with shorter telomere length in white blood cells [84]. A recent study found that increased expression of pro-inflammatory genes in laboratory samples was also linked to shorter telomere length in immune cells called peripheral blood mononuclear cells. Inflammation can accelerate the shortening of telomeres by increasing oxidative stress and activating certain transcription factors like nuclear factor-kappa B (NF-κB). When TNF-α is administered in vitro to human lymphocytes, it triggers the movement of TERT into the cell nucleus and enhances telomerase activity. This effect is mediated through the signaling pathway of NF-κB. Conversely, TERT can regulate the expression of specific genes that are dependent on NF-κB. The interaction between TERT and the p65 subunit of NF-κB, as well as the recruitment of TERT to certain gene promoters controlled by NF-κB, like IL-6 and TNF-α, suggests that telomerase can establish a positive feedback loop within the immune system by promoting the expression of NF-κB-dependent genes [1].

4.4.4.3 Telomere alterations in inflammatory responses

While several studies have examined the relationship between inflammation and telomere length in adults, there is limited research exploring the potential connection between maternal prenatal inflammation and TL in newborns. Early research has provided initial support for the significant influence of maternal inflammation on the programming of TL in offspring [81]. In a 2015 study, pregnant mice were administered TNF-α via intraperitoneal injection resulting in telomere shortening in various cells, including blood cells, in their offspring [85]. Recently, another study in mice replicated these findings and further substantiated the role of TNF-α in inducing the expression of activation transcription factor 7 (ATF7), which contributes to telomere shortening [81].

4.4.5 Gestational Hypertension and Further High Blood Pressure Complications

Gestational Hypertension, also known as Pregnancy-Induced Hypertension (PIH), is a condition characterized by high blood pressure during pregnancy. The measurements for both chronic and gestational hypertension typically refer to systolic blood pressure greater than 140 mmHg and/or diastolic blood pressure greater than 90 mmHg [86]. The exact pathophysiology of hypertension during pregnancy is not fully understood, but it has been associated with significant increases in total peripheral resistance, heightened responsiveness to angiotensin II, and notable reductions in renal blood flow and glomerular filtration rate [87]. Recent research has also highlighted the role of antiangiogenic factors released by placental tissue contributing to systemic endothelial dysfunction and resulting in systemic hypertension [88].

4.4.5.1 Gestational hypertension can lead to pre-eclampsia during pregnancy

Pre-eclampsia (PE) is a pregnancy-related syndrome that typically occurs after 20 weeks of gestation [89]. It is characterized by the presence of gestational hypertension and abnormal protein excretion in the urine with values equal to or exceeding 300 mg/day or a protein/creatinine ratio equal to or greater than 0.3 [88]. PE is a complex and diverse disorder that can be categorized as mild, severe, or superimposed depending on the severity of its symptoms. When pre-eclampsia develops before the 34th week of pregnancy, it is referred to as early-onset PE, while PE that occurs after the 34th week is known as late-onset PE [89]. In cases of pre-eclampsia, maternal high blood pressure leads to reduced blood supply to the fetus, which can result in decreased oxygen and nutrients [90]. If left untreated, PE can progress to a more severe condition called eclampsia. Eclampsia is characterized by generalized tonic–clonic seizures and poses a serious threat to the life of the mother [88].

4.4.5.2 Correlation between hypertensive disorders and fetal telomere length

Cardiovascular diseases, including hypertension, have been previously associated with shorter telomeres, and recent studies have delved into the influence that these complications have on fetal telomeres. Arterial hypertension seems to be a critical factor in the modulation of newborn telomere length. In a study conducted by Tellechea et al., it was found that newborn leukocyte telomere length was significantly and inversely associated with the arterial blood pressure of the mothers during the current pregnancy as well as with a history of arterial hypertension in previous pregnancies [91]. In addition, the length of telomeres that neonates are born with seems to be related to their renal fetal growth which affects the number of nephrons they have in each kidney and their blood pressure early in childhood which are both associated with later-life hypertension [92].

Regarding pre-eclampsia, even though women with shorter telomeres are more prone to developing this pregnancy complication [93], there have been conflicting results regarding whether pre-eclampsia truly affects fetal telomere length [94–96]. What seems to be related is the oxidative stress status that has been described as increased, decreased, or unchanged in pregnancies where pre-eclampsia occurs [80]. The difference in oxidative stress between fetuses of preeclamptic women may be one of the factors contributing to the differences in telomere length as measured from placental cells during fetal growth. Furthermore, it is currently unknown whether the telomere length in cord blood or placental tissue can provide insights into the specific telomere shortening that occurs in cardiac cells and other tissues at birth or later in life [92].

4.5 Post-utero Life: The Role of Postnatal Conditions on Infant Telomeres

In the previous section, we analyzed how intrauterine life can shape telomere dynamics and determine the telomere length that neonates will be born with. Although each person is born with varying lengths due to a combination of internal and external factors, it is widely recognized that TL is at its peak during birth. The subsequent rate of telomere shortening is heavily influenced by a combination of genetic predisposition, environmental conditions, and early-life experiences.

During the first years of a child's life, rapid cellular turnover and physiological changes lead to significant telomere shortening [97]. Research suggests that the rate of telomere attrition is not consistent, with the most rapid shortening occurring in the first years of life, followed by a more gradual reduction over time [98]. A study conducted by Zeichner et al. (1999) showed an average telomere length reduction rate of 270 base pairs per year from birth to 36 months, which was considerably higher than the rate of 50 base pairs per year telomere loss in adult blood cells [99]. Additionally, Frenck et al. (1998) revealed three identifiable phases of telomere loss. An initial stage marked by a rapid decrease in average TL spanning from birth to the age of 4, followed by a phase of stability in TL from the age of 4 until adulthood (indicating little change in average TL), and a third phase, associated with advancing

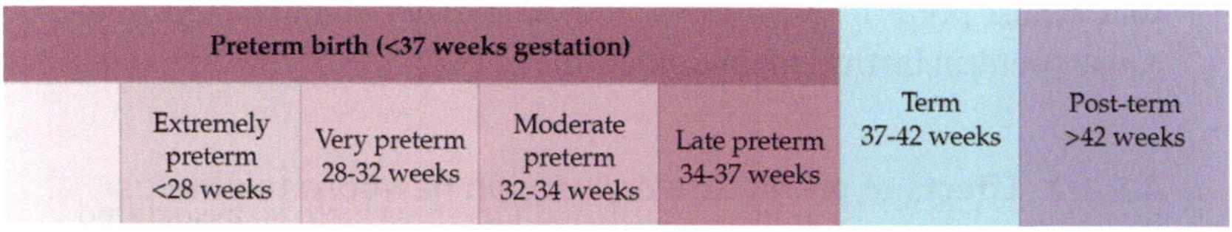

Figure 4.3 The classification of preterm birth in relation to total weeks of gestation.

age, that showed a gradual decline in mean TL [97]. These findings suggest that telomeres experience a distinct pattern of changes throughout their lifespan, with a rapid decline taking place during the first 2–3 years of life. In the upcoming sections, we will explore the primary determinants that impact infant telomeres and their attrition rate during the first years following birth.

4.5.1 Impact of Premature Birth on Neonatal Telomeres

The typical duration of a human pregnancy is usually between 37 and 42 gestational weeks during which the developing fetus undergoes cell differentiation and organ formation, which are necessary for survival outside the womb. When the gestation period is disrupted and childbirth occurs before 37 weeks (or 259 days from the last day of menstruation), childbirth is characterized as premature (Fig. 4.3) [100].

4.5.1.1 Causes and characteristics of preterm delivery

Preterm birth is a multifactorial phenomenon, and its potential causes might arise from the mother, the fetus, or the environment in which it develops (the placenta, the uterus, and the amniotic fluid). Multiple pregnancies, diabetes mellitus, thyroiditis, obesity, alcohol use during pregnancy, and smoking are the main maternal factors that appear to affect premature pregnancy [101–109]. It is more prevalent among male infants, with approximately 55% of preterm births occurring in boys [110], and mortality rates are also higher among premature boys compared to premature girls [111]. Infants with congenital abnormalities have an increased likelihood of being born prematurely, although they are often excluded from studies that report preterm birth rates, and, as a result, many factors that cause preterm birth remain unidentified [112].

4.5.1.2 Effects of premature delivery on newborn telomeres

Studies have indicated that after birth and until the age of two, preterm infants displayed greater TL compared to full-term infants, although there was no noticeable distinction in the rate of telomere attrition between these two groups [113]. Colatto et al. conducted a study in which they examined TL using fetal membrane samples obtained from pregnant women undergoing various conditions: term in labor, term not in labor, preterm premature rupture of membranes, and spontaneous preterm labor with intact membranes [114]. They showed that fetal membranes from the term labor group exhibited a reduction in telomere length in comparison to those from the other groups. Other studies have indicated conflicting results as low birth weight neonates (1500–2500 grams) had shorter telomeres in comparison to term ones [115].

It should be noted that premature birth (as well as low birth weight newborns) may have an impact on telomere length due to the immaturity of various biological systems that are influenced by both the intrauterine and extrauterine environment. One notable difference, in comparison to full-term infants, is the difference in oxygen levels between the environment inside and outside the womb. During the final weeks of pregnancy, the fetus gradually increases its antioxidant enzyme levels in an attempt to prepare for the transition to the relatively oxygen-rich external environment. However, in the case of preterm delivery, especially before 32 weeks, this preparation can remain incomplete, rendering the fetus susceptible to oxidative stress that can imbalance the normal rates of telomere shortening [116].

4.5.2 Postnatal Newborn Nutrition

There has been a recent emphasis in the scientific community on the significance of proper nutrition throughout the initial 1000 days of life, encompassing early pregnancy and breastfeeding. Indeed, insufficient nourishment among expectant mothers, particularly a lack of crucial nutrients, seems to be connected to adverse health effects for both the mother and the child [117].

4.5.2.1 Benefits of breastfeeding

Breast milk serves as the exclusive and highly beneficial source of nourishment for infants during the initial 4–6 months of life [118]. It primarily consists of water (87%) along with macronutrients (fatty acids, carbohydrates, proteins), micronutrients (vitamins), and bioactive substances (immune factors, hormones, etc.) [119]. The composition of these elements varies depending on the breastfeeding stage and environment. Breast milk provides essential nutrients crucial for the proper growth and development of infants. It contains fatty acids such as lauric acid and palmitic acid as well as enzymes like lipase and cholesterol that aid in digestion and brain development [120]. Proteins found in breast milk include casein, alpha-lactalbumin, lactoferrin, secretory IgA, and lysozyme which gradually decrease in concentration in the first few weeks of life [121–123]. The presence of sugars, particularly lactose, contributes to milk production and helps regulate the intestinal flora [124]. Moreover, breast milk intake offers protection against various diseases and infections thanks to its immune-boosting and antioxidant properties [125].

It is worth mentioning that breast milk has more benefits than any other milk formula due to a combination of factors. Breastfed infants have also been shown to have a lower risk of childhood obesity and metabolic syndrome in comparison to formula-fed ones. Infant formula contains more protein per serving compared to breast milk, which can potentially trigger unhealthy insulin secretion and contribute to the higher obesity rates that have been noticed [126]. Additionally, the biological response to breast milk differs from that of formula. Breast milk prompts the release of a protein from the baby's liver, which aids in regulating metabolism. In contrast, formula feeding leads to increased insulin concentrations in the baby's bloodstream, prolonging the insulin response [127].

Breastfeeding can have a significant impact on newborn telomeres by providing essential nutrients that support cellular replication and DNA repair ultimately influencing TL. Research by

Wojcicki et al. (2016) revealed that exclusively breastfed children had longer telomeres, approximately 5% longer or between 350 and 450 DNA base pairs, compared to children who were not exclusively breastfed [128]. In contrast, poor nutrition for children, lack of breastfeeding, and/or nutrient deficiencies within the first years of life can contribute to increased oxidative stress and inflammation leading to accelerated telomere shortening via mechanisms that have already been discussed in this chapter [129]. Breast milk, being the optimal source of infant nutrition, contains bioactive components such as growth factors and hormones that influence cellular processes including telomere maintenance. Some of these factors, like insulin-like growth factor 1 (IGF-1) have been associated with longer telomeres in newborns potentially promoting cellular longevity and healthy aging [130]. Human milk also possesses antioxidant properties due to the presence of vitamins C and E as well as enzymes like catalase and glutathione peroxidase [131]. These antioxidants protect against the harmful effects of oxidative stress, which can lead to accelerated telomere shortening.

4.5.2.2 Introduction to solid food

According to the World Health Organization (WHO) and UNICEF, it is recommended to exclusively breastfeed infants for the first six months of their lives. After six months, it is advised to introduce nutritionally suitable and safe solid foods along with continued breastfeeding until the age of two or beyond [132]. This way, it is ensured that babies will receive sufficient nutrition as they transition from breast milk to a regular family diet. Early introduction to solid foods seems to heighten the chances of developing diarrheal diseases and food allergies [133]. One possible reason is that the immune system's response to these foods is specific to each type. For instance, research has shown that introducing foods like wheat, rye, oats, fish, peanuts, and eggs early on can reduce the likelihood of developing allergic sensitivities during childhood [134]. Additionally, a high intake of calories and the frequent consumption of carbohydrates and proteins, while low in fiber during the critical stages of childhood care are also linked to higher chances of developing childhood obesity [127, 134].

The impact of specific foods on newborns is an area of ongoing research, and the direct effects of individual foods on their telomeres and their influence on overall health have not been definitively established, although they seem to correlate with the influence that proper nutrition has later in life. Adequate intake of food like leafy green vegetables, citrus fruits, legumes, and fortified grains has been linked with decreased mortality rates and telomere preservation [135]. Omega-3 fatty acids, found in fatty fish such as salmon and sardines, have also been linked with a positive effect on fetal telomere length [136]. Phenolic compounds found in plant-based foods offer potential advantages to human health due to their ability to interact with and regulate various cellular signaling pathways and molecules, contributing to their beneficial effects from in utero development to adulthood [137] Additionally, foods rich in antioxidants like berries, nuts, and colorful fruits and vegetables contain compounds that can reduce oxidative stress and protect the body from the negative impact of free radicals, thus, supporting telomere length [138].

4.5.3 Postnatal Exposure to Toxins

Research has provided increasing evidence that exposure to common environmental toxins, including heavy metals, pesticides, and industrial chemicals, can have negative effects on fetal development and the maturation of organs beyond birth. Newborns and infants are particularly vulnerable to the detrimental effects of environmental toxins, especially on their immune and respiratory systems, which undergo extensive physical development from the early embryonic stages to early postnatal life [139]. This vulnerability is attributed to the complex signaling pathways involved in regulating cell proliferation and differentiation among the diverse cell types within these systems.

4.5.3.1 Pathways of toxic exposure

Postnatal and early-life exposure to harmful chemicals can occur through various pathways. In terms of exposure to environmental toxins, the primary pathways to consider are inhalation, ingestion, and absorption through the skin. Breathing in pollutants is likely the most common pathway for toxin intake, and newborns can inhale a range of pollutants, including particulate matter and indoor air pollutants [140]. Particulate matter consists of fine particles containing harmful substances that can lead to oxidative stress and inflammation potentially affecting telomeres. Indoor air pollutants, such as volatile organic compounds (VOCs), can also be inhaled and contribute to cellular damage and telomere shortening [141].

Exposure patterns to ingested and inhaled toxicants differ between children and adults. Children consume more water relative to their body weight than adults, resulting in potentially higher exposure to chemicals in drinking water including those used in infant food preparation [142]. Furthermore, infants and young children have a higher resting metabolic rate and oxygen consumption per unit of body weight. This means that, on a body weight basis, a larger volume of air passes through their lungs compared to adults. However, their lung surface area is relatively smaller, and their narrower airways make them more susceptible to air pollution-induced irritation, which can even lead to diseases like asthma later in life [143].

4.5.3.2 Endocrine-disrupting compounds and infant's health

We already discussed that breastfeeding is widely recognized as the best source of nutrition for infants offering numerous benefits for their overall health, growth, and development. However, it is important to acknowledge that breastfeeding infants can still be exposed to endocrine-disrupting compounds present in the mother's body. These compounds, which imitate or disrupt natural hormones, can enter the mother's bloodstream and accumulate in her breast milk [144]. Consequently, when an infant consumes breast milk containing these endocrine disruptors (EDs), they can be exposed to these substances.

Apart from breastfeeding, EDs can enter the infant's body through inhalation, skin contact, and ingestion [139]. These compounds, which resemble natural hormones, interfere with normal hormonal functions. More specifically, they can activate, interact with, and antagonize hormone receptors, alter specific signal transduction in hormone-responsive cells, induce epigenetic modifications, and affect hormone synthesis metabolism as transport across cells [145]. EDs can be found in the environment, food, household products, kids' toys, and everyday products like canned goods, plastic bottles, cosmetics, and medications [146]. Some common groups of substances with proven endocrine-disrupting effects include parabens, triclosan, phthalates, dichlorodiphenyltrichloroethane (DDTs), Polychlorinated biphenyls (PCBs) and bisphenols. The specific mechanisms through which they directly or indirectly affect human telomeres are not fully understood. However, they have been associated with various health issues later in life, including cardiovascular diseases, obesity, allergies, diabetes, asthma, and neurological disorders [147–152].

4.5.4 Supporting Caregiving for Newborns and Infants

During early childhood, the interactions and experiences between infants and caregivers play a significant role in shaping behavior and brain development [153]. Supporting caregiving actions like attachment and bonding impacts infants in various ways. Attachment refers to a specific aspect of the child–caregiver relationship that focuses on providing safety, security, and protection for the child. It involves the child using the primary caregiver as a secure base for exploration and as a source of comfort and safety when needed. On the other hand, bonding, a concept first mentioned by Klaus and Kennell, suggests that parent–child bonding depends on early skin-to-skin contact during early life such as the breastfeeding period. Until today, these two terms are still often used interchangeably [154].

Supporting caregiving helps in promoting the infant's overall well-being and development. It plays a major role in regulating the infant's emotions, promoting self-regulation skills, and enhancing their social and cognitive abilities [155].

4.5.4.1 Can parental caregiving truly affect an infant's telomere?

Research has shown that infants who encounter stress and adversity within their caregiving environment have a higher likelihood of developing psychiatric disorders [156]. At the same time, other studies have shown a correlation between caregiving and telomere length in newborns. In a study conducted by Asok et al., it was observed that experiencing nurturing or aversive caregiving environments during infancy can result in lasting alterations in TL. Specifically, they found that female brain regions such as the amygdala and prefrontal cortex exhibited longer telomeres as a result of caregiving treatment [157].

These pieces of evidence, among others, emphasize the importance of caregiving for the infant's health. Currently, the World Health Organization has released guidelines for caregiving and nutrition during the initial three years of an infant's life. These guidelines aim to offer evidence-based recommendations on enhancing early childhood development by promoting responsive caregiving [158].

4.6 Summary and Future Perspectives

Throughout our discussions, we delved into the intricate connection between telomere dynamics and the factors that influence TL alterations both during fetal development and after birth. The area of research that investigates the relationship between telomere length and developmental programming is relatively new. However, there is an increasing volume of scientific literature indicating a connection between fetal programming and fetal telomere length.

Maternal lifestyle factors, including diet, physical activity, and exposure to stress, can impact the intrauterine environment affecting fetal development and its telomere length, mainly due to oxidative stress. Possible pregnancy complications, such as preeclampsia or gestational diabetes, are known to alter the placental environment influencing fetal telomere dynamics. Simultaneously, infant nutrition and early-life exposure to toxins appear to have different yet substantial influences on telomere length, mediated by nutrients and molecules that are transported to the infant. Yet, the precise mechanisms linking adverse events regarding TL shaping during the first 1000 days of a person's life remain unclear and require additional investigation.

As our understanding of telomere biology continues to evolve, researchers are actively investigating potential interventions to modulate TL and preserve cellular health. Continued research and exploration of telomeres hold the promise of shedding further light on the complex interplay between the early telomere programming that takes place even before birth and the long-term pattern of telomere loss during early life.

References

1. Entringer, S., de Punder, K., Buss, C., & Wadhwa, P. D. (2018). The fetal programming of telomere biology hypothesis: an update, *Philosophical Transactions of the Royal Society of London. Series B, Biological Sciences*, **373**(1741), pp. 20170151.
2. Entringer, S., Buss, C., & Wadhwa, P. D. (2012). Prenatal stress, telomere biology, and fetal programming of health and disease risk, *Science Signaling*, **5**, pp. 12.
3. Entringer, S., Buss, C., & Wadhwa, P. D. (2010). Prenatal stress and developmental programming of human health and disease risk: concepts and integration of empirical findings, *Current Opinion in Endocrinology, Diabetes, and Obesity*, **17**, pp. 507–516.
4. Martens, D. S., Van Der Stukken, C., Derom, C., Thiery, E., Bijnens, E. M., & Nawrot, T. S. (2021). Newborn telomere length predicts later life telomere length: tracking telomere length from birth to child- and adulthood, *EBioMedicine*, **63**, pp. 103164.
5. Arima, Y., & Fukuoka, H. (2020). Developmental origins of health and disease theory in cardiology, *Journal of Cardiology*, **76**, pp. 14–17.
6. Holmes, D. K., Bellantuono, I., Walkinshaw, S. A., Alfirevic, Z., Johnston, T. A., Subhedar, N. V., *et al.* (2009). Telomere length dynamics differ in foetal and early post-natal human leukocytes in a longitudinal study, *Biogerontology*, **10**, pp. 279–284.
7. Monaghan, P., & Ozanne, S. E. (2018). Somatic growth and telomere dynamics in vertebrates: relationships, mechanisms and consequences. *Philosophical Transactions of the Royal Society of London, Series B, Biological Sciences*, **373**, pp. 20160446.
8. Glade, M. J., & Meguid, M. M. (2015). A glance at ... telomeres, oxidative stress, antioxidants, and biological aging, *Nutrition (Burbank, Los Angeles County, Calif.)*, **31**, pp. 1447–1451.

9. Zhang, J., Rane, G., Dai, X., Shanmugam, M. K., Arfuso, F., Samy, R. P., *et al.* (2016). Ageing and the telomere connection: an intimate relationship with inflammation, *Ageing Research Reviews*, **25**, pp. 55–69.
10. Prasad, K. N., Wu, M., & Bondy, S. C. (2017). Telomere shortening during aging: attenuation by antioxidants and anti-inflammatory agents, *Mechanisms of Ageing and Development*, **164**, pp. 61–66.
11. Jia, P., Her, C., & Chai, W. (2015). DNA excision repair at telomeres, *DNA Repair*, **36**, pp. 137–145.
12. Wright, W. E., Piatyszek, M. A., Rainey, W. E., Byrd, W., & Shay, J. W. (1996). Telomerase activity in human germline and embryonic tissues and cells, *Developmental Genetics*, **18**, pp. 173–179.
13. Fujisawa, M., Tanaka, H., Tatsumi, N., Okada, H., Arakawa, S., & Kamidono, S. (1998). Telomerase activity in the testis of infertile patients with selected causes, *Human Reproduction (Oxford, England)*, **13**, pp. 1476–1479.
14. Liu, J. P., & Li, H. (2010). Telomerase in the ovary, *Reproduction (Cambridge, England)*, **140**, pp. 215–222.
15. Else, T. (2009). Telomeres and telomerase in adrenocortical tissue maintenance, carcinogenesis, and aging, *Journal of Molecular Endocrinology*, **43**, pp. 131–141.
16. Ulaner, G. A., & Giudice, L. C. (1997). Developmental regulation of telomerase activity in human fetal tissues during gestation, *Molecular Human Reproduction*, **3**, pp. 769–773.
17. Duhig, K., Chappell, L. C., & Shennan, A. H. (2016). Oxidative stress in pregnancy and reproduction, *Obstetric Medicine*, **9**, pp. 113–116.
18. Physical activity and exercise during pregnancy and the postpartum period: ACOG Committee Opinion, Number 804. (2020). *Obstetrics and Gynecology*, **135**, pp. e178–e188.
19. Berghella, V., & Saccone, G. (2017). Exercise in pregnancy! *American Journal of Obstetrics and Gynecology*, **216**, pp. 335–337.
20. Flor-Alemany, M., Acosta-Manzano, P., Migueles, J. H., Varela-López, A., Baena-García, L., Quiles, J. L., *et al.* (2023). Influence of an exercise intervention plus an optimal Mediterranean diet adherence during pregnancy on the telomere length of the placenta, The GESTAFIT project, *Placenta*, **136**, pp. 42–45.
21. Bauer, I., Hartkopf, J., Kullmann, S., Schleger, F., Hallschmid, M., Pauluschke-Fröhlich, J., *et al.* (2020). Spotlight on the fetus: how physical activity during pregnancy influences fetal health: a narrative review, *BMJ Open Sport & Exercise Medicine*, **6**, pp. e000658.

22. Davenport, M. H., Sobierajski, F., Mottola, M. F., Skow, R. J., Meah, V. L., Poitras, V. J., *et al.* (2018). Glucose responses to acute and chronic exercise during pregnancy: a systematic review and meta-analysis, *British Journal of Sports Medicine*, **52**, pp. 1357–1366.
23. Hinman, S. K., Smith, K. B., Quillen, D. M., & Smith, M. S. (2015). Exercise in pregnancy: a clinical review, *Sports Health*, **7**, pp. 527–531.
24. Cai, M., Zhang, B., Yang, R., Zheng, T., Dong, G., Lin, H., *et al.* (2021). Association between maternal outdoor physical exercise and the risk of preterm birth: a case-control study in Wuhan, China, *BMC Pregnancy and Childbirth*, **21**, pp. 206.
25. Lowensohn, R. I., Stadler, D. D., & Naze, C. (2016). Current concepts of maternal nutrition, *Obstetrical & Gynecological Survey*, **71**, pp. 413–426.
26. Burton, G. J., Jauniaux, E., & Charnock-Jones, D. S. (2007). Human early placental development: potential roles of the endometrial glands, *Placenta*, **28** (Suppl A), pp. S64–S69.
27. Habibi, N., Bianco-Miotto, T., Phoi, Y. Y., Jankovic-Karasoulos, T., Roberts, C. T., & Grieger, J. A. (2021). Maternal diet and offspring telomere length: a systematic review, *Nutrition Reviews*, **79**, pp. 148–159.
28. Marshall, N. E., Abrams, B., Barbour, L. A., Catalano, P., Christian, P., Friedman, J. E., *et al.* (2022). The importance of nutrition in pregnancy and lactation: lifelong consequences, *American Journal of Obstetrics and Gynecology*, **226**, pp. 607–632.
29. Salihu, H. M., Adegoke, K. K., King, L. M., Daas, R., Paothong, A., Pradhan, A., *et al.* (2018). Effects of maternal carbohydrate and fat intake on fetal telomere length, *Southern Medical Journal*, **111**, pp. 591–596.
30. Zhou, M., Zhu, L., Cui, X., Feng, L., Zhao, X., He, S., *et al.* (2016). Influence of diet on leukocyte telomere length, markers of inflammation and oxidative stress in individuals with varied glucose tolerance: a Chinese population study, *Nutrition Journal*, **15**, pp. 39.
31. Office of Dietary Supplements – Folate. https://ods.od.nih.gov/factsheets/Folate-HealthProfessional/
32. Entringer, S., Epel, E. S., Lin, J., Blackburn, E. H., Buss, C., Shahbaba, B., *et al.* (2015). Maternal folate concentration in early pregnancy and newborn telomere length, *Annals of Nutrition & Metabolism*, **66**, pp. 202–208.
33. Folic acid vs. folate - what's the difference? https://www.healthline.com/nutrition/folic-acid-vs-folate

34. Folate https://lpi.oregonstate.edu/mic/vitamins/folate#
35. Zhou, D., Li, Z., Sun, Y., Yan, J., Huang, G., & Li, W. (2022). Early life stage folic acid deficiency delays the neurobehavioral development and cognitive function of rat offspring by hindering de novo telomere synthesis, *International Journal of Molecular Sciences*, **23**, pp. 6948.
36. Office of Dietary Supplements - Vitamin D. https://ods.od.nih.gov/factsheets/VitaminD-HealthProfessional/
37. Ashley, B., Simner, C., Manousopoulou, A., Jenkinson, C., Hey, F., Frost, J. M., *et al.* (2022). Placental uptake and metabolism of 25(OH) vitamin D determine its activity within the fetoplacental unit, *eLife*, **11**, pp. e71094.
38. Kim, J. H., Kim, G. J., Lee, D., Ko, J. H., Lim, I., Bang, H., *et al.* (2018). Higher maternal vitamin D concentrations are associated with longer leukocyte telomeres in newborns, *Maternal & Child Nutrition*, **14**, pp. e12475.
39. Wagner, C. L., Taylor, S. N., Johnson, D. D., & Hollis, B. W. (2012). The role of vitamin D in pregnancy and lactation: emerging concepts. *Women's Health (London, England)*, **8**, pp. 323–340.
40. Griffin, I., Ibrahimou, B., Navejar, N., Aggarwal, A., Myers, K., Mauck, D., *et al.* (2020). Maternal caffeine consumption and racial disparities in fetal telomere length, *International Journal of MCH and AIDS*, **9**, pp. 14–21.
41. World Health Organization. (2016). *WHO Recommendations on Antenatal Care for a Positive Pregnancy Experience.*
42. Gallagher, D., Heymsfield, S. B., Heo, M., Jebb, S. A., Murgatroyd, P. R., & Sakamoto, Y. (2000). Healthy percentage body fat ranges: an approach for developing guidelines based on body mass index, *The American Journal of Clinical Nutrition*, **72**, pp. 694–701.
43. Dolatian, M., Sharifi, N., Mahmoodi, Z., Fathnezhad-Kazemi, A., Bahrami-Vazir, E., & Rashidian, T. (2020). Weight gain during pregnancy and its associated factors: A Path analysis, *Nursing Open*, **7**, pp. 1568–1577.
44. Martens, D. S., Plusquin, M., Gyselaers, W., De Vivo, I., & Nawrot, T. S. (2016). Maternal pre-pregnancy body mass index and newborn telomere length, *BMC Medicine*, **14**, pp. 148.
45. Wei, B., Shao, Y., Liang, J., Tang, P., Mo, M., Liu, B., *et al.* (2021). Maternal overweight but not paternal overweight before pregnancy is associated with shorter newborn telomere length: evidence from

Guangxi Zhuang birth cohort in China, *BMC Pregnancy and Childbirth*, **21**, pp. 283.

46. Howell, M. P., Jones, C. W., Herman, C. A., Mayne, C. V., Fernandez, C., Theall, K. P., *et al.* (2022). Impact of prenatal tobacco smoking on infant telomere length trajectory and ADHD symptoms at 18 months: a longitudinal cohort study, *BMC Medicine*, **20**, pp. 153.
47. Osorio-Yáñez, C., Clemente, D. B. P., Maitre, L., Vives-Usano, M., Bustamante, M., Martinez, D., *et al.* (2020). Early life tobacco exposure and children's telomere length: The HELIX project, *The Science of the Total Environment*, **711**, pp. 135028.
48. Anblagan, D., Jones, N. W., Costigan, C., Parker, A. J., Allcock, K., Aleong, R., *et al.* (2013). Maternal smoking during pregnancy and fetal organ growth: a magnetic resonance imaging study, *PloS One*, **8**, pp. e67223.
49. Mirzakhani, H., De Vivo, I., Leeder, J. S., Gaedigk, R., Vyhlidal, C. A., Weiss, S. T., *et al.* (2017). Early pregnancy intrauterine fetal exposure to maternal smoking and impact on fetal telomere length, *European Journal of Obstetrics, Gynecology, and Reproductive Biology*, **218**, pp. 27–32.
50. Marchetto, N. M., Glynn, R. A., Ferry, M. L., Ostojic, M., Wolff, S. M., Yao, R., *et al.* (2016). Prenatal stress and newborn telomere length, *American Journal of Obstetrics and Gynecology*, **215**, pp. 94.e1–94.e948.
51. Leistner, C., & Menke, A. (2020). Hypothalamic-pituitary-adrenal axis and stress, *Handbook of Clinical Neurology*, **175**, pp. 55–64.
52. Lin, J., & Epel, E. (2022). Stress and telomere shortening: Insights from cellular mechanisms, *Ageing Research Reviews*, **73**, pp. 101507.
53. Epel E. S. (2009). Psychological and metabolic stress: a recipe for accelerated cellular aging? *Hormones (Athens, Greece)*, **8**, pp. 7–22.
54. Entringer, S., Epel, E. S., Lin, J., Buss, C., Shahbaba, B., Blackburn, E. H., *et al.* (2013). Maternal psychosocial stress during pregnancy is associated with newborn leukocyte telomere length, *American Journal of Obstetrics and Gynecology*, **208**, pp. 134.e1–134.e1347.
55. Izano, M. A., Cushing, L. J., Lin, J., Eick, S. M., Goin, D. E., Epel, E., *et al.* (2020). The association of maternal psychosocial stress with newborn telomere length, *PloS One*, **15**, pp. e0242064.
56. Leddy, M. A., Power, M. L., & Schulkin, J. (2008). The impact of maternal obesity on maternal and fetal health, *Reviews in Obstetrics & Gynecology*, **1**, pp. 170–178.
57. Akay, G. G. (2022). Telomeres and psychological stress: perspective on psychopathologies, *Noro Psikiyatri Arsivi*, **59**, pp. 330–337.

58. Burton, G. J., & Fowden, A. L. (2015). The placenta: a multifaceted, transient organ, *Philosophical Transactions of the Royal Society of London, Series B, Biological Sciences*, **370**, pp. 20140066.
59. Knöfler, M., Haider, S., Saleh, L., Pollheimer, J., Gamage, T. K. J. B., & James, J. (2019). Human placenta and trophoblast development: key molecular mechanisms and model systems, *Cellular and Molecular Life Sciences: CMLS*, **76**, pp. 3479–3496.
60. Burton, G. J., Charnock-Jones, D. S., & Jauniaux, E. (2009). Regulation of vascular growth and function in the human placenta, *Reproduction (Cambridge, England)*, **138**, pp. 895–902.
61. Kohlrausch, F. B., & Keefe, D. L. (2020). Telomere erosion as a placental clock: from placental pathologies to adverse pregnancy outcomes, *Placenta*, **97**, pp. 101–107.
62. Hutter, D., Kingdom, J., & Jaeggi, E. (2010). Causes and mechanisms of intrauterine hypoxia and its impact on the fetal cardiovascular system: a review, *International Journal of Pediatrics*, **2010**, pp. 401323.
63. Gilbert, J.S., Nijland, M.J., Knoblich, P. (2008). Placental ischemia and cardiovascular dysfunction in preeclampsia and beyond: making the connections, *Expert Rev. Cardiovasc. Ther.* **6**, pp. 1367–1377.
64. Tal, R., Shaish, A., Barshack, I., Polak-Charcon, S., Afek, A., Volkov, A., *et al.* (2010). Effects of hypoxia-inducible factor-1alpha overexpression in pregnant mice: possible implications for preeclampsia and intrauterine growth restriction, *The American Journal of Pathology*, **177**, pp. 2950–2962.
65. Guan, J. Z., Guan, W. P., Maeda, T., & Makino, N. (2012). Different levels of hypoxia regulate telomere length and telomerase activity, *Aging Clinical and Experimental Research*, **24**, pp. 213–217.
66. Ravlić, S., Škrobot Vidaček, N., Nanić, L., Laganović, M., Slade, N., Jelaković, B., *et al.* (2018). Mechanisms of fetal epigenetics that determine telomere dynamics and health span in adulthood, *Mechanisms of Ageing and Development*, **174**, pp. 55–62.
67. Sharma, D., Shastri, S., & Sharma, P. (2016). Intrauterine growth restriction: antenatal and postnatal aspects, clinical medicine insights, *Pediatrics*, **10**, pp. 67–83.
68. Toutain, J., Prochazkova-Carlotti, M., Cappellen, D., Jarne, A., Chevret, E., Ferrer, J., *et al.* (2013). Reduced placental telomere length during pregnancies complicated by intrauterine growth restriction, *PloS One*, **8**, pp. e54013.

69. Plows, J. F., Stanley, J. L., Baker, P. N., Reynolds, C. M., & Vickers, M. H. (2018). The Pathophysiology of Gestational Diabetes Mellitus, *International Journal of Molecular Sciences*, **19**, pp. 3342.
70. Alfadhli E. M. (2015). Gestational diabetes mellitus, *Saudi Medical Journal*, **36**, pp. 399–406.
71. Chu, S. Y., Callaghan, W. M., Kim, S. Y., Schmid, C. H., Lau, J., England, L. J., *et al.* (2007). Maternal obesity and risk of gestational diabetes mellitus, *Diabetes Care*, **30**, pp. 2070–2076.
72. Padayachee, C., & Coombes, J. S. (2015). Exercise guidelines for gestational diabetes mellitus, *World Journal of Diabetes*, **6**, pp. 1033–1044.
73. Dolatkhah, N., Hajifaraji, M., & Shakouri, S. K. (2018). Nutrition therapy in managing pregnant women with gestational diabetes mellitus: a literature review, *Journal of Family & Reproductive Health*, **12**, pp. 57–72.
74. Garcia-Martin, I., Penketh, R. J. A., Janssen, A. B., Jones, R. E., Grimstead, J., Baird, D. M., *et al.* (2018). Metformin and insulin treatment prevent placental telomere attrition in boys exposed to maternal diabetes, *PloS One*, **13**, pp. e0208533.
75. Biron-Shental, T., Sukenik-Halevy, R., Naboani, H., Liberman, M., Kats, R., & Amiel, A. (2015). Telomeres are shorter in placentas from pregnancies with uncontrolled diabetes, *Placenta*, **36**, pp. 199–203.
76. Li, P., Tong, Y., Yang, H., Zhou, S., Xiong, F., Huo, T., *et al.* (2014). Mitochondrial translocation of human telomerase reverse transcriptase in cord blood mononuclear cells of newborns with gestational diabetes mellitus mothers, *Diabetes Research and Clinical Practice*, **103**, pp. 310–318.
77. Gilfillan, C., Naidu, P., Gunawan, F., Hassan, F., Tian, P., & Elwood, N. (2016). Leukocyte telomere length in the neonatal offspring of mothers with gestational and pre-gestational diabetes, *PloS One*, **11**, pp. e0163824.
78. Cross, J. A., Temple, R. C., Hughes, J. C., Dozio, N. C., Brennan, C., Stanley, K., *et al.* (2010). Cord blood telomere length, telomerase activity and inflammatory markers in pregnancies in women with diabetes or gestational diabetes, *Diabetic Medicine: A Journal of the British Diabetic Association*, **27**, pp. 1264–1270.
79. Gielen, M., Hageman, G., Pachen, D., Derom, C., Vlietinck, R., & Zeegers, M. P. (2014). Placental telomere length decreases with gestational age

and is influenced by parity: a study of third trimester live-born twins, *Placenta*, **35**, pp. 791–796.

80. Xu, J., Ye, J., Wu, Y., Zhang, H., Luo, Q., Han, C., *et al.* (2014). Reduced fetal telomere length in gestational diabetes, *PloS One*, **9**, pp. e86161.
81. Lazarides, C., Epel, E. S., Lin, J., Blackburn, E. H., Voelkle, M. C., Buss, C., *et al.* (2019). Maternal pro-inflammatory state during pregnancy and newborn leukocyte telomere length: a prospective investigation, *Brain, Behavior, and Immunity*, **80**, pp. 419–426.
82. Tung, K. T. S., Hung, C. M. W., Chan, K. L., Wong, R. S., Tsang, H. W., Wong, W. H. S., *et al.* (2021). Influence of maternal infection and pregnancy complications on cord blood telomere length, *Oxidative Medicine and Cellular Longevity*, **2021**, pp. 3339456.
83. Auriti, C., De Rose, D. U., Santisi, A., Martini, L., Piersigilli, F., Bersani, I., *et al.* (2021). Pregnancy and viral infections: mechanisms of fetal damage, diagnosis and prevention of neonatal adverse outcomes from cytomegalovirus to SARS-CoV-2 and Zika virus, *Biochimica et Biophysica Acta, Molecular Basis of Disease*, **1867**, pp. 166198.
84. Ghosh, A., Saginc, G., Leow, S. C., Khattar, E., Shin, E. M., Yan, T. D., *et al.* (2012). Telomerase directly regulates NF-κB-dependent transcription, *Nature Cell Biology*, **14**, pp. 1270–1281.
85. Liu, B., Maekawa, T., Chatton, B., & Ishii, S. (2016). In utero TNF-α treatment induces telomere shortening in young adult mice in an ATF7-dependent manner, *FEBS Open Bio*, **6**, pp. 56–63.
86. Braunthal, S., & Brateanu, A. (2019). Hypertension in pregnancy: Pathophysiology and treatment, *SAGE Open Medicine*, **7**, 2050312 119843700.
87. Granger, J. P., Alexander, B. T., Bennett, W. A., & Khalil, R. A. (2001). Pathophysiology of pregnancy-induced hypertension, *American Journal of Hypertension*, **14**, pp. 178S–185S.
88. Luger RK, Kight BP. Hypertension in pregnancy. [Updated 2022 Oct 3]. In: *StatPearls* [Internet]. Treasure Island (FL): StatPearls Publishing; 2023 Jan-. Available from: https://www.ncbi.nlm.nih.gov/books/NBK430839/Jan-.
89. Yang, X., Benny, P. A., Cervera-Marzal, E., Wu, B., Lassiter, C. B., Astern, J., *et al.* (2022). Placental telomere length shortening is not associated with severe preeclampsia but the gestational age, *Aging*, **15**, pp. 353–370.
90. Pre-eclampsia and eclampsia. https://www.nichd.nih.gov/health/topics/preeclampsia

91. Tellechea, M., Gianotti, T., Alvariñas, J. *et al.* (2015). Telomere length in the two extremes of abnormal fetal growth and the programming effect of maternal arterial hypertension, *Sci Rep,* **5**, pp. 7869.
92. Martens, D. S., Sleurs, H., Dockx, Y., Rasking, L., Plusquin, M., & Nawrot, T. S. (2022). Association of newborn telomere length with blood pressure in childhood, *JAMA Network Open*, **5**, pp. e2225521.
93. Abu-Awwad, S. A., Craina, M., Gluhovschi, A., Ciordas, P. D., Marian, C., Boscu, L., *et al.* (2023). Linking pregnancy and long-term health: the impact of cardiovascular risk on telomere shortening in pregnant women, *Medicina (Kaunas, Lithuania)*, **59**, pp. 1012.
94. Akkad, A., Hastings, R., Konje, J. C., Bell, S. C., Thurston, H., & Williams, B. (2006). Telomere length in small-for-gestational-age babies, *BJOG: An International Journal of Obstetrics and Gynaecology*, **113**, pp. 318–323.
95. Okuda, K., Bardeguez, A., Gardner, J. P., Rodriguez, P., Ganesh, V., Kimura, M., *et al.* (2002). Telomere length in the newborn, *Pediatric Research*, **52**, pp. 377–381.
96. Biron-Shental, T., Sukenik-Halevy, R., Sharon, Y., Goldberg-Bittman, L., Kidron, D., Fejgin, M. D., *et al.* (2010). Short telomeres may play a role in placental dysfunction in preeclampsia and intrauterine growth restriction, *American Journal of Obstetrics and Gynecology,* **202**, pp. 381.e1–381.e3817.
97. Gorenjak, V., Petrelis, A. M., Stathopoulou, M. G., & Visvikis-Siest, S. (2020). Telomere length determinants in childhood, *Clinical Chemistry and Laboratory Medicine*, **58**, pp. 162–177.
98. Frenck, R. W., Jr, Blackburn, E. H., & Shannon, K. M. (1998). The rate of telomere sequence loss in human leukocytes varies with age, *Proceedings of the National Academy of Sciences of the United States of America*, **95**, pp. 5607–5610.
99. Zeichner, S. L., Palumbo, P., Feng, Y., Xiao, X., Gee, D., Sleasman, J., *et al.* (1999). Rapid telomere shortening in children, *Blood*, **93**, pp. 2824–2830.
100. Samuel, T. M., Sakwinska, O., Makinen, K., Burdge, G. C., Godfrey, K. M., & Silva-Zolezzi, I. (2019). Preterm birth: a narrative review of the current evidence on nutritional and bioactive solutions for risk reduction, *Nutrients*, **11**, pp. 1811.
101. Christiaan Monden, Gilles Pison, Jeroen Smits. (2021). Twin peaks: more twinning in humans than ever before, *Human Reproduction,* **36**, pp. 1666–1673.

102. Buchanan, T. A., Xiang, A. H., & Page, K. A. (2012). Gestational diabetes mellitus: risks and management during and after pregnancy, *Nature Reviews, Endocrinology*, **8**, pp. 639–649.

103. Hawthorne, G. (2011). Maternal complications in diabetic pregnancy: best practice & research, *Clinical Obstetrics & Gynaecology*, **25**, pp. 77–90.

104. Gheorghiu, M. L., Bors, R. G., Gheorghisan-Galateanu, A. A., Pop, A. L., Cretoiu, D., & Varlas, V. N. (2021). Hyperthyroidism in pregnancy: the delicate balance between too much or too little antithyroid drug, *Journal of Clinical Medicine,* **10**, pp. 3742.

105. De Groot, L., Abalovich, M., Alexander, E. K., Amino, N., Barbour, L., Cobin, R., *et al.* (2012). Management of thyroid dysfunction during pregnancy and postpartum: an endocrine society clinical practice guideline, *J Clin Endocrinol Metab.*, **97**, pp. 2543–65.

106. de Jongh, B. E., Paul, D. A., Hoffman, M., & Locke, R. (2014). Effects of pre-pregnancy obesity, race/ethnicity and prematurity, *Maternal and Child Health Journal,* **18**, pp. 511–517.

107. Heslehurst, N., Simpson, H., Ells, L. J., Rankin, J., Wilkinson, J., Lang, R., *et al.* (2008). The impact of maternal BMI status on pregnancy outcomes with immediate short-term obstetric resource implications: a meta-analysis, *Obesity Reviews: An Official Journal of the International Association for the Study of Obesity*, **9**, pp. 635–683.

108. McCarthy, F. P., O'Keeffe, L. M., Khashan, A. S., North, R. A., Poston, L., McCowan, L. M. E., *et al.* (2013). Association between maternal alcohol consumption in early pregnancy and pregnancy outcomes, *Obstetrics and Gynecology*, **122**, pp. 830–837.

109. Shah, N. R., & Bracken, M. B. (2000). A systematic review and meta-analysis of prospective studies on the association between maternal cigarette smoking and preterm delivery, *American Journal of Obstetrics and Gynecology,* **182**, pp. 465–472.

110. Haghighi, L., Najmi, Z., Barzegar, S. H., & Barzegar, N. (2013). Twin's sex and risk of pre-term birth, *The Journal of the Institute of Obstetrics and Gynaecology*, **33**, pp. 823–826.

111. Kent, A. L., Wright, I. M., Abdel-Latif, M. E., & New South Wales and Australian Capital Territory Neonatal Intensive Care Units Audit Group (2012). Mortality and adverse neurologic outcomes are greater in preterm male infants, *Pediatrics*, **129**, pp. 124–131.

112. Blencowe, H., Cousens, S., Chou, D., Oestergaard, M., Say, L., Moller, A. B., *et al.* (2013). Born too soon: the global epidemiology of 15 million preterm births, *Reproductive Health*, **10** (Suppl 1), pp. S2.

113. Henckel, E., Landfors, M., Haider, Z., Kosma, P., Hultdin, M., Degerman, S., *et al.* (2020). Hematopoietic cellular aging is not accelerated during the first 2 years of life in children born preterm, *Pediatric Research*, **88**, pp. 903–909.

114. Colatto, B. N., de Souza, I. F., Schinke, L. A. A., Noda-Nicolau, N. M., da Silva, M. G., Morceli, G., *et al.* (2020). Telomere length and telomerase activity in foetal membranes from term and spontaneous preterm births, *Reproductive Sciences* (Thousand Oaks, Calif.), **27**, pp. 411–417.

115. Friedrich, U., Schwab, M., Griese, E. U., Fritz, P., & Klotz, U. (2001). Telomeres in neonates: new insights in fetal hematopoiesis, *Pediatric Research*, **49**, pp. 252–256.

116. Ramírez-Vélez R. (2012). Programación Fetal in utero y su impacto en la salud del adulto [In utero fetal programming and its impact on health in adulthood]. *Endocrinologia y Nutricion: Organo De La Sociedad Espanola de Endocrinologia y Nutricion*, **59**, pp. 383–393.

117. Aparicio, E., Jardí, C., Bedmar, C., Pallejà, M., Basora, J., Arija, V., & The Eclipses Study Group (2020). Nutrient intake during pregnancy and post-partum: ECLIPSES study, *Nutrients*, **12**, pp. 1325.

118. Pham, Q., Patel, P., Baban, B., Yu, J., & Bhatia, J. (2020). Factors affecting the composition of expressed fresh human milk, *Breastfeeding Medicine: The Official Journal of the Academy of Breastfeeding Medicine*, **15**, pp. 551–558.

119. Lönnerdal, B., Erdmann, P., Thakkar, S. K., Sauser, J., & Destaillats, F. (2017). Longitudinal evolution of true protein, amino acids and bioactive proteins in breast milk: a developmental perspective, *The Journal of Nutritional Biochemistry*, **41**, pp. 1–11.

120. Ballard, O., & Morrow, A. L. (2013). Human milk composition: nutrients and bioactive factors, *Pediatric Clinics of North America*, **60**, pp. 49–74.

121. Nommsen, L. A., Lovelady, C. A., Heinig, M. J., Lönnerdal, B., & Dewey, K. G. (1991). Determinants of energy, protein, lipid, and lactose concentrations in human milk during the first 12 mo of lactation: the DARLING study, *The American Journal of Clinical Nutrition*, **53**, pp. 457–465.

122. Bauer, J., & Gerss, J. (2011). Longitudinal analysis of macronutrients and minerals in human milk produced by mothers of preterm infants, *Clinical Nutrition* (Edinburgh, Scotland), **30**, pp. 215–220.

123. Lönnerdal B. (2004). Human milk proteins: key components for the biological activity of human milk, *Advances in Experimental Medicine and Biology*, **554**, pp. 11–25.

124. Romero-Velarde, E., Delgado-Franco, D., García-Gutiérrez, M., Gurrola-Díaz, C., Larrosa-Haro, A., Montijo-Barrios, E., *et al.* (2019). The importance of lactose in the human diet: outcomes of a mexican consensus meeting, *Nutrients,* **11**, pp. 2737.

125. Lyons, K. E., Ryan, C. A., Dempsey, E. M., Ross, R. P., & Stanton, C. (2020). Breast milk, a source of beneficial microbes and associated benefits for infant health, *Nutrients,* **12**, pp. 1039.

126. Liotto N. (2020). Protein content of infant formula for the healthy full-term infant, *The American Journal of Clinical Nutrition,* **111**, pp. 946–947.

127. Trandafir, L. M., & Temneanu, O. R. (2016). Pre- and post-natal risk and determination of factors for child obesity, *Journal of Medicine and Life,* **9**, pp. 386–391.

128. Wojcicki, J. M., Heyman, M. B., Elwan, D., Lin, J., Blackburn, E., & Epel, E. (2016). Early exclusive breastfeeding is associated with longer telomeres in Latino preschool children, *The American Journal of Clinical Nutrition*, **104**, pp. 397–405.

129. Meshkani, S. E., Kooshki, A., Alahabadi, A., Lari Najafi, M., Rad, A., Riahimanesh, F., *et al.* (2021). Dietary pattern and telomere length in preschool children in a middle-income country, *Maternal & Child Nutrition*, **17**, pp. e13146.

130. York, D. J., Smazal, A. L., Robinson, D. T., & De Plaen, I. G. (2021). Human milk growth factors and their role in NEC prevention: a narrative review, *Nutrients,* **13**, pp. 3751.

131. Xavier, A. M., Rai, K., & Hegde, A. M. (2011). Total antioxidant concentrations of breastmilk—an eye-opener to the negligent, *Journal of Health, Population, and Nutrition*, **29**, pp. 605–611.

132. World Health Organization. (2009). *Infant and Young Child Feeding.* NCBI Bookshelf, PMID: 23905206 Bookshelf ID: NBK14896.

133. Yu, C., Binns, C. W., & Lee, A. H. (2019). The early introduction of complementary (solid) foods: a prospective cohort study of infants in Chengdu, China, *Nutrients,* **11**, pp. 760.

134. Mathias, J. G., Zhang, H., Soto-Ramirez, N. *et al.* (2019). The association of infant feeding patterns with food allergy symptoms and food allergy in early childhood, *Int Breastfeed J*, **14**, pp. 43.

135. Huh, S. Y., Rifas-Shiman, S. L., Taveras, E. M., Oken, E., & Gillman, M. W. (2011). Timing of solid food introduction and risk of obesity in preschool-aged children, *Pediatrics,* **127**, pp. e544–e551.

136. Tucker L. A. (2021). Fruit and vegetable intake and telomere length in a random sample of 5448 U.S. Adults, *Nutrients*, **13**, pp. 1415.

137. Ali, S., Scapagnini, G., & Davinelli, S. (2022). Effect of omega-3 fatty acids on the telomere length: a mini meta-analysis of clinical trials, *Biomolecular concepts*, **13**, pp. 25–33.

138. Santangelo, C., & Masella, R. (2021). *Molecular Aspects of Dietary Polyphenols in Pregnancy*, Academic Press, pp. 233–264.

139. Rahaman, M. M., Hossain, R., Herrera-Bravo, J., Islam, M. T., Atolani, O., Adeyemi, O. S., *et al.* (2023). Natural antioxidants from some fruits, seeds, foods, natural products, and associated health benefits: an update, *Food Science & Nutrition*, **11**, pp. 1657–1670.

140. Dai, Y., Huo, X., Cheng, Z., Faas, M. M., & Xu, X. (2020). Early-life exposure to widespread environmental toxicants and maternal-fetal health risk: a focus on metabolomic biomarkers, *The Science of the Total Environment*, **739**, pp. 139626.

141. Lin, Li-Zi., Chen, Jin-Hui., Yu, Yun-Jiang., Dong, Guang-Hui. (2023). Ambient air pollution and infant health: a narrative review, *eBiomedicine, THE LANCET Discovery Science*, **93**, pp. 104609.

142. Rosário Filho, N. A., Urrutia-Pereira, M., D'Amato, G., Cecchi, L., Ansotegui, I. J., Galán, C., *et al.* (2021). Air pollution and indoor settings, *The World Allergy Organization Journal*, **14**, pp. 100499.

143. Moya, J., Bearer, C. F., & Etzel, R. A. (2004). Children's behavior and physiology and how it affects exposure to environmental contaminants, *Pediatrics*, **113**, pp. 996–1006.

144. Carroquino, M. J., Posada, M., & Landrigan, P. J. (2012). Environmental toxicology: children at risk, *Environmental Toxicology: Selected Entries from the Encyclopedia of Sustainability Science and Technology*, pp. 239–291.

145. Heinzow, B.G.L. (2009). Endocrine disruptors in human milk and the health-related issues of breastfeeding, *Woodhead Publishing Series in Food Science, Technology and Nutrition*, **13**, pp. 322–355.

146. La Merrill, M. A., Vandenberg, L. N., Smith, M. T., Goodson, W., Browne, P., Patisaul, H. B., *et al.* (2020). Consensus on the key characteristics of endocrine-disrupting chemicals as a basis for hazard identification, *Nature Reviews, Endocrinology*, **16**, pp. 45–57.

147. Martin, L., Zhang, Y., First, O., Mustieles, V., Dodson, R., Rosa, G., *et al.* (2022). Lifestyle interventions to reduce endocrine-disrupting phthalate and phenol exposures among reproductive age men and

women: a review and future steps, *Environment International*, **170**, pp. 107576.

148. Fu, X., Xu, J., Zhang, R., & Yu, J. (2020). The association between environmental endocrine disruptors and cardiovascular diseases: a systematic review and meta-analysis, *Environmental Research*, **187**, pp. 109464.
149. Dodson, R. E., Nishioka, M., Standley, L. J., Perovich, L. J., Brody, J. G., & Rudel, R. A. (2012). Endocrine disruptors and asthma-associated chemicals in consumer products, *Environmental Health Perspectives*, **120**, pp. 935–943.
150. Darbre, P. D. (2017). Endocrine disruptors and obesity, *Current Obesity Reports*, **6**, pp. 18–27.
151. Predieri, B., Bruzzi, P., Bigi, E., Ciancia, S., Madeo, S. F., Lucaccioni, L., *et al.* (2020). Endocrine disrupting chemicals and type 1 diabetes, *International Journal of Molecular Sciences*, **21**, pp. 2937.
152. Kato, T., Tada-Oikawa, S., Wang, L., Murata, M., & Kuribayashi, K. (2013). Endocrine disruptors found in food contaminants enhance allergic sensitization through an oxidative stress that promotes the development of allergic airway inflammation, *Toxicology and Applied Pharmacology*, **273**, pp. 10–18.
153. Gee, D. G., & Cohodes, E. M. (2021). Caregiving influences on development: a sensitive period for biological embedding of predictability and safety cues, *Current Directions in Psychological Science*, **30**, pp. 376–383.
154. Benoit D. (2004). Infant-parent attachment: definition, types, antecedents, measurement and outcome, *Paediatrics & Child Health*, **9**, pp. 541–545.
155. Dosman, C., & Andrews, D. (2012). Anticipatory guidance for cognitive and social-emotional development: birth to five years, *Paediatrics & Child Health*, **17**, pp. 75–80.
156. Blaze, J., Asok, A., & Roth, T. L. (2015). The long-term impact of adverse caregiving environments on epigenetic modifications and telomeres, *Frontiers in Behavioral Neuroscience*, **9**, pp. 79.
157. Asok, A., Bernard, K., Rosen, J. B., Dozier, M., & Roth, T. L. (2014). Infant-caregiver experiences alter telomere length in the brain, *PloS One*, **9**, pp. e101437.
158. Improving Early Childhood Development: WHO Guideline [Internet]. Geneva: World Health Organization; 2020. Available from: https://www.ncbi.nlm.nih.gov/books/NBK555073/

Chapter 5

Diet as a Strategy to Lengthen Life Expectancy

Konstantinos Xenos[a] and Evgenia Alexandrou[b]

[a]*Clinical Dietitian, Nutrigenetics Department, Athens Euroclinic Hospital, D. Soutsou, Athens, Greece*

[b]*Dietitian–Nutritionist, Athens Euroclinic Hospital, D. Soutsou, Athens, Greece*

kxdiet@gmail.com, alexandrou.diet@gmail.com

5.1 Introduction

The proportion of the elderly in the world is expanding rapidly. The percentage of people 60 years and over in the world is anticipated to surpass 20% by 2050, exceeding the number of children globally.

As aging is defined by a progressive loss of physiological integrity, which results in diminished function and autonomy, it has significant social and economic repercussions.

This functional decline is the greatest risk factor for the majority of chronic diseases, including type 2 diabetes, Alzheimer's disease, and various cancers, along with other conditions that restrict health span (Fig. 5.1).

Telomeres: Biomarkers of a Healthy Life and Successful Aging
Edited by Aristidis Tsatsakis

ISBN 978-981-5129-49-6 (Hardcover), 978-1-003-56809-4 (eBook)
www.jennystanford.com

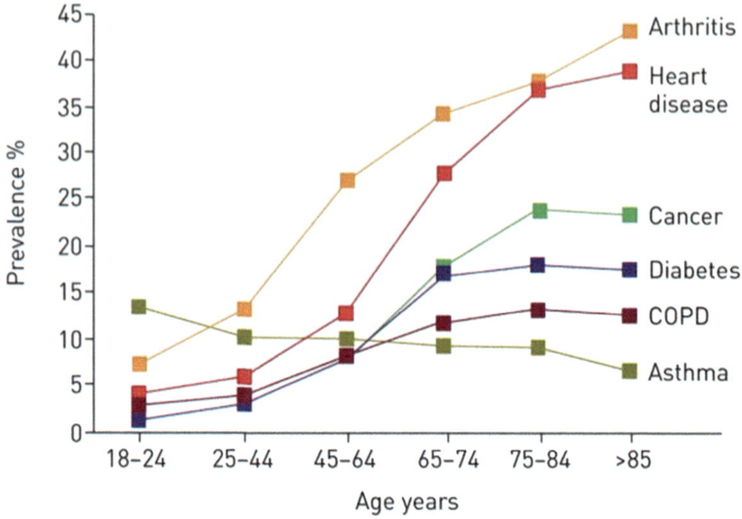

Figure 5.1 Prevalence of particular chronic diseases in relation to age [1].

Notably, aging has surpassed all other risk factors for death in developed countries, and as a result, the preservation of health and independence during old age becomes particularly crucial. Today more than ever, increasing awareness of age-related illness prevention strategies is a major public health concern.

Genomic instability, telomere attrition, epigenetic changes, proteostasis loss, and alterations in intercellular communication are just a few examples of genetic pathways and biochemical processes that regulate the rate of aging and in recent years also led to major research breakthroughs. Although biological aging can be measured using several biomarkers, "telomere shortening" is regarded as a key aging characteristic, due to its critical involvement in cellular senescence and organism aging.

Telomere length (TL) is one of the most often utilized aging biomarkers in clinical and epidemiological studies, a reliable biomarker of aging, morbidity, and death. Pathological conditions linked to aging as type 2 diabetes, cardiovascular disease, or chronic renal diseases were linked to a shorter TL.

The research on aging has revealed that lifestyle factors, such as stress, physical activity, obesity, and diet, affect health, biological longevity, and TL dynamics [2]. Moreover, the significance of controlling telomere length and integrity during aging, proposed potential therapies to lengthen life expectancy, like maintaining a healthy diet. Studies have shown that poor dietary choices have been related to shorter "leukocyte telomere length (LTL)," a biomarker of the "biological age" of cells, as opposed to the "chronological age." Some studies have discovered a connection between diet or the consumption of certain foods and leukocyte telomere length. **To note, the rates of telomere shortening are significantly similar in leukocytes and somatic cells, so that telomere length in leukocytes is now considered to be representative of global telomere length in somatic cells.**

5.2 Association Among Oxidative Stress, Diet, and Telomere Length

As oxidative stress strongly influences TL shortening, studies have focused on examining the association between TL and a diet high in antioxidant capacity. The consumption of fruits and vegetables, certain antioxidant substances, or healthy eating patterns like the Mediterranean diet were all linked to longer TL according to some recent systematic reviews [2].

On the other hand, unhealthy eating patterns have been connected to an inflammatory condition, which accelerates telomere degradation. It is likely that bad eating habits have an impact on telomere erosion by increasing the oxidation of telomeric DNA, as these habits enhance the formation of reactive oxygen species (ROS). This is supported by the finding that, at least in vitro tests, telomeric sequences are especially susceptible to oxidation into 8-oxoG, due to their high content in guanine residues. When present at telomeres, 8-oxoG residues probably reduce shelterin proteins' affinity for telomeric DNA and disrupt the G-quadruplex structures of telomeres, which perform important functions at telomeres such as controlling telomerase activity. Therefore, it is believed that nutrients control the health of telomeres through controlling oxidative stress and systemic inflammation. Generally, it is possible to anticipate that any anti-inflammatory or antioxidant diet may protect telomeres by reducing their shortening and delaying aging. At least in mice, consumption of foods with anti-inflammatory and antioxidant characteristics, such as vitamin C or E, polyphenols, curcumin, or omega-3 fatty acids, have been linked to longer telomeres.

In animal models, calorie restriction has been shown to have a positive effect on telomere length and to generally delay the onset of aging and age-related diseases, such as diabetes, cardiovascular diseases, various neurological disorders, cancer, and obesity, possibly via a reduction in oxidative stress. The statistics for humans are less convincing possibly because it is very difficult for the human population to reduce caloric consumption by a third or a half over the long term [3].

5.3 Importance of a Healthy Diet in the Early Years of Life

Even though research on TL in adults has provided useful insights, there is increased interest in research on TL in the formative years of life as it may play a causative role in the emergence of negative consequences in later adulthood. Some researchers have hypothesized that TL in childhood shortens much quicker than in adulthood, especially during the first 20 years of life.

The systematic review of Valera-Gran et al. examined the association between intake of nutrients, certain foods, or food groups, and dietary patterns and TL in childhood and adolescence [2]. According to this review, a higher intake of fruits and vegetables, nuts and seeds, fish, olives, and legumes may be linked to a longer TL in middle childhood and adolescence. On the other hand, this review also discovered that factors related to TL shortening included higher consumption of dairy products, simple sugar between 5 and 7 years of age as well as cereals, particularly white bread, and a diet high in glycemic load between 6 and 18 years.

Similar to earlier studies on adults, it was discovered in Iranian children aged 5–7 that eating more nuts and seeds was associated with having a longer TL. In addition, preliminary results from recent randomized controlled trials have indicated that eating walnuts and pistachio nuts can help maintain LTL and reduce DNA oxidative damage. However, the evidence that is currently available on the effects of nuts on the TL has also revealed negative or null results indicating that further study is needed [2].

The study by Meshkani et al. also revealed that olive intake, particularly olive oil, was associated with a longer TL along with the consumption of nuts [4]. Polyunsaturated fatty acids (PUFA) and total antioxidant capacity (TAC) were two additional dietary intake parameters that were found in this review to be favorably linked with TL in the young population. The evidence that is now available indicates that omega-3 PUFA intake was primarily responsible for the beneficial effect of PUFA on TL. The relationship between omega-3 PUFA, and TL cannot be conclusively established, much alone the influence of omega-6 PUFA or the role of overall PUFA intake regarding TL, even though PUFA may play a role in regulating gene expression implicated in metabolic changes and chronic illnesses. Therefore, more investigation into this dietary component is required to determine how it affects telomere biology. In terms of nutritional epidemiology research using dietary TAC as a general indicator of antioxidant status is innovative for examining how it affects the maintenance of TL.

There are various methods to evaluate the total antioxidant capacity which can be divided into three major technique groups: chromatography, electrochemical tests, and spectrometry. Each category includes several antioxidant capacity tests (ORAC—oxygen radical absorption capacity, HORAC—hydroxyl radical antioxidant capacity, TRAP—total peroxyl radical trapping antioxidant parameter, etc.), which can be further divided into two categories depending on the potential chemical reactions: reaction-based procedures for hydrogen atom transfer (HAT) and single electron transfer (SET). Despite the reaction mechanism, the outcome is the same even though the kinetics and reaction phases may vary. The evaluation of the total antioxidant capacity should not be conducted by just one method. To ascertain the antioxidant properties of the target sample, several antioxidant tests should be carried out in vitro.

García-Calzón et al. have demonstrated that dietary TAC is associated with a longer TL in kids and adolescents [5]. The authors hypothesized, based on prior research on the Mediterranean diet pattern, that dietary TAC as opposed to individual food groups may have a higher impact on TL because of its synergistic effect brought on by the overall interaction of the antioxidants. It is interesting to note that this diet-based approach has sparked new interest in the potential effects of a diet high in antioxidants on the biological stability of TL.

The study by Meshkani et al. was the first to examine the direct impact of simple sugar on TL in children [4]. Although Basking et al. looked at the impact of sugar and fast-food intake in kids of a similar age, no correlation was found with TL. However, the results of a study examining the greater glycemic load (GL) through cereals and white bread reported by García-Calzón et al. in a sample of 287 Spanish children and adolescents are consistent with the negative effect of the higher GL on TL [5].

White bread, refined cereals, and sugar are foods with a high glycemic load according to the official reference values. Although the information from other studies suggests that the evidence in this area is still unclear, the limited results from this study are consistent with earlier research done in other adult populations. This review also emphasizes the need for more research to identify potential nutritional determinants of TL in childhood and adolescence with a focus on longitudinal studies and randomized controlled trials.

5.4 Specific Diet Pattern Impact on Telomere Length

While it is vital to understand how particular substances affect telomere length, it is even more crucial to evaluate the overall impact of the nutrient in a specific diet as this reflects reality more accurately.

In 2015, Lee et al. compared the influence of the dietary pattern on leukocyte telomere length [6]. Dietary data were collected from a semi-quantitative food frequency questionnaire at baseline and leukocyte telomere length was assessed using qPCR 10 years later. A total of 1958 middle-aged and older Korean adults aged 40–69 years were included in the study. The authors identified two major dietary patterns: "the prudent dietary pattern" was characterized by a high intake of whole grains, fish and seafood, legumes, vegetables, and seaweed; whereas, the "western dietary pattern" included a high intake of refined grain, red meat or processed meat, and sweetened carbonated beverages. Using a multiple linear regression model adjusted for age, sex, body mass index, and other potentially confounding variables, the "prudent dietary pattern" was found to be positively associated with leukocyte telomere length; whereas, the "western dietary pattern" showed a negative correlation. These findings imply that the degree of biological aging in middle-aged and older people may be influenced by diet.

One of the best models of healthy eating is the Mediterranean diet, which is characterized by a high intake of vegetables, legumes, nuts, fruits, and cereals (mainly unrefined); a moderate to high intake of fish; a low intake of saturated lipids but high intake of unsaturated lipids, particularly olive oil; and a regular but moderate intake of alcohol, specifically wine. A high level of adherence to the Mediterranean diet has consistently been associated with several health benefits including a decrease in overall mortality, a decrease in the incidence of chronic diseases, particularly serious cardiovascular diseases, and an increased likelihood of healthy aging.

As a result, higher adherence to the Mediterranean diet would be linked to longer telomere length because fruits, olive oil, vegetables, and nuts—essential components of the Mediterranean diet—have well-known antioxidant and anti-inflammatory effects. Therefore, the primary goal of the Nurses' Health Study cohort was to investigate the relationship between higher Mediterranean diet adherence and leukocyte telomere length in US women. This study also looked at the relationship between leukocyte telomere length comparing various dietary patterns (prudent pattern, Western pattern, and Alternative Healthy Eating Index).

Higher scores on the Mediterranean diet, as determined by food frequency questionnaires, were linked to longer leukocyte telomere length in 4676 healthy women aged 42–70. Notably, while a higher Alternate Mediterranean Diet score was significantly associated with longer leukocyte telomere length, none of the individual components showed any association with leukocyte telomere length, underlines the significance of looking at the relationship between dietary patterns and health in addition to individual dietary factors. This shows that the association might be a result of the Mediterranean diet's overall impact. Longer telomere length was also linked to the Alternative Healthy Eating Index; however, the largest correlation was found among women who adhered more closely to the Mediterranean diet [7].

Similarly, Canudas et al. showed that higher adherence to a Mediterranean diet was linked to longer leukocyte telomere length and higher peripheral blood mononuclear cell telomerase activity in 217 men and women aged 71–87 years [8].

Several studies have shown that the Mediterranean diet may have a protective antioxidant and anti-inflammatory effect on telomeres. In the study of Marin et al., the serum of 20 elderly subjects (age >65 years; 10 men and 10 women) was collected before and after they randomly followed each of the following diets for 4 weeks: a Mediterranean diet, a saturated fatty acid diet, and a low fat–high carbohydrate diet [9]. This study sought to determine whether the Mediterranean diet could delay endothelial cellular senescence by controlling oxidative stress. Incubation of human endothelial cells with serum collected after consuming the Mediterranean diet resulted in decreased intracellular ROS, unavoidable byproducts of aerobic metabolism, and a smaller percentage of cells with telomere shortening than baseline and the two other intervention diets. The findings, according to the authors, may have been influenced by antioxidant-rich foods found in the Mediterranean diet.

In 2015, a study followed a group of people with a high risk of cardiovascular disease, discovering a direct correlation between telomere shortening and the pro-inflammatory capability of the diet. After a five-year follow-up period, the diets with the higher pro-inflammatory scores were linked to a higher chance of having shorter telomeres and a two-fold risk of accelerated telomere shortening. Tumor necrosis factor-alpha (TNF), a pro-inflammatory factor, causes human leukemic cells to enter a senescent state at the molecular level. This state was characterized by a prolonged growth arrest, elevated beta-galactosidase activity, activated cyclin-dependent kinase inhibitor 1 (p21), decreased telomerase activity, telomeric activity, telomeric disturbances, such as shortening, losses, and fusions as well as additional chromosomal aberrations. These findings suggest that TNF modifies telomere maintenance. **Additionally, individuals who followed completely the Mediterranean diet had lower plasmatic levels of the inflammatory markers C-reactive protein (CRP), interleukin 6 (IL-6), TNF, and nitrotyrosine.**

The Mediterranean diet may protect telomere stability by reducing oxidative stress and inflammation, which are known to speed up the telomere attrition (or telomere shortening) rate.

Even though a healthy diet may generally have a good impact on telomeres, it appears that the advantage may be diminished in some people with particular genetic backgrounds. For instance, it has been demonstrated that the Mediterranean diet interacts with the rs1800629 polymorphism at the TNF gene to modify triglyceride metabolism and inflammatory status in patients with metabolic syndrome [2]. In comparison to patients with the GA or AA alleles, patients with the GG alleles showed increased fasting and postprandial triglyceride and C-reactive protein plasma levels at baseline. However, after following the Mediterranean diet for a year, the differences between the polymorphisms seen at baseline disappeared indicating that the GG carriers were extremely sensitive to this particular diet. **Recognizing the function of gene-diet connections may be an effective method for treating particular illnesses such as metabolic syndrome with individualized care.**

5.5 Particular Food Group Impact on Telomere Length

According to studies, telomere length is positively associated with the consumption of legumes, nuts, seaweed, fruits, 100% fruit juice, dairy products, and coffee; whereas, it is inversely associated with the consumption of alcohol, red meat, or processed meat [3]. Telomere attrition may represent a mechanism by which high sugar intake accelerates cardiometabolic disease. According to several studies, reducing the intake of sugary beverages may be associated with extended telomere length regardless of other factors like age, sex, or body mass index [3]. These findings suggest that the maintenance of leukocyte telomere length may be vulnerable to the long-term metabolic effects of high sugar intake.

Leung et al. examined the associations between the consumption of sugar-sweetened beverages (including soda, soft drinks, fruit-flavored drinks, sports drinks, and energy drinks), diet soda, and fruit juice, and leukocyte telomere length in 5309 American adults aged 20–65 years who had no prior history of diabetes or cardio-vascular disease [10]. After adjustment for sociodemographic and health-related characteristics, the consumption of sugar-sweetened beverages was associated with shorter telomeres; whereas, the consumption of 100% fruit juice was associated with a higher telomere length.

Due to the omega-3 PUFA content of fatty fish, a significant body of epidemiological research has demonstrated that fish consumption has a protective effect on chronic diseases involving systemic inflammation processes. It has probably been suggested that the anti-inflammatory characteristics of omega-3 PUFA, which are found in fish, may help maintain TL. There is evidence supporting the preventive activity of marine omega-3 PUFA against telomere attrition, even though the connection between diet rich in fish and TL is still unclear [2].

Numerous studies have shown that dietary fiber significantly affects aging and health. More specifically the risk of illness and early mortality decreases as fiber consumption increases. NHANES study, which was published in Nutrients in 2018, showed that 1 gram increase in fiber intake per 1000 kcal was linked to an increase in telomere length of 8.3 bases (human cells start at conception with an average telomere length of 15.000 base pairs – a unit of measurement of telomeres length, abbreviation bps), indicating a positive and linear association between the two variables [11]. Researchers noted that a 10-gram increase in fiber consumption per 1000 kcal would be equivalent to telomeres that were 83 base pairs longer corresponding to 5.4 fewer years of biological aging as each year of chronological age was related with a shortening of telomeres by 15.5 base pairs. It was also reported that even after the results were corrected for smoking, BMI, alcohol usage, and physical activity, each 10-gram increase in fiber per 1000 kcal corresponded to telomeres that were 67 base pairs longer leading to 4.3 fewer years of biological aging.

5.6 Nutrients and Telomere Length

Telomere length has been linked to nutritional status in both human and animal research indicating processes through which different nutrients may affect telomere length (Fig. 5.2).

5.6.1 Omega-3 Fatty Acids

High consumption of omega-3 fatty acids and more specifically docosahexaenoic acid and eicosapentaenoic acid have been found to be positively associated with decreased telomere length attrition in research subjects over a period of 5–8 years [12]. Plasma levels of omega-3 fatty acids are linked to low levels of pro-inflammatory indicators and high levels of anti-inflammatory markers. A diet rich in omega-3 fatty acids prolonged the life span of mice and improved the activity of the antioxidant enzymes catalase, glutathione peroxidase, and superoxide dismutase. Omega-3 fatty acids' anti-inflammatory and antioxidant effects have an impact on DNA damage, which may reduce telomere shortening [13].

5.6.2 Polyphenols

It has been suggested that polyphenols in tea and grape seeds contain anti-inflammatory and antioxidant properties. Biomarkers of inflammation are inversely correlated with tea consumption. Regular tea drinkers had longer telomeres than individuals who consume tea less frequently. When compared to the control group,

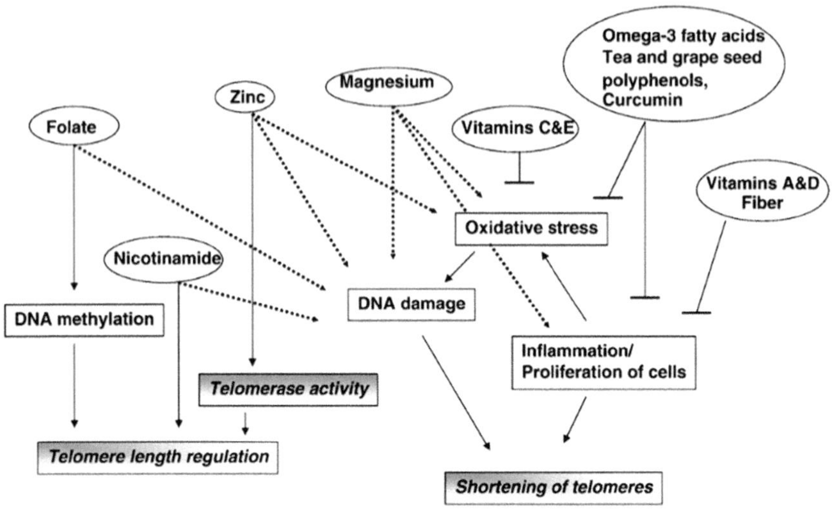

Figure 5.2 Possible pathways underlying how nutrients affect telomere length [13].

mice that consumed grape seed polyphenols showed a tendency toward having longer telomeres [14].

5.6.3 Curcumin

The anti-inflammatory compound curcumin increases the production of glutathione while decreasing the release of interleukin-8 and the stimulation of the nuclear transcription factor NF-kappa B. Studies in mice showed that a diet rich in curcumin resulted in reduced DNA damage and a tendency for longer telomeres [13].

5.7 Supplements and Telomere Length

5.7.1 Folate

Telomere length and plasma concentration of folate have been correlated in several studies on both genders. Folate is essential for maintaining DNA integrity and DNA methylation; two processes that affect telomere length. The average folate intake requirement is 250 μg/day in both genders [15].

Low folate availability leads to the incorrect inclusion of uracil in place of thymidine in DNA because folate serves as a precursor for the synthesis of thymidylate. Strand breaks are created in DNA when these uracil nucleotides are eliminated by excision repair enzymes. In the presence of folate deficiency, thymidine may be replaced by uracil resulting in telomeric DNA damage. As a result, short telomeres are caused by low folate nutritional status possibly as a result of DNA damage. Nucleotide pools in the cell would become unbalanced as a result of a folate deficiency. This imbalance has the ability to shorten telomeres and disrupt replication forks independently of DNA damage brought on by uracil misincorporation [13].

Low folate status is associated with genomic DNA hypomethylation. During low folate status in cell culture chromosome rearrangements have been observed. One of the ways that folate influences disease risk is through telomere dysfunction-induced genomic instability.

Folate supplementation can change DNA methylation and influence the expression of genes [16].

5.7.2 Vitamin B12

Despite the significance of vitamin B12 in producing methyl groups for methylation processes, neither vitamin B12 consumption nor plasma concentration has been linked to telomere length. However, compared to non-users, women who used vitamin B12 supplements had longer telomeres. The recommended intake of vitamin B12 is 4 μg/day for both genders (EFSA-dietary reference values), which may be more than 400 times higher in vitamin B12 supplements than in food or in multivitamins, which deliver higher amounts of this vitamin [15]. Due to its potent capabilities and ability to save the reactive oxygen species (ROS) scavenger glutathione, vitamin B12 helps lower oxidative stress. Additionally, supplements containing higher amounts of vitamin B12 can inhibit nitric oxide synthase and may decrease inflammation. Longer telomeres have been observed in people who took vitamin B12 supplements, which may be explained by the reduced oxidative stress and inflammation brought on by the high amount of vitamin B12 [13].

5.7.3 Vitamin A

The average vitamin A intake requirement is 490 μg/day for women and 570 μg/day for men [15]. Vitamin A deficiency exposes individuals to the risk of infections that might shorten telomeres. Vitamin A supplementation decreased the plasma concentration of the pro-inflammatory cytokine tumor necrosis factor-alpha and enhanced the plasma levels of the anti-inflammatory cytokine interleukin-10 in individuals with vitamin A insufficiency [13].

5.7.4 Vitamin D

The average vitamin D intake requirement is 15 μg/day for both genders [15]. According to Richards et al., there is a correlation between telomere length in women's peripheral leukocytes and serum vitamin D concentration [17]. Immunosuppressive characteristics can be found in 1,25 dihydroxyvitamin D3 (calcitriol), which is the physiologically active version of vitamin D. The inverse correlation between plasma vitamin D levels and the inflammatory marker CRP reflects this. The plasma levels of CRP are inversely linked with telomere length. The proliferation of lymphocytes is decreased when 1,25-dihydroxyvitamin D3 is added to the cell culture medium because it inhibits the expression of the growth factor granulocyte-macrocyte colony-stimulating factor, which is essential for the proliferation of all the lines of hematopoietic cells. The expression of the inflammatory mediators, interleukin-2 and interferon-gamma, is also decreased by vitamin D. Vitamin D's anti-inflammatory and anti-proliferative characteristics reduce cell turnover, which may slow the erosion of telomere length [16].

5.7.5 Vitamins C and E

It is well known that vitamins C and E have antioxidant properties. The average vitamin C requirement for women is 80 mg/day and for men 90 mg/day while the average intake for vitamin E is 11 mg/day for women and 13 mg/day for men [15]. In women, dietary or multivitamin intake of vitamins C and E is positively correlated with considerably longer telomeres. By introducing physiological amounts of vitamin C or E, age-dependent telomere shortening and a decline in telomerase activity can be slowed down and life span can be enhanced in cell cultures. Vitamin E's ability to scavenge ROS resulted in a decrease in ROS. This procedure might prevent telomeric DNA from suffering oxidative damage, which would otherwise result in telomere length reduction. Vitamin C's beneficial impact on telomere length may potentially result from a similar ROS scavenging mechanism [13].

5.7.6 Magnesium

Numerous enzymes, such as those responsible for DNA repair and RNA synthesis depend on magnesium for catalytic activity. The average magnesium intake for women is 300 mg/day and for men 350 mg/day [15]. Telomere length in women has been shown to be favorably correlated with dietary magnesium consumption. In animal and cell cultures, shortened telomeres appeared as a result of chronic magnesium deficiency. The increase in oxidative stress that occurs along with the reduction in telomere length following magnesium deficiency is another mechanism that contributes to telomere attrition. High levels of the inflammatory marker CRP are also correlated with low levels of serum magnesium. Another theory states that impaired genomic integrity results from magnesium ions' decreased availability. DNA polymerase needs to attach to magnesium ions to function effectively. Furthermore, chromosome abnormalities are brought on by magnesium deficiency resulting in reduced ability to repair DNA. Therefore, scientists speculate that magnesium in addition to its potential function in oxidative stress and inflammation regulates telomere length through impacting DNA integrity and repair [13].

5.7.7 Zinc

Reverse transcriptases, DNA polymerases, and RNA polymerases are a few of the cell's zinc-dependent enzymes. Reverse transcriptase telomerase's activity is increased by adding more zinc to the culture medium [18]. The DNA repair enzyme poly (ADP-ribose) polymerase requires zinc to be activated at DNA damage sites. Zinc deficiency has been linked to DNA damage, which is associated with critically shorter telomeres. Moreover, zinc offers protection against oxidative stress. Although zinc is not directly involved in neutralizing ROS, zinc deficiency has been linked to oxidative damage. The average zinc intake requirement for women is 7.6 mg/day and for men is 9.3 mg/day [15]. Zinc supplementation has been shown to reduce inflammation and oxidative stress. Also, taking zinc supplements reduces the risk of infection, which is another condition responsible for telomere attrition. As a result, zinc may have an important impact on telomere length through the ability to regulate telomerase activity, DNA stability, oxidative stress, and infection susceptibility [13].

5.7.8 Iron

As opposed to other nutrient supplements, iron supplementation is strongly associated with shorter telomeres [19]. Iron binds to cysteine residues in proteins to create hydroxyl free radicals. The ability of iron to produce free radicals may be the cause of the shortened telomeres observed in those who take iron supplements. The average daily iron intake requirement is 7 mg/day in women and 6 mg/day in men [15].

5.7.9 Nicotinamide

Nicotinamide supplementation reduces telomere attrition while enhancing the ability of human fibroblasts to replicate in culture. The precursor for poly (ADP-ribose) polymerases (PARPs) to synthesize poly (ADP-ribose) onto acceptor proteins is nicotinamide adenine dinucleotide. The function of the acceptor proteins, which are mostly involved in nucleic acid metabolism, DNA repair, and chromosome integrity maintenance, is modulated by the addition of negatively charged ADP-ribose polymers by PARP. In reaction to DNA damage, nicotinamide adenine dinucleotide is used more frequently, increasing the activity of PARPs and the production of poly (ADP-ribose). The prevalence of micronuclei in lymphocytes, a sign of genetic instability, is inversely correlated with nicotinamide consumption. Because PARPs are involved in telomere extension nicotinamide may also have an impact on telomere length. The ADP-ribosylation of telomere repeat binding factor-1, a negative regulator of telomere elongation, causes telomere length to be positively controlled by the PARPs tankyrases 1 and 2. Even while telomere repeat binding factor-2's ADP-ribosylation does not affect telomere length, it is crucial for preserving telomere integrity. Since nicotinamide itself has no antioxidant characteristic, it is likely that the way in which the addition of nicotinamide reduced telomere attrition also affected cellular components that are involved in reducing ROS production. As a result, nicotinamide may affect telomere length via various mechanisms involving DNA stability and telomere length regulation via PARPs [13].

5.7.10 Spermidine

Spermidine, a naturally occurring polyamine has been found to improve the lifespan of worms, flies, and mice [20]. In both animal and human models, endogenous spermidine levels decrease with aging. Spermidine action has been connected to the control of reactive oxygen species, DNA replication, transcription and translation, anti-inflammatory effects, mitochondrial function, proteostasis, increased hypusination, and induction of autophagy. Moreover, research in aging mice has demonstrated that spermidine treatment not only increases lifespan but also has cardioprotective effects as well as protective effects on the synaptic and mitochondrial status of aging animals [21]. The exact methods by which spermidine supplementation could prevent telomere erosion are still unknown [22].

5.8 Discussion

A major public health priority today more than ever is highlighting methods to combat age-related disorders. We examined information from recently released research investigating the impact of lifestyle factors such as diet on one of the most significant markers of aging: the telomere length.

Most of the research shows a significant impact of nutrition on the rate of biological aging. In fact, a balanced diet that prioritizes dietary fiber and unsaturated fats has been shown to protect telomere health; whereas, a diet high in sugar and saturated fats has been shown to accelerate telomere attrition. Since longer telomeres relate to antioxidant and anti-inflammatory properties of foods, these effects are probably mediated by oxidative stress and inflammation.

In children and adolescents, a longer TL was associated with an increased intake of fruits and vegetables, nuts and seeds, fish, olives, and legumes. Risk factors for TL shortening at these ages included a larger intake of dairy products, sugar, cereals, white bread, and a diet with a high glycemic load. Although the information from other studies suggests that the evidence in this area is still unclear, these limited results are consistent with earlier studies conducted in other adult populations. Therefore, there is a need for additional research to identify potential nutritional factors influencing TL in childhood and adolescence, preferably from longitudinal studies and randomized controlled trials.

Numerous nutrients have a serious impact on telomere length through mechanisms related to their participation in cellular processes, such as DNA methylation, inflammation, oxidative stress, and activity of the enzyme telomerase, which contributes to the addition of telomeric repeats. Telomeric repeat attrition is a result of additional cell divisions brought on by inflammatory mechanisms that accelerate cell turnover. Telomeres shorten as a result of damage to telomeric DNA brought on by oxidative stress or decreased availability of nucleotide precursors. As a result, nutrients with anti-inflammatory and antioxidant properties can slow telomere degradation. The regulation of telomere length may also be influenced by nutrients, such as folate, vitamins A, D, C, E, nicotinamide, spermidine, and more.

We suggest that maintaining a healthy diet is an effective way to protect telomere maintenance and lengthen life expectancy.

However, further research is required to fully comprehend how various diets and particular foods affect biological aging to create effective dietary plans tailored to diverse populations.

References

1. MacNee, W., Rabinovich, R. A., Choudhury, G. (2014). Ageing and the border between health and disease, *Eur. Respir. J.*, **44**, pp. 1332–52.
2. Valera-Gran, D., Prieto-Botella, D., Hurtado-Pomares, M., Baladia, E., Petermann-Rocha, F., Sánchez-Pérez, A., *et al.* (2022). The impact of foods, nutrients, or dietary patterns on telomere length in childhood and adolescence: a systematic review, *Nutrients*, **14**, pp. 3885.
3. Balan, E., Decottignies, A., Deldicque, L. (2018). Physical activity and nutrition: two promising strategies for telomere maintenance? *Nutrients*, **10**, pp. 1942.
4. Meshkani, S. E., Kooshki, A., Alahabadi, A., *et al.* (2021). Dietary pattern and telomere length in preschool children in a middle-income country, *Matern. Child. Nutr.*, **17**, pp. e13146.
5. García-Calzón, S., Martínez-González, M. A., Razquin, C., Arós, F., Lapetra, J., Martínez, J. A., *et al.* (2016). Mediterranean diet and telomere length in high cardiovascular risk subjects from the PREDIMED-NAVARRA study, *Clin. Nutr.*, **35**, pp. 1399–1405.
6. Lee, J. Y., Jun, N. R., Yoon, D., Shin, C., Baik, I. (2015). Association between dietary patterns in the remote past and telomere length, *Eur. J. Clin. Nutr.*, **69**, pp. 1048–52.
7. Crous-Bou, M., Fung, T. T., Prescott, J., Julin, B., Du, M., Sun, Q., *et al.* (2014). Mediterranean diet and telomere length in Nurses' Health Study: population-based cohort study, *BMJ*, **349**, pp. 6674.
8. Canudas, S., Becerra-Tomás, N., Hernández-Alonso, P., Galié, S., Leung, C., Crous-Bou, M. *et al.* (2020). Mediterranean diet and telomere length: a systematic review and meta-analysis, *Advances in Nutrition*, **11**, pp. 1544–1554.
9. Marin, C., Delgado-Lista, J., Ramirez, R., Carracedo, J., Caballero, J., Perez-Martinez, P., *et al.* (2012). Mediterranean diet reduces senescence-associated stress in endothelial cells, *Age (Dordr)*, **34**, pp. 1309–16.
10. Leung, C. W., Laraia, B. A., Needham, B. L., Rehkopf, D. H., Adler, N. E., Lin, J., *et al.* (2014). Soda and cell aging: associations between sugar-sweetened beverage consumption and leukocyte telomere length in healthy adults from the National Health and Nutrition Examination Surveys, *Am. J. Public Health,* **104**, pp. 2425–31.
11. Tucker, L. A. (2018). Dietary fiber and telomere length in 5674 U.S. adults: an NHANES study of biological aging, *Nutrients*, **10**, pp. 400.

12. Farzaneh-Far, R., Lin, J., Epel, E. S., Harris, W. S., Blackburn, E. H., Whooley, M. A. (2010). Association of marine omega-3 fatty acid levels with telomeric aging in patients with coronary heart disease, *JAMA*, **303**, pp. 250–7.
13. Ligi, Paul. (2011). Diet, nutrition and telomere length, *J Nutr Biochem.* **22**, pp. 895–901.
14. Galilea-Zabalza, I., Buil-Cosiales, P., Salas-Salvadó, J., Toledo, E., Ortega-Azorín, C., Díez-Espino, J., *et al*; PREDIMED-PLUS Study Investigators. (2018). Mediterranean diet and quality of life: baseline cross-sectional analysis of the PREDIMED-PLUS trial, *PLoS One*, **13**, pp. e0198974.
15. European Food Safety Authority – EFSA. Dietary reference values. (2019). https://multimedia.efsa.europa.eu/drvs/index.htm.
16. Galiè, S., Canudas, S., Muralidharan, J., García-Gavilán, J., Bulló, M., Salas-Salvadó, J. (2020). Impact of nutrition on telomere health: systematic review of observational cohort studies and randomized clinical trials, *Adv Nutr.*, **11**, pp. 576–601.
17. Valdes, A. M., Richards, J. B., Gardner, J. P., Swaminathan, R., Kimura, M., Xiaobin, L., *et al.* (2007). Telomere length in leukocytes correlates with bone mineral density and is shorter in women with osteoporosis, *Osteoporos Int.*, **18**, pp. 1203–10.
18. Sharif, R., Thomas, P., Zalewski, P., Fenech, M. (2015). Zinc supplementation influences genomic stability biomarkers, antioxidant activity, and zinc transporter genes in an elderly Australian population with low zinc status, *Mol. Nutr. Food Res.*, **59**, pp. 1200–12.
19. Liu, B., Sun, Y., Xu, G., Snetselaar, L. G., Ludewig, G., Wallace, R. B., *et al.* (2019). Association between body iron status and leukocyte telomere length, a biomarker of biological aging, in a nationally representative sample of US adults, *Journal of the Academy of Nutrition and Dietetics*, **119**, pp. 617–625, ISSN 2212–2672.
20. Wirth, A., Wolf, B., Huang, C. K., Glage, S., Hofer, S. J., Bankstahl, M., *et al.* (2021). Novel aspects of age-protection by spermidine supplementation are associated with preserved telomere length, *Geroscience*, **43**, pp. 673–690.
21. Ni, Y. Q., Liu, Y. S. (2021). New insights into the roles and mechanisms of spermidine in aging and age-related diseases, *Aging Dis.*, **12**, pp. 1948–1963.
22. Madeo, F., Carmona-Gutierrez, D., Keep, O., Kroemer, G. (2018). Spermidine delays aging in humans, *Aging (Albany NY)*, **10**, pp. 2209–2211.

Chapter 6

The First Steps toward Balanced Eating

Evangelos Zoumpaneas
Founder, diatrofi.gr
Master Practitioner in Eating Disorders & Obesity, www.keadd.gr
CEO, Eating Disorders Education & Treatment Center, Nea Ionia, Athens, Greece
diatrofioe@gmail.com

6.1 A True Story About Surviving the Day

Since the past centuries, scientists have come across a big puzzlement. They wondered why the primitive people would regularly leave their safe caves to venture outside into the dangerous jungle and hunt occasionally even very large animals, like the humungous mammoths.

In the following characteristic image of a rock inscription, there is a depiction of such a hunting scene, next to the 1870 painting of Ernest Griset with a similar theme (Fig. 6.1).

Imagine, if you may, a group of 30 primitive hunters devising plans of attack to get hold of the giant mammoth, which might even weigh 10 tons. The project was, for sure, a difficult one, and by the time they killed it, they could have lost half the men in the process. However, that same night, the ones who had survived were back in

Telomeres: Biomarkers of a Healthy Life and Successful Aging
Edited by Aristidis Tsatsakis

ISBN 978-981-5129-49-6 (Hardcover), 978-1-003-56809-4 (eBook)
www.jennystanford.com

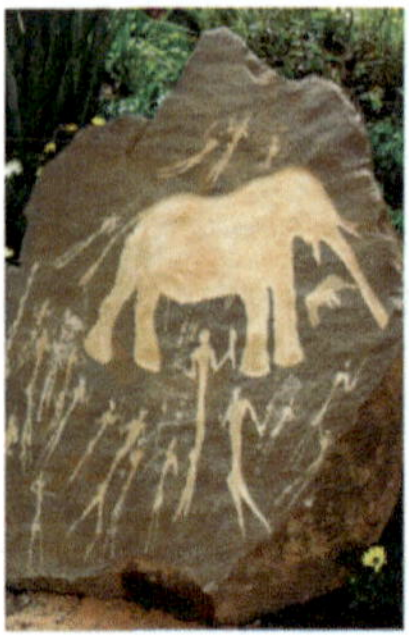

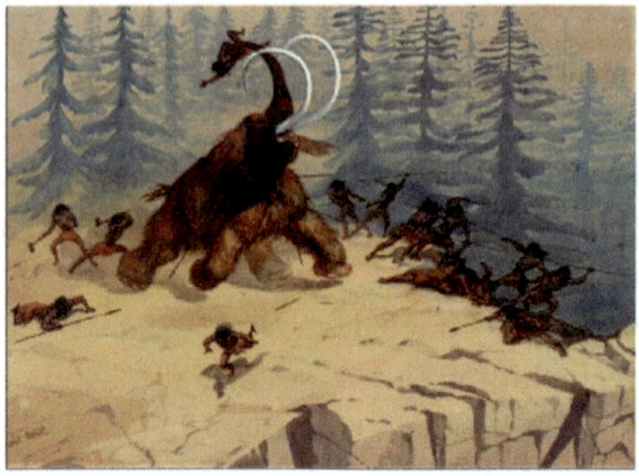

Figure 6.1 Example of hunting scenes. Rock inscription of a hunting scene. Ernest Griset's painting of a hunting scene.

their safe caves with plenty of meat for themselves and their women and children. That quiet night, they would all eat well sitting around the fire, until the dawn of the next hunting day. . .

The big question that troubled the first scientists was exactly that: why would the primitive people put their own lives in danger in search of meat, when they could have survived on the mere collection of fruits, nuts, and vegetables, as monkeys did?

6.2 The Protein-Eating Humans

The answer was soon discovered. Humans are basically protein eaters. We need animal-based proteins for the following basic daily functions:

1. To renew all damaged cells and make new ones, restore damaged muscle groups, and constantly replenish calcium for the bones and other things. Our bodies renew almost all their cells every three years. We can proudly assume that every three years, we are brand new from head to toe.
2. To replenish the blood supply by creating new blood. When we donate blood to a fellow human being, we are instructed at the end that, if we wish to repeat this wonderful act, we will have to wait patiently for about 4–6 months until our body manages to remake the blood that was given.

3. To constantly produce antibodies in order to protect ourselves from various infections as well as any external viruses.
4. To constantly renew the production of all the necessary hormones for the proper function of our organisms, such as those of the thyroid and the brain, and to produce special hormones for the effective management of daily stressors, such as the hormones of adrenaline and cortisol.

All of the above are part of the protein-based functions of our body, which require adequate amounts of animal-based protein foods daily for the time-effective completion of those functions.

But what does it mean for the human body to have adequate proteins from animal sources, so as to manage the demanding task of homeostasis day in and day out?

For example, if a person consumes a glass of milk for breakfast, a steak for lunch, and a piece of cheese for dinner, then he will have covered, for the most part, their protein needs for the day (Fig. 6.2)

For the sake of simplicity, from now on, we will name this category of animal-based protein foods "animal proteins." But what will happen, if someday someone misses their protein portion like many people who begin their day in haste without breakfast?

If we take a closer look at the meat of a steak, we will notice that it is formed by very small fibers looking like thick lines, which are piling up parallel to each other. The meat of the steak we eat is nothing other than the muscle of an animal, due to its fibrous nature, is called "striated muscle." Similar striated muscles are found in the human body.

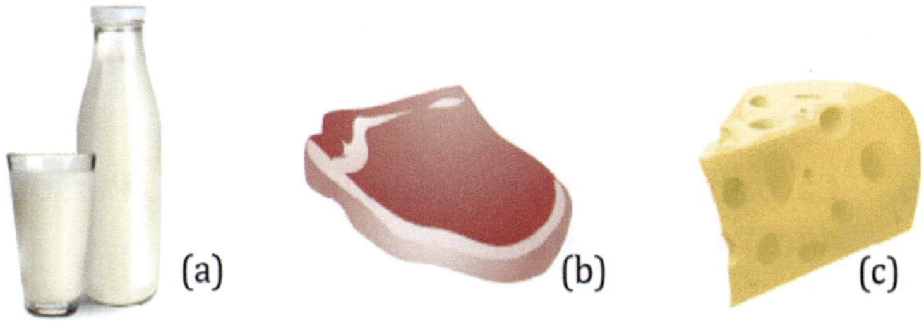

Figure 6.2 Examples of protein-containing food to fulfill our protein needs during the day: a glass of milk (a), and a steak (b), a piece of cheese (c).

When our daily diet does not contain adequate amounts of animal-based proteins, which will provide our body with the necessary amount of protein, something incredible will happen. Our body will use a small piece of its muscles — like burning a small muscle fiber to perform different functions, i.e., producing new blood, antibodies, and hormones — and cell renewal will take place at a later stage. That day somehow, we will have aged a day.

If the inadequacy in animal protein intake continues for long, it will soon exhaust a substantial part of our muscle tissue, and the consequences of this will be sagging muscles. Moreover, more negative functions will take place, like anemia, the exhaustion of our immune system, and the disruption of the harmonic production of hormones with first and foremost the deregulation of the thyroid gland.

An added consequence of the prolonged inadequacy of protein intake will be the decrease of basic metabolism because the thyroid will significantly decrease our daily needs in calories to prevent the abrupt and damaging degradation of muscle tissue. The results will show that we begin to put on weight despite consuming fewer calories.

But what does a portion of protein mean for each person? Is it, for example, a small pork steak or a whole piglet?

There are several smart ways in which someone can estimate the portions of various foods, and there are abundant examples on the internet. Depending on the body structure of each person and his daily activities, people will have different needs in the amounts of nutrients from various food groups, but this will be further analyzed later. For the time being, I want the reader to understand the basic steps, which will lead you to manage your daily diet.

6.3 Carbohydrate-Dependent Industrious Person and Thinking Brain

Often in my lectures, and particularly so, when I speak to parents, toward the end of my presentation, I ask them to give me an answer to the following dilemma:

If, for some reason, a child had to choose just one type of food among a steak, potatoes, and salad, which one would I encourage them to choose? Most people respond, "the salad." However, those who paid close attention to my presentation responded correctly to the steak.

The adequacy of protein intake is the first and foremost important element in the conservation and survival of the human organism. Once the body has secured its protein needs, then what it needs next is the proper groups of food, which will give it the energy to move, think, and realize anything else that requires physical activity.

Beyond the needs for movement which require muscle activity, even internal vital functions (like breathing, heart beating, and thinking) require their smaller or bigger energy fuel represented in the glorious molecule of glucose.

The availability of glucose depends directly on the adequate daily consumption of foods, which contain what we all know as carbohydrates. Familiar foods that contain these great nutrients are cereal, pulses, starchy vegetables, dairy products, and fruits. Let's see now how we can add our carbohydrates, which, for the sake of simplicity, will be named "starch."

Next to a glass of milk, a portion of cereal could be added for breakfast (Fig. 6.3).

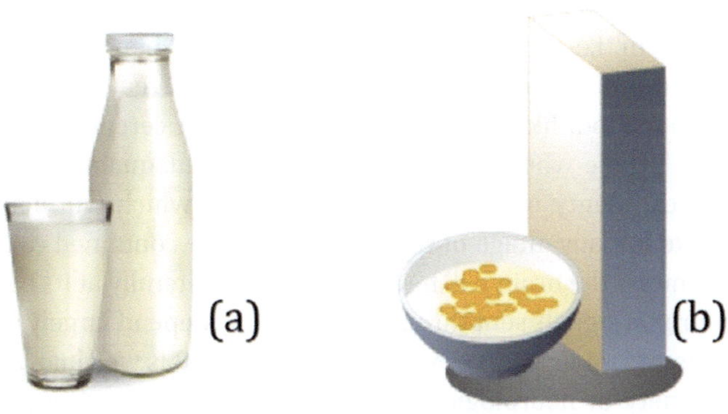

Figure 6.3 Example of foods combining protein with carbohydrates in order to create our breakfast: milk (a) and a portion of cereal (b).

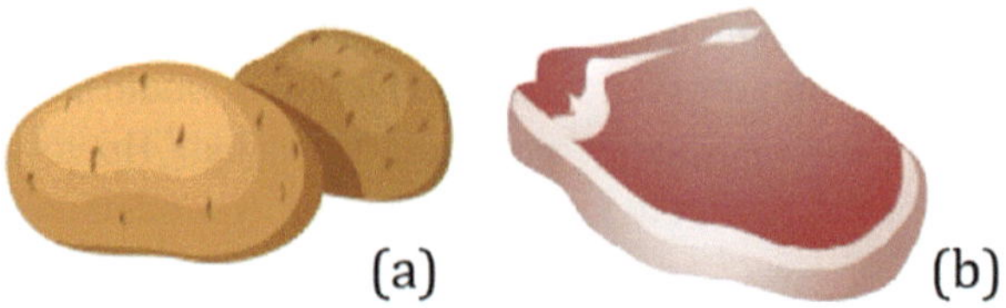

Figure 6.4 Example of foods combining protein with carbohydrates to create our lunch: a portion of potatoes (a) and a steak (b).

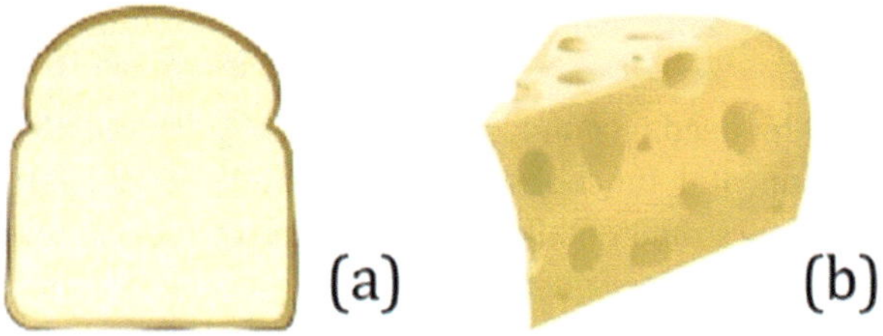

Figure 6.5 Example of foods combining protein with carbohydrates in order to create our dinner: a toast (a) and a piece of cheese (b).

The steak could be combined with a portion of potatoes for lunch (Fig. 6.4).

Cheese could be combined with a barley rusk or two slices of bread for dinner (Fig. 6.5).

Thus, we succeeded in adding a good source of "starch" to all our meals.

If we try to add portions of "starch" as close as possible to their natural form, i.e., not much processed, then the benefits multiply. Even more so, when it comes to products of cereal flours, if we choose our food, like bread, pasta, or breakfast cereal to be what is called "whole wheat," we will have secured adequacy in vitamin B complex, plenty of minerals, and nutrients, which will help the body take full advantage of the energy from the contained calories. Furthermore, the brain will be able to function literally at its best, as the neuronal signals sent throughout the body depend largely on the vitamins and minerals from whole wheat cereal. It is well known that for a variety of neurological problems often diagnosed in people, as well as for mental illnesses, among the first aids subscribed to patients are supplements based on B complex vitamins. The adequate consumption of the appropriate sources of "starch" surely functions as the best shield against such illnesses.

Without a doubt, it is the whole wheat cereal along with fruits and vegetables that provide us with the precious microscopic but miraculous dietary fibers that help our body discard anything unnecessary and useless through the regular bowel movement.

6.4 Beauty and Youth Are Multi-Vitamin-Based

If someone asks about the secret of remaining young and beautiful-looking, there is only one answer ready to spring out: fresh fruits and vegetables. And that is well said. Because beauty and youthful looks do not come alone. They need to walk on endless carpets of deep red, bright yellow, all green, orange, and many other multicolored fresh fruits and vegetables that only nature knows how to abundantly offer at the altar of radiance and charm. For the sake of simplicity, we will from now on call the category of fresh fruits and vegetables "the fresh."

Vitamins, minerals, and all sorts of antioxidants contained within fruits and vegetables will complete our story. This is, anyway, what we have been trying to get at, what is rightly called "a full meal."

So, let's see how we can nicely match them all together.

Next to the glass of milk and our breakfast cereal, we could add an apple (Fig. 6.6).

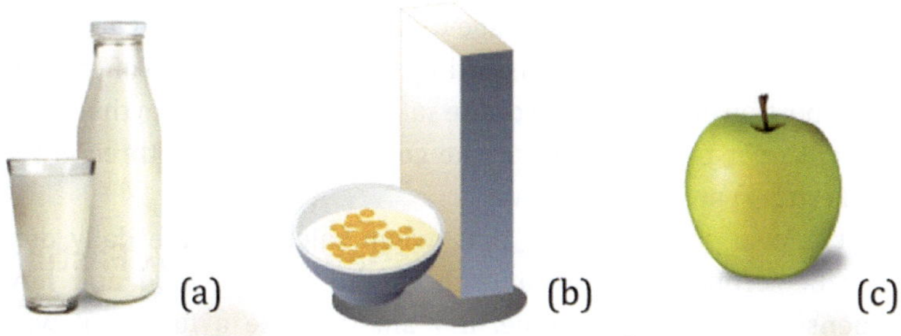

Figure 6.6 Example of combining fresh fruit in our breakfast to absorb our vitamins, minerals, and antioxidants: a glass of milk (a), a portion of cereal (b), and an apple (c).

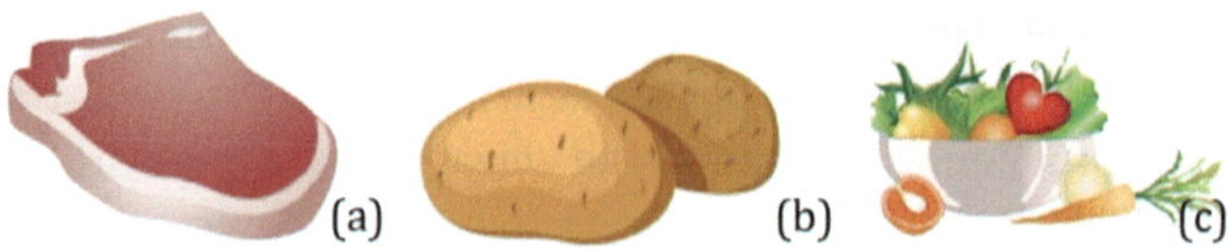

Figure 6.7 Example of combining fresh salad in our lunch in order to absorb our vitamins and antioxidants: a steak (a), a portion of potatoes (b), and a colorful salad (c).

Figure 6.8 Example of combining fresh vegetables in our dinner to absorb our vitamins, minerals, and antioxidants: a piece of cheese (a), a slice of bread (b), and a tomato (c).

With our steak and potatoes, we could match a colorful salad (Fig. 6.7).

And next to our cheese and bread, we could add a tomato (Fig. 6.8).

6.5 A Triad in Your Meal

As we will see next, which foods you will put together does not really matter. It is important to manage to include all three food groups in every basic or full meal, i.e., a portion of protein, a portion of "starch," and a portion of fresh food. For the sake of simplicity, from this point, we will refer to "full meal" as the combination of the three group foods (triad) mentioned above.

It is also good to know that, when calculating the daily diet, it is of secondary significance both the kind of food and how expensive it is. For example, if I am to make a full meal with shrimp (animal food), quinoa cereal from Latin America (starch), and brussels sprouts (fresh), the cost of my meal goes up to 50 euros, a cheaper alternative would be sardine (animal food), rusk (starch), and tomato (fresh), which will cost 2 euros, and there will be no difference at all for the body. For the human organism, what matters is that after the food has been broken down into its basic elements reaching the small intestine, proteins, carbohydrates, fat, vitamins, and minerals will be recognized and absorbed for the maintenance of homeostasis.

6.6 Management of Hunger Requires a Strategic Plan

If there have ever been times during which you feel like a wild animal that wants to devour whatever it may come across, but somewhere at a corner of your brain there is an urge not to do it, then the following paragraph will help you understand which factors create this situation, and how you may manage such difficult cases.

First, we may start with the simple notion that, even if there was nothing for you to eat at a certain time, you are not about to die, since you live in some part of the so-called modern western world. The abundance of food you had at your disposition the previous days, months, and years, can sustain you for about 7–10 days for every kilogram of fat in you. Imagine that, if you have 10 kg more than the normal range, these may suffice to survive for about three months, and this is something to consider regarding your body's capabilities.

The second important fact that you need to keep in mind is that, if the human organism remains without food for more than 4 hours, what will be affected is not primarily the basic body functions, but mainly the functioning of the brain. Imagine that under such conditions, you function as an animal which, upon waking up in the morning, the first thing it wants to do is search for food. If time passes and the animal cannot find food, it starts to become angry and, when it finally finds some, it devours it like a wild beast having as much of it as possible. Humans, being creatures of the same natural environment such as animals, may well react in a similar manner under conditions of prolonged hunger.

The human brain uses all the glucose reserves available in the blood every 4 hours or so. Then, in order to find alternative sources of energy, it sends a message to the liver ordering it: "Send glucose now…". The liver, being itself a docile organ, starts immediately a process called "gluconeogenesis." The body's demand for glucose is met through this biochemical process when the carbohydrate intake is inadequate.

Studies have shown that, under conditions of scarcity in glucose, the brain's ability to handle situations, such as making the right choices, dealing with stress, and memorizing a paragraph, is as high as having to do similar activities, while having a severe headache.

But from the moment the brain sends out the specific order for glucose production, it has already experienced a severe condition of stress. You must never forget that your body functions mainly with its basic survival instincts. At any time, during which the body experiences the ultimate hunger, it cannot know that you have money in your pocket to buy food at a given chance, or that upon returning home after many working hours, there will be a plate of food set on the table for you. For every second that goes by, the brain interprets the absence of available energy as a condition of starvation. The sensation of starvation and uncontrollable hunger becomes second to the sensation of imminent danger from external attacks, the most stressful situation it may experience. Besides, the condition of death from starvation is registered deeply inside the human DNA. Every form of intense hunger is experienced by humans as a close or remote chance that they may cease to exist. Therefore, we could rightly accept that in extreme conditions of biological hunger, we would attempt to fill up our stomachs with as much food as we could possibly fit. Furthermore, under such conditions, the sense of having filled up the stomach will not result from quietly chewing the food, but rather from quickly swallowing it. This is so because the alleged threat that denied us the food so far may also contain further danger to our physical safety. We will consume very fast all we can, and we will seek a place to hide and digest. The devouring of the food is also a process deeply ingrained in our DNA.

The difference between humans and other animals in the handling of hunger is that humans can predict situations. The timely and appropriate meals that cover the necessary variety of nutrients are our unique weapon in coming out victorious against our hunger.

The knowledge of how the fundamental biochemical mechanisms in the body work as well as the amounts and kinds of nutrients we need in our daily diet may help us secure better quality in our life and respond optimally to our daily needs and hassles.

6.7 Right Snacks at the Right Moment

The human brain, as I explained earlier, consumes approximately every 4 hours all reserves of glucose available in the blood. So, before the completion of those 4 hours, one must ensure that the brain still has energy reserves, so when the time for the next basic meal comes, one will have the ability to handle appropriately their hunger.

There are hours after a 3-course meal, you will need a smaller meal in a combination of two, a dyad.

You will need:

a. A small portion of fruit whether fresh or dried; for example, a small apple, a pear, two dried fruits, a prune, a spoonful of raisins, blueberries, etc., immediately provides the brain with an excellent source of glucose (Fig. 6.9).
b. At the same time, a small portion of a snack that contains adequate plant fibers, such as a spoonful of dried nuts (almonds, walnuts, or other combinations) or a small cereal snack bar, snack bar with dried nuts, a digestive biscuit, a small cookie, a whole wheat breadstick, and so on (Fig. 6.10).

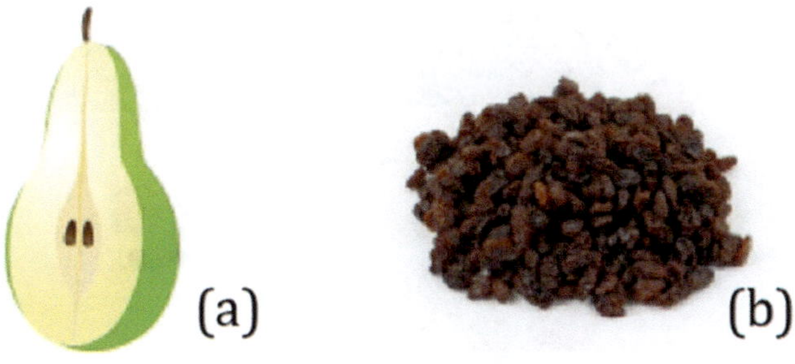

Figure 6.9 Example of fresh or dried fruit: a pear (a) and a spoonful of raisins (b).

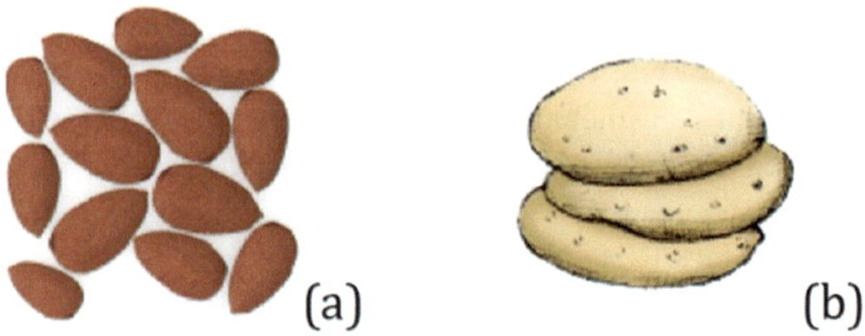

Figure 6.10 Example of snacks that contain adequate plant fibers: almonds (a) and digestive biscuits (b).

The plant fibers contained in these food combinations will help the body manage better the glucose received from the fresh or dried fruits, to avoid big fluctuations in the blood sugar concentration. From this point, for the sake of simplicity, we will refer to every small intermediate meal as a "dyad" (two foods). A fruit and a snack, in other words, are the inseparable allies against hunger.

An excellent example of a dyad is a mixture of dried nuts and fruits, as shown below, which includes raw, unsalted almonds, walnuts, cashews, raisins, or a snack bar made of dried nuts, cereal, and dried fruits (Fig. 6.11).

The more plant fibers contained within this small, intermediate meal, the more feeling of satiation will last because the body will manage to keep the blood sugar levels stable for the next 2–3 hours

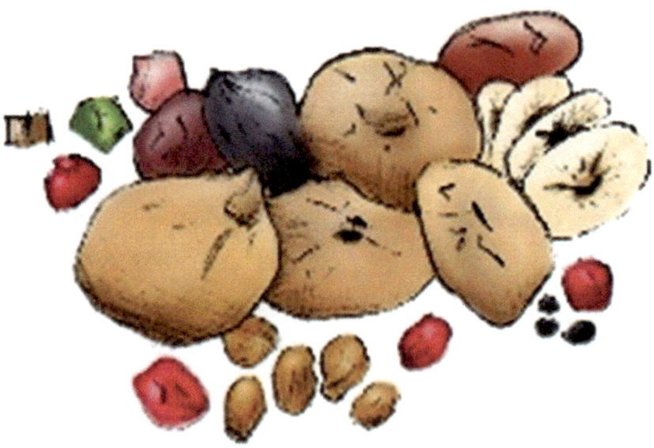

Figure 6.11 Example of a snack using a dyad: nuts with dried fruits.

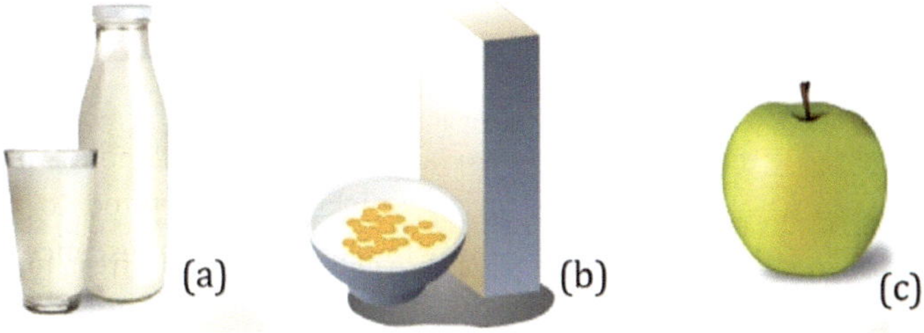

Figure 6.12 Example of breakfast using a triad that contains protein, starch, and fresh food: a glass of milk (a), a portion of cereal (b), and an apple (c).

until you consume either your next basic meal (your triad) or your next small snack (your dyad).

6.8 Scheduling the Daily Diet

The first thing you ought to think about, before you start planning your daily diet, is to organize in terms of time your basic meals for the day.

To make things easy, let's use as examples the meals pictured above. Next, many more alternative ideas and solutions for food combinations will be suggested, so that you will have at your disposal many tastier and nutritional suggestions.

For example, your "morning triad" consists of milk as animal-based protein, cereal as starch, and an apple as fresh food, that you have your breakfast at 8 am (Fig. 6.12).

Let us assume that your "lunch triad" consists of a steak as animal-based protein, a potato as starch, and a bowl of salad as fresh food, which you take your lunch at 2 pm (Fig. 6.13).

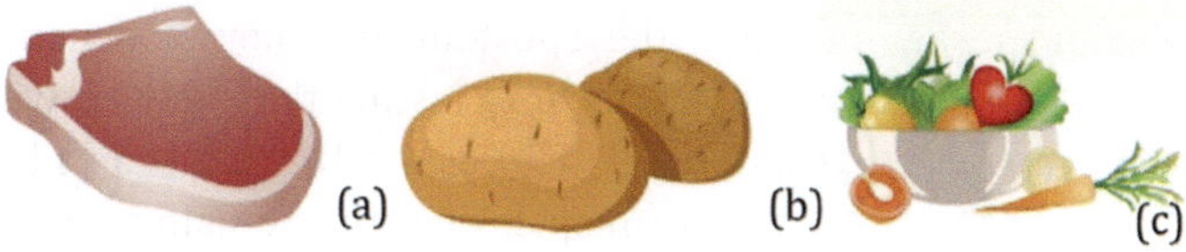

Figure 6.13 Example of lunch-containing protein, starch, and fresh food: a steak (a), a portion of potatoes (b), and a fresh colorful salad (c).

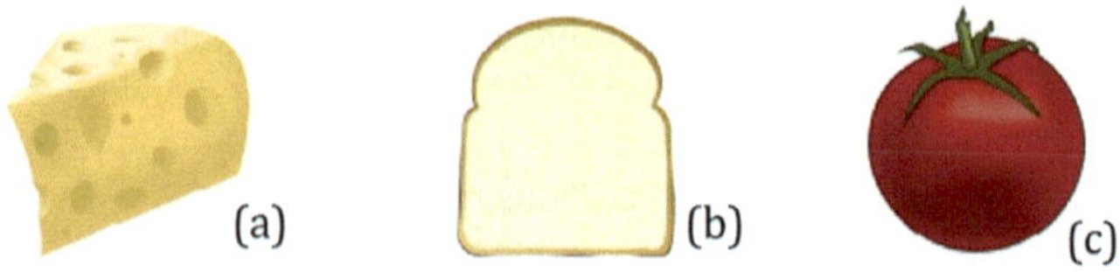

Figure 6.14 Example of dinner using a triad that contains protein, starch, and fresh food: a piece of cheese (a), a slice of bread (b), and a fresh tomato (c).

Finally, your "dinner triad" consists of cheese as animal-based protein, bread as starch, and a tomato as fresh food, that you have your dinner at 10 pm (Fig. 6.14).

6.9 Finding the Right Time for Your Brunch

Using as a starting point, your first meal for the day, scheduled for 8 am, you calculate that in 3 hours, you will need the first small intermediate meal, the so-called brunch. The ideal time for it will be at (8 + 3 =) 11 am. At that time, you will need to eat a dyad, which means a small portion of fresh food and a small snack; for example, as a dyad, you may have a pear and a spoonful of almonds at 11 am (Fig. 6.15).

Starting at 11 am, another snack might be needed before lunch. Therefore, we calculate 11 am + 3 hours = 2 pm. However, this is

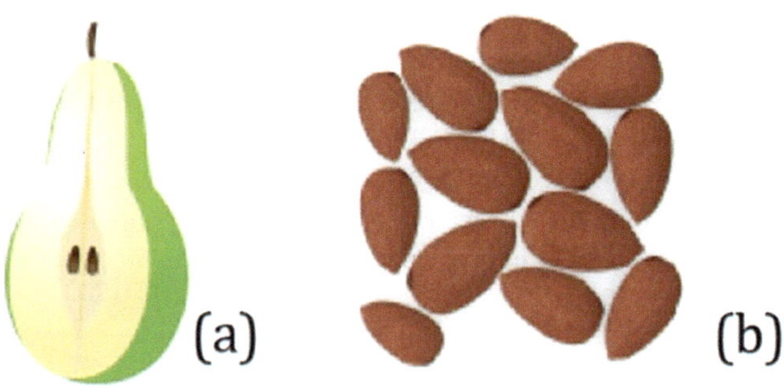

Figure 6.15 Example of snack using a dyad: an apple (a) and a portion of almonds (b).

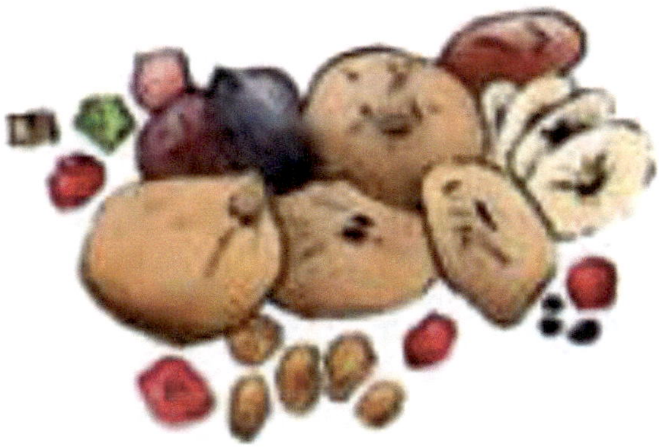

Figure 6.16 Example of snack using a dyad: a mixture of dried nuts and fruits.

the time for your lunch, which means that you do not need to add another snack.

6.10 Finding the Right Time for Afternoon Snack

After you consume your lunch at 2 pm, you start counting again and adding 3 hours, you find that the ideal time for your afternoon snack is exactly 5 pm.

As a dyad, you may have a mixture of dried nuts and fruits at 5 pm (Fig. 6.16).

6.11 Another Intermediate Snack Out of Necessity

If your dinner is scheduled for 8 pm, then, obviously, you do not need another intermediate snack. If you have that, you are fine. However, some people may be so busy at that time that they will remain without food for more than 4–5 hours until they finish with all their daily chores and projects. In this case, two things usually happen; they either engage in nibbling at food with little or no nutritional value, or when they eventually relax later at night, instead of having

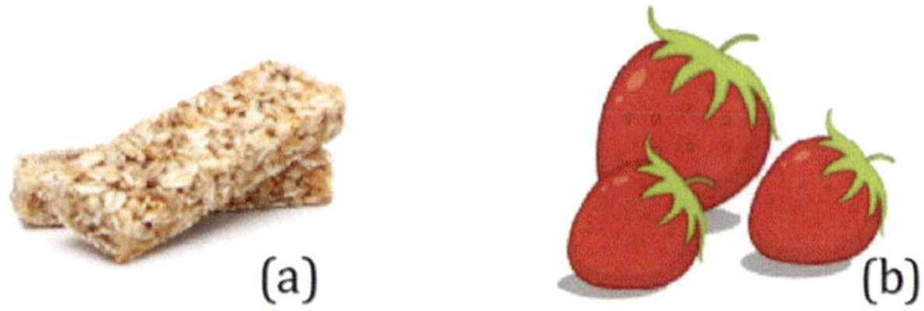

Figure 6.17 Example of snack using a dyad: a snack bar with dried nuts (a) and strawberries (b).

a normal meal, they devour big portions of food. During those night hours, people tend to overindulge in food.

Programming another small intermediate meal before the scheduled dinner functions as a shield against late afternoon or evening overeating. The ideal time is calculated again as before, i.e., 3 hours after the previous meal, whether main meal or snack.

So, if you had your afternoon snack at 5 pm, and you did not have another meal after that, you will need to calculate a small meal at 8 pm.

As a dyad, you may have a snack bar with dried nuts and dried fruits and you could accompany that with a small fruit, like a few strawberries, at 8 pm (Fig. 6.17).

Given that dinner has been scheduled for some reason for 10 pm, even if it is not 3 hours since your last meal, you will have it as scheduled. As I explained earlier, first we program our three basic meals (breakfast, lunch, and dinner) in triads, and then based on their times, we calculate the rest of the intermediate snack in dyads for every 3 hours.

6.12 What to Do if You Miss One of the Basic Meals

If for any reason, you miss a scheduled basic meal, you substitute it, temporarily, with a small, intermediate one, always based on the dyad. Smart combinations in dyads, such as snack bars with dried nuts and dried fruits, but also other combinations mentioned next, may get you out of the difficult situation. From the time you have eaten your dyad, you will have another 3 hours to go until your next basic meal.

6.13 What to Do if You Miss One of Your Intermediate Snacks

If, for any reason, you miss a scheduled small intermediate snack, then you make sure you have it at the first chance you get, even if that is 10 minutes before the basic meal (triad). Even at that moment, it will function as a break in front of the great hunger that will have started to develop despite your best intentions for self-restraint. It is a mistake to think that since it has passed its time, I will overlook it and pass over its calories, as well. If I overlook it, the calories that I will consume next will be cumulatively many more (Fig. 6.18).

6.14 What to Do if You Do Not Have Enough Time to Have Your Basic Meal for Lunch

The pleasure of eating is an important thing for every person. If at the time when you desire to have your meal, you are required to be up and about answering phones, responding to emails, expediting projects, and carrying on in a demanding professional environment, then the matter of taste is a lost cause.

Food, indeed, means to provide our body with all necessary energy and nutrients, so that it can function properly. In theory, no matter how you manage to do so, your body should find a way to make the best of it and keep on. But the situation is different. When the body functions under conditions of stress; for example, in a highly demanding and stressful working environment, it will change its biochemical functions to adjust to the new condition.

The adrenal glands, which are located close to the kidneys, as soon as they sense a hint of stress, begin to produce two hormones in large quantities: adrenaline and cortisol. These so-called "stress hormones" have one thing as their goal; to prepare us for "fight or flight" when in a stressful situation. The body, which

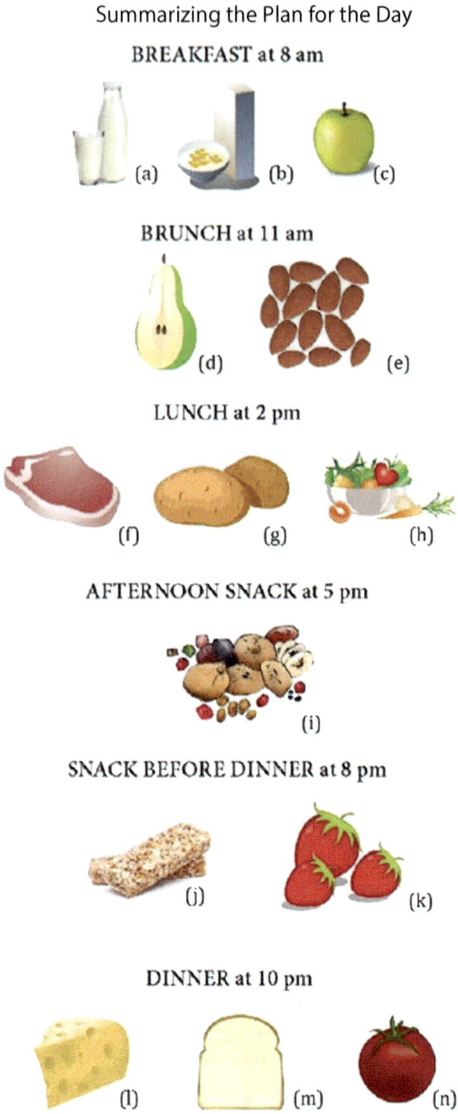
Summarizing the Plan for the Day
BREAKFAST at 8 am
(a)
(b)
(c)
BRUNCH at 11 am
(d)
(e)
LUNCH at 2 pm
(f)
(g)
(h)
AFTERNOON SNACK at 5 pm
(i)
SNACK BEFORE DINNER at 8 pm
(j)
(k)
DINNER at 10 pm
(l)
(m)
(n)

Figure 6.18 Example of a daily plan of nutrition: a glass of milk (a), a portion of cereal (b), an apple (c), a pear (d), a portion of almonds (e), a steak (f), a portion of potatoes (g), a fresh salad (h), a mixture of dried nuts and fruits (i), a snack bar (j), strawberries (k), a piece of cheese (l), a slice of bread (m), and a tomato (n).

always functions with its primitive instincts, cannot recognize if the situation that causes the stress is; for example, encountering a snake or your need to deliver an urgent professional project with a tight deadline.

6.15 "Squeezed" by the Snake of Nutrition

Unless you are a snake charmer to deal with the snake, you will have to run. Your only allies in this effort will be the adrenaline that will give super strength in your legs and the cortisol that will provide you with much oxygen and clear thinking, so that your reactions will be accurate and effective. Or we could say that: the anecdotal expression "relieving myself in my pants" is not random. In order to be able to run for your life, the stress hormones will try to relieve the body of all unnecessary weight. At that moment, food remaining in the stomach will be considered unnecessary weight. Then the body will put on hold anything related to digestion and will cause spasms in the stomach, in order to expel all food through self-induced diarrhea. Anecdotal sources mention that there were cases in which, when the Spartan troops in Ancient Greece would line up in front of other cities' armies, it was a common phenomenon that their opponents would succumb to massive diarrhea at the sight and reputation of the fearsome Spartans.

The constant pressure in the workplace may, at some point, affect the gastrointestinal system. It is a fact that, under such conditions, you literally feel like the food is "sitting" in your stomach. As time goes by, the process of digestion takes longer and longer, as the secretion of gastric fluids is slowed down or suspended, and symptoms like the sensations of swelling, flatulence, heartburn, and alternations between constipation and diarrhea are waiting just ahead.

6.16 Siesta: Do It Like the Mexicans

Those who have served in the army know that even there, the time for meals is considered sacred. Peacefulness and concentration are very important during eating time. Appropriate chewing, tasteful presentation of the food on the table, sitting with good posture on the chair, and the ceasing of worrying and calculating chores in the mind are all essential for the attainment of an appropriate nutritional and digestive result.

If you cannot have your lunch (basic meal) in peace and then take a short nap, like Mexicans are known to do, then reverse it with your dinner. The light meal of the day, i.e., dinner, is better consumed at lunchtime. Therefore, you can switch your basic meal for whatever time you return home or the time you believe you will be able to relax and enjoy it. Schedule your siesta at a time that best fits your daily routine.

By switching your lunch meal with your lighter dinner meal, you will be able to gain not just time, but also a better nutritional result, which will not burden your digestive system.

This is one of my favorite small meals that I usually eat for lunch in the office. It is light, full of nutrients, and most importantly, it provides me with all the energy I need to continue working without thinking about food (Fig. 6.19).

And during all this time, I can hear the question buzzing in my ears, like a bee around my head, again and again: "But does not dinner add to weight?"

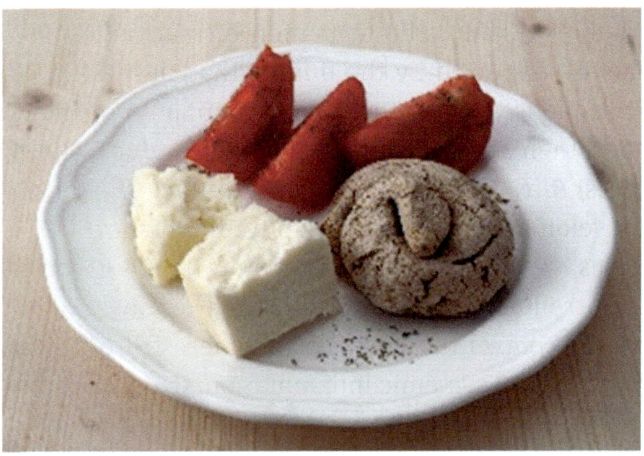

Figure 6.19 Example of lunch combining a protein food, a starchy food, and a fresh food: a piece of cheese, a rusk, and a tomato.

6.17 It Is Not That Food Makes You Fat. It Is How Much of It You Have...

One should definitely have dinner. Surely dinner contributes to weight increase, especially when the stomach has remained empty for more than 3–4 hours without any snacks. Then, the amount of food consumed is so much more than it would be normally which leads to putting on weight.

6.18 The "Offence" of Hypoglycemia

If you have starved yourself to the point that blood glucose has reached low limits, it means that the amount of food you will end up consuming will be much more than expected. This means more calories.

The following picture is an excellent suggestion for an afternoon coffee with a snack (Fig. 6.20).

On the other hand, if you have had all your necessary meals, from the very first up to the last small intermediate snack, you will be able to manage your hunger and your body will be satisfied with the right amount of food.

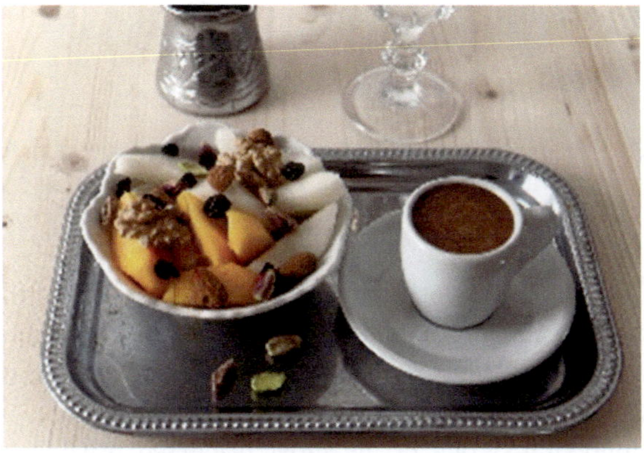

Figure 6.20 Example of an afternoon snack: a coffee with dried nuts and fruits.

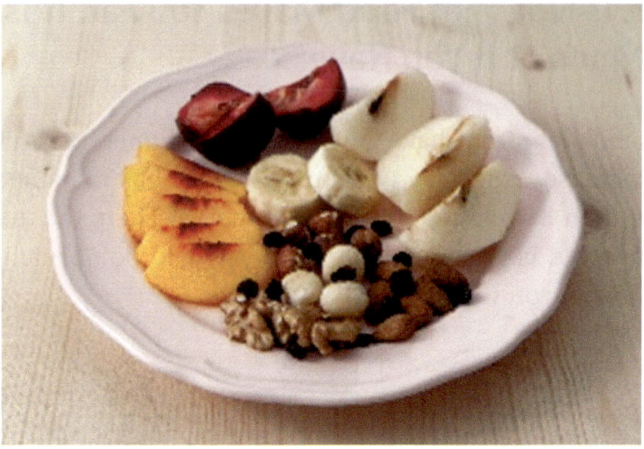

Figure 6.21 Example of the small intermediate meal at the office combining a mixture of fresh fruits, dried nuts, and dried fruit.

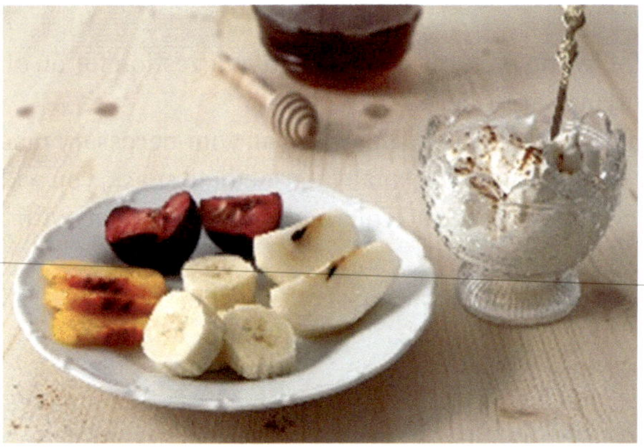

Figure 6.22 Example of breakfast that contains a triad. This breakfast contains yogurt with honey, cinnamon, dry nuts, and fresh fruit.

This is one of my favorite small intermediate meals at the office, where the only thing changing is the kind of fruits according to the seasons. It is something like a stimulant between the basic meals (Fig. 6.21).

The following is one of my most preferred breakfasts in the triad: yogurt with honey and cinnamon as well as pieces of fruit and moistened dry nuts (Fig. 6.22).

Examples of Right Combinations (Tables 6.1–6.4)

Table 6.1 Triads for breakfast

Animal-based proteins	Starch–nuts	Fruits–vegetables
Milk	Breakfast cereal	Apple
Yogurt	Oatmeal	Pear
Gouda cheese	Bread	Banana
Egg	Rusk	Orange juice
Feta cheese	Whole wheat biscuit	Dried fruits
Buttermilk - Kefir	Whole wheat cake	Tomato
Soy milk	Dried nuts	Peach

Table 6.2 Triads for basic meals

Animal-based proteins	Starch–nuts	Vegetables
Meat	Pasta	Lettuce
Chicken	Rice	Cabbage
Burger	Potato	Tomato
Egg	Rusk	Green peas
Fish	Bread	Beans
Feta cheese	Corn	Beets
Seafood	Legumes	Greens

Table 6.3 Triads for light meals

Animal-based proteins	Starch–nuts	Fruits–vegetables
Gouda cheese	Bread	Lettuce
Yogurt	Dried nuts	Apple
Feta cheese	Rusk	Tomato
Egg	Potato	Cucumber
Chicken	Pasta	Cabbage
Tuna	Corn	Carrots
Turkey	Rice	Greens

Table 6.4 Dyads for small intermediate meals

Snacks	Fruits–vegetables
Snack bar with dried nuts	Apple
Barley rusk	Cherries
Cereal bar	Pear
Whole wheat biscuits	Banana
Digestive biscuits	Apricot
Crackers	Dried fruits
Digestive bar	Dried prunes
Dried nuts	Peach
Whole wheat cake	Strawberries
Breadsticks	Raisins
2 tbsp of hummus	Carrot sticks
Vegetable chips	Blueberries

6.19 Basic Guidelines to Organize Our Daily Nutrition

An essential requirement for uplifting your body, in combination with the proper nutrition suggested later in this chapter, is sufficient, which will be achieved with at least 6 hours of continuous night-time sleep. Before each meal, always drink a glass of water; during the meal, drink a cup of green tea or other beverages that significantly aid digestion and act as a diuretic.

6.20 During the Day You Can Eat the Following Snacks

A tablespoon of raw, unsalted nuts, such as walnuts, pecan walnuts, raw, unsalted almonds, cashews, macadamia, pistachios, Brazilian walnuts, etc., which you should first have soaked in water for 30–60 minutes.

A good idea is to soak them with a spoonful of dried fruit, such as raisins, dried cherries, oatmeal, blackberries, or two dried fruits or plums. You can pour the water into a pot that you want to fertilize. You may also prepare larger quantities and store them in the refrigerator.

This way, you will achieve the maximum intake of nutrients and beneficial fats from the fruits. The softer fiber will allow for better deconstruction and absorption of the nutrients from the body.

Other snacks you can use are:

- Two small digestive biscuits with no sugar
- Half of a small wholegrain bun
- A bar of Honey Oatmeal from honey-oat-tahini
- Two wholegrain crackers or two small rusks

A wide variety of balanced combinations can also be found on the Instagram account: #diatrofi.gr founded by Evangelos Zoumbaneas.

Drink mountain tea or green tea with each meal and preferably accompany your dinner with chamomile.

An essential prerequisite for any diet program's success is to accompany it with physical activity, such as exercising, walking, etc., for at least 30 minutes, 5–6 times a week.

6.21 What Is a Serving of Food?

Using the methods described in more detail in the book "THIN... Positive: Secrets to Control Hunger and Nutrition," we will guide you on exactly how to eat and understand how much food you need without help.

The optimal way to do this is to organize your meals in at least three triads and two intermediate pairs to help you get a "personal regulator" of appetite and satiety.

But for some foods, such as meat, fish, or cheese, it would be useful to have a sense of the quantity needed. Because we consider food weighing an unnecessarily strict method, we will give you a way to calculate servings based on your body. For example, if we were to serve pork steaks to a 1.85-m tall man and a 1.60-m tall woman, we can safely assume that we would choose a larger one for the former and a smaller one for the latter. A practical way to calculate servings based on our physique is to calculate a portion of meat by forming a circle with both our palms' thumbs and index fingers. The circle formed, about the thickness of the index finger, is about the size of a medium boneless steak. This is also the volume of two or three small burgers or a small or large chicken breast always depending on each person's fingers' size. In the same way, we can calculate the amount of a serving of fish. Only this time, we will use the larger circle formed by our thumbs and middle fingers instead of index fingers. Imagine this size as a fish without its head or tail, or a perch, swordfish, or salmon fillet. Simply put, because fish has much less fat than red meat does, we can always eat a little more. We can calculate our serving of cheese using a different finger formation. If we bring our index, middle, and ring fingers together, from the base of the fingers to the top, a rectangular shape is formed, the volume of which is our individual cheese serving. If the cheese contains more fat, we calculate the serving based on the volume occupied by the index and middle fingers. This is because the harder a cheese is, the more fat it contains.

The size of a potato, when mentioned, will be considered as occupying the volume of a tennis ball. The amount of "a cup" will refer to the same volume as an individual yogurt container, weighing 200–220 g. All other quantities will be measured in teaspoons or tablespoons.

6.22 Shopping List

- Medium-sized flatbreads or tortillas (preferably made with wholegrain flour)
- Whole meal or Zeas flour bread (sourdough)
- Barley rusks, small-sized 40 g, and medium-sized 60 g
- Fresh fruit
- Fresh vegetables (lettuce, cabbage, carrots, peppers, spinach, broccoli, cauliflower, etc.)
- Frozen vegetables (green beans, peas)
- Pre-made salads
- Dried nuts
- Dried fruit
- Tahini, peanut butter
- Honey
- Vegetable milk (almond, soy, or coconut)
- Cheese

- Yogurt
- Kefir
- Legumes
- Fresh or frozen corn
- Brown rice

6.23 How to Have Proper Meals?

Our body is a perfect machine, which is tuned to work correctly even in conditions of food shortage, to keep us alive. However, this ideal setup for our survival comes at odds with today's society of abundance, often leading us to over-eating. Of course, all this would serve the primitive man to store the energy needed to survive, even in adverse conditions. However today, even in "adverse conditions," or when we are stressed, we still have access to food, particularly the harsher the circumstances, the more calorie-laden the food we crave is. This is why, we continue to store fat without using it. Thus, we need to adjust our satiety mechanism with clever tricks to teach our bodies to be satiated with the proper servings.

It is crucial to remember the "magic 20-minute time frame." The human body cannot realize whether it has been satiated before 20 minutes have passed from the beginning of the meal, no matter how much food we have consumed. It is not a perfect computer that we provide with input, press a button, and get a result. From the moment the first bite enters the mouth, touching the sublingual capillaries, the body begins to perceive the input of food. Still, to ensure our survival, the message of satiety has been programmed to reach the brain along with the rise in blood glucose levels, the synthesis of neurotransmitters and neuropeptides, and serotonin, which is after 20 minutes have passed.

Because of this mechanism, we should only serve one serving, proper for our body and needs, chew our food well (at least 10 times), and give our body time to enjoy this process, tastes, textures, and smells. If we are hungry after 20 minutes, then the body really needs more food.

6.24 There Are Some Tricks to Help Our Body Get Full

- Consuming a glass of water or fresh juice about 20–30 minutes before a meal and having a cup of tea or other digestive beverage with our food is very beneficial. We will continue drinking after the meal is over.
- As a first dish, we can have a warm or cold, light vegetable soup, low in calories, with no cream and fat to cover our stomach volume. Also, a cup of meat broth helps eat less and enhances good gastrointestinal health. We could also use ready-made organic soups with glutamine monosodium.
- Before starting our meal, we can also eat half an apple and the other half after the meal, thus signaling the end of food ingestion and assisting its digestion. The same can be done with another fruit or with some yogurt or a glass of kefir.
- Other tools for signaling the end of a meal could be a cup of coffee, tea, or cocoa beans, chewing gum or candy, or even a spoonful of nuts with little honey or dried fruit.
- Finally, one method that helps signal the end of a meal is tooth brushing. Brushing off the meal removes any food residue. This is how the brain is instructed that our meal is over.

6.25 Diet and Its Secrets for Controlling Hunger and Safety

For those who have tried every "diet" available in the market, the prospect of learning to eat properly, minding the hunger and satiety mechanisms again, is a great challenge. Another significant point is remaining in good spirits while you are on a diet, watching your body improve day by day, observing changes in your clothes, and learning to take care of yourself without depending on the scales. Providing yourself with what you need and not much more and aiming at taking care of yourself, your health improves, your self-esteem increases along with your self-image, and you experience delayed aging while your body regains its ideal weight. All these are the benefits of this restorative process.

For this to happen, we need to ensure two things: (a) the proper production of serotonin by our body throughout the day and (b) the balance of glucose in our blood. Serotonin, the hormone of joy, boosts positive mood — which is why most antidepressants artificially increase its concentration in the brain — and conveys three messages:

1. I'm OK.
2. I got it under control.
3. I have had ENOUGH.

To produce serotonin, our body's complex mechanisms require every major meal (breakfast, lunch, and dinner) to contain: (a) a serving of fresh food, e.g., a cup of fresh fruit or vegetable, or 1–2 tablespoons of dried fruit or juice, mainly for vitamin C; (b) a serving of protein food, e.g., three fingers of soft cheese or two fingers of hard cheese, yogurt, egg, one palm of meat or fish, seafood, etc., for amino acids and especially tryptophan; and (c) a serving of starch, preferably whole grain, e.g., a potato soup, rice, legumes, corn, pasta, etc., for carbohydrates, fiber, magnesium, and B complex vitamins. One of the main meals should be lighter, e.g., salad with chicken and rusk or yogurt with nuts and fruit.

Provided that the serotonin produced requires a "magic 20-minute time frame" to act, we need to eat slowly, chewing well so that each meal lasts at least 20 minutes. After 20 minutes, we can see whether we have had enough. If not, one or two tablespoons of nuts or dried fruit can save us! Serotonin levels in the brain drop slowly and are depleted within 8 hours, so at most every 8 hours, we need to renew the food triad to produce serotonin again and maintain its positive effect throughout our day.

As for glucose, we must remember that after 3–3.5 hours of fasting or after 1 hour of exercise, glucose blood levels fall below 0.8 mg, causing slight hypoglycemia, which wakes up a "beast" in our body. This has a negative effect on our mood and concentration and causes nervousness, drowsiness, and a feeling of fatigue. When stress levels fall, and we regain access to food, we eat uncontrollably. If we consume foods rich in simple sugars, with no nutritional value, e.g., chocolate, we cannot stop — we wake up another beast — and we are even hungrier.

That is why no one can eat just one sweet. If one has been on an empty stomach since breakfast (e.g., at 9 am) having eaten nothing all day (only coffee, cigarettes, or fast food), then at 9 pm he will have four "beasts" to satisfy and is very likely to consume food for all four of them at once. We can weaken hypoglycemic "beasts" smartly by feeding them a proper source of glucose, such as fresh fruit, along with some snacks high in fiber, e.g., soaked nuts, cereal bars, or nuts and cereal bars, etc., to avoid reactive hypoglycemia and feel satiated for longer.

We should not forget to drink 10 glasses of water as, for each glass, our metabolism works at 10%, and not miss opportunities for bitter or sour flavors that boost our metabolism (e.g., black coffee, bitter greens, lemon, etc.). When we want something extra, e.g., sweet, we eat normally, before and after, and preferably consume it with or even better after nutrition, e.g., fruit and nuts, and then the sweet.

Finally, physical activity is indispensable in all its forms that are possible and pleasurable (walking, yoga, fitness, dancing, etc.) enhancing our good mood with the produced "endorphins" and giving up to 60% success of a diet program as "the loss of extra body fat is a matter of athletic time."

6.26 Ideas for Three-Course Meal Combinations

Triads for breakfast

- Oatmeal porridge and chopped fruit
- Two tablespoons of tahini or peanut butter with one fresh fruit and one glass of almond milk
- Milk with two small oat biscuits and one fruit
- Yogurt with oats, honey, and raisins
- Yogurt with oat jam and ground-dried nuts
- Toast with cottage cheese, jam, dried nuts, and fruits
- Toast with tahini, honey, fruit, dried nuts, and a glass of almond milk or kefir

- A slice of bread, an egg, and a glass of juice
- Cherry tomatoes with cheese and a rusk
- Baked nutmeg and fruit
- Almond milk with oat honey and raisins
- Smoothie with banana, kefir, oats, honey, and cocoa

Triads for lunch with legumes

All legumes are combined with a serving of animal food, such as cheese or a small serving of fish, and can be accompanied by five large or ten small olives and a fresh salad.

- Black-eyed peas with spinach
- Black-eyed peas with tuna made in a pot
- Chickpea soup
- Chickpeas with red pepper and mushrooms
- Baked chickpeas with onions and carrots
- Falafel made with chickpeas
- Grilled beans with turkey
- Bean soup
- Lentil soup
- Peas made in a pot with a little potato

Triad for lunch with cooked vegetables

Cooked vegetables are combined with a serving of protein, such as cheese or a small serving of fish, a moderate serving of nuts or a two-slice bread or wholegrain breadcrumbs, and a fresh salad.

- Mushroom fricassee
- Grilled mushrooms with gruyere
- Mushroom soup
- Mushrooms stuffed with minced meat
- Beans
- Baked okra
- Green celery with rice
- Cabbage with rice
- Vegetarian burger
- Vegetable risotto with feta cheese

- Stuffed vegetables with rice
- Eggplants stuffed with rice, onions, and tomato
- Omelet with vegetables
- Spinach with rice
- Eggplant with potatoes made in a pot
- Baked potatoes
- Cannelloni stuffed with minced eggplants

Triad for minced meat

They are almost always combined with a fresh salad and a medium-sized rusk, two thin slices of bread, or a cup of potato, rice, corn, or other cooked starch.

- Cabbage rolls with lemon sauce
- Meatballs with rice boiled in a lemony broth (Greek dish called "Giouvarlakia")
- Mince roll in the oven with roasted vegetables
- Light pasticcio
- Pasta with minced meat or spaghetti
- Mushrooms stuffed with minced meat
- Aubergines stuffed with minced meat, mozzarella, or gruyere
- Meatballs made in a saucepan with lemon, carrots, potatoes, mustard
- Grilled burgers with sauce and rice
- Burger with potato salad

Triads for dinner

- Tortilla with roasted vegetables Philadelphia, ham, and turkey
- Oatmeal porridge
- Milk, oats, honey, and raisins
- Potato salad, feta cheese, tomatoes, and olives
- Potherb with a serving of cheese and a medium-sized rusk
- Egg, salad, cherry tomatoes, and rusk
- Sandwiches with gouda, ham, mustard, tomato, mushrooms
- Sandwiches with cream cheese, salmon, and lettuce

- Egg sandwich with cucumber, tomato, and light mayonnaise
- Pitta-based pizza
- Tuna salad with tomato, cucumber, carrot, and rusk
- Tuna salad with lettuce, dill, light mayonnaise, and cucumber
- Skewer with tomato, pitta baked without oil, and yogurt
- Pitta, salad, and meat skewers
- Greek salad with tomato, feta cheese, cucumber, and rusks
- Rusks with cottage cheese, turkey, and tomato
- Trahana with feta cheese and cucumber
- Roasted eggs with chopped tomatoes and a slice of toasted bread
- Egg tortilla, yogurt, pickles, mustard, grated carrot chef salad with lettuce, cherry tomatoes, cucumber, egg, ham, gouda, and a little sauce

Reference

1. Zoumpaneas, E. (2013). *THIN... POSITIVE: Secrets to Control Hunger and Appetite + Diet Coaching*. [EKPEDEFTIKO KENTRO DIATROFIKON DIATARACHON M.EPE. (Contributor), Eleni Achilleopoulou (Series Editor)].

Chapter 7

Fasting and Telomeres

Antonis Tsintarakis,[a] Michael Stroumpakis,[b] Maria Sifaki,[c] Dimitra Nikolopoulou,[d,e] Vassilis Zoumpourlis,[a] and Aristidis Tsatsakis[d,e]

[a]*Biomedical Applications Unit, Institute of Chemical Biology, National Hellenic Research Foundation, Athens, Greece*
[b]*Historical Byzantine Musicology, Patriarchal University Ecclesiastical Academy of Crete, Greece*
[c]*Skin Clinic, Heraklion, Crete, Greece*
[d]*Laboratory of Toxicology and Forensic Sciences, Medical School, University of Crete, Heraklion, Greece*
[e]*Lifeplus S.A., Science & Technological Park of Crete, Vassilika Vouton, Heraklion, Crete, Greece*
d.nikolopoulou@uoc.gr

7.1 Introduction

Fasting is a universal practice, endorsed by numerous religions worldwide [1], involving abstinence from certain foods and serving as a means of spiritual growth, self-discipline, and a means of connecting with the divine. The term "fasting" in Greek derives from the negative prefix "νη" (Nu/ˈnjuː/ Greek: νι ni [ni] nee) and the verb ἐσθίω (esthíō) = to eat, signifying "not to eat" [2, pp.

Telomeres: Biomarkers of a Healthy Life and Successful Aging
Edited by Aristidis Tsatsakis

ISBN 978-981-5129-49-6 (Hardcover), 978-1-003-56809-4 (eBook)
www.jennystanford.com

21]. The etymological analysis implies that fasting is the complete (starvation) or partial abstinence from particular foods during recurring intervals.

One of the earliest instances of religious fasting can be traced back to the Hellenistic mystery religions, particularly the "healing cult" of Asclepius, the ancient Greek God of medicine. Additionally, in the pre-Columbian societies of Peru, fasting frequently constituted a prerequisite for penance following the confession of sins before a priest [3].

Several studies have been undertaken to examine the influence of religious beliefs on the preservation of one's health through dietary patterns [1, 4]. In particular, several basic or even complex religious directives concerning a great variety of dietary practices have evolved over the centuries, all aimed at cultivating both body and spirit. In other words, the regulations governing food consumption, commonly referred to as diet, exhibit variability based on individual preferences, religious affiliations, or tenets. Such dietary practices are introduced as integral components of an individual's way of life as well as a method of attaining spiritual and physical benefits [5].

While fasting may vary in form and duration depending on the faith, the core principles remain consistent, which are abstinence from food, drink, or specific activities for a set period of time, to strengthen one's connection to faith and fortify inner resolve [1, 5]. The intervals of refraining from specific types of food along with the adherence to designated dietary regimens during fasting have been correlated with a plethora of health benefits. These include weight management, improved blood pressure and cholesterol levels, modulation of insulin levels and sensitivity as well as overall cardiovascular health [5].

Accumulated data from studies conducted in the last two decades in various fields of biomedical sciences reveal the profound implications of diverse dietary patterns on critical cellular processes, such as inflammation, oxidative stress, autophagy, and cell senescence. Considering this data, new "key players" emerge at the forefront of these cellular processes governing our longevity and well-being. These key players are none other than "telomeres."

7.2 Fasting Across Diverse Cultures and Religions

Fasting has been associated with religious rites and national historical memories and, in some cases, with the expression of social or political views. Most of the time, fasting is observed in the context of mourning and contemplation [3]. A brief retrospective examination of the history of various civilizations, including the ancient Asian societies, the ancient Greeks, the Egyptians, and other peoples of Africa, prominently reveals this correlation. This becomes even more apparent when fasting serves as a conduit of religious expression, as exemplified among Muslims, Jews, Hindus, Buddhists, and Christians.

In **Islam**, fasting (As-Saum) during the holy month of Ramadan constitutes one of the Five Pillars [1, 6]. Muslims around the world fast from dawn to dusk abstaining from food, drink, and other bodily needs. Fasting during Ramadan is considered not only a sign of obedience to God but also a way to reflect on one's life and strengthen self-discipline [6]. It is a period of increased spirituality, increased prayer, and deeper empathy for those suffering from poverty and hunger [5]. In addition to obligatory fasting during Ramadan, various non-mandatory fasting practices exist within the Islamic faith, such as sunnah and nafl. A characteristic example of such practice is Sannah Monday and Thursday fasting [7].

In **Judaism**, Yom Kippur, the Day of Atonement, is the most sacred day in the Jewish calendar. During this solemn occasion, the Jews refrain from food and drink for 25 hours. This fasting ritual is not solely a way of seeking forgiveness and atonement but also a time for reflection and spiritual self-observation [1, 4, 8]. In addition to Yom Kippur, other days of fasting that exist within the Jewish calendar include Tisha B'Av, Seventeenth of Tammuz, Fast of Gedaliah, Fast of Esther, and Ten Tevet [6, 9].

Within the context of **Buddhism**, fasting assumes a crucial role in various traditions. Monks and nuns adhere to a strict dietary code, which includes periods of fasting to support their meditation and sustain mindfulness [10]. Furthermore, fasting can be observed on Uposatha days, which occur four times a month and serve as a way to purify the mind and maintain discipline [4, 10].

In **Hinduism**, fasting (Vrat and Upvaas) constitutes a common practice among adherents and becomes apparent in various forms. Some individuals choose to fast on specific days of the week like Ekadashi, while others fast on religious festivals or auspicious occasions such as the month of Shravan [6, 11]. Fasting is regarded as a way to purify body and mind, seek divine blessing, and demonstrate devotion to various deities.

7.3 Fasting in Christian Orthodox Church

Since the emergence of the Church, the Christian doctrine demonstrated an interest in dealing with man in a holistic approach. Thus, man is regarded as an indivisible psychosomatic whole, whose balance, if disturbed, affects the entirety of the individual [6, 12, 13]. Fasting has been a common practice deeply rooted in the Orthodox Christian tradition for centuries since the first followers of Christianity (known as Apostles or Fathers of the Church) recognized the importance of dietary practices, a feature that can be traced back to Jesus Christ, the founder of the Christian Church. According to texts found in the Gospels, Christ adhered to specific dietary habits, thereby setting an example to the faithful for the consumption or avoidance of certain foods [6, 14]. Furthermore, the tradition of abstaining from particular foods during a certain period of time is considered a sacred duty by the adherents as it resembles Christ's forty-day fast in the desert.

Religious fasting in the Christian church was established during the first apostolic times and was reshaped over the centuries reaching its multi-leveled form we currently observe, encompassing from the complete abstinence from food to the consumption of all edible varieties [6, 12, 15, 16]. For simplification purposes, the various fasting regimens adhered to within Orthodox Christianity can be categorized according to Table 7.1.

The aforementioned dietary regimens, in most cases, are not random dietary choices and are implemented at annual recurring intervals. In this sense, fasting practices can be distinguished into regular and extraordinary.

Table 7.1 Various levels of fasting restrictions observed in the Christian Orthodox religion

FASTING LEVEL	Fasting restrictions
A) STARVATION	During starvation, fasting focuses on complete abstinence from food consumption, and if possible, from water. This type of fasting is practiced by monks during the first three days of Great Lent.
B) DRY EATING	During dry fasting, an individual may consume strictly plant-based foods, such as bread, vegetables, nuts, olives (but not oil), and fruits. Water consumption is permissible, but alcoholic beverages are excluded.
C) OIL-FREE FASTING	During oil-free fasting, the adherent may consume water-boiled plant-based foods without the addition of oil.
D) WINE AND OIL CATALYSIS	During this type of catalysis, the adherent may eat plant-based foods cooked with oil or other vegetable fats. The consumption of wine and seafood (mollusks, shellfish, fish, eggs/roe) is allowed.
E) FISH CATALYSIS	In addition to the conditions of wine and oil catalysis, during this type of fasting, fish is also allowed for consumption, but not dairy products or eggs.
F) CHEESE AND EGG CATALYSIS	At this level of fasting, all the aforementioned foods are allowed along with dairy products, eggs, and their derivatives.
G) CATALYSIS OF ALL	During the last level of Orthodox fasting, all restrictions are lifted, allowing for the consumption of plant and animal products as well as meat.

Regular fasting occasions include the following [15, 16]:

- ***Fasting on Wednesdays and Fridays.*** During these days, fasting encompasses dry eating (level B, Table 7.1) provided that the food is taken after the ninth Byzantine hour, equivalent to three in the afternoon. This specific regimen resembles the 18:6 fasting scheme. Notably, for the monks of Mount Athos, an additional day, Monday, is incorporated into the aforementioned two days. While for the general population, the 5:2 scheme is followed (consumption of regular food for five days and restriction to minimal food intake for two days), for the monks of Mount Athos the 4:3 scheme is implemented (limited food consumption over a portion of the week). It is worth noting that the fasting schemes apply to healthy individuals while for the sick, the scheme is modified according to needs.

- ***The Observance of Great Lent (duration: 40 days).*** Great Lent is a movable period, and its commencement is determined by the onset of the Triodion, which is also a movable period. Fasting during Great Lent commences on Clean Monday and concludes the day after the Divine Liturgy of the Resurrection of Christ. During this period, a dry eating regimen is followed on Wednesdays and Fridays (and Mondays for monks, level B, Table 7.1) and an oil-free regimen on Mondays, Tuesdays, and Thursdays (level C, Table 7.1). During the weekends wine and oil consumption is permissible (Level D, Table 7.1). Throughout the holidays of the Annunciation and Palm Sunday, which coincide with the period of Great Lent, the consumption of fish is permitted (level E, Table 7.1). Triodion, which precedes the Great Lent period, marks a three-week preparatory phase during which preparations for the observance of Great Lent are made. During the initial week of Triodion, there are no restrictions on food consumption (level G, Table 7.1). During the second week consumption of food without restrictions is retained (level G, Table 7.1) except for Wednesday and Friday (level B, Table 7.1). In the third week, dairy products, eggs, and fish along with all their derivatives are permitted (level F, Table 7.1).
- ***The Christmas Fasting (duration: 40 days).*** Christmas fasting commences on November 15th and concludes on December 25th (Christmas) after the liturgy for the Nativity of Christ. During this particular period, fasting on Wednesday and Friday (and Monday for monks, B level,

Table 7.1) is retained, while for the rest of the days, the regimen of wine and oil catalysis is followed (D level, Table 7.1). Additionally, fish consumption (E level, Table 7.1) is permitted for most individuals, except for Wednesdays and Fridays, and for the most ascetic it is limited only to holidays within this timeframe. Finally, fish catalysis is applicable for some until December 12th, while for others, it is extended until December 17th.

- ***The Dormition Fast (13 days).*** The Dormition Fast encompasses fasting on Wednesdays and Fridays (and Mondays for monks, level B, Table 7.1), wine and oil catalysis (level D, Table 7.1) during the weekends, and oil-free fasting (level C, Table 7.1) for the rest of the days. Within this period, the celebration of the Transfiguration of Christ is celebrated (6th of August), during which the adherents are permitted to consume fish (level E, Table 7.1).
- ***The Fast of the Holy Apostles (not a fixed duration).*** The observance of this fast commences the day after All Saints' Sunday and concludes on the 29th of June (Feast of Saints Peter and Paul). Throughout this period, fasting on Wednesday and Friday (and Monday for monks, level B, Table 7.1) is observed along with the consumption of fish for the rest of the week (level E, Table 7.1).
- ***The Eve of Epiphany/Theophany (5th January, 1 day).*** During the eve of the Epiphany, a regimen of dry eating is followed, unless this day coincides with a Saturday or Sunday, in which case oil consumption is permissible (level D, Table 7.1).
- ***The Exaltation/Elevation of the Holy Cross (September 14, 1 day).*** The feast of the Exaltation (or Elevation) of the Holy Cross involves adhering to dry eating practices (level B, Table 7.1), unless this day coincides with a Saturday or Sunday, in which case oil consumption is permissible (level D, Table 7.1).
- ***The Commemoration of the Beheading of St. John the Baptist (August 29, 1 day).*** This day of fasting, associated with the commemoration of the Beheading of St. John the Baptist, involves adhering to dry eating practices (level B,

Table 7.1), unless this day coincides with a Saturday or Sunday, in which case oil consumption is permissible (level D, Table 7.1).

Extraordinary fasting refers to voluntary decisions and is supplementary to regular or customary fasting practices.

7.4 General Observations on the Fasting Regimens of Orthodox Christians

The fasting practices of the Orthodox Church pay close attention to the nutritional aspects of an individual's way of life. According to the teachings of the Christian Orthodox Church, the health of the body contributes to the health of the soul and vice versa. Thus, fasting practices should be implemented in everyday life, on a daily or weekly basis, and for the entirety of one's life, from childhood to old age. In contrast to the occasional fasting regimens followed periodically in the form of a diet, the Orthodox Church advocates for a lifelong commitment to healthier dietary practices.

The fasting practices observed by the Orthodox Church adhere to the 5:2 intermittent diet scheme. Individuals following this program are encouraged to engage in intermittent fasting two days a week (Wednesdays and Fridays). For the monks of Mount Athos, the daily and weekly schedule is stricter, and thus a 4:3 intermittent scheme is implemented (Mondays, Wednesdays, and Fridays). Consequently, it can be deduced that throughout the Orthodox fasting periods, the human body consistently experiences a state of refraining from overeating.

In monastic circles, particularly those of Mount Athos, the distance between meals ranges from 10 to 12 hours daily (except Mondays, Wednesdays, and Fridays) and the dietary practices incorporate a well-balanced and time-consistent dietary plan [17, 18, pp. 178–181].

Finally, the fasting practices of the Orthodox Church can be characterized as partially vegetarian, given that the days of meat consumption are limited to 52 per year [19].

7.5 Health Benefits Related to Christian Orthodox Fasting

The enduring health benefits associated with fasting have been extensively recognized, as documented in various sources [20, 21], and testimonies in support of the benefits of fasting can also be found in the texts of the "Fathers of the Church," like the speech given by Bishop Asterios of Amasea (end of the 4th century, 415 AD) [22, pp. 15–17].

According to scientific studies [1, 16, 23–29], the benefits of fasting are multiple (Fig. 7.1):

- **Improved cardiovascular health:** The adoption of a plant-based diet, as observed during fasting periods, is associated with lower levels of saturated fat and cholesterol, contributing to a reduced risk of cardiovascular diseases. The consumption of a variety of vegetables and legumes provides essential nutrients and fiber contributing to overall cardiovascular health.
- **Weight management:** Fasting periods can facilitate weight loss or assist an individual in maintaining a healthy weight by restricting the intake of high-calorie and high-fat foods. An emphasis on a plant-based diet can also enhance metabolism and maintain energy balance.
- **Enhanced mental clarity:** Fasting is believed to contribute to mental clarity and heightened focus. Some adherents report increased mental clarity and an elevated sense of self-discipline during the fasting period, potentially leading to improved decision-making and stress management.
- **Healthier Digestive System:** The adoption of a plant-based diet can benefit the digestive system resulting in improved gut health and reduced risk of digestive disorders. Additionally, individuals with irritable bowel syndrome (IBS) may experience symptom relief.
- **Improved blood sugar control:** Fasting periods encourage the consumption of whole grains, which contain a lower glycemic index and can aid in the regulation of blood sugar levels. This effect can be particularly advantageous for

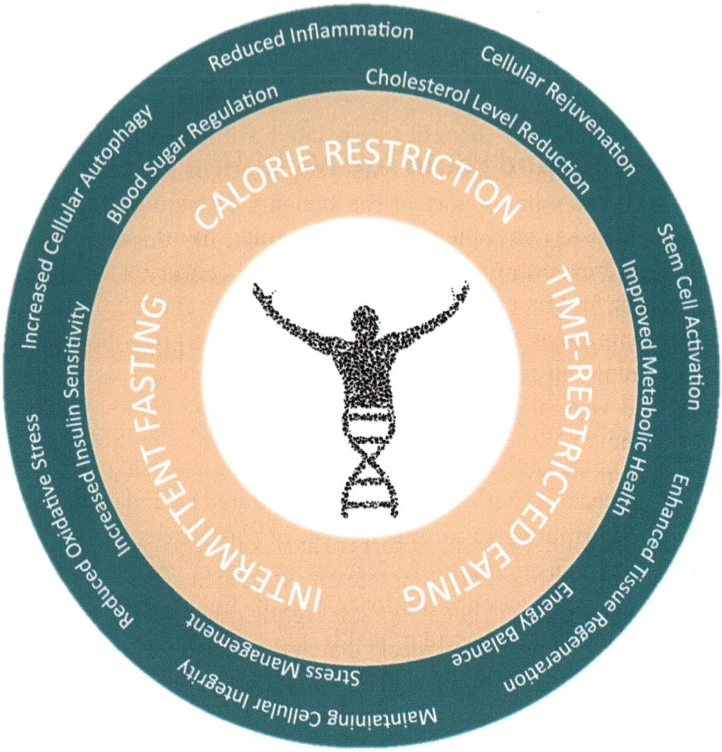

Figure 7.1 The multifaceted effects of Christian Orthodox Fasting.

individuals with diabetes or those at risk of developing the condition.

7.6 Potential Effect of Christian Orthodox Fasting on Telomeres

Our genetic material, our DNA, is what defines us at the biological level providing the instructions for our genetic traits, our physical characteristics, development, functioning, and much more. The information encoded in our genetic material, expressed in the form of proteins, constitutes our cells, tissues, organs, and whole organisms.

Chromosomes are structures within the nucleus of our cells formed by the condensation and organization of different linear molecules of DNA. In our somatic cells, chromosomes come in 23 pairs (46 chromosomes in total), with each chromosome in a pair inherited from our parents. At the ends of each chromosome are located repetitive DNA sequences that form conserved structures (T-loops) [30], protecting the internal chromosomal regions. These particular sequences are known as telomeres deriving from the Greek words "τέλος" (end) and "μέρος" (part) [31].

Our cells possess the ability to divide, wherein one cell gives rise to two identical daughter cells. During cellular division, our DNA is replicated and divided equally between the newly forming cells in such a way that genetic stability is maintained. However, due to a phenomenon known as "the end replication problem," during every cycle of DNA replication a fraction of genetic information is lost, resulting in the progressive shortening of the telomeric regions. Once telomere length reaches a critical point, cells experience replicative senescence, where they are unable to divide any further. Telomere shortening and the subsequent replicative senescence have been associated with loss of tissue function, organismal aging, and the development of age-related diseases [30, 32].

Ongoing scientific research indicates that various factors, such as chronic inflammation, oxidative stress levels, metabolic syndrome as well as other lifestyle-related parameters, seem to exert an influence on telomere length and aging [29, 32–34]. Interestingly, as discussed in previous sections of this chapter, these factors can, in turn, be influenced by various dietary practices such as fasting. This raises the following question: Is there a plausible association between intermittent fasting or caloric restriction and telomere length?

7.6.1 Effect of Fasting-Stimulated Autophagy on Telomeres

Autophagy is a process crucial in the maintenance of cellular homeostasis and health involving an intricate intracellular network of membranous structures and a variety of proteins. Three types of autophagy have been identified: macroautophagy, microautophagy, and chaperone-mediated autophagy. All of them facilitate, in various manners, the lysosomal degradation and recycling of damaged or malfunctioning cellular components, such as proteins and organelles. These processes are performed constantly and under any conditions in our cells [35, 36].

Nutrient availability constitutes a critical factor in the initiation or inhibition of autophagy. Under non-starvation (nutrient availability) conditions, the mammalian target of rapamycin (mTOR) is activated, suppressing a major initiator of autophagy, the Unc-51-like kinase (ULK) complex. However, under nutrient deficit, mTOR is inactivated allowing the activating phosphorylation of ULK complex by the 5′-adenosine monophosphate (AMP)-activated protein kinase (AMPK). Activation of the ULK complex commences a signaling cascade that recruits secondary complexes for the initiation of autophagy (Fig. 7.2) [36–38].

Mitophagy is a subset of autophagy, responsible for the selective removal of damaged or unnecessary mitochondria. Although mitochondria serve as the primary energy producers in cells, on some occasions, an excess quantity or malfunctioning of these organelles leads to increased levels of reactive oxygen species (ROS); a phenomenon mitigated by mitophagy. Numerous pathways that commence mitophagy have been elucidated, and among these, one pathway that implicates ULK1 and nutrient deficiency has been identified [39, 40]. In nutrient-stressed cells, ULK1 could promote mitophagy by protecting from proteasomal degradation and phosphorylating the mitochondrial cargo receptor BNIP3 leading to its association with microtubule-associated protein 1 light chain 3 (LC3) (Fig. 7.2) [39].

Several studies over the years have highlighted that autophagic (and mitophagic) activity declines with age resulting in the accumulation of cellular debris, dysfunctional mitochondria, and the increase of oxidative stress; phenomena closely associated with aging and the development and progression of age-related diseases [36, 40]. Interestingly, other studies focused on the intricate interplay between telomere maintenance and autophagy/mitophagy suggest the existence of a link between them [35, 41]. Studies on mouse embryos elucidated that dysfunctional mitochondria were sufficient to promote telomere shortening and loss as well as genomic instability [35, 42].

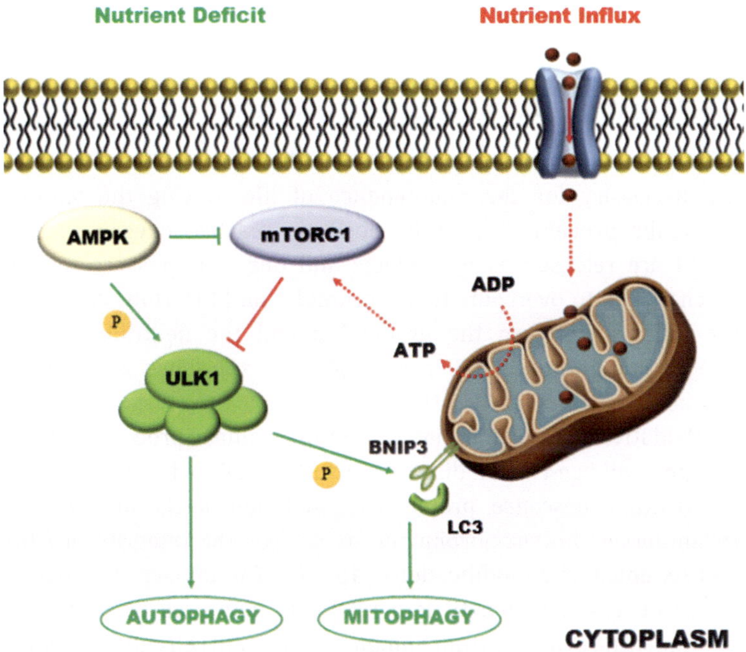

Figure 7.2 Autophagy and mitophagy during nutrient influx and deficit. During nutrient influx, the energy produced by mitochondria in the form of ATP activates mTORC1 which suppresses the ULK complex from initializing autophagy or mitophagy. During nutrient deficit the conversion of ADP to ATP seizes leading to the inactivation of mTORC1 and the activation of AMPK which phosphorylates ULK1, allowing for the activation of autophagy or BNIP3/LC3 mediated mitophagy.

Although a conclusive correlation between fasting-induced autophagy and telomere length has not been detected yet, there seem to be plausible mechanisms by which enhanced autophagy and mitophagy could influence telomeres. Fasting in the form of prolonged, as well as intermittent fasting or caloric restriction, creates an environment of nutrient deficit, which, in turn, has been shown to stimulate autophagy or mitophagy in cells [36–40, 43].

In conclusion, during fasting and nutrient deficit, cells adapt by prioritizing the recycling of cellular components and removing malfunctioning proteins and organelles, thereby creating a potential substrate for cellular rejuvenation and maintenance of genomic integrity.

7.6.2 Fasting, Oxidative Stress, and Telomeres

Cellular metabolism comprises a set of biochemical reactions that are necessary for the maintenance of life. During the various metabolic processes our cells perform, reactive oxygen species (ROS) are released as byproducts and our cells possess several mechanisms to overcome their accumulation [44]. However, when the balance between the production and the neutralization of ROS is compromised, the cells begin to experience a condition characterized as oxidative stress [44, 45].

Oxidative stress can influence multiple cellular processes linked to aging and age-related diseases including cell cycle, proliferation, cell death, senescence, proteostasis, metabolism, the intracellular inflammatory microenvironment, as well as the integrity of DNA and its epigenetic modifications [45, 46]. The impact of oxidative stress on telomere length is a relatively new area of study, but accumulating evidence from human, murine, and cell culture models suggests a strong inverse correlation between oxidative stress levels and telomere length [46]. Reduced levels of oxidative stress typically correlate with less DNA damage and by extension less telomere damage. Consequently, the reduction of oxidative stress levels may potentially slow down the rate of telomere shortening.

From this perspective, the dietary nutrients during fasting may exert a positive impact on cellular health. Although there are not many studies concerning the effect of Christian fasting on oxidative stress levels, Orthodox fasting incorporates healthy, plant-based dietary plans [19], resembling in many aspects the Mediterranean diet [47]. It is rich in antioxidants (vitamin E, retinol, carotene precursors) and essential nutrients that have the potential to minimize oxidative stress, therefore ensuring reduced telomere shortening and contributing to a longer life span [47–50]. Additionally, Orthodox fasting incorporates various intermittent fasting schemes, and while not conclusively proven, intermittent fasting appears to exert an effect on oxidative stress [51]. Interestingly, two studies on individuals observing Ramadan diurnal intermittent fasting revealed that this type of intermittent fasting could ameliorate the expression of antioxidant genes (TFAM, SOD2, and Nrf2) and reduce oxidative stress [52, 53].

7.6.3 Correlation Between Fasting, Inflammation, and Telomeres

Inflammation is the physiological process during which our immune system responds to a variety of harmful stimuli, including damaged cells, toxic compounds, irradiation, as well as invading pathogens. It is a multifaceted process involving numerous cells of the immune system, even more secretory proteins, and complex signaling networks. The three major pathways governing and mediating inflammation include nuclear factor-κB (NF-κB), Janus kinase/signal transducer and activator of transcription (JAK/STAT), and mitogen-activated protein kinase (MAPK) [54].

Acute inflammation is crucial for the restoration of damaged tissue and the combating of pathogens. However, uncontrolled inflammatory responses that remain unresolved for great periods of time give rise to chronic inflammation, which can be harmful to the organism and increase the incidence of developing age-related diseases [54, 55]. Lifestyle factors, including dietary habits, contribute decisively to the development of chronic inflammation [49, 56]. Furthermore, the gut microbiome exerts its influence on inflammatory conditions. During dietary fiber deficit, it begins to utilize the host's mucus glycoproteins as an energy source leading to degradation of the colonic mucus barrier and subsequent inflammation [56, 57].

It is important to note that chronic inflammation and aging might be intertwined creating a vicious cycle. The constant release of proinflammatory cytokines can accelerate cellular senescence. Subsequently, senescent cells present a senescence-associated secretory phenotype (SASP), expressing even more proinflammatory cytokines, a phenomenon that leads to constant senescence of cells of the immune system [58]. Interestingly, one important feature of senescent cells is telomere shortening.

In recent years, a significant body of research has begun to focus on the relationship between inflammation and telomere attrition

[49, 55, 59]. In vivo and ex vivo data indicated that neutrophils, a subset of innate immunity cells, which were recruited to sites of inflammation, released ROS inducing premature senescence and accelerating telomere dysfunction [60]. Other studies observed a significant correlation between leukocyte telomere length (LTL) and the consumption of proinflammatory food groups [49]. Moreover, studies on participants who adhered to higher proinflammatory-capacity diets demonstrated an elevated risk of accelerated telomere shortening compared to the low-fat diet control group or the Mediterranean-based diet group [59]. Moreover, obesity and insulin resistance were associated with changes in adipocytokines and inflammatory mediators, that could, in turn, accelerate aging and telomere shortening [34].

Conclusively, it appears that individual dietary habits exert direct and indirect influence on the various inflammatory processes. A time-restricted dietary scheme and a healthier plant-based nutritional plan could potentially mitigate instances of inflammation and subsequent telomere shortening by reducing the total body fat and insulin levels, providing the organism with anti-inflammatory elements, and supplying the gut microbiome with the necessary plant fibers.

7.7 Conclusions

Fasting constitutes a longstanding tradition, among peoples with historical roots spanning millennia. It has been practiced for diverse purposes, including the spiritual and mental benefits it provides. Religious fasting is a form of fasting that evolved within the doctrines of all major religions. Despite the intra- and inter-religious variability, the core principles of fasting remain consistent: abstinence from food for a defined period and adherence to specific dietary regimens.

The fasting practices of the Christian Orthodox Church generally adhere to the 5:2 intermittent fasting scheme and on several auspicious occasions range from complete abstinence from food to consumption of all edible varieties. The dietary nutrition plan of the adherents resembles that of the Mediterranean diet incorporating numerous vegetarian elements.

Several studies revealed that the benefits of adhering to such dietary regimens can be multiple, including improved cardiovascular health, weight management, improved blood sugar control, enhanced mental clarity, and a healthier digestive system. Additional data from research conducted in the last two decades indicate that dietary patterns, such as calorie restriction, intermittent fasting, or time-restricted fasting can influence cellular processes like inflammation, oxidative stress, and autophagy.

Oxidative stress, arising from the production of free radicals, exerts a negative effect on numerous cellular processes and appears to have the potential to stimulate cellular senescence and reduce telomere length. Similarly, inflammation acts as a complementary process to oxidative stress, initiating a vicious cycle during which the existing inflammatory environment enhances itself. Cells of the immune system that are implicated in this vicious cycle experience cell senescence, potentially due to telomere shortening, an increase in the production of ROS, and inflammation. Furthermore, the decline in the autophagy and mitophagy activity of the cells, which comes with age, results in the accumulation of cellular debris and malfunctioning or excess mitochondria contributing to increased ROS accumulation, oxidative stress, and telomere attrition.

Dietary interventions associated with intermittent fasting and calorie restriction appear to mitigate both oxidative stress and inflammation while promoting cellular autophagy and mitophagy. Christian Orthodox dietary practices and Mediterranean dietary patterns share common elements as they are both abundant in antioxidants and anti-inflammatory substances that alleviate oxidative stress and inflammation, respectively. Additionally, they are rich in plant-based fibers, which enhance gut health and microbiome balance, reducing oxidative stress and inflammation even more.

While fasting offers numerous health benefits, it is critical to carefully assess every individual's medical background, current health status, and nutritional needs, before adhering to one, since such practices may not affect everyone to the same extent or in the same manner.

In conclusion, while there is a growing interest in the potential impact of fasting on cellular processes and telomere maintenance, several aspects of this relationship remain still unexplored.

References

1. Trabelsi, K., Ammar, A., Boujelbane, M. A., Puce, L., Garbarino, S., Scoditti, E., et al. (2022). Religious fasting and its impacts on individual, public, and planetary health: fasting as a "religious health asset" for a healthier, more equitable, and sustainable society, *Front. Nutr.*, **9**, pp. 1036496.
2. Spiliotis, G.M. (2009). *The Diet of the God. The Diet of the Orthodox Church* (G. Spiliotis Publications).
3. "The Catholic Columbian, Volume 27, Number 22, 31 May 1902." The Catholic Columbian, May 1902. JSTOR, https://jstor.org/stable/community.35614917. Accessed 29 Feb. 2024.
4. Sarri, K., Higgins, S., Kafatos, A. (2006). Are religions "healthy"? A review on religious recommendations on diet and lifestyle, *J. Hum. Ecol. Special Issue*, **14**, pp. 7–20.
5. Trepanowski, J. F., Bloomer, R. J. (2010). The impact of religious fasting on human health. *Nutr. J.*, **9**, pp. 57.
6. Visioli, F., Mucignat-Caretta, C., Anile, F., Panaite, S. A. (2022). Traditional and medical applications of fasting, *Nutrients*, **14**, pp. 433.
7. Reza, I. F., Magfiroh, M., Novianto, A., Ilham, A., Ningsih, E. A. dan Rezi Tiana Permatasari, F. R. P. (2019). Fasting on Mondays and Thursdays as a factor increases the emotional intelligence of young Moslem, *Jurnal Studia Insania*, **7**, pp. 108–121.
8. Yom Kippur (2023) Wikipedia, The free encyclopedia. Available at: https://en.wikipedia.org/wiki/Yom_Kippur (Accessed: 15 November 2023).
9. Tisha B'Av (2023) Wikipedia, The free encyclopedia. Available at: https://en.wikipedia.org/wiki/Tisha_B%27Av (Accessed: 15 November 2023).
10. Gaikwad, S. (2017). Apprehending concept, canons and types of fasting in Buddhism, *Journal of Innovative Research and Creative Technology*, **2**, pp. 164–168.
11. Kannan, S., Mahadevan, S., Seshadri, K., Sadacharan, D., Velayutham, K. (2016). Fasting practices in Tamil Nadu and their importance for patients with diabetes, *Indian J. Endocrinol. Metab.*, **20**, pp. 858–862.

12. Faros, F. (2003). *Healing as Part of Holistic Health. Holistic Medicine as an Ecclesiastical Tradition and a Scientific Innovation* (Athens: Armos Publications).
13. Faros, F. (2017). *Being of Good Health. The Meaning of Health and Disease* (Athens: Armos Publications).
14. Colbert, D. (2002) *What Would Jesus Eat?* (Nashville: Thomas Nelson Publishers).
15. Kalamaras, Meletios (Metropolitan of Preveza) (2019). *The Fasting of the Saints* (Ionas Publications).
16. Giaginis, C., Mantzorou, M., Papadopoulou, S. K., Gialeli, M., Troumbis, A. Y., Vasios, G. K. (2023). Christian Orthodox fasting as a traditional diet with low content of refined carbohydrates that promotes human health: a review of the current clinical evidence, *Nutrients*, **15**, pp. 1225.
17. Spiliotis, T. (2018) Διατροφική Ηγεσία. Τι τρώνε οι μοναχοί του Αγίου 'Ορους. το μυστικό για μια μακρά και υγιή ζωή, LinkedIn. Available at: https://www.linkedin.com/pulse/ηγεσιά-και-διατροφή-τι-τρώνε-οι μοναχοί-του-αγίου-το-spiliotis-mba/ (Accessed: 30 September 2023).
18. Spiliotis, G.M. (2023). *The Monk Who Became CEO. 1000 Years of Management of Athos* (Athens: Kaktos Publications).
19. Sarri, K., Linardakis, M., Codrington, C., Kafatos, A. (2007). Does the periodic vegetarianism of Greek Orthodox Christians benefit blood pressure? *Prev. Med.*, **44**, pp. 341–8.
20. ΝΗΣΤΕΙΑ: ΠΟΙΑ ΕΙΝΑΙ ΤΑ ΟΦΕΛΗ ΤΗΣ (ΜΕΡΟΣ Α) (2021) GRDiscovery. Available at: https://grdiscovery.com/nisteia-poia-einai-ta-ofeli-tis-meros-a/ (Accessed: 03 October 2023).
21. ΠΟΙΑ ΕΙΝΑΙ ΤΑ ΟΦΕΛΗ ΤΗΣ ΝΗΣΤΕΙΑΣ (ΜΕΡΟΣ b) (2021) GRDiscovery. Available at: https://grdiscovery.com/ta-ofeli-tis-nisteias-meros-b/ (Accessed: 03 October 2023).
22. Korakidis, A. (2005). *The Supremacy of Church Fasting for Mental and Physical HealthThe Supremacy of Church Fasting for Mental and Physical Health* (Athens: Armos Publications).
23. Koufakis, T., Karras, S. N., Antonopoulou, V., Angeloudi, E., Zebekakis, P., Kotsa, K. (2017). Effects of Orthodox religious fasting on human health: a systematic review, *Eur. J. Nutr.*, 56, pp. 2439–2455.
24. Sarris, K. (2006). The nutritional value of fasting in the Orthodox Church and its effect on lipid metabolism and other biochemical and biological factors, University of Crete, School of Medicine. Department of Social Medicine. Preventive Medicine and Nutrition Clinic, Heraklion, Crete.

25. Michael, A., Baye, K. (2023). Ethiopian orthodox fasting is associated with weight reduction and body composition changes among healthy adults: a prospective cohort study, *Sci Rep*, **13**, pp. 7963.
26. Karras, S. N., Persynaki A., Petróczi, A., Barkans, E., Mulrooney, H., Kypraiou, M. (2017). Health benefits and consequences of the Eastern Orthodox fasting in monks of Mount Athos: a cross-sectional study, *Eur. J. Clin. Nutr.*, **71**, pp. 743–749.
27. Papadaki, A., Vardavas, C., Hatzis, C., Kafatos, A. (2008). Calcium, nutrient and food intake of Greek Orthodox Christian monks during a fasting and non-fasting week, *Public Health Nutr.*, **11**, pp. 1022–9.
28. Basilakis, A., Kiprouli, K., Mantzouranis, S., Konstantinidis, T., Dionisopoulou, M., Hackl, J. M., et al. (2002). Nutritional study in Greek-Orthodox Monasteries - effect of a 40-day religious fasting, *Aktuelle Ernährungsmedizin*, **27**, pp. 250–255.
29. Most, J., Tosti, V., Redman, L. M., Fontana, L. (2017). Calorie restriction in humans: an update, *Ageing Res. Rev.*, **39**, pp. 36–45.
30. Shay, J. W., Wright, W. E. (2019). Telomeres and telomerase: three decades of progress, *Nat. Rev. Genet.*, **20**, pp. 299–309.
31. Muller, H. J. (1938). The remaking of chromosomes, *The Collecting Net*, **8**, pp. 182–195.
32. Heba, A. C., Toupance, S., Arnone, D., Peyrin-Biroulet, L., Benetos, A., Ndiaye, N. C. (2021). Telomeres: new players in immune-mediated inflammatory diseases? *J. Autoimmun.*, **123**, pp. 102699.
33. Longo, V. D., Anderson, R. M. (2022). Nutrition, longevity and disease: from molecular mechanisms to interventions, *Cell*, **185**, pp. 1455–1470.
34. Al-Attas, O. S., Al-Daghri, N. M., Alokail, M. S., Alfadda, A., Bamakhramah, A., Sabico, S., et al. (2010). Adiposity and insulin resistance correlate with telomere length in middle-aged Arabs: the influence of circulating adiponectin, *Eur. J. Endocrinol.*, **163**, pp. 601–7.
35. Barbosa, M. C., Grosso, R. A., Fader, C. M. (2018). Hallmarks of aging: an autophagic perspective, *Front. Endocrinol. (Lausanne)*, **9**, pp. 790.
36. Aman, Y., Schmauck-Medina, T., Hansen, M., Morimoto, R. I., Simon, A. K., Bjedov, I., et al. (2021). Autophagy in healthy aging and disease, *Nature Aging*, **1**, pp. 634–650.
37. Zachari, M., Ganley, I. G. (2017). The mammalian ULK1 complex and autophagy initiation, *Essays Biochem*, **61**, pp. 585–596.
38. Cheon, S. Y., Kim, H., Rubinsztein, D. C., Lee, J. E. (2019). Autophagy, cellular aging and age-related human diseases, *Exp. Neurobiol.*, **28**, pp. 643–657.

39. Poole, L. P., Bock-Hughes, A., Berardi, D. E., Macleod, K. F. (2021). ULK1 promotes mitophagy via phosphorylation and stabilization of BNIP3, *Sci. Rep.*, **11**, pp. 20526.
40. Um, J. H., Yun, J. (2017). Emerging role of mitophagy in human diseases and physiology, *BMB Rep*, **50**, pp. 299–307.
41. Kaushik, S., Tasset, I., Arias, E., Pampliega, O., Wong, E., Martinez-Vicenteet, M., et al. (2021). Autophagy and the hallmarks of aging, *Ageing Res Rev*, **72**, pp. 101468.
42. Liu, L., Trimarchi, J. R., Smith, P. J. S., Keefe, D. L. (2002). Mitochondrial dysfunction leads to telomere attrition and genomic instability, *Aging Cell*, **1**, pp. 40–6.
43. Shabkhizan, R., Haiaty, S., Moslehian, M. S., Bazmani, A., Sadeghsoltani, F., Bagheri, H. S., et al. (2023). The beneficial and adverse effects of autophagic response to caloric restriction and fasting, *Adv. Nutr.*, **14**, pp. 1211–1225.
44. Snezhkina, A. V., Kudryavtseva, A. V., Kardymon, O. L., Savvateeva, M. V., Melnikova, N. V., Krasnovet, G. S., et al. (2019). ROS generation and antioxidant defense systems in normal and malignant cells, *Oxid. Med. Cell Longev.*, **2019**, pp. 6175804.
45. de Almeida, A. J. P. O., de Oliveira, J. C. P. L., da Silva Pontes, L. V., de Souza Júnior, J. F., Gonçalves, T. A. F., Danta, S. H., et al. (2022). ROS: basic concepts, sources, cellular signaling, and its implications in aging pathways, *Oxid. Med. Cell Longev.*, **2022**, pp. 1225578.
46. Barnes, R. P., Fouquerel, E., Opresko, P. L. (2019). The impact of oxidative DNA damage and stress on telomere homeostasis, *Mech. Ageing Dev.*, **177**, pp. 37–45.
47. Boccardi, V., Esposito, A., Rizzo, M. R., Marfella, R., Barbieri, M., Paolisso, G. (2013). Mediterranean diet, telomere maintenance and health status among elderly, *PLoS One*, **8**, pp. e62781.
48. del Río, L. F., Gutiérrez-Casado, E., Varela-López, A., Villalba., J. M. (2016). Olive oil and the hallmarks of aging, *Molecules*, **21**, pp. 163.
49. Galiè, S., Canudas, S., Muralidharan, J., García-Gavilán, J., Bulló, M., Salas-Salvadó, J. (2020). Impact of nutrition on telomere health: systematic review of observational cohort studies and randomized clinical trials, *Adv. Nutr.*, **11**, pp. 576–601.
50. Sarri, K., Bertsias, G., Linardakis, M., Tsibinos, G., Tzanakis, N., Kafatos, A. (2009). The effect of periodic vegetarianism on serum retinol and alpha-tocopherol levels, *Int. J. Vitam. Nutr. Res.*, **79**, pp. 271–80.
51. Mohr, A. E., McEvoy, C., Sears, D. D., Arciero, P. J., Sweazea, K. L. (2021). Impact of intermittent fasting regimens on circulating markers

of oxidative stress in overweight and obese humans: A systematic review of randomized controlled trials, *Advances in Redox Research*, **3**, pp. 100026.

52. Madkour, M. I., El-Serafi, A. T., Jahrami, H. A., Sherif, N. M., Hassan, R. E., Awadallah, S. (2019). Ramadan diurnal intermittent fasting modulates SOD2, TFAM, Nrf2, and sirtuins (SIRT1, SIRT3) gene expressions in subjects with overweight and obesity, *Diabetes Research and Clinical Practice*, **155**, pp. 107801.
53. Faris, M. A. I. E., Jahrami, H. A., Obaideen, A. A., Madkour, M. I. (2019). Impact of diurnal intermittent fasting during Ramadan on inflammatory and oxidative stress markers in healthy people: Systematic review and meta-analysis, *Journal of Nutrition & Intermediary Metabolism*, **15**, pp. 18–26.
54. Chen, L., Deng, H., Cui, H., Fang, J., Zuo, Z., Deng, J. (2018). Inflammatory responses and inflammation-associated diseases in organs, *Oncotarget*, **9**, pp. 7204–7218.
55. O'Donovan, A., Pantell, M. S., Puterman, E., Dhabhar, F. S., Blackburn, E. H., Yaffel., K. (2011). Cumulative inflammatory load is associated with short leukocyte telomere length in the health, aging and body composition study, *PLoS One*, **6**, pp. e19687.
56. Wagenaar, C. A., van de Put, M., Bisschops, M., Walrabenstein, W., de Jonge, C. S., Herrema, H., et al. (2021). The effect of dietary interventions on chronic inflammatory diseases in relation to the microbiome: a systematic review, *Nutrients*, **13**, pp. 3208.
57. Desai, M.S., Seekatz, A. M., Koropatkin, N. M., Kamada, N., Hickey, C. A., Wolter, M., et al. (2016). A dietary fiber-deprived gut microbiota degrades the colonic mucus barrier and enhances pathogen susceptibility, *Cell*, **167**, pp. 1339–1353.e21.
58. Fülöp, T., Larbi, A., Witkowski, J. M. (2019). Human inflammaging, *Gerontology*, **65**, pp. 495–504.
59. García-Calzón, S., Zalba, G., Ruiz-Canela, M., Shivappa, N., Hébert, J. R., Martínez, J. A., et al. (2015). Dietary inflammatory index and telomere length in subjects with a high cardiovascular disease risk from the PREDIMED-NAVARRA study: cross-sectional and longitudinal analyses over 5 y, *Am. J. Clin. Nutr.*, **102**, pp. 897–904.
60. Lagnado, A., Leslie, J., Ruchaud-Sparagano, M-H., Victorelli, S., Hirsova, P., Ogrodnik, M., et al. (2021). Neutrophils induce paracrine telomere dysfunction and senescence in ROS-dependent manner, *EMBO J.*, **40**, pp. e106048.

Chapter 8

The Impact of Exercise on Telomere Length

Stella Baliou,[a,b] Petros Ioannou,[c] Vassilis Zoumpourlis,[d] Demetrios Spandidos,[e] and Aristidis Tsatsakis[a,b]

[a] *Laboratory of Toxicology, Medical School, University of Crete, Heraklion, Greece*
[b] *Lifeplus S.A., Science & Technological Park of Crete, Vassilika Vouton, Heraklion, Crete, Greece*
[c] *School of Medicine, University of Crete, Heraklion, Greece*
[d] *Biomedical Applications Unit, Institute of Chemical Biology, National Hellenic Research Foundation, Athens, Greece*
[e] *Laboratory of Clinical Virology, Medical School, University of Crete, Heraklion, Greece*
tsatsaka@uoc.gr

8.1 Introduction

Telomeres are nucleoprotein structures located at the repetitive regions of chromosomes in which protein structures are assembled preventing errors and ensuring chromosomal stability [1]. During each cell division, telomeres gradually shorten, and telomere length can reach a critical threshold at advanced aging [1]. Critical short telomeres induce permanent damage and, eventually, cell death

Telomeres: Biomarkers of a Healthy Life and Successful Aging
Edited by Aristidis Tsatsakis

ISBN 978-981-5129-49-6 (Hardcover), 978-1-003-56809-4 (eBook)
www.jennystanford.com

[2]. The telomere shortening can be reversed through telomerase activity. There are two main components of telomerase: telomerase reverse transcriptase (TERT) and telomerase RNA component (TERC). The TERC is coated with DNA nucleotides complementary to telomeres in order to proceed to telomere elongation through reverse transcription [3].

In aging research, critical advances have been accomplished in recent years, and novel insights into aging emerge through the evaluation of telomere length. Nowadays, it is irrefutable that aging is a significant risk factor for many age-related complications as manifested by the accumulation of DNA damage in aged cells [5]. Undoubtedly, telomere length is genetically regulated through each cell division [4]. However, it should be noted that there is a plausible interplay between lifestyle and telomere length of every individual [6, 7]. When telomere length was measured in six blood cell types from 1046 individuals using the Flow-FISH methodology, it was proven that the determination of telomere length depended on lifestyle apart from its genetic regulation [6]. Indeed, an unhealthy lifestyle can accelerate telomere length elimination [8]. When an unhealthy lifestyle is adopted through sedentary behavior or metabolic disorders, oxidative stress and inflammation are predominant mechanisms that induce telomere shortening [9, 10]. Besides, telomere length in leukocytes is considered representative of all cell types through mitotic inheritance [11].

In contrast, a healthy lifestyle and exercise significantly sustain a health span in every individual throughout life [12]. Over the last decades, exercise has emerged as an effective approach to restoring distortion of organ or tissue functions during aging. In essence, exercise seems to reverse accelerated biological aging conferring a lower risk of malignancies [13], cardiovascular diseases [14], and chronic metabolic syndromes [13].

More specifically, exercise benefits every organ expressing its effect by regulating signaling cascades in the cardiovascular, musculoskeletal, pulmonary, central, and peripheral nervous systems [14, 15]. In particular, the cardiovascular benefits of exercise are mediated by the renewal of endothelial progenitor cells and the reduction of endothelial oxidative stress, which are crucial in injuries. Exercise is considered an intervention with positive effects on neurogenesis, gluconeogenesis, glucagon secretion, fatty acid metabolism, insulin-independent glucose uptake, and muscle endurance [16–18]. Enhancement of these processes contributes to the protective effect of exercise upon different organs in the human body. Regarding the skeletal system, exercise increases bone mass to the greatest extent and reduces the potential for osteoporosis or sarcopenia [19, 20]. Concerning the nervous system, the effects of exercise are of utmost importance delaying the onset of Alzheimer's disease and other degenerative diseases [21]. Compared to the beneficial effect of exercise in the battle against age-related diseases, a sedentary life has been reported to account for the increased occurrence of cardiometabolic diseases like type 2 diabetes (T2D) [22].

Since the longevity of an individual is reflected by telomere dynamics [23], the prevalence of aging and age-related diseases is linked to telomere shortening [24]. In this context, the rate of telomere shortening can be reversed through exercise, which delays the onset of age-related disorders [24]. Indeed, exercise emerges as the first preventive lifestyle intervention to attenuate the risk of aging-related diseases by reducing the characteristics of aging [25, 26]. Concurrently, exercise is the most significant factor in lowering mortality irrespective of the cause [27].

There is irrefutable evidence that exercise is positively associated with telomere length. In most studies, telomere shortening is moderated through exercise [9]. Notably, Vyas et al. studied the effect of exercise on TL in 3 groups: Hispanic (n = 247), Black (n = 248), and non-Hispanic White (n = 254) US subjects. Men and women were in equal distribution in the studied population. The study showed that as the age increased, TL became shorter. Higher physical activity was associated with longer telomeres. Moreover, a stronger association between exercise and telomere length was more prominent for the non-Hispanic White group rather than the two other groups, which indicated that race/ethnicity affects the impact of exercise on TL [28]. Ekelund et al. did a systematic review and a harmonized meta-analysis of 8 studies (n = 36 383; mean age 62.6 years; 72.8% women), where the effect of total physical activity, different intensities of physical activity, and sedentary time on all-cause mortality was assessed. It was shown that an increase in exercise at any intensity significantly reduced the risk for premature mortality in middle-aged and older adults [29]. As a result, depending on the level of exercise, an individual's life gain can be between two and four years [29, 30]. A study examining the effect of aerobic exercise versus time-restricted feeding (TRF) in diet-induced aged obese mice has shown that these factors have a beneficial effect on the health span of those mice even if they are introduced at a later stage in life. Both factors, aerobic exercise and TRF, have had a positive effect on the mice's body composition, metabolism, physical function, daily living behavior, and liver pathology (all factors related to obesity and aging). However, TRF might have a negative impact on lean mass and vascular function. This leads to the conclusion that exercise is safe for aged obese mice, but the efficacy of TRF to improve health span in late life stage still needs further clarification [31].

Based on the significance of exercise in well-being, epidemiological evidence supports that exercise is tightly linked to telomere length maintenance [32]. In this direction, several systematic reviews have highlighted the positive association of exercise with telomere dynamics. Firstly, Valente et al. conducted a systematic review with meta-analysis of 30 studies and 7418 participants concluding that physical activity is associated with elongation of telomere length but there is a low certainty for that effect. Therefore, he suggests contrary to the authors above that the effect of the exercise on telomere length is probably overestimated [33]. On the other hand, Aguiar et al. supported that master athletes ($n = 240$) who followed a healthy lifestyle accompanied by controlled exercise were characterized by longer telomeres compared to physically inactive controls after a meta-analysis of eleven studies [34]. The master athletes (100 m to marathon) were used as models of biological aging because of their metabolic profile and physical fitness associated with respective adaptation in their pulmonary system [35]. From a molecular perspective, they had low inflammation, high antioxidant defense, increased recruitment of shelterin complex proteins, and increased mitochondrial biogenesis and telomerase activity contributing to telomere length elongation [34]. Master athletes showed upregulation of critical enzymes implicated in antioxidant defense, such as catalase and superoxide dismutase/thiobarbituric acid reactive substances (SOD/TBARS) ratio [34]. However, the risk of bias in studies included in the systematic review was moderate [34]. Accordingly, Song et al. reported that aerobic exercise for more than six months protected telomeres from their deterioration than other types of exercise and durations as concluded by seven randomized controlled trials (RCTs) with 939 participants [36]. The heterogeneity of all included studies in the meta-analysis was low (13%). However, the results of a systematic review concerning the impact of exercise on telomere length arose from five of the eight RCTs. The differences among the three studies depended on population characteristics such as sex, body mass index (BMI), age, and extent of exercise [36]. Another systematic review of 20 studies with 2995 participants proved that a healthy lifestyle and exercise contributed to telomere length elongation irrespective of individuals' traits [8]. The most recent conclusions came from three systematic reviews of twenty-seven observational studies, eight randomized controlled studies (RCTs), and eight interventional studies with small groups of individuals [37]. Those systematic reviews showed that aerobic and moderate-intensity exercise profoundly affected telomere length maintenance [37]. As it was observed by all studies of systematic reviews, exercise cannot be considered the cause or consequence of telomere length elongation.

Exercise delays the pace of aging through the inhibition of telomere shortening. There are several mechanisms by which exercise contributes to telomere length maintenance or elongation. Exercise increases the expression levels of telomeric repeat-binding factor 2 (TRF2), which is a protein of the shelterin complex. The primary function of this complex is to prevent telomeres from being detected as double-strand breaks (DSBs), hindering the deficient repair mechanisms and the erosion of telomeres [38]. Accordingly, the DNA repair pathway's proteins seem to increase in middle-aged individuals in response to exercise. It has been highlighted that exercise protects telomeres from shortening induced by inflammation and oxidative bursts. Exercise is supposed to reduce inflammation by reducing the expression levels of pro-inflammatory mediators [tumor necrosis factor-alpha (TNF-a), interleukin-6 (IL-6), nuclear factor kappa B, poly (ADP-ribose) polymerase 1 (PARP-1), repressor-activator protein 1 (RAP-1), and TERT] since inflammation plays a critical role in telomere

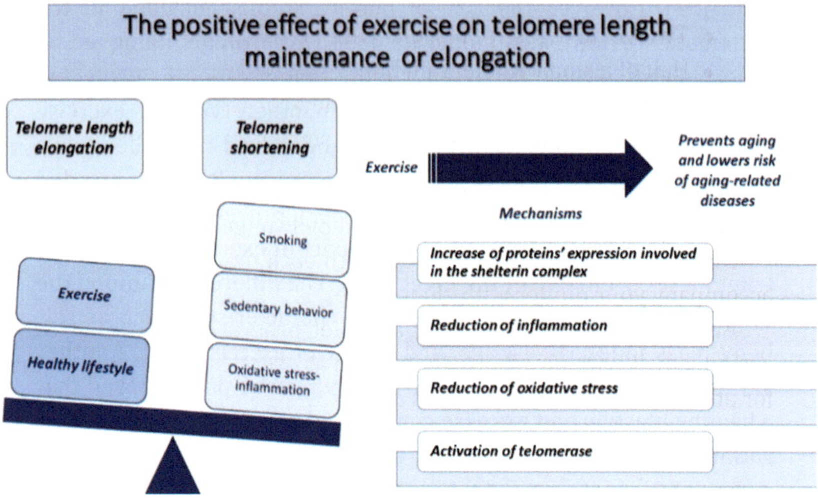

Figure 8.1 Exercise exerts a beneficial effect on telomere length maintenance or elongation by hindering oxidative stress accompanied by inflammation and enhancing telomerase action as well as the protein abundance of the shelterin complex.

shortening [39]. The protective effect of exercise lies in increasing the antioxidants and reducing the formation of reactive oxygen species (ROS) (Fig. 8.1) [40].

Even though exercise is positively associated with maintaining good human health, several parameters like duration, frequency, intensity, and type of exercise determine the impact of exercise on telomere maintenance (Fig. 8.2).

8.2 Exercise Duration Effect on Telomere Length

There is substantial evidence that acute exercise (high-intensity exercise at a single session) activates a sustainable inflammation impairing the function of every organ in the human body and simulating processes implicated in aging and aging-related diseases. Importantly, it has been observed that molecular adaptations of aging parallel those triggered by acute exercise [41]. Indeed, acute exercise upregulates glucose uptake through increased translocation of glucose transporter type 4 (GLUT4) to the plasma membrane

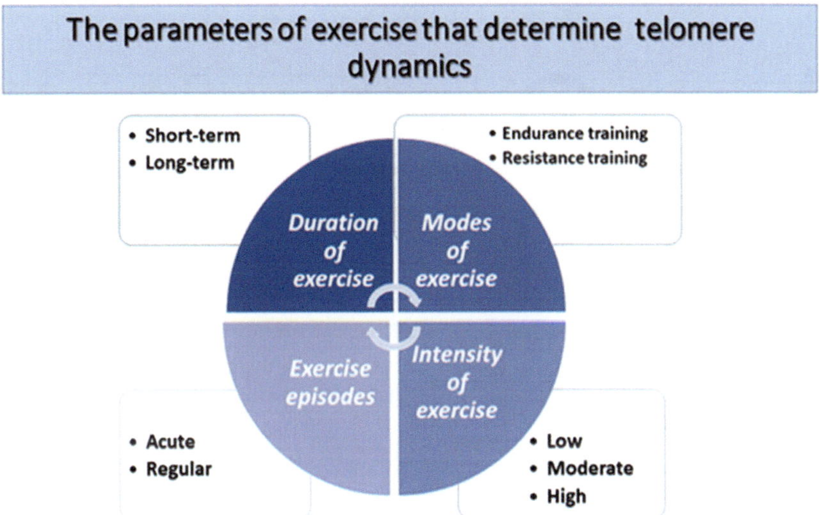

Figure 8.2 The chart shows that the effect of exercise on telomere dynamics is determined by the duration, frequency, intensity, and types of exercise.

which is mediated by the activation of the AMP-activated protein kinase (AMPK) signaling cascade and accumulation of intracellular calcium (Ca^{+2}) pools [42]. The processes mentioned earlier are explained by acute bouts of exercise since muscle cell contraction relies on increasing ROS formation [42]. In acute exercise, oxygen is needed and consumed at high levels, translated in a molecular setting with the activation of mitochondrial activity and accumulation of superoxide ions in the skeletal muscle [43]. This redox disequilibrium mediated by acute exercise leads to preventing the action of plasma membrane Ca^{+2}ATPase, which, in turn, contributes to increased intracellular pools of Ca^{+2} and membrane translocation of the GLUT-4 transporter [44]. As a result, acute exercise negatively affects the redox balance resulting in cellular damage [45]. Besides, the protective effects of exercise have been seen in even 30 minutes of treadmill running that contributed to sustaining telomere length through increasing RNA expression levels of TERT and of sirtuin-6 (SIRT-6) deacetylase, thus regulating gene expression [46].

Long-term exercise reorganizes the functions of several organs including neurological, cardiorespiratory, endocrine, musculoskeletal, and immune systems [47]. In parallel, chronic moderate exercise

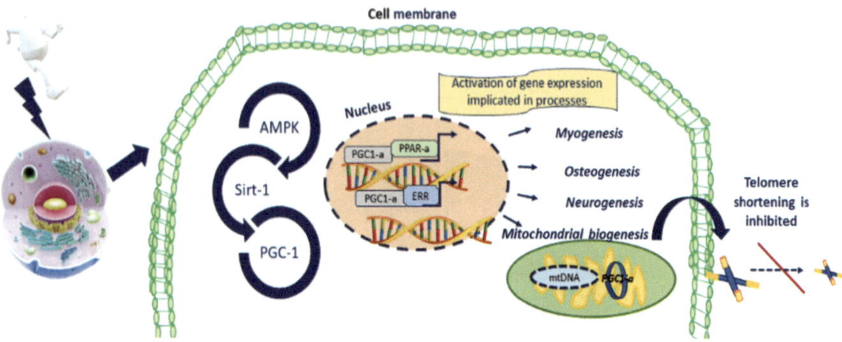

Figure 8.3 The impact of long-term exercise through activation of the AMPK/SIRT1/PGC-1α signaling pathway, thus triggering myogenesis, osteogenesis, neurogenesis, and mitochondrial biogenesis and finally preventing telomere shortening.

is beneficial in hindering age-related telomere shortening [48]. From a molecular perspective, exercise is essential in increasing muscle mitochondrial activity, upregulating peroxisome proliferator-activated receptor co-activator (PGC-1α), a marker of mitochondrial biogenesis [49, 50]. Overexpression of PGC-1α has also been considered a vital regulator in osteogenesis, neurogenesis, and myogenesis. More precisely, the increased adenosine monophosphate/adenosine triphosphate (AMP/ATP) ratio creates activation of AMPK and Sirt1 allowing the nuclear translocation of PGC-1α. Then, PGC-1a assembles with either peroxisome proliferator activator-a (PPAR-a) or estrogen-related receptor (ERR) activating mitochondrial biogenesis, myogenesis, neurogenesis, and osteogenesis (Fig. 8.3) [51–55].

In this manner, chronic exercise ameliorates mitochondrial quality and quantity attenuating the risk of cardiovascular diseases [56]. Furthermore, long-term exercise has been shown to increase telomerase activity in a broad spectrum of tissues including human peripheral blood mononuclear cells (PBMCs) [57], mouse skeletal muscle [48], heart [58], aorta [38], and hippocampi [59]. Besides, the activation of telomerase depends on TERT and endothelial nitric oxide synthase (eNOS) protein expression since telomerase is not stimulated in knock-out mice for TERT and eNOS (TERT-/- eNOS -/-) [58]. It should be noted that chronic moderate exercise can mediate vascular protective effects through eNOS activation [38]. Despite the inverse relationship of TERT and eNOS with telomerase, research findings have shown the boosting impact of insulin growth factor-1 (IGF-1) on telomerase action as observed in the cardiac myocytes of exercised mice [38].

In patients with myocardial infarction, 8-week-training provided benefits in maintaining telomere length through increasing the proteins of shelterin complex [telomeric repeat binding factor 1 (TRF1), telomeric repeat binding factor 2 (TRF2)] at the ends of chromosomes and upregulating telomerase in a statistically significant manner [60].

8.3 Exercise Intensity Effect on Telomere Length

The benefits of exercise are different depending on the intensity of exercise. Focusing on the intensity, the exercise is positively associated with telomere length as an inverted U-shaped curve. In an RCT that had recruited elderly, physically inactive, and overweight individuals, regular exercise greatly impacted telomere length maintenance [61]. Firstly, Fretts et al. also highlighted the positive relationship of regular exercise with telomere length elongation in a feedforward loop [62]. Secondly, Savela et al. have shown that moderate exercise caused telomere length elongation compared to other exercise intensities in 782 midlife men [63]. Thirdly, Ludlow et al. have illustrated that energy expenditure of 991 up to 2340 kcals per week was favorable to telomere length preservation [64]. Accordingly, the most remarkable evidence about the beneficial impact of moderate exercise on telomere dynamics came from a 12-year study in over 400,000 individuals who moderately exercised at least 15 min a day, thereby displaying reduced risk for all-cause mortality [65]. Exercise intensity can also play a crucial role in disease conditions. For example, postmenopausal women with stage I–III breast cancer who were physically active at moderate to vigorous exercise presented telomere length elongation compared to their inactive controls [66]. The results mentioned above were consistent with those of the cross-sectional study, showing that postmenopausal women had longer telomeres, owing to their continuous exercise for nineteen months [67].

The protective effect of moderate exercise relies on reducing age-related immunosenescence in specific CD8+ CD28+ T-cell populations, thereby maintaining telomere length [68]. Another proposed mechanism for moderate intensity mediated protective effects is age-dependent stimulation of telomerase action [37]. As a result, moderate-intensity exercise has been proven beneficial on telomere length compared to low and vigorous exercise [69]. Indeed, the higher amounts of exercise do not provide additional benefits on telomere dynamics [70]. Vigorous exercise has been reported to exert detrimental effects on homeostasis [37]. It should be noted that even courses of intermittent exercise effectively alleviate health problems [71].

8.4 Regular Exercise Effect on Telomere Length

It has been substantiated that regular exercise reduces the potential for mortality [72]. Prospective cohort studies have shown that regularly exercised individuals exhibited a 70% mortality risk, which was exacerbated in an age-dependent manner [29, 30]. Moreover, regular exercise has brought a surge of research into disease conditions. In a study with enrolled prostate cancer patients, a 3-month intervention composed of regular exercise for three months (30 minutes of walking per 6 days of the week) combined with a well-controlled lifestyle offered considerable benefits on telomere length [73]. Notably, the benefits of regular exercise with a healthy diet were evidenced by longer telomeres in exercised individuals compared to physically inactive age-matched controls 5 years after the onset of a healthy lifestyle [73]. The proposed principle for telomere length elongation has been attributed to the activation of telomerase in PBMCs [57].

It is well established that regularly active individuals are characterized by better fitness in all their organs attenuating the possibility of diseases [72]. Those results corroborate the findings of a 1-year randomized controlled study showing that regular exercise can improve the cardiorespiratory profile and mitigate age-dependent brain atrophy in the elderly delaying memory dysfunction for one up to 2 years [74].

Another suggested mechanism underlying regular exercise's protective effects seems to be targeting oxidative stress [75]. Regular physical exercise regulates the redox state upregulating the levels of antioxidants, thus, in turn, reducing oxidative DNA damage and sustaining telomere length [75]. In addition to the above, regular exercise exerts its protective effects by lowering inflammatory cytokine levels and increasing anti-inflammatory cytokine levels [76]. Regular exercise has been shown to attenuate all the characteristics of inflammation by reducing the population of exhausted and senescent cells while significantly contributing to the elevation of the T-cell population, natural killer (NK)-mediated cytotoxicity, and neutrophil phagocytosis [77]. Those results were concordant with those of Sousa et al. showed that the level of exercise in master athletes was positively related to sustaining telomere length through reduction of inflammation [78]. Besides, the rate of telomere shortening can be exacerbated through inflammation [39].

Reinforcing the beneficial impact of regular exercise on telomere length, it has also been shown that regular exercise increases the expression of shelterin complexes like TRF1 and TRF2 proteins [60]. Accordingly, telomerase has been identified as an important player in mediating protective effects mediated by regular exercise [46, 70]. Remarkably, continuous regular exercise for at least 10 years was sufficient to cause telomere length elongation as proved by a meta-analysis of elite athletes aged above 45 years old [79].

8.5 Effect of Type of Exercise on Telomere Length

In addition to the above, there are two types of exercise, endurance and resistance training, which affect the rate of telomere shortening in a distinct manner. Endurance, called aerobic exercise, often includes distance running, swimming, and cycling. The required energy for endurance exercise is provided by mitochondrial respiration, so the heart function and breathing are high [80]. Notably, the maximum oxygen consumption can be increased from 10% up to 15% [81]. In contrast, resistance exercise is characterized by the capacity of muscles to work against weight or force.

Some activities of resistance exercise are the following: bicep curls, leg extensions, sprinting, and powerlifting. Every individual who engages in resistance exercise takes energy from anaerobic glycolysis and creatine phosphate (CP), which are not based on oxygen consumption [82].

Exploring the different modes of exercise on telomere dynamics, only one RCT showed that participants who engaged in endurance exercise had longer leukocyte telomere length than their controls who did resistance training [83]. Concerning endurance exercise, a landmark study has shown that ultra-endurance athletes presented telomere length elongation by 11% more than their controls with a sedentary lifestyle providing a gain of biological age at sixteen years [84]. One benefit of endurance to athletes compared to master sprinters has been attributed to finetuning endothelial function through increasing nitric oxide (NO) levels. In contrast, sprinter athletes conferred had lower levels of oxidative stress and inflammation [85]. Telomere shortening could also be attenuated in endurance athletes by increasing telomerase action and proteins of the shelterin complex [38]. Regarding resistance exercise, there are conflicting results about its impact on telomere length [86]. The most recent study supported the positive association of 12-week resistance exercise on telomere length for a follow-up of 12 months [83, 86–88]. The inconsistencies throughout the research findings can be attributed to the different genetic profiles of individuals, age ranges, DNA extraction methods, ways of evaluating exercise and measuring telomere length, and other confounding factors (like nutrition, psychological stress, and lifestyle of the individual) (Table 8.1). In summary, endurance exercise significantly improves telomere length compared to resistance exercise.

8.6 Conclusions

Undoubtedly, exercise is fundamental for maintaining good health for every individual throughout life, offering myriads of benefits. The consensus from the above studies is that physically active individuals sustain or elongate their telomere length compared to sedentary peers. This chapter concludes that long-term moderate-

Table 8.1 The effects of exercise on telomere length and their underlying molecular mechanisms

Parameters of exercise	Exercise effect on TL	Molecular mechanisms of exercise
Acute exercise	Negative	Induction of oxidative stress and cellular damage
Long-term exercise	Positive	Activation of myogenesis, osteogenesis, neurogenesis, mitochondrial biogenesis
Moderate exercise	Positive	Reduction of immunosenescence
Regular exercise	Positive	Activation of telomerase, reduction of oxidative stress and inflammation, increased proteins' expression involved in the shelterin complex
Endurance exercise	Positive	Increase of mitochondrial respiration, telomerase, proteins' expression involved in the shelterin complex, reduction of inflammation and oxidative stress
Resistance exercise	Negative	Anaerobic glycolysis

intensity endurance exercise appears to be the most effective in elongating telomere length compared to another type of exercise, shedding light on its underlying molecular mechanisms.

Abbreviations

Adenosine monophosphate (AMP)
Adenosine triphosphate (ATP)
AMP-activated protein kinase (AMPK)
Body mass index (BMI)
Creatine phosphate (CP)
Double-strand breaks (DSBs)
Endothelial nitric oxide synthase (eNOS)
Estrogen-related receptor (ERR)
Glucose transporter type 4 (GLUT4)
Insulin growth factor-1 (IGF-1)
Interleukin 6 (IL-6)
Nitric oxide (NO)

Peripheral blood mononuclear cells (PBMCs)
Peroxisome proliferator activator-a (PPAR-a)
Peroxisome proliferator-activated receptor co-activator (PGC-1α)
Poly (ADP-ribose) polymerase 1 (PARP-1)
Randomized controlled trials (RCTs)
Reactive oxygen species (ROS)
Repressor-activator protein 1 (RAP-1)
Sirtuin-6 (SIRT-6)
Superoxide dismutase (SOD)
Telomerase reverse transcriptase (TERT)
Telomerase RNA component (TERC)
Telomeric repeat binding factor 1 (TRF1)
Telomeric repeat binding factor 2 (TRF2)
Telomeric repeat-binding factor 2 (TRF2)
Thiobarbituric acid reactive substances (TBARS)
Tumor necrosis factor-alpha (TNF-a)
Type 2 diabetes (T2D)

References

1. López-Otín, C., Blasco, M. A., Partridge, L., Serrano, M. and Kroemer, G. (2013). The hallmarks of aging, *Cell*, **153**, pp. 1194–217.
2. Sanders, J. L. and Newman, A. B. (2013). Telomere length in epidemiology: a biomarker of aging, age-related disease, both, or neither? *Epidemiol. Rev.*, **35**, pp. 112–131.
3. Feng, J., Funk, W.D., Wang, S.S., Weinrich, S.L., Avilion, A.A., Chiu, C.P., *et al.* (1995). The RNA component of human telomerase, *Science*, **269**, pp. 1236–1241.
4. Vaiserman, A. and Krasnienkov, D. (2021). Telomere length as a marker of biological age: state-of-the-art, open issues, and future perspectives, *Front. Genet.*, **11**, pp. 630186.
5. Kakridonis, F., Pneumatikos, S. G., Vakonaki, E., Berdiaki, A., Tzatzarakis, M. N., Fragkiadaki, P., *et al.* (2023). Telomere length as a predictive biomarker in osteoporosis (review), *Biomed. Rep.*, **19**, pp. 87.
6. Andreu-Sánchez, S., Aubert, G., Ripoll-Cladellas, A., Henkelman, S., Zhernakova, D.V., Sinha, T., *et al.* (2022). Genetic, parental and lifestyle factors influence telomere length, *Commun. Biol.*, **5**, pp. 565.

7. Tsoukalas, D., Fragkiadaki, P., Docea, A. O., Alegakis, A. K., Sarandi, E., Vakonaki, E., *et al.* (2019). Association of nutraceutical supplements with longer telomere length, *Int. J. Mol. Med.*, **44**, pp. 218–226.

8. Buttet, M., Bagheri, R., Ugbolue, U. C., Laporte, C., Trousselard, M., Benson, A., *et al.* (2022). Effect of a lifestyle intervention on telomere length: a systematic review and meta-analysis, *Mech. Ageing Dev.*, **206**, pp. 111694.

9. Navarro-Ibarra, M. J. Hernández, J., and G. Caire-Juvera, G. (2019). Diet, physical activity and telomere length in adults, *Nutr. Hosp.*, **36**, pp. 1403–1417.

10. Starkweather, A. R., Alhaeeri, A. A., Montpetit, A., Brumelle, J., Filler, K., Montpetit, M., *et al.* (2014). An integrative review of factors associated with telomere length and implications for biobehavioral research, *Nurs. Res.*, **63**, pp. 36–50.

11. Demanelis, K., Jasmine, F., Chen, L. S., Chernoff, M., Tong, L., Delgado, D., *et al.* (2020). Determinants of telomere length across human tissues, *Science*, **369**, pp. eaaz6876.

12. Longo, V. D., Antebi, A., Bartke, A., Barzilai, N., Brown-Borg, H. M., Caruso, C., *et al.* (2015). Interventions to slow aging in humans: are we ready? *Aging Cell*, **14**, pp. 497–510.

13. Gulsin, G. S., Henson, J., Brady, E. M., Sargeant, J. A., Wilmot, E. G., Athithan, L., *et al.* (2020). Cardiovascular determinants of aerobic exercise capacity in adults with type 2 diabetes, *Diabetes Care*, **43**, pp. 2248–2256.

14. Buchman, A. S., Boyle, P. A., Yu, L., Shah, R. C., Wilson, R. S. and Bennett, D. A. (2012). Total daily physical activity and the risk of AD and cognitive decline in older adults, *Neurology*, **78**, pp. 1323–1329.

15. Egan, B. and Zierath, J. R. (2013). Exercise metabolism and the molecular regulation of skeletal muscle adaptation, *Cell Metab.*, **17**, pp. 162–184.

16. Roh, J. D., Houstis, N., Yu, A., Chang, B., Yeri, A., Li, H., *et al.* (2020). Exercise training reverses cardiac aging phenotypes associated with heart failure with preserved ejection fraction in male mice, *Aging Cell*, **19**, pp. e13159.

17. Xia, W. H., Li, J., Su, C., Yang, Z., Chen, L., Wu, F., *et al.* (2012). Physical exercise attenuates age-associated reduction in endothelium-reparative capacity of endothelial progenitor cells by increasing CXCR4/JAK-2 signaling in healthy men, *Aging Cell*, **11**, pp. 111–119.

18. Pierce, G. L., Donato, A. J., La Rocca, T. J., Eskurza, I., Silver, A. E., and Seals, D. R. (2011). Habitually exercising older men do not demonstrate

age-associated vascular endothelial oxidative stress, *Aging Cell*, **10**, pp. 1032–1037.

19. Santos, L., Elliott-Sale, K. J. and Sale, C. (2017). Exercise and bone health across the lifespan, *Biogerontology*, **18**, pp. 931–946.
20. Crane, J. D., MacNeil, L. G., Lally, J. S., Ford, R. J., Bujak, A. L., Brar, I. K., *et al.* (2015). Exercise-stimulated interleukin-15 is controlled by AMPK and regulates skin metabolism and aging, *Aging Cell*, **14**, pp. 625–634.
21. Radak, Z., Hart, N., Sarga, L., Koltai, E., Atalay, M., Ohno, H. *et al.* (2010). Exercise plays a preventive role against Alzheimer's disease, *J. Alzheimers Dis. JAD*, **20**, pp. 777–783.
22. Patterson, R., McNamara, E., Tainio, M., de Sá, T.H., Smith, A.D., Sharp, S.J., *et al.* (2018). Sedentary behaviour and risk of all-cause, cardiovascular and cancer mortality, and incident type 2 diabetes: a systematic review and dose response meta-analysis, *Eur. J. Epidemiol.*, **33**, pp. 811–829.
23. Babizhayev, M. A., Savel'yeva, E. L., Moskvina, S. N.and Yegorov, Y. E. (2011). Telomere length is a biomarker of cumulative oxidative stress, biologic age, and an independent predictor of survival and therapeutic treatment requirement associated with smoking behavior, *Am. J. Ther.*, **18**, pp. e209–226.
24. Shammas, M. A. (2011). Telomeres, lifestyle, cancer and aging, *Curr. Opin. Clin. Nutr. Metab. Care*, **14**, pp. 28–34.
25. Bennie, J. A., Shakespear-Druery, J. and De Cocker, K. (2020). Muscle-strengthening exercise epidemiology: a new frontier in chronic disease prevention, *Sports Med. - Open*, **6**, pp. 40.
26. Rebelo-Marques, A., De Sousa Lages, A., Andrade, R., Ribeiro, C.F., Mota-Pinto, A., Carrilho, F. *et al.* (2018). Aging hallmarks: the benefits of physical exercise, *Front. Endocrinol.*, **9**, pp. 258.
27. Katzmarzyk, P. T., Church, T. S., Craig, C. L. and Bouchard, C. (2009). Sitting time and mortality from all causes, cardiovascular disease, and cancer, *Med. Sci. Sports Exerc.*, **41**, pp. 998–1005.
28. Vyas, C. M, Ogata, S., Reynolds, C. F., Mischoulon, D., Chang, G., Cook N.R., *et al.* (2021). Telomere length and its relationships with lifestyle and behavioural factors: variations by sex and race/ethnicity, *Age Ageing*, **50**, pp. 838–846.
29. Ekelund, U., Tarp, J., Steene-Johannessen, J., Hansen, B. H., Jefferis, B., Fagerland, M. W., *et al.* (2019). Dose-response associations between accelerometry measured physical activity and sedentary time and all-cause mortality: systematic review and harmonised meta-analysis, *BMJ*, **366**, pp. l4570.

30. Semeraro, M.D., Smith, C., Kaiser, M., Levinger, I., Duque, G., Gruber, H.J. and Herrman, M. (2020). Physical activity, a modulator of aging through effects on telomere biology, *Aging (Albany NY)*, **12**, pp. 13803–13823.
31. Schafer, M. J., Mazula, D. L., Brown, A. K., White, T. A., Atkinson, E., Pearsall, V. M., *et al.* (2019). Late-life time-restricted feeding and exercise differentially alter healthspan in obesity, *Aging Cell*, **18**, pp. e12966.
32. Semeraro, M. D, Smith, C., Kaiser, M., Levinger, I., Duque, G., Gruber, H. J. *et al.* (2020). Physical activity, a modulator of aging through effects on telomere biology, *Aging*, **12**, pp. 13803–13823.
33. Valente, C., Andrade, R., Alvarez, L., Rebelo-Marques, A., Stamatakis, E. and Espregueira-Mendes, J. (2021). Effect of physical activity and exercise on telomere length: systematic review with meta-analysis, *J. Am. Geriatr. Soc.*, **69**, pp. 3285–3300.
34. Aguiar, S. S., Sousa, C. V., Santos, P. A., Barbosa, L. P., Maciel, L. A., Coelho-Júnior, H. J., *et al.* (2021). Master athletes have longer telomeres than age-matched non-athletes. A systematic review, meta-analysis and discussion of possible mechanisms, *Exp. Gerontol.*, **146**, pp. 111212.
35. Kusy, K. and Zieliński, J. (2015). Sprinters versus long-distance runners: how to grow old healthy, *Exerc. Sport Sci. Rev.*, **43**, pp. 57–64.
36. Song, S., Lee, E. and Kim, H. (2022). "Does exercise affect telomere length? A systematic review and meta-analysis of randomized controlled trials, *Med. Kaunas Lith.*, **58**, pp. 242.
37. Schellnegger, M., Lin, A. C., Hammer, N. and Kamolz, L.-P. (2022). Physical activity on telomere length as a biomarker for aging: a systematic review, *Sports Med. - Open*, **8**, pp. 111.
38. Werner, C., Fürster, T., Widmann, T., Pöss, J., Roggia, C., Hanhoun, M., *et al.* (2009). Physical exercise prevents cellular senescence in circulating leukocytes and in the vessel wall, *Circulation*, **120**, pp. 2438–2447.
39. Zhang, J., Rane, G., Dai, X., Shanmugam, M.K., Arfuso, F., Samy, R.P., *et al.* (2016). Ageing and the telomere connection: an intimate relationship with inflammation, *Ageing Res. Rev.*, **25**, pp. 55–69.
40. Radak, Z., Chung, H. Y., Koltai, E., Taylor, A. W. and Goto, S. (2008). Exercise, oxidative stress and hormesis, *Ageing Res. Rev.*, **7**, pp. 34–42.
41. Lefferts, W. K., Davis, M. M. and Valentine, R. J. (2022). Exercise as an aging mimetic: a new perspective on the mechanisms behind exercise as preventive medicine against age-related chronic disease, *Front. Physiol.*, **13**, pp. 866792.

42. Stanford, K. I., Goodyear, L. J. (2014). Exercise and type 2 diabetes: molecular mechanisms regulating glucose uptake in skeletal muscle, *Adv. Physiol. Educ.*, **38**, pp. 308–14.
43. Urso, M. L. and Clarkson, P. M. (2003). Oxidative stress, exercise, and antioxidant supplementation, *Toxicology*, **189**, pp. 41–54.
44. Wright, D. C. Hucker, K. A., Holloszy, J. O. and Han, D. H. (2004). Ca2+ and AMPK both mediate stimulation of glucose transport by muscle contractions, *Diabetes*, **53**, pp. 330–335.
45. He, F., Li, J., Liu, Z., Chuang, C.-C., Yang, W. and Zuo, L. (2016). Redox mechanism of reactive oxygen species in exercise, *Front. Physiol.*, **7**, pp. 486.
46. Chilton W. L., Marques F. Z., West J., Kannourakis G., Berzins S. P., O'Brien B. J. *et al.* (2014). Acute exercise leads to regulation of telomere-associated genes and microRNA expression in immune cells, *PloS One*, **9**, pp. e92088.
47. Timmons, J. A., Knudsen, S., Rankinen, T., Koch, L. G., Sarzynski, M., Jensen, T., *et al.* (2010). Using molecular classification to predict gains in maximal aerobic capacity following endurance exercise training in humans, *J. Appl. Physiol. Bethesda Md 1985*, **108**, pp. 1487–1496.
48. Ludlow, A. T., Witkowski, S., Marshall, M. R., Wang, J., Lima, L. C., Guth, L. M., *et al.* (2012). Chronic exercise modifies age-related telomere dynamics in a tissue-specific fashion, *J. Gerontol. A. Biol. Sci. Med. Sci.*, **67**, pp. 911–926.
49. Meex, R. C., Schrauwen-Hinderling, V. B., Moonen-Kornips, E., Schaart, G., Mensink, M., Phielix, E., *et al.* (2010). Restoration of muscle mitochondrial function and metabolic flexibility in type 2 diabetes by exercise training is paralleled by increased myocellular fat storage and improved insulin sensitivity, *Diabetes*, **59**, pp. 572–579.
50. Mu, J., Brozinick, J. T., Valladares, O., Bucan, M. and Birnbaum, M. J. (2001). A role for AMP-activated protein kinase in contraction- and hypoxia-regulated glucose transport in skeletal muscle, *Mol. Cell*, **7**, pp. 1085–1094.
51. Herzig, S. and Shaw, R. J. (2018). AMPK: guardian of metabolism and mitochondrial homeostasis, *Nat. Rev. Mol. Cell Biol.*, **19**, pp. 121–135.
52. Garcia, D. and Shaw, R. J. (2017). AMPK: mechanisms of cellular energy sensing and restoration of metabolic balance, *Mol. Cell*, **66**, pp. 789–800.
53. Handschin, C. (2009). The biology of PGC-1α and its therapeutic potential, *Trends Pharmacol. Sci.*, **30**, pp. 322–329.

54. Wang, S., Dougherty, E. J. and Danner, R. L. (2016). PPARγ signaling and emerging opportunities for improved therapeutics, *Pharmacol. Res.*, **111**, pp. 76–85.

55. McMeekin L. J., Joyce K. L., Jenkins L. M., Bohannon B. M., Patel K. D., Bohannon A. S., *et al.* (2021). Estrogen-related receptor alpha (ERRα) is required for PGC-1α-dependent gene expression in the mouse brain, *Neuroscience*, **479**, pp. 70–90.

56. Chen, L. and Knowlton, A. A. (2010). Mitochondria and heart failure: new insights into an energetic problem, *Minerva Cardioangiol.*, **58**, pp. 213–229.

57. Ornish, D., Lin, J., Daubenmier, J., Weidner, G., Epel, E., Kemp, C., *et al.* (2008). Increased telomerase activity and comprehensive lifestyle changes: a pilot study, *Lancet Oncol.*, **9**, pp. 1048–1057.

58. Werner, C., Hanhoun, M., Widmann, T., Kazakov, A., Semenov, A., Pöss, J., *et al.* (2008). Effects of physical exercise on myocardial telomere-regulating proteins, survival pathways, and apoptosis, *J. Am. Coll. Cardiol.*, **52**, pp. 170–82.

59. Wolf, S. A., Melnik, A. and Kempermann, G. (2011). Physical exercise increases adult neurogenesis and telomerase activity and improves behavioral deficits in a mouse model of schizophrenia, *Brain. Behav. Immun.*, **25**, pp. 971–980.

60. Saki, B., Bahrami, A., Ebrahim, K., Abedi-Yekta, A. and Hedayati, M. (2016). Effect of concurrent training on telomere length in patients with myocardial infarction: randomised clinical trial of cardiac rehabilitation, *Gene Rep.*, **4**, pp. 264–268.

61. Sjögren, P., Fisher, R., Kallings, L., Svenson, Roos, U. G. and Hellénius, M.-L. (2014). Stand up for health-avoiding sedentary behaviour might lengthen your telomeres: secondary outcomes from a physical activity RCT in older people, *Br. J. Sports Med.*, **48**, pp. 1407–1409.

62. Fretts, A. M., Mete, M., Howard, B. V., Best, L. G., Siscovick, D. S., Eilat-Adar, S. *et al.* (2018). Physical activity and telomere length in American Indians: the strong heart study, *Eur. J. Epidemiol.*, **33**, pp. 497–500.

63. Savela, S. L., Saijonmaa, O., Strandberg, T. E., Koistinen, P.O.I., Strandberg, A. Y., Tilvis, R. S. *et al.* (2012). Physical activity in midlife and telomere length measured in old age, *Experimental Gerontology*, **48**, pp. 81–84.

64. Ludlow, A. T., Zimmerman, J. B., Witkowski, S., Hearn, J. W., Hatfield, B. D. and Roth, S. M. (2008). Relationship between physical activity level, telomere length, and telomerase activity, *Med. Sci. Sports Exerc.*, **40**, pp. 1764–1771.

65. Wen, C. P., Wai, J. P., Tsai, M. K., Yang, Y. C., Cheng, T. Y., Lee M. C., *et al.* (2011). Minimum amount of physical activity for reduced mortality and extended life expectancy: a prospective cohort study, *Lancet Lond. Engl.*, **378**, pp. 1244–1253.
66. Garland, S. N., Johnson, B., Palmer, C., Speck, R. M., Donelson, M., Xie, S. X., *et al.* (2014). Physical activity and telomere length in early-stage breast cancer survivors, *Breast Cancer Res. BCR*, **16**, pp. 413. doi: 10.1186/s13058-014-0413-y.
67. Kim, J.-H., Ko, J.-H., Lee, D., Lim, I. and Bang, H. "Habitual physical exercise has beneficial effects on telomere length in post-menopausal women, *Menopause N. Y. N*, **19**, pp. 1109–1115. doi: 10.1097/gme.0b013e3182503e97.
68. Bastos, M. F., Matias, M. S. T., Alonso, A. C., Silva, L. C. R., de Araújo, A. L., Silva, P. R., *et al.* (2020). Moderate levels of physical fitness maintain telomere length in non-senescent T CD8+ cells of aged men, *Clin. Sao Paulo Braz.*, **75**, pp. e1628.
69. Mundstock, E., Zatti, H., Louzada, F. M., Oliveira, S. G., Guma, F. T., Paris, M. M., *et al.* (2015). Effects of physical activity in telomere length: systematic review and meta-analysis, *Ageing Res. Rev.*, **22**, pp. 72–80.
70. Denham, J., O'Brien, B. J., Prestes, P. R., Brown, N. J. Charchar, F. J. (2016). Increased expression of telomere-regulating genes in endurance athletes with long leukocyte telomeres, *J. Appl. Physiol. Bethesda Md 1985*, **120**, pp. 148–158.
71. O'Donovan, G., Lee, I.-M., Hamer, M. and Stamatakis, E. (2017). Association of 'Weekend Warrior' and Other Leisure Time Physical Activity Patterns with Risks for All-Cause, Cardiovascular Disease, and Cancer Mortality, *JAMA Intern. Med.*, **177**, pp. 335–342.
72. Arem, H., Moore, S. C., Patel, A., Hartge, P., Berrington de Gonzalez, A., Visvanathan, K., *et al.* (2015). Leisure time physical activity and mortality: a detailed pooled analysis of the dose-response relationship, *JAMA Intern. Med.*, **175**, pp. 959–967.
73. Ornish, D., Lin, J., Chan, J. M., Epel, E., Kemp, C., Weidner, G., *et al.* (2013). Effect of comprehensive lifestyle changes on telomerase activity and telomere length in men with biopsy-proven low-risk prostate cancer: 5-year follow-up of a descriptive pilot study, *Lancet Oncol.*, **14**, pp. 1112–1120.
74. Erickson K. I., Voss, M. W., Prakash, R. S., Basak, C., Szabo, A., Chaddock, L., *et al.* (2011). Exercise training increases size of hippocampus and improves memory, *Proc. Natl. Acad. Sci. U. S. A.*, **108**, pp. 3017–3022.

75. Gomes, M. J., Martinez, P. F., Pagan, L. U., Damatto, R. L., Cezar, M. D. M., Lima, A. R. R., *et al.* (2017). Skeletal muscle aging: influence of oxidative stress and physical exercise, *Oncotarget*, **8**, pp. 20428–20440.
76. Pedersen, B. K. and Febbraio, M. A. (2012). Muscles, exercise and obesity: skeletal muscle as a secretory organ, *Nat. Rev. Endocrinol.*, **8**, pp. 457–465.
77. Simpson, R. J., Lowder, T. W., Spielmann, G., Bigley, A. B., LaVoy, E. C., and Kunz, H. (2012). Exercise and the aging immune system, *Ageing Res. Rev.*, **11**, pp. 404–420.
78. Sousa, C. V., Silva Aguiar, S., Deus, L. A., Barbosa, L. P., Dos Santos, P. A., Neves, R. V. P., *et al.* (2020). Faster and healthier: relationship between telomere and performance in master athletes, *Int. J. Sports Med.*, **41**, pp. 339–344.
79. Saßenroth, D., Meyer, A., Salewsky, B., Kroh, M., Norman, K., Steinhagen-Thiessen, E. *et al.* (2015). Sports and exercise at different ages and leukocyte telomere length in later life-data from the berlin aging study II (BASE-II), *PloS One*, **10**, pp. e0142131.
80. Harber, M.P., Konopka, A.R., Undem, M.K., Hinkley, J.M., Minchev, K., Kaminsky, L.A., *et al.* (2012). Aerobic exercise training induces skeletal muscle hypertrophy and age-dependent adaptations in myofiber function in young and older men, *J. Appl. Physiol. Bethesda Md 1985*, **113**, pp. 1495–1504.
81. Carapeto, P. V. and Aguayo-Mazzucato, C. (2021). Effects of exercise on cellular and tissue aging, *Aging*, **13**, pp. 14522–14543.
82. Seynnes, O. R., de Boer, M. and Narici M. V. (2007). Early skeletal muscle hypertrophy and architectural changes in response to high-intensity resistance training, *J. Appl. Physiol. Bethesda Md 1985*, **102**, pp. 368–373.
83. Werner, C. M., Hecksteden, A., Morsch, A., Zundler, J., Wegmann, M., Kratzsch, J., *et al.* (2019). Differential effects of endurance, interval, and resistance training on telomerase activity and telomere length in a randomized, controlled study, *Eur. Heart J.*, **40**, pp. 34–46.
84. Denham, J., Nelson, C. P., O'Brien, B. J., Nankervis, S. A., Denniff, M., Harvey J. T., *et al.* (2013). Longer leukocyte telomeres are associated with ultra-endurance exercise independent of cardiovascular risk factors, *PLoS ONE*, **8**, pp. e69377.
85. Rosa, F. T., Freitas, E. C., Deminice, R., Jordão, A. A. and Marchini, J. S. (2014). Oxidative stress and inflammation in obesity after taurine supplementation: a double-blind, placebo-controlled study, *Eur. J. Nutr.*, **53**, pp. 823–830.

86. Nickels, M., Mastana, S., Hunter, D., Denniff, M., Codd, V. and Akam E. (2020). The effect of a 12week resistance training intervention on leukocyte telomere length, *Heliyon*, **6**, pp. 04151.

87. Dimauro, I., Scalabrin, M., Fantini, C., Grazioli, E., Reyes Beltran Valls, M., Mercatelli, N., *et al.* (2016). Resistance training and redox homeostasis: Correlation with age-associated genomic changes, *Redox Biology*, **10**, pp. 34–44.

88. Tosevska, A., Franzke, B., Hofmann, M., Vierheilig, I., Schober-Halper, B., Oesen, S., *et al.* (2016). Circulating cell-free DNA, telomere length and bilirubin in the Vienna Active Ageing Study: exploratory analysis of a randomized, controlled trial. *Sci Rep.*, **6**, pp. 38084.

Chapter 9

Telomere Shortening: A Link between Substances of Abuse and Accelerated Senescence

Lina Solange Matos,[a,b] João Pedro Silva,[a,b] and Félix Carvalho[a,b]

[a]*Associate Laboratory i4HB—Institute for Health and Bioeconomy, Faculty of Pharmacy, University of Porto, Porto, Portugal*
[b]*UCIBIO, REQUIMTE, Laboratory of Toxicology, Department of Biological Sciences, Faculty of Pharmacy, University of Porto, Porto, Portugal*
jpmsilva@ff.up.pt, felixdc@ff.up.pt

9.1 Introduction

Substance abuse remains a major global public health, social, and economic burden. The 2022 World Drug Report published by the United Nations Office on Drugs and Crime (UNODC) showed that substance abuse (including alcohol, tobacco, and drugs) accounted for about 11.9 million deaths worldwide in 2019 and was responsible for 359 million years of healthy life loss due to disability and premature death [1]. These drug-use disorders were mostly associated with opioid abuse, although cannabis remained the most

Telomeres: Biomarkers of a Healthy Life and Successful Aging
Edited by Aristidis Tsatsakis

ISBN 978-981-5129-49-6 (Hardcover), 978-1-003-56809-4 (eBook)
www.jennystanford.com

abused psychoactive substance. At the same time, cocaine use has been widely spread all over Europe in recent years [1, 2].

Substances of abuse mainly target the central nervous system (CNS), altering normal brain activity, frequently associated with the disruption of neurotransmitter release, increased oxidative stress, mitochondrial dysfunction, neuronal cell death, neurogenesis, or neuroinflammation. Along with impaired brain function, substance abuse has been also associated with irreversible functional changes in the heart, lungs, kidney, liver, or bone, which altogether may ultimately lead to premature senescence [3]. Notably, exposure to drug-induced oxidation or inflammation has been reported to cause telomere attrition, which could account for the accelerated biological senescence observed in some drug users [4].

9.2 Drugs of Abuse and Telomere Shortening

In recent years, there has been accumulating evidence that some psychoactive substances (e.g., methamphetamine, cocaine, heroin, and alcohol) may lead to accelerated senescence with substance-induced telomere shortening, a specific aging biomarker, likely contributing to such an effect [3, 5]. Telomere length can be affected by several factors including environmental factors, unhealthy lifestyle (e.g., drug abuse, smoking, sedentarism), and/or psychological stress [6]. Telomere shortening is one of the main reasons for cell senescence to occur [7]. Indeed, short telomeres have been reported in different pathologies (e.g., Alzheimer's disease, obesity, and liver disorders) [8–10].

While running an association study in the Chinese Han population, Yang et al. observed that drug abusers presented shorter leukocyte telomere length (LTL) when compared to non-abusers (Fig. 9.1). This effect was especially evident for abusers taking depressant drugs acting on the CNS (e.g., opioids, benzodiazepines, and cannabis), in particular heroin and diazepam, compared to users of stimulants (e.g., cocaine, ketamine, and MDMA) and hallucinogenic (e.g., triazolam) drugs [11]. Interestingly, in this study, ketamine abusers also tended to present longer LTLs. Data from the same study suggested that the route of administration

Type of drug	Number of drug abusers	T/S ratio (mean ± SD)	P value	
Depressant drugs				0.038
Heroin	281	0.763 ± 0.167	0.018	
Opium	8	–	–	
Dolantin	21	0.739 ± 0.214	0.198	
Morphine	9	–	–	
Methadone	83	0.771 ± 0.154	0.935	
Dihydroetorphine	3	–	–	
Buprenorphine	3	–	–	
Diazepam	58	0.736 ± 0.195	0.009	
Secobarbital	3	–	–	
Tramadol	102	0.757 ± 0.196	0.051	
Marijuana	37	0.816 ± 0.225	0.339	
Bucinperazine	3	–	–	
Stimulant drugs				0.525
Somedon	35	0.806 ± 0.236	0.601	
MDMA	63	0.808 ± 0.241	0.582	
Methamphetamine	168	0.789 ± 0.198	0.798	
Cocaine	7	–	–	
Ephedrine	4	–	–	
Ketamine	105	0.819 ± 0.220	0.094	
Hallucinogenic drugs				0.086
Triazolam	62	0.753 ± 0.198	0.086	
CNB	1	–	–	

Figure 9.1 Association of distinct types of drugs with leukocyte telomere length obtained in an association study performed in a cohort of 415 Han Chinese drug abusers. T/S ratio: telomere/single copy gene ratio; MDMA: methylenedioxymethamphetamine; CNB: Caffeine and sodium benzoate. Reproduced from Yang et al. (2013) [11] with permission from Springer Nature (CC BY-NC-ND 3.0).

could influence LTL as abusers taking drugs by sniffing displayed longer LTLs than abusers using other methods (e.g., intravenous, oral, and opium pipe).

Polydrug exposure has also been reported to decrease telomere length. For example, Vakonaki et al. compared LTL in individuals concomitantly abusing different drugs (e.g., heavy cannabis, amphetamines, benzodiazepines, opiates, and cocaine) with a control group comprising healthy individuals noticing significantly shorter telomeres in leukocytes from drug abusers, which was most evident in cannabis and opioid users [5]. Notably, these authors also found that the biological age of polydrug abusers was higher than their chronological age indicating premature senescence.

Although studies on polydrug abusers suggest the involvement of substance abuse in alterations of telomere length, they do not allow the correlation of a specific substance with such effects on telomere shortening. Nevertheless, a few studies have already reported the impact of specific substances on telomere length. Here, we review the available data about the potential effects of the abuse of such substances on telomere length.

Acknowledging the long-term impact of these substances on premature senescence is considered of major relevance to the implementation of more effective drug prevention policies contributing to healthier aging.

9.2.1 Alcohol

Binge drinking has been shown to hasten the senescence process, with the toxicological consequences of alcohol depending on the time of exposure and the levels of its reactive metabolite acetaldehyde (AcH) in the blood [12, 13].

The analysis of alcohol consumption in two different longitudinal cohort studies after considering confounding factors (e.g., age, race, comorbidities, and drinking patterns) found no evidence of a relationship between any amount of alcohol consumed (e.g., moderate and binge drinking) and changes in telomere length. Nevertheless, this analysis was limited by (1) using self-reported data as a measure of alcohol consumption, (2) missing longitudinal data on the participants' alcohol consumption pattern, thus assuming that the baseline drinking represented their typical pattern, and (3) telomere length being measured in older individuals (participants with extremely harmful drinking patterns and/or very short telomeres may have died prematurely) [14]. Also, in a cross-sectional study analyzing the effects of different factors (i.e., alcohol consumption, cigarette smoking, and physical activity) on relative LTL, the authors found no association between alcohol consumption and changes in telomere length [15].

In contrast, data from a cross-sectional study including 1771 middle-aged and elderly Korean participants showed that heavy alcohol consumption (considered as $>$ 30 g of average daily alcohol ingestion) significantly decreased LTL among carriers of the mutant alleles (CT and TT) of rs2074356, a surrogate marker of the aldehyde dehydrogenase 2 (ALDH2) polymorphism. Interestingly, light and moderate alcohol consumption was associated with longer LTL, especially in individuals carrying the wild-type (CC) allele, suggesting a potential benefit of light-to-moderate alcohol drinking [16]. Pavanello et al. measured the telomere length in the peripheral blood leukocytes of 457 Caucasian males, of which 200 represented drunk-driving traffic offenders diagnosed as alcohol abusers (according to the Diagnostic and Statistical Manual of Mental Disorders IV criteria) and 257 social drinkers (considered as controls) concluding that the LTL in alcohol abusers was about half of the telomere length in the control group [17]. The authors further reported that alcohol abusers had a higher prevalence of the ADH1B1*1/*1 genotype and displayed shorter telomeres than individuals with other ADH1B1 genotypes. Yamaki et al. also reported that men with alcohol dependence had shorter telomeres than the healthy control individuals. However, in this case, telomere shortening occurred regardless of the presence of the alcohol dehydrogenase ADH1B (which metabolizes alcohol to AcH) and ALDH2 (responsible for acetaldehyde elimination) genotypes. Since the combination of ADH1B and ALDH2 genotypes results in AcH accumulation, the lack of contribution of these genotypes to the shorter telomeres in alcohol users suggested that alcohol, rather than AcH, was responsible for telomere shortening in the alcohol users [13]. However, since this was a cross-sectional study, no causal relationship between alcohol and telomere shortening could be established.

Aida et al. have also observed a marked telomere shortening in the esophageal epithelium of alcoholic patients, compared to a control group of age-matched non-alcoholic individuals suggesting that reduced telomere length in that tissue could account for the increased risk of esophageal cancer in alcohol addicts [18].

Harpaz et al. observed a decrease in the telomere length of immortalized human foreskin fibroblasts, primary human foreskin fibroblasts, and human hepatocellular carcinoma cells exposed to either 25 mM ethanol or 25 mM AcH for one week. Interestingly, cell exposure to 4-methylpyrazole, an inhibitor of alcohol dehydrogenase, shortened telomeres to a lesser extent (compared to alcohol and AcH) suggesting a key role played by AcH in ethanol-mediated telomere shortening [19]. The authors further observed an increase in the binding of TRF2 and TRF2-associated proteins (e.g., XPF and PARP1) to telomeric regions in ethanol-treated cells suggesting their involvement in ethanol-related telomere shortening. Interestingly, telomerase activity was not affected by ethanol.

Only a few studies have explored the mechanisms underlying telomere shortening in alcohol users. For example, alcohol binge drinking has been associated with a substantial decrease in the levels of NAD^+, a cofactor used by several enzymes including sirtuin 1 (SIRT1), a class III histone deacetylase associated with the regulation of telomere stability via NFkB signaling [20]. Also, AcH has been shown to form adducts with DNA, which are closely associated with the ALDH2 genotype in individuals exposed to high AcH levels due to alcohol binge drinking [21].

9.2.2 Cannabis and Cannabinoids

Cannabis (*Cannabis Sativa* sp.) is the most used psychoactive substance worldwide with about 192 million estimated users [1]. It is composed of many chemical substances, among which D^9-tetrahydrocannabinol (D^9-THC) and cannabidiol (CBD) are the most studied. Cannabis has been shown to decrease telomerase activity (an enzyme that plays a key role in maintaining telomere length) through the inhibition of the telomerase reverse transcriptase (TERT) gene [22] suggesting its possible involvement in telomere shortening. Moreover, CBD (an inverse agonist of CB1 and CB2 receptors) has been shown to extend the lifespan of *C. elegans* protecting it against autophagy and neuronal senescence in a process involving sir-2.1, the *C. elegans* ortholog of SIRT1 [23].

However, to the best of our knowledge, the effects of cannabis and cannabinoids on telomere length remain questionable mostly due to the presence of other confounding factors such as the concomitant use of other substances, or reduced sample size. For example, in a study comprising 90 individuals divided into three groups (30 in a control group of healthy non-smokers, 30 tobacco smokers, and 30 tobacco and marijuana smokers), Mohamed et al. observed a notorious degradation of telomeres in the group of both cannabis and heavy tobacco smokers compared to the non-smokers [24]. However, no group of only cannabis users was included in that study. Similarly, Vakonaki et al. reported a reduction in LTL in blood samples from individuals with a history of concomitant heavy cannabis and opiate abuse compared to a control group of healthy individuals [25]. Also, in this case, cannabis was not the sole substance consumed.

Moreover, while addressing the impact of human immunodeficiency virus (HIV) infection on LTL and whole blood mitochondrial DNA, Hsieh et al. observed that cannabis use did not change LTL compared to non-cannabis users in both HIV-positive and HIV-negative groups [26]. However, due to the several confounding factors involved in this study (e.g., age, ethnicity, HIV, and tobacco smoking), it was not possible to assess the independent contribution of cannabis to LTL.

9.2.3 Cocaine

Cocaine belongs to the stimulants class and it is the second most used illicit drug worldwide [1]. The consumption of this substance has hazardous consequences including psychological (e.g., agitation and paranoia) and physiological (e.g., reduction of grey matter, liver disease, and immunodeficiency) changes, which are most pronounced in the elderly (e.g., cognitive failure, brain degeneration, and immunodeficiency) [27]. Nonetheless, Ersche et al. observed that middle-aged cocaine addicts globally presented a higher grey matter volume loss per year, compared with healthy volunteers, suggesting that cocaine accelerates brain senescence [28]. These data were further supported by a cross-sectional study carried out by Levandowski et al., who compared telomere length in the peripheral blood of 34 crack (the crystalized form of cocaine)-dependent women with 49 healthy elderly women (used as a reference for cellular senescence) [29]. The authors observed that crack users had shorter telomeres than the control group, despite being younger (between 18 and 55 years old) (Fig. 9.2).

Cocaine use is commonly associated with the use of other substances, including alcohol. Recently, Tannous et al. found no statistically significant differences between telomere length in individuals with both cocaine use disorder and alcohol use disorder ($n = 22$), and healthy control participants ($n = 25$) [30]. However, the reduced sample size and lack of proper controls (i.e., individuals with only cocaine use disorders) may have contributed to the absence of such differences.

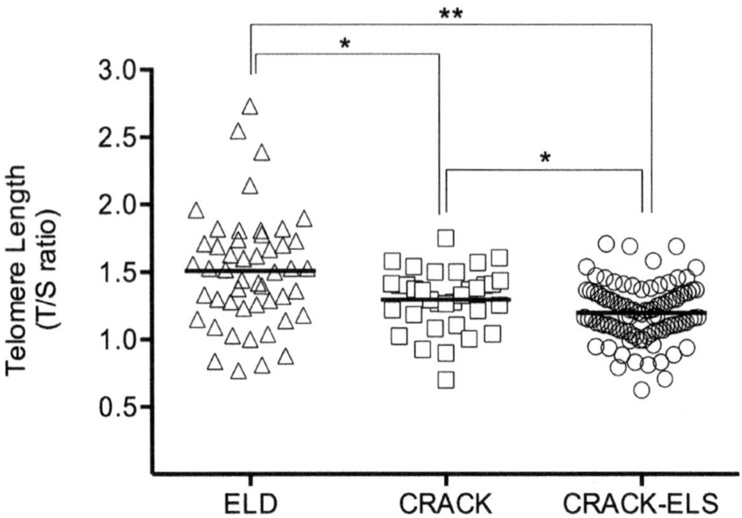

Figure 9.2 Comparison of telomere length in the peripheral blood from 49 healthy elderly women (ELD) with 127 crack-dependent young women (aged 18–55) with (CRACK-ELS, n = 93) or without (CRACK, n = 34) history of early life stress (ELS). Horizontal lines represent mean values. $^{**}p < 0.001$. $^{*}p < 0.05$. Reprinted from Levandowski et al. [29], with permission from Elsevier (license number 5510300027689).

Lai et al. addressed whether cocaine use accelerated telomere shortening in HIV-positive users. For such purpose, telomere length was measured in 147 HIV-positive individuals, 125 of whom were cocaine users. Telomere length was then measured in a follow-up study in 93 of those 147 participants. It should be emphasized that a large share of the participants were also alcohol users (47.3%) and/or cigarette smokers (64.5%). Both cross-sectional and longitudinal data analyses showed that cocaine use was independently associated with telomere shortening in HIV-positive individuals, besides accelerating alcohol-induced telomere shortening in those patients [31].

9.2.4 Methamphetamine

Methamphetamine is a widely used stimulant drug [32]. A few studies have already demonstrated that this substance may affect telomere length. For example, a study assessing the LTL in 187 methamphetamine young adult users (being methamphetamine the main substance used at least once per month) showed that these individuals had shorter telomeres than their healthy counterparts [33]. Moreover, the authors observed that the longer the duration of methamphetamine use, the more pronounced the decrease in telomere length [33]. Similarly, in a cross-sectional study involving 29 methamphetamine users and 50 control participants, Mehta et al. observed that the use of this substance was associated with shorter LTL [34]. A recent study conducted on 370 Thai individuals, 185 of whom had used methamphetamine more than 10 times during their lifetime, 118 were methamphetamine-dependent and 67 were diagnosed with methamphetamine-induced psychosis, no differences were detected in LTL among these three groups [35]. However, no control group composed of healthy non-methamphetamine users was considered in this study, preventing the assessment of a possible effect of this substance on telomere length.

9.2.5 Opioids

Opioid consumption has been linked to the acceleration of telomere shortening [5]. Cheng et al. analyzed the link between heroin use and senescence by measuring telomerase activity in peripheral blood samples and assessing cerebral function with magnetic resonance imaging. The authors observed that the telomerase activity was lower in heroin users compared to a control group (non-heroin users) suggesting heroin-induced premature senescence [36]. Moreover, they further noted that changes in telomerase activity caused a loss of integrity of the right dorsal prefrontal cortex, the brain area related to addiction, as indicated by modifications in the connectivity between the right dorsal prefrontal cortex and regions responsible for senescence. Yang et al. also reported a reduction in the length of telomeres in leukocytes from blood samples collected from heroin consumers (Fig. 9.1) [11]. By assessing a possible association between the method of consumption (i.e., intravenous, olfactory, and smoking) and the length of the telomeres, the authors also showed that telomeres were longer in the leukocytes of heroin addicts who inhaled heroin as a preferential method.

No studies have been performed to evaluate the mechanisms responsible for opioid-induced telomere shortening. However, increased oxidative stress, which has been reportedly associated with telomere shortening, could account for the observations in heroin abusers. Indeed, while analyzing the plasma of 114 heroin abusers and 100 healthy volunteers, Zhou et al. concluded that oxidative stress was higher in heroin abusers compared to healthy individuals, as determined by increased levels of lipoperoxides and nitric oxide, and decreased antioxidant enzyme activity (e.g., superoxide dismutase, catalase, and glutathione peroxidase) [37].

Interestingly, it was recently shown that maternal opioid use may also affect the relative telomere length in leukocytes of male, but not female, newborns [38]. Indeed, male newborns from mothers who regularly used opioids ($n = 30$) including opium, sookhteh, shire, and/or heroin displayed longer relative LTL than newborns from non-drug-using mothers ($n = 27$). Such a difference was not observed in the female newborns (Fig. 9.3). Interestingly, only maternal age and maternal education level were controlled as potential confounding factors. Also, the authors were not able to provide any explanation as to the mechanisms underlying their observations.

9.2.6 Tobacco

Tobacco is associated with the onset of chronic diseases, as well as with premature senescence mostly due to the accumulation of oxidative stress and inflammation caused by cigarette smoking, which may ultimately lead to premature death [39]. The telomere length in leukocytes from smokers has been found to decrease when compared to non-smokers. For example, by analyzing the DNA from leukocytes in the blood samples collected from 1122 white women aged between 18 and 76 years, Valdes et al. observed that cigarette smoking represented a major risk factor for premature senescence. Moreover, smokers or ex-smokers appeared to be approximately 4.6 years older compared to non-smokers [40]. A prospective cohort

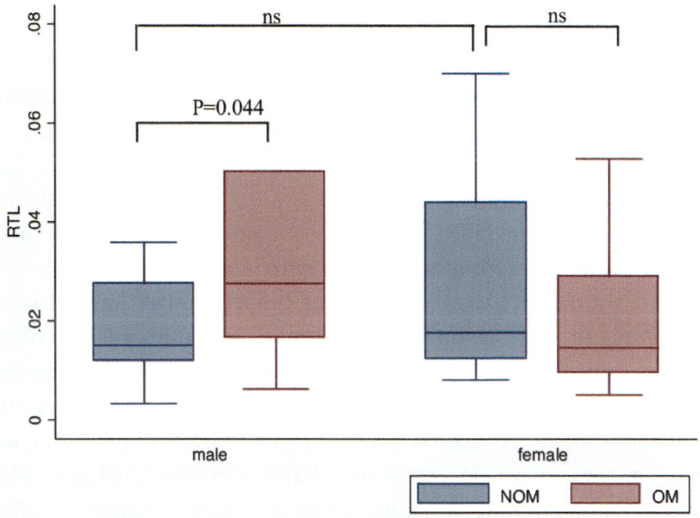

Figure 9.3 Relative telomere length (RTL) in male and female offspring from opioid-using (OM, n = 30) and non-opioid-using (NOM, n = 27) mothers. The horizontal bar within the box represents the median; the upper and lower horizontal lines of the box correspond to the 75th and 25th percentiles, respectively. The upper and lower horizontal bars outside the box represent the maximum and minimum values, respectively, except for outliers. ns: not significant. Reproduced, without modifications, from Abad et al. [38] with permission from PLoS One (CC BY 4.0).

study comprising 8074 individuals from the Prevention of Renal and Vascular End-stage Disease (PREVEND), in which LTL was measured on three different occasions (at the beginning of the study and after 4.3 and 6.6 years), showed a near three-fold increased telomere attrition rate in active smokers compared to non-smokers [41]. In a cross-sectional study comprising 477 healthy volunteers that also assessed the effects of alcohol consumption and physical activity on relative LTL, Latifovic et al. observed an association between cigarette smoking and shorter telomeres [15]. The comparison between LTL in 30 tobacco smokers and 30 healthy non-smokers showed shorter telomeres in the leukocytes of tobacco smokers [24]. Interestingly, such telomere shortening was accompanied by increased malondialdehyde and urinary 8-hydroxydeoxyguanosine suggesting the involvement of oxidative stress in tobacco-mediated telomere shortening.

Khan et al. analyzed the role played by several factors associated with cigarette smoking (e.g., smoking status, smoking intensity, type of filter, second-hand smoke, and serum cotinine levels) in telomere length. The authors observed that heavy smokers (i.e., individuals who smoked an average of 20 cigarettes per day) from a US population of 5800+ individuals comprising different races, presented shorter lymphocytes' telomere length [39].

Notably, distinct meta-analyses of cohort studies have reached contradicting conclusions. For example, a meta-analysis of 30 studies revealed that telomeres were shorter among smokers compared to non-smokers, and among current smokers compared to never or former smokers. It also showed that the number of pack-years of smoking was inversely correlated with telomere length [42]. Interestingly, smoking cessation seemed to have a beneficial effect on LTL [26, 42]. Recently, another meta-analysis of 18 longitudinal cohorts (including a total of 4678 smokers and 7901 non-smokers followed-up over a mean interval of 8.6 years) found no causal effect of smoking on telomere shortening, rather suggesting that individuals with shorter telomeres may be more prone to start smoking [43].

9.3 Conclusions

The abuse of some substances has been reportedly associated with accelerated senescence. Although increased oxidative stress and inflammation induced by such substances have been accounted for such an effect, the mechanisms underlying substance-induced biological senescence have been mostly underexplored. Despite research on the impact of these substances on telomere length being in its infancy, accumulating evidence suggests that telomere shortening could help bridge the knowledge gap between drug-induced oxidative stress and inflammation, and accelerated senescence. Psychoactive substances like alcohol, tobacco, cannabis, heroin, cocaine, or methamphetamine, which have been associated with increased oxidative stress [11], have also been reported to promote telomere shortening especially in chronic users. Acknowledging the long-term impact of these substances on premature senescence assumes extreme relevance for forensic and clinical toxicologists and for the implementation of more effective drug prevention policies contributing to healthier aging.

Acknowledgments

This work was funded by FEDER – *Fundo Europeu de Desenvolvimento Regional* through the COMPETE 2020 – Operational Programme for Competitiveness and Internationalisation (POCI), and by Portuguese funds through FCT – *Fundação para a Ciência e a Tecnologia*, I. P. in the framework of the projects POCI-01-0145-FEDER-029584; UIDP/04378/2021 and UIDB/04378/2021 of the Research Unit on Applied Molecular Biosciences – UCIBIO; and LA/P/0140/2021 of the Associate Laboratory Institute for Health and Bioeconomy – i4HB. J.P.S. is supported by FCT via research contract 2021.01789.CEECIND/CP1662/CT0014 (under the Scientific Employment Stimulus).

References

1. United Nations Office on Drugs and Crime (UNODC), (2022). World drug report 2022. United Nations Publications, Vienna, Austria.
2. European Monitoring Center for Drugs and Drug Addiction (EMCDDA), (2022). European drug report 2021: Trends and developments. Publications Office of the European Union, Luxembourg.
3. Bachi, K., Sierra, S., Volkow, N. D., Goldstein, R. Z., Alia-Klein, N. (2017). Is biological aging accelerated in drug addiction? *Curr. Opin. Behav. Sci.*, **13**, pp. 34–39.
4. Lindqvist, D., Epel, E. S., Mellon, S. H., Penninx, B. W., Révész, D., Verhoeven, J. E., *et al.* (2015). Psychiatric disorders and leukocyte telomere length: Underlying mechanisms linking mental illness with cellular aging, *Neurosci. Biobehav. Rev.*, **55**, pp. 333–364.

5. Vakonaki, E., Tzatzarakis, M., Tsiminikaki, K., Nathena, D., Fragkiadaki, P., Kalliantasi, K., *et al.* (2019). Effect of chronic and heavy drug abuse on biological aging, *World Acad. Sci. J*, **1, Issue 2**, pp. 67–73.
6. Srinivas, N., Rachakonda, S., Kumar, R. (2020). Telomeres and telomere length: A general overview, *Cancers*, **12**, pp. 558.
7. Fathi, E., Charoudeh, H. N., Sanaat, Z., Farahzadi, R. (2019). Telomere shortening as a hallmark of stem cell senescence, *Stem Cell Investig.*, **6**, pp. 7.
8. Arsenis, N., C., You, T., Ogawa,E. F. , Tinsley G. M., Zuo L. (2017). Physical activity and telomere length- impact of aging and potential mechanisms of action, *Oncotarget*, **8**, pp. 45008–45019.
9. Barnes R. P., Fouquerel E., Opresko P. L. (2019). The impact of oxidative DNA damage and stress on telomere homeostasis, *Mech. Ageing Dev.*, **177**, pp. 37–45.
10. Hirota, K. S., K. S., Lambert, D. G. (1999). Interaction of ketamine with μ2 opioid receptors in sh-sy5y human neuroblastoma cells, *J. Anesth.* **13**, pp. 107–109.
11. Yang, Z., Ye, J., Li, C., Zhou, D., Shen, Q., Wu, J., *et al.* (2013). Drug addiction is associated with leukocyte telomere length, *Sci. Rep.*, **3**, pp. 1542.
12. Martins de Carvalho, L., Wiers, C. E., Manza, P., Sun, H., Schwandt, M., Wang, G.-J., *et al.* (2019). Effect of alcohol use disorder on cellular aging, *Psychopharmacol.*, **236**, pp. 3245–3255.
13. Yamaki, N., Matsushita, S., Hara, S., Yokoyama, A., Hishimoto, A., Higuchi, S. (2019). Telomere shortening in alcohol dependence: Roles of alcohol and acetaldehyde, *J. Psychiatr. Res.*, **109**, pp. 27–32.
14. Dixit, S., Whooley, M. A., Vittinghoff, E., Roberts, J. D., Heckbert, S. R., Fitzpatrick, A. L., *et al.* (2019). Alcohol consumption and leukocyte telomere length, *Sci. Rep.*, **9**, pp. 1404.
15. Latifovic, L., Peacock, S. D., Massey, T. E., King, W. D. (2016). The influence of alcohol consumption, cigarette smoking, and physical activity on leukocyte telomere length, *Cancer Epidemiol. Biomarkers Prev.*, **25**, pp. 374–380.
16. Shin, C., Baik, I. (2016). Associations between alcohol consumption and leukocyte telomere length modified by a common polymorphism of aldh2, *Alcohol: Clin. Exp. Res.*, **40**, pp. 765–771.
17. Pavanello, S., Hoxha, M., Dioni, L., Bertazzi, P. A., Snenghi, R., Nalesso, A., *et al.* (2011). Shortened telomeres in individuals with abuse in alcohol consumption, *Int. J. Cancer*, **129**, pp. 983–992.

18. Aida, J., Yokoyama, A., Izumiyama, N., Nakamura, K.-i., Ishikawa, N., Poon, S. S., *et al.* (2011). Alcoholics show reduced telomere length in the oesophagus, *J. Pathol.*, **223**, pp. 410–416.
19. Harpaz, T., Abumock, H., Beery, E., Edel, Y., Lahav, M., Rozovski, U., *et al.* (2018). The effect of ethanol on telomere dynamics and regulation in human cells, *Cells*, **7**, pp. 169.
20. French, S. W. (2016). Chronic alcohol binging injures the liver and other organs by reducing NAD+ levels required for sirtuin's deacetylase activity, *Exp. Mol. Pathol.*, **100**, pp. 303–306.
21. Matsuda, T., Kawanishi, M., Matsui, S., Yagi, T., Takebe, H. (1998). Specific tandem gg to tt base substitutions induced by acetaldehyde are due to intra-strand crosslinks between adjacent guanine bases, *Nucleic Acids Res.*, **26**, pp. 1769–1774.
22. Hussein, N. A. E. M., El-Toukhy, M. A. E.-F., Kazem, A. H., Ali, M. E.-S., Ahmad, M. A. E.-R., Ghazy, H. M. R., *et al.* (2014). Protective and therapeutic effects of cannabis plant extract on liver cancer induced by dimethylnitrosamine in mice, *Alexandria J. Med.*, **50**, pp. 241–251.
23. Wang, Z., Zheng, P., Chen, X., Xie, Y., Weston-Green, K., Solowij, N., *et al.* (2022). Cannabidiol induces autophagy and improves neuronal health associated with sirt1 mediated longevity, *GeroSci.*, **44**, pp. 1505–1524.
24. Mohamed, M. A., Ibrahim, K. S., Mahdy-Abdallah, H., Mohamed, H. A. (2016). Leukocyte telomere length in heavy tobacco and marijuana Egyptian smokers, *Int. J. ChemTech Res.*, **9**, pp. 501–508.
25. Vakonaki, E., Fragkiadaki, P., Tsoukalas, D., Alegkakis, A., Vaki, G., Tsiminikaki, K., *et al.* (2017). Telomere length in opiates and cannabis abusers as a marker of early aging, *Toxicol. Lett.*, **280**, pp. S242.
26. Hsieh, A. Y. Y., Kimmel, E., Pick, N., Sauvé, L., Brophy, J., Kakkar, F., *et al.* (2020). Inverse relationship between leukocyte telomere length attrition and blood mitochondrial DNA content loss over time, *Aging*, **12**, pp. 15196–15221.
27. Karila, L., Petit, A., Lowenstein, W., Reynaud, M. (2012). Diagnosis and consequences of cocaine addiction, *Curr. Med. Chem.*, **19**, pp. 5612–5618.
28. Ersche, K. D., Jones, P. S., Williams, G. B., Robbins, T. W., Bullmore, E. T. (2013). Cocaine dependence: A fast-track for brain ageing? *Mol. Psychiatry*, **18**, pp. 134–135.
29. Levandowski, M. L., Tractenberg, S. G., de Azeredo, L. A., De Nardi, T., Rovaris, D. L., Bau, C. H., *et al.* (2016). Crack cocaine addiction,

early life stress and accelerated cellular aging among women, *Prog. Neuropsychopharmacol. Biol. Psychiatry*, **71**, pp. 83–89.

30. Tannous, J., Mwangi, B., Hasan, K. M., Narayana, P. A., Steinberg, J. L., Walss-Bass, C., *et al.* (2019). Measures of possible allostatic load in comorbid cocaine and alcohol use disorder: Brain white matter integrity, telomere length, and anti-saccade performance, *PloS One*, **14**, pp. e0199729.
31. Lai, S., Heaphy, C. M., Rizzo, A. J., Celentano, D. D., Gerstenblith, G., Li, J., *et al.* (2018). Cocaine use may induce telomere shortening in individuals with HIV infection, *Prog. Neuro-Psychoph.*, **84**, pp. 11–17.
32. United Nations Office on Drugs and Crime (UNODC), (2021). Drug market trends: Cocaine, amphetamine-type stimulants. United Nations Publications, Vienna, Austria.
33. Lin, Y.-F., Chen, P.-Y., Liu, H.-C., Chen, Y.-L., Chou, W.-H., Huang, M.-C. (2021). Shortened leukocyte telomere length in young adults who use methamphetamine, *Transl. Psychiatry*, **11**, pp. 519.
34. Mehta, S. R., Iudicello, J. E., Lin, J., Ellis, R. J., Morgan, E., Okwuegbuna, O., *et al.* (2021). Telomere length is associated with HIV infection, methamphetamine use, inflammation, and comorbid disease risk, *Drug Alcohol Depend.*, **221**, pp. 108639.
35. Rungnirundorn, T., Krusong, K., Kalayasiri, R., Maes, M. (2022). Leukocyte telomere length is not shortened in methamphetamine dependence or methamphetamine-induced psychosis but is increased following traumatic events, *World J. Biol. Psychiatry*, **23**, pp. 613–621.
36. Cheng, G. L., Zeng, H., Leung, M. K., Zhang, H. J., Lau, B. W., Liu, Y. P., *et al.* (2013). Heroin abuse accelerates biological aging: A novel insight from telomerase and brain imaging interaction, *Transl. Psychiatry*, **3**, pp. e260.
37. Zhou, J. F., Yan, X. F., Ruan, Z. R., Peng, F. Y., Cai, D., Yuan, H., *et al.* (2000). Heroin abuse and nitric oxide, oxidation, peroxidation, lipoperoxidation, *Biomed. Environ. Sci.*, **13**, pp. 131–139.
38. Rahimi Mehdi Abad, F., Khalili, P., Jalali, F., Pirsadeghi, A., Esmaeili Nadimi, A., Manshoori, A., *et al.* (2021). Maternal opioid use is reflected on leukocyte telomere length of male newborns, *PloS One*, **16**, pp. e0261013.
39. Khan, R. J., Gebreab, S. Y., Gaye, A., Crespo, P. R., Xu, R., Davis, S. K. (2019). Associations of smoking indicators and cotinine levels with telomere length: National health and nutrition examination survey, *Prev. Med. Rep.*, **15**, pp. 100895.

40. Valdes, A. M., Andrew, T., Gardner, J. P., Kimura, M., Oelsner, E., Cherkas, L. F., *et al.* (2005). Obesity, cigarette smoking, and telomere length in women, *Lancet*, **366**, pp. 662–664.
41. Huzen, J., Wong, L. S. M., van Veldhuisen, D. J., Samani, N. J., Zwinderman, A. H., Codd, V., *et al.* (2014). Telomere length loss due to smoking and metabolic traits, *J. Intern. Med.*, **275**, pp. 155–163.
42. Astuti, Y., Wardhana, A., Watkins, J., Wulaningsih, W. (2017). Cigarette smoking and telomere length: A systematic review of 84 studies and meta-analysis, *Environ. Res.*, **158**, pp. 480–489.
43. Bateson, M., Aviv, A., Bendix, L., Benetos, A., Ben-Shlomo, Y., Bojesen, S. E., *et al.* (2019). Smoking does not accelerate leucocyte telomere attrition: A meta-analysis of 18 longitudinal cohorts, *R. Soc. Open Sci.*, **6**, pp. 190420.

Chapter 10

Telomere Length as Potential Metal Exposure Biomarker: State of the Art and Perspectives

Anatoly Skalny,[a] Michael Aschner,[b] Aristidis Tsatsakis,[c] Petr Litvitsky,[a] Andrey Svistunov,[a] Monica Paoliello,[d] Abel Santamaria,[e] Ji-Chang Zhou,[f] and Alexey Tinkov[g]

[a]*IM Sechenov First Moscow State Medical University, Sechenov University, Moscow, Russia*
[b]*Department of Molecular Pharmacology, Albert Einstein College of Medicine, Bronx, New York, USA*
[c]*Laboratory of Toxicology, Medical School, University of Crete, Voutes, Heraklion, Crete, Greece*
[d]*Department of Molecular Pharmacology, Albert Einstein College of Medicine, Bronx, New York, USA*
[e]*Facultad de Ciencias, Universidad Nacional Autónoma de México, Mexico City, Mexico*
[f]*School of Public Health (Shenzhen), Sun Yat-sen University, Shenzhen, China*
[g]*Laboratory of Ecobiomonitoring and Quality Control, Yaroslavl State University, Yaroslavl, Russia*
tinkov.a.a@gmail.com

10.1 Introduction

Telomeres are terminal parts of linear chromosomes consisting of repeated nucleotide sequences and six proteins termed shelterin

Telomeres: Biomarkers of a Healthy Life and Successful Aging
Edited by Aristidis Tsatsakis

ISBN 978-981-5129-49-6 (Hardcover), 978-1-003-56809-4 (eBook)
www.jennystanford.com

complex that caps telomeric DNA from degradation [1]. Telomere shortening occurs with each mitotic cycle, due to the end replication problem [2]. The reduction of telomere length may be counteracted by telomerase, an enzyme consisting of RNA subunit and catalytic subunit telomerase reverse transcriptase (TERT), which elongates telomeric DNA. Alternative telomere lengthening may also occur due to recombination-based DNA replication [3]. Concomitantly, telomerase is active only in actively dividing cells like germ or cancer cells, whereas in differentiating cells its expression is down-regulated. Therefore, somatic cells have a predetermined number of divisions subsequently [4]. When telomeres are shortened to a critical length, the cell becomes senescent and dysfunctional and undergoes apoptosis. The rate of telomere shortening has increased in aging and a number of age-related diseases [5].

The results of meta-analyses demonstrated a significant association between telomere shortening and cardiovascular diseases (CVDs) [6], especially coronary heart disease [7], diabetes mellitus type 2 [8], stroke [9], obesity [10], neurodegeneration in Alzheimer's disease [11], chronic obstructive pulmonary disease (COPD) [12], etc. Although the association of telomere length with a wide spectrum of diseases may appear contradictory, the existing data clearly demonstrate the relationship of telomere length with certain types of cancer [13]. In addition, telomere length was shown to be associated not only with cancer risk [14] but also with cancer prognosis [15]. A tight association with tissue telomere shortening was demonstrated for bladder, esophageal, gastric, and kidney cancers [16].

In addition to the association of telomere length with physiological factors including disease development, environmental factors were also found to possess a significant impact on telomere shortening and expression of telomere-related genes [17]. Specifically, laboratory and epidemiological studies revealed a significant impact of air pollution on telomere length [18]. The results of a recent meta-analysis demonstrated that polyaromatic hydrocarbon (PAH) and long-term PM2.5 exposure are associated with shorter telomeres, whereas polychlorinated biphenyls (PCBs) and short-term PM2.5 exposure are characterized by direct association with telomere length in exposed subjects [19]. Due to the involvement of telomere regulation in the pathogenesis of a wide spectrum of pathologies and the significant impact of environmental pollutants on telomere length, the latter may be considered as the functional exposure biomarker [20]. At the same time, the association patterns were found to be strongly dependent on the dose, duration, and route of exposure [21].

In the present chapter, we provide a PubMed-based review of studies demonstrating the potential usefulness of telomere length as a metal exposure biomarker and discuss the potential underlying mechanisms.

10.2 Cadmium

Cadmium (Cd) is a toxic metal that primarily affects the kidney, bones, and reproductive system, although it possesses toxicity for other organs. Although the level of Cd in the organism's biosamples like blood/plasma, urine, hair, and nails could be indicative of Cd exposure [22], certain limitations exist, and kidney-specific biomarkers may provide more accurate information on Cd burden in the body [23]. Certain studies also demonstrated that Cd interferes with telomere length and the latter could be considered as a functional, although not specific, biomarker of Cd toxicity.

Epidemiological studies demonstrated that the association between Cd exposure and telomere length strongly depends on exposure doses. Specifically, both blood and urinary Cd levels were significantly associated with 5.54% (95% CI: −8.70, −2.37) and 4.50% (95% CI: −8.79, −0.20) shorter leukocyte telomere length in US adults from the National Health and Nutrition Examination Survey (1999–2002) [24]. Analysis of the same dataset demonstrated that in adult Americans with mean blood Cd levels of 0.40–0.51 μg/L every increase in Cd concentration by 1 μg/L was significantly ($p < 0.001$) associated with 3.74% (95% CI: 5.35, 2.10%) reduction in telomere length [25]. At the same time, in American Indians from the Strong Heart Study Urinary Cd levels (mean 1.01 μg/g creatinine) were only border significantly ($p = 0.05$) associated with leukocyte telomere length in the adjusted model [26].

Urinary Cd levels with the mean value of 0.33 ± 0.33 μg/g creatinine were inversely associated with salivary telomere length in Nepalese adolescents ($\beta = -0.24$, 95% CI: −0.42, −0.07; $p = 0.01$) [27]. A similar association between urinary Cd and telomere shortening was revealed in adults from Northern Laos [28]. Artificial neural network demonstrated that urinary Cd levels (mean 0.31 ng/ml) exerted the most significant negative effect on telomere length as compared to barium (Ba), cobalt (Co), cerium (Ce), molybdenum (Mo), lead (Pb), antimony (Sb), and thallium (Tl) in American adults and especially those in advanced age [29]. At the same time, in Japanese female university students with a mean level of Cd in urine of 0.402 μg/L (0.312 μg/g creatinine), urinary Cd levels were not associated significantly with telomere length [30].

A number of studies demonstrated that prenatal Cd exposure as assessed by maternal urinary Cd levels is associated with cord blood telomere shortening. A study performed in Wuhan (China) demonstrated that doubling of maternal urinary Cd levels (mean 0.68 μg/g creatinine) is associated with 6.83% (95% CI: −11.44%, −1.97%; $p = 0.006$) shorter cord blood telomeres in regression models adjusted for newborn and maternal characteristics, as well as maternal zinc (Zn) and selenium (Se) levels [31]. Similar associations were revealed in Myanmar at higher maternal urinary Cd levels (0.9 μg/g creatinine) [32]. These observations generally correspond to the observation of an inverse correlation between placental Cd content and placental telomere length in pregnant women living in a Chinese city near an electronic waste recycling site [33]. It is noteworthy that certain dietary factors may affect the association between prenatal Cd exposure and newborn telomere length. Specifically, urinary Se levels were also shown to modulate the association between maternal Cd levels and umbilical cord blood telomere length, which was significant only in mothers with low urinary Se [34].

In addition to a direct relationship between Cd exposure and telomere length, it has been demonstrated that telomere shortening may at least partially contribute to Cd-induced adverse health effects, being indicative of the role of telomere length as a functional biomarker of Cd exposure. In Cd-exposed subjects from Taiyuan (Shanxi, China), both urinary Cd levels (OR = 2.092, 95% CI: 1.179–3.710) and leukocyte telomere length (OR = 0.105, 95% CI: 0.025–

0.453) were found to be significant predictors of hypertension, whereas the association between Cd and hypertension was partially mediated by telomere shortage [35]. Correspondingly, in adults participating in the 2019 Iwaki Health Promotion Project, leukocyte telomere shortening was significantly associated with higher systolic and diastolic blood pressure only in subjects with high urinary Cd levels [36]. In addition to the observed higher urinary Cd levels in subjects with lower telomere length, both parameters were significantly associated with impaired renal tubular function in adults living in Shaanxi (China) [37]. It is also noteworthy that blood Cd levels (0.358–1.066 ppm) were found to be inversely associated with serum telomerase activity in patients with COPD. Moreover, the reduction of telomerase activity was also shown to mediate from 19% to 38% of the inverse association between blood Cd levels and pulmonary function [38].

Nonetheless, despite a significant negative correlation between urinary Cd and telomere length in US adults, telomere shortage did not mediate the association between Cd exposure and osteoarthritis [39].

In vivo and in vitro laboratory studies demonstrated that Cd exposure may affect telomere length as well as telomerase activity. Exposure of embryonic stem cells to cigarette smoke condensate as well as Cd, being its constituent, resulted in apoptotic cell damage upon acute exposure (20 μM Cd) and increased DNA damage with telomere shortage in chronic treatment groups (5 μM Cd) [40]. It has been also demonstrated that Cd exposure to mouse embryos induced oxidative stress, apoptosis, and impaired embryo development, altogether associated with telomere shortening and loss, whereas these effects were attenuated by antioxidant (N-acetylcysteine) treatment, being indicative of the role of oxidative stress in Cd-induced telomere shortening (Fig. 10.1). Moreover, these adverse developmental effects of Cd exposure were more pronounced in telomerase RNA component knockout (TercKO) mouse embryos [41].

At the same time, in rat hepatocytes $CdCl_2$ exposure (5–20 μmol/kg) significantly increased telomerase activity and mRNA expression in parallel with an increase in p53 and c-myc expression, which may contribute to the carcinogenic effect of Cd [42]. In agreement with this hypothesis, it has been demonstrated that

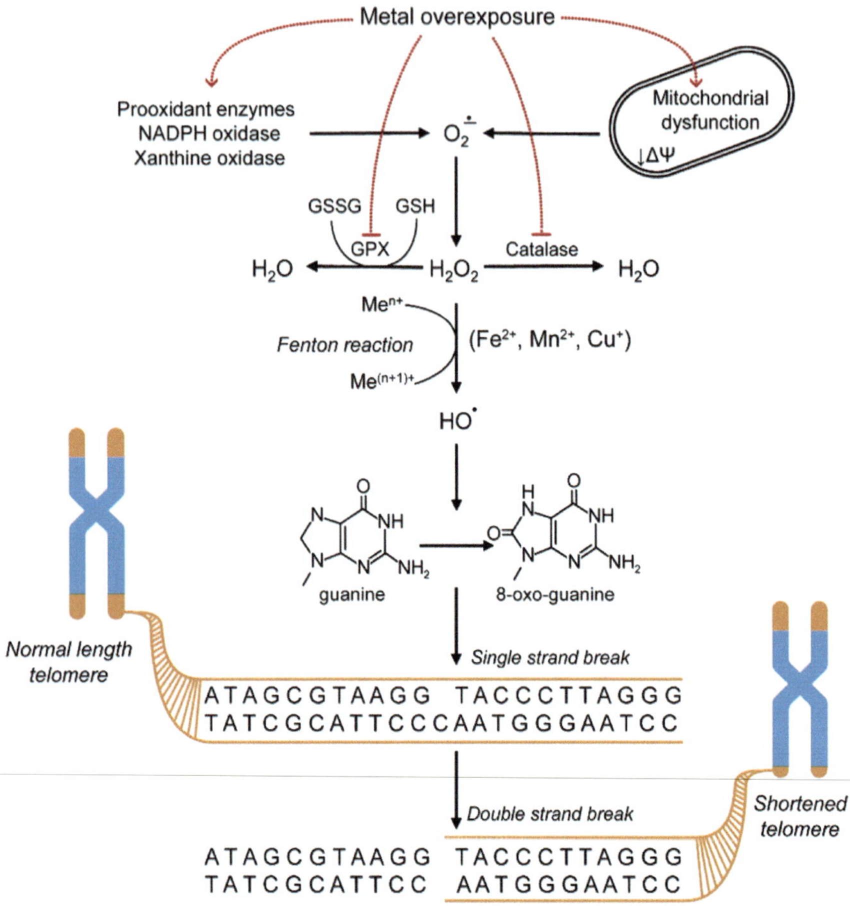

Figure 10.1 A simplified scheme of the role of metal-induced oxidative stress in telomere shortening. Briefly, metal overexposure results in mitochondrial dysfunction and activation of prooxidant enzymes, as well as inhibition of antioxidant enzymes, altogether contributing to the formation of reactive oxygen species. Moreover, redox-active metals like Fe, Cu, and Mn are known to be involved in the Fenton reaction resulting in hydroxyl radical generation.

human telomerase reverse transcriptase (hTERT) mRNA expression increased with the progression of malignant transformation in Cd-transformed 16HBE cells as compared to normal cells [43]. In MCF-7 human breast cancer cells, Cd exposure significantly increased transactivation at the hTERT promoter in parallel with up-regulation of estrogen receptor α (ERα) signaling [44]. Similarly, in ovarian epithelial cells, Cd exposure (10 mM for 24 h) induced a nearly twofold increase in telomerase activity [45].

Taken together, the existing data demonstrate that environmental Cd exposure is associated with telomere shortening at high exposure doses associated with habitation in polluted environments, although at lower doses of exposure, this relationship is less profound. Maternal Cd exposure was also shown to be inversely associated with telomere length in newborns and children. Moreover, certain studies demonstrated that telomere shortening may at least partially mediate adverse effects of Cd exposure including kidney damage, hypertension, and COPD. In vitro studies also corroborate epidemiological data demonstrating a reduction of telomere length upon Cd exposure. At the same time, the up-regulation of telomerase activity in Cd-exposed cells may be indicative of the potential carcinogenic effect of Cd. Therefore, current epidemiological evidence indicates the potential utility of telomere length as a biomarker of Cd exposure.

10.3 Lead

Lead (Pb) is a neurotoxic metal that also affects the kidneys, cardiovascular system, and liver to name a few. Lead blood (Pb) level is considered the most widely used biomarker of Pb exposure [46]. Assessment of metal levels in other biosamples including urine, hair, and teeth were also used as criteria of Pb exposure, although certain limitations for using these biosamples exist. Functional biomarkers of Pb toxicity may include the activity of δ-aminolevulinic acid dehydratase (ALAD), δ-aminolevulinic acid levels in blood and urine, as well as activity of blood pyrimidine nucleotidase (P5'N), and nicotinamide adenine dinucleotide synthetase (NADS) that are indicative of toxic effects of the metal [47]. Current findings from occupationally and environmentally exposed subjects, including prenatally exposed children, demonstrate that telomere length may be also indicative of Pb toxicity as discussed further.

High-dose Pb exposure associated with occupational involvement in industrial processes was significantly related to telomere shortening. In Pb-acid storage battery plant workers' blood, Pb levels increased from 17.4 μg/dl in 2016 to 20.8 μg/dl in 2018, being associated with increased DNA damage and telomere shortage but not phosphatidylinositol glycan class A mutation [48]. In a similar group of workers' peripheral white blood cells, telomere length was found to be 13% lower in subjects with abnormal blood (2.91 ± 0.92 μmol/l) or urinary (0.26 ± 0.01 μmol/l) Pb levels as compared to the examinees with normal Pb levels in blood (1.49 ± 0.35 μmol/l) and urine (0.101 ± 0.001 μ mol/l). Moreover, telomere length was inversely associated with both blood and urinary Pb levels as well as working length and body mass index (BMI) [49]. While examining 1896 workers of Pb-acid battery plant, it has been demonstrated that the benchmark dose of Pb obtained from relative telomere length (35 μg/L) was significantly lower than that estimated using red blood cells (RBC), Hb, and micronuclei frequency values [50] being indicative of higher sensitivity of telomere length as a biomarker of Pb exposure. Pb-exposed workers of Pb smelters were also characterized by 18% shorter relative telomere length in comparison to control values. That value was independently associated with blood Pb levels and oxidative stress markers (hemolysate thiobarbituric acid-reactive species, TBARS) after adjustment for age, anthropometric parameters, and smoking status, indicative of the potential contribution of oxidative stress in telomere shortening upon Pb exposure (Fig. 10.1). In turn, no association between Pb exposure and telomerase expression was observed [51]. Correspondingly, in subjects working at a large-scale electronics manufacturer, Pb blood levels (mean 28.57 μg/dL) were inversely associated with relative telomere length [52]. It is notable that in Pb-exposed workers, elevated blood Pb levels (mean 266.1 μg/L) inversely correlated not only with relative telomere length but also with telomere-binding protein protection of telomeres protein 1 (POT1)-interacting protein 1 (TPP1) mRNA expression that may be responsible for altered telomere repair [53].

At the same time, certain contradictions regarding the association between Pb exposure and telomere length exist. Rohr et al. revealed a positive association between Pb exposure and telomere length in workers exposed to a construction environment [54]. In occupationally non-exposed US adults from the National Health and Nutrition Examination Survey (1999–2002), lead levels in blood

(1.67 μg/dL) were not associated with leukocyte telomere length [27].

In addition to occupational exposure, environmental Pb overload due to habitation near Pb pollution sources may also affect telomere length. Specifically, lead blood levels (mean 3.28 μg/dl) in children living near industrial lead emitters were associated with lower relative telomere length irrespective of maternal smoking status [55]. At the same time, in children attending a school located in the industrial zone of Salamanca in Mexico, lead blood levels (mean 3.78 μg/dL) were inversely associated with mitochondrial DNA copy number (mtDNAcn) ($r = -0.39$; $p = 0.002$), although correlation with telomere length was only nearly significant ($r = -0.212$; $p = 0.062$) [56].

In contrast to occupational exposure, existing data on the association between prenatal Pb overload and altered telomere length are limited. PROGRESS (2007–2011) study in Mexico failed to reveal any significant associations between lead levels in maternal blood at delivery (mean 3.33 μg/dl) and lead levels in bone one month postpartum (4.96–5.41 μg/g) with cord blood telomere length as well as Horvath's DNA methylation age [57]. An examination involving pregnant women and their newborns in Myanmar failed to reveal a significant association between maternal urinary Pb levels (1.8μg/g creatinine) and cord blood telomere shortening [34]. At the same time, the association between maternal Pb exposure markers and cord blood telomere length was shown to be significantly modified by Se status with a lack of significance in the high Se group [58].

Laboratory studies corroborate the existing epidemiological data being also indicative of Pb-induced telomere shortening. Specifically, an in vitro study using B3 cells demonstrated that Pb exposure as 100 μM $Pb(NO_3)_2$ significantly increased the number of telomere dysfunction-induced foci leading to telomere loss due to altered telomere replication on the lagging DNA strand [59]. Furthermore, exposure to 10–50 μg/mL Pb acetate significantly increased oxidative DNA damage, DNA strand break frequency, misrepair, as well as telomere end fusion in lymphocyte culture [60]. It is also notable that response to Pb exposure may be dependent on the cell types. It has been demonstrated that exposure to 0.5 μM Pb acetate resulted in significant telomere shortening in L-02 hepatocytes; whereas in SMMC-7721 hepatoma cells, Pb induced an increase in telomere length [61].

Generally, the existing epidemiological data demonstrate that telomere length is inversely associated with occupational and environmental high-dose Pb exposure agreeing with the results of laboratory studies. Pb-induced telomere shortening was also shown to be associated with markers of oxidative stress and genotoxicity in exposed subjects. At the same time, data on the association between maternal Pb exposure and cord blood telomere length are rather contradictory. Therefore, telomere length may be considered as a potential biomarker of environmental and occupational but not maternal Pb exposure.

10.4 Arsenic

Arsenic (As) is a toxic metalloid that possesses a broad spectrum of adverse health effects with the kidney, liver, and cardiovascular systems being the primary targets. Moreover, As is ranked by the International Agency for Research on Cancer (IARC) as a human carcinogen. Biomarkers of As exposure are generally represented by the detected levels of the metalloid in blood, urine, hair, and nails [62]. In addition to an assessment of metalloid levels in biosamples, markers of As-induced genotoxicity may be also considered as the potential biomarkers of As toxicity [63]. In view of epidemiological and laboratory indications of the association between As exposure and telomere length, the application of the latter as a biomarker of As exposure is of particular interest.

Most epidemiological findings are obtained from cohorts environmentally exposed to As through drinking water. A study originating from Bangladesh revealed that urinary As levels (median 158.02 μg/g creatinine) were directly associated not only with telomere length but also telomeric repeat-binding factor 2 (TERF2), dyskerin pseudouridine synthase 1 (DKC1), TERF2IP (TERF2-interacting protein), and OB Fold-containing Protein 1 (OBFC1) gene expression, whereas relationship with Werner syndrome helicase/exonuclease protein expression was inverse [64]. The examination of children living in West Bengal (India) exposed to As through drinking water (50.8 vs 6.2 μg/L As in controls) revealed the elevation of urinary As levels (74.7 vs 25.4 μg/L in controls) along with a non-significant tendency to increased telomere length, although markers of genetic damage were observed in lymphocytes, buccal, and urothelial cells [65]. Urinary As levels (10.1–1251 μg/L) in As-exposed women living in Northern Argentina were directly associated with telomere length as well as hTERT expression, while the association with telomere length was stronger for inorganic As compared to monomethylarsonic acid (MMA) [66]. Correspondingly, in indigenous Bolivian people urinary (mean 88 μg/L) and blood (mean 2.4 ng/g) arsenic levels were associated with higher telomere length in parallel with oxidative damage marker levels [67]. It is also notable that a significant correlation between urinary As levels and telomere length ($r_2 = 0.47$; $p = 0.039$) was found to be significant only in As-exposed subjects from Coahuila (Mexico) with mean urinary As levels of 497.5 μ g/g creatinine, whereas in the control group (urinary As −151.1 μ g/g creatinine), this association was not significant ($r_2 = 0.09$; $p = 0.062$) [68]. It is noteworthy that As exposure is associated with higher telomere length in subjects with impaired As metabolism characterized by higher inorganic As^{3+} levels [69]. At the same time, the examination of Bangladeshi children aged 5–7 years old demonstrated a negative relationship between urinary As (143.85 μg/L or 228.28 μg/g creatinine) and relative telomere length in whole blood [70].

Generally, consistent data were obtained from studies involving mother–child pairs upon environmental As exposure. Specifically, examination of 762 mother–newborn pairs from Wuhan demonstrated that maternal urinary As level in the third trimester (mean 27.1 μg/g creatinine) was positively associated with cord blood telomere length, and doubling of maternal As levels was related to 5.75% longer cord blood telomeres [71]. As levels in placenta (8.4 μg/kg), blood (0.16 μg/L), and urine (13-2450 μg/L) were found to be directly associated with placental relative telomere length in a mother–child cohort in northern Argentina [72]. In contrast to these findings, a study performed in Matlab (Bangladesh) demonstrated that both maternal (8th week of gestation) and child urinary As levels higher than 45 μg/L were inversely associated with blood telomere length in 9-year-old children [73].

In view of the role of arsenic overexposure in the development of skin lesions and carcinogenesis [74], several studies assessed the potential association of this relationship with telomere length. In a study performed in West Bengal (India) subjects with As-induced skin, lesions were characterized by telomerase-independent increase in telomere length due to increased expression telomeric repeat-binding factors 1 and 2 (TRF-1 and TRF-2) that are responsible for alternative telomere elongation [75]. Srinivas et al. revealed a significant interactive effect of As exposure and telomere length on skin basal cell carcinoma when the highest carcinogenic risk was observed in subjects with drinking water high in As levels and short telomeres [76].

Laboratory studies also indicate that telomere length may significantly modulate cellular response to As exposure. It has been demonstrated that cells with altered telomere states are characterized by higher susceptibility to As toxicity [77]. Significant telomere shortening along with telomerase deficiency was shown to increase the susceptibility of mouse embryos to As toxicity associated with oxidative stress [78] (Fig. 10.1). In addition, sodium meta-arsenite was shown to induce DNA damage and telomere erosion in cells with short telomeres, but not with the long ones [79].

The impact of As on telomere maintenance mechanisms was also studied in laboratory studies to reveal its potential contribution to As-induced carcinogenesis [80] or the anticancer effects of arsenicals [81].

Valuable data were obtained from studies of dose-dependent effects of As on telomerase activity and expression. Specifically, a study in the HaCaT keratinocyte cell line revealed a U-shaped association between As exposure and hTERT mRNA expression that increased from 0 to 1.0 μM and further decreased from 2.5 to 10 μM of the exposing As dose [82]. Correspondingly, incubation of human cord blood cells with different doses of As revealed a significant up-regulation of telomerase mRNA and protein expression, as well as increased mRNA expression of the oncogenes ras and c-Myc upon low dose As exposure (0.0001 μM), whereas high doses of As (1 μM) significantly reduced telomerase expression, telomere length, as well as induced apoptotic and necrotic cell death in a reactive oxygen species (ROS)-dependent manner [83]. Zhang et al. (2003) also demonstrated increased telomerase activity and proliferation in HL-60 human leukemia cells and HaCaT keratinocytes upon exposure to low doses of As (< 1 μM), whereas high As doses induced a ROS-dependent decrease in telomerase activity and telomere length in parallel with apoptosis [84].

Generally, As was shown to inhibit telomerase activity and hTERT mRNA expression in a broad spectrum of cancer cell lines including human leukemia HL-60 cells [85], mammary adenocarcinoma MA-891 cells [86], myelogenous leukemia K562 cells [87], human colorectal carcinoma LS-174T cells [88], liver cancer HepG2 cells [89], colon adenocarcinoma LS-174T cells [90], endometrial carcinoma cell lines [91], multiple myeloma cell line KM3 [92], and human nasopharyngeal carcinoma CSNE-1 xenografts [93].

As-induced inhibition of telomerase activity was closely associated with significant modulation of cell cycle regulation. In HL-60 leukemia cells arsenic trioxide treatment significantly suppressed hTERT mRNA and protein expression in parallel with reduction of specificity protein 1 (Sp1), c-Myc, nuclear factor kappa B (NF-κB), and upstream stimulatory factor 2 (USF2) expressions, altogether resulting in growth inhibition and apoptosis [94]. The role of down-regulated Sp1 and c-Myc activity was also shown to mediate As-induced inhibition of hTERT gene expression in leukemia cell line, NB4 [95]. Inhibition of telomerase activity by As_2O_3 was also associated with altered expression of proteins involved in cell cycle regulation, namely B-cell lymphoma 2 protein (Bcl-2), retinoblastoma protein (Rb), P16 tumor suppressor, apoptosis-associated caspase-3, and cell cycle regulators cyclin A and E in leukemia cell lines NB4 [96]. Despite As-induced down-regulation of telomerase activity, such an inhibitory effect was shown to be indirect [97]. As-induced telomerase translocation [79], ROS overproduction [98], oxidative DNA damage [99], ROS-dependent c-Jun N-terminal kinase (JNK) activation [100], and alteration of NF-kB signaling [101] may at least partially mediate telomerase inhibition in As-exposed cancer cell lines.

Taken together, these findings are indicative of up-regulation of telomerase activity with stimulation of cellular proliferation that may underlie the carcinogenic effect of low-dose As exposure, whereas high doses of As down-regulate telomerase activity and expression thus promoting apoptosis and possessing anticancer effects.

In contrast to Cd or Pb, As body burden was shown to be associated with longer telomeres in populations environmentally exposed to high doses of As, although certain contradictions exist due to differences in dose of exposure, age, and other factors [102]. Moreover, an induced increase in telomere length was shown to be associated with the development of As-induced skin lesions and skin cancer. Correspondingly, laboratory studies demonstrated that arsenic exposure significantly increases telomerase activity, although this effect may be observed only in low doses. In contrast, in cancer cell lines high dose As treatment led to an inhibitory effect on telomerase activity that may be considered as the potential mechanism of anticancer effect. Therefore, the impact of As on telomerase activity may be indicative of proliferative or antiproliferative response in the exposed cells. Increased telomere length may be considered as the potential biomarker of As exposure and risk of carcinogenic effect in environmental studies, but not for assessment of prenatal As exposure.

10.5 Other Toxic Metals

In addition to Cd, Pb, and As possessing a significant influence on telomere length, single studies demonstrated that exposure to other toxic metals is also associated with altered telomere length and impaired telomerase activity. Although the existing data are insufficient to consider telomere length as a biomarker of exposure to mercury (Hg), hexavalent chromium (Cr(VI)), titanium, thallium, and antimony, further studies are required to assess the dose-response relationship and potential usefulness of telomere length as a marker of exposure.

10.5.1 Mercury

Given the role of prenatal mercury (Hg) exposure in adverse neurodevelopmental effects of the metal, single studies assessed the relationship between prenatal metal exposure and telomere length. Cord blood Hg level was positively associated with cord blood telomere length in children born in proximity to a local coal-burning power plant [103]. At the same time, examination of 229 mother–child pairs within the Seychelles Child Development Study involving subjects with high dietary seafood intake failed to reveal any significant associations between maternal and children hair Hg content and telomere length in maternal and cord blood as well as blood samples from children of 5 years old [104]. Although these findings are highly inconsistent, these contradictions may occur due to differences in the dose and the route of exposure, as well as particular Hg species.

Laboratory studies demonstrated the impact of methylmercury on telomerase expression. It has been demonstrated that intraperitoneal injection of methylmercury (MeHg) (2.5 mg/kg daily for 4 days) significantly reduced brain TERT mRNA expression in mice [105]. At the same time, MeHg exposure did not affect splenic TERT mRNA expression, neither in wild type nor in apolipoprotein E (APOE) knockout mice, despite the significant induction of oxidative stress, dyslipidemia, and cytogenetic abnormalities [106].

10.5.2 Hexavalent Chromium

The impact of isolated hexavalent chromium [Cr(VI)] exposure on telomere length was studied only in laboratory in vitro models. Specifically, human fibroblasts exposed to Cr(VI) were characterized by telomere loss and sister chromatid fusions that were reduced by both telomerase and Werner syndrome helicase/exonuclease protein activity [107]. Correspondingly, sensitivity to cytotoxic effects of Cr(VI) was dependent on telomerase activity. Specifically, long-term Cr(VI) exposure to BJ-fibroblasts resulted in chromosome damage, genomic instability, and apoptosis only in telomerase-deficient cells, but not in those expressing hTERT [108].

10.5.3 Titanium

In vivo and in vitro laboratory studies also demonstrated that titanium (Ti) exposure has a significant impact on telomere length. Specifically, exposure to titanium dioxide (500 mg/kg/week) for 10 weeks induced significant telomere shortening in rat lungs, but not the liver or spleen [109]. In another study in pulmonary epithelial cells TiO_2, exposure resulted in a trend to lower telomere length and increased percentage of short telomeres, although this effect was not significant despite a significant increase in G1-phase cell fraction and apoptotic and necrotic cell death [110]. The impact of titanium dioxide (TiO_2) nanoparticles (NPs) on telomere length was strongly dependent on cell type. Specifically, TiO_2 NPs-reduced telomere length along with down-regulation of nuclear factor erythroid 2-related factor 2 (Nrf-2), TRF1, TRF2, and POT1 mRNA expression in L-02 hepatocytes, whereas the impact of TiO_2 on Nrf2 and three core shelterin components mRNA expression in QGY hepatocarcinoma cells appeared to be stimulatory [111].

10.5.4 Thallium

The association between thallium (Tl) exposure and telomere length was addressed by Wu et al. (2021) through analysis of data of 746 mother–newborn pairs from Wuhan Children Hospital (2013–2015). A significant inverse relationship between prenatal Tl exposure and relative telomere length was revealed. Specifically, each 25% increase in maternal urinary Tl levels during delivery was associated with 1.85% shorter cord blood leukocyte telomeres, whereas no significant relationship was revealed with urinary Tl levels assessed during three trimesters of pregnancy [112].

10.5.5 Antimony

Analysis of NHANES 1999–2002 data demonstrated a significant inverse association between urinary Sb and leukocyte telomere length especially in middle-aged subjects and elderly [113].

10.6 Essential Metals with the Risk of Overexposure

Essential metals that are involved in multiple metabolic processes may also possess toxic effects at overload. Dietary intake of essential metals like Mg, Cu, and Fe within the recommended ranges was found to be associated with longer telomeres in US adults [114]. In contrast to toxic metals, an increased body burden of essential metals may be associated both with environmental overexposure and dysregulation of metal handling in the organism that may be associated with genetic disorders like hemochromatosis or Wilson's disease, as well as other non-heritable diseases.

10.6.1 Iron

Data from the Hemochromatosis and Iron (Fe) Overload Screening Study demonstrate that phenotypic iron overload is characterized by a significant association with a higher risk of telomere shortening than the HFE genotype [115]. Findings from this study also demonstrated that elevated transferrin saturation is associated with shorter telomere length as well as worse general and mental health status as compared to subjects with normal transferrin saturation (< 45% in females and < 50% in males) [116]. Moreover, Shin and Baik demonstrated that subjects with high-normal transferrin saturation percentage (35–45%) had shorter relative leukocyte length than those with low-normal values (< 30%) and this difference was more pronounced in obese examinees [117]. It has also been demonstrated that patients with hemochromatosis and iron overload have 39% shorter telomeres as compared to those without manifest iron overload, whereas the difference in comparison to healthy examinees was more than twofold [118]. Hemodialysis patients with hyperferritinemia indicative of iron overload were characterized by 12% shorter telomere length as compared to patients with normal ferritin levels. Moreover, both circulating ferritin levels and hemodialysis duration were inversely associated with relative telomere length [119]. One nutritional study was aimed at the assessment of iron supplementation on telomere length. However, despite the observation of mitochondrial damage following ferrous sulfate supplementation in Cambodian women, this intervention did not lead to a significant impact on relative leukocyte telomere length [120].

In a rat model of iron overload telomerase activity was found to be increased without any significant differences in TERT mRNA or protein expression in the liver in parallel with increased hepatic reduced glutathione and cysteine levels, as well as glutamate-cysteine ligase activity, altogether being indicative of a compensatory response to iron overload [121].

Taken together, these findings demonstrate that iron overload is associated with telomere shortening, although these data were obtained only from patients with disease-associated iron dysregulation.

10.6.2 Copper

Copper (Cu) overload was shown to be associated with multiple adverse health effects due to its toxicity. However, data on the impact of either genetically or environmentally induced Cu overload on telomere length appears to be limited. In contrast, the relationship between dietary Cu and telomere length was studied. Specifically, analysis of NHANES 1999–2002 data revealed a direct association between dietary Cu intake and leukocyte telomere length after adjustment for multiple confounders including smoking status, BMI, and CVD to name a few [122]. Higher dietary copper intake was shown to be associated with longer telomeres in a general cohort of patients with hypertension as well as in patients of age $>$45 years old and taking antihypertensive medications [123].

An in vitro study demonstrated that Raji cells exposed to Cu(II) and ascorbic acid were characterized by telomere shortening and oxidative DNA strand breaks, whereas Asp-Ala-His-Lys (DAHK), a specific copper chelator being an analog to N-terminus of human albumin, completely attenuated Cu-induced damage [124], corresponding to the role of Cu as a redox-active metal (Fig. 10.1).

10.6.3 Manganese

Examination of 762 mother–newborn pairs in Wuhan (China) revealed a significant positive relationship between maternal urinary manganese (Mn) levels and cord blood telomere length, when doubling of maternal Mn levels was associated with a 2.1% increase in telomere length in the second, but not first or third trimesters [125]. At the same time, we have demonstrated that null mutation of telomerase catalytic subunit in *Caenorhabditis elegans* (*trt-1*) is associated with lower susceptibility to dopaminergic neurotoxicity and improved survival upon acute Mn exposure [126].

10.7 Metal Mixtures

Although most studies were focused on the relationship between overload of one particular metal and telomere length, exposure to a single metal is more characteristic for habitation in specific geochemical provinces characterized by its high content in the environment (e.g., As overload in Bangladesh) or dietary intake of products that accumulate particular metals (e.g., Hg in seafoods). In turn, environmental exposure to multiple metals is much more common due to similar sources of metal emissions. Even industrial processes associated with the processing of a single metal (e.g., lead smelters) are shown to be the sources of environmental pollution with other metals like Cd, As, Cu, and Sb to name a few [127, 128]. Therefore, investigation of the association between multiple metal exposure and telomere length is of particular interest.

Interesting findings were obtained from subjects occupationally exposed to multiple metals and other pollutants. Welders are constantly exposed to welding fumes that contain multiple metals like Fe, Cr, Ni, and Pb [129], although Mn is considered the key hazardous factor [130]. The examination of welders working in fitness equipment manufacture demonstrated that blood Cr, Co, and As levels were inversely correlated with telomere length, although in multiple regression models only a negative association between telomere length and As concentrations remained significant after adjustment for age, smoking status, and the level of other metals [131]. The effects of welding fumes on telomere length and telomerase activity were also investigated in laboratory studies. In contrast to occupationally exposed humans, exposure of Fischer-344 (F-344) rats to welding fumes was associated with increased cerebral telomere length without any significant changes in telomerase activity, although TRF1 and TRF2 mRNA and protein expression was found to be reduced. Alterations of telomere length were also associated with amyloidogenic pathway up-regulation and α-synuclein accumulation [132]. It was also demonstrated that metal content in welding fumes has a significant impact on telomere length. Specifically, intratracheal instillation of welding fume NPs containing 41% Fe, 29% Cr, 17% Mn, and 3% Ni induced a more profound increase in telomere length in parallel with oxidative stress and inflammation as compared to Sprague-Dawley rats exposed to welding NPs containing 85% Fe and 14% Mn [133].

In 842 workers of a coke-oven plant exposed to multiple metals, plasma Mn levels were shown to be the key positive predictor of exposure-associated changes in telomere length, although significant direct associations were also revealed for plasma aluminum (Al), antimony (Sb), chromium (Cr), nickel (Ni), titanium (Ti), and vanadium (V) concentrations. Moreover, the association between manganese (Mn) exposure and higher telomere length is also potentiated by TERT and cleft lip and palate transmembrane protein 1-like cluster on chromosome 5p15.33 (TERT-CLPTM1L) variants [134]. At the same time, analysis of data from the Dongfeng-Tongji cohort consisting of retired motor corporation workers demonstrated that plasma vanadium (V), copper (Cu), arsenic (As), aluminum (Al), and nickel (Ni) levels were associated with shorter leukocyte telomeres, whereas manganese (Mn) and zinc (Zn) concentrations were directly associated with telomere length. Moreover, the association between metal mixture, and especially circulating vanadium and aluminum levels with telomere shortening was more profound in overweight and obese subjects [135].

Habitation near large industrial centers is also associated with exposure to metal mixtures. In subjects living near an e-waste recycling plant or occupationally involved workers' blood, As, Ni, lanthanum (La), silver (Ag), and cerium (Ce) levels as well as telomere length and mtDNAcn were found to be elevated, whereas only blood Ni concentration was positively associated with telomere length in occupationally exposed examinees that may be indicative of increased carcinogenic risk [136]. Exposure to rare earth elements due to habitation near rare earth mines was associated with increased blood lanthanum (La), cerium (Ce), dysprosium (Dy), yttrium (Y), praseodymium (Pr), neodymium (Nd), samarium (Sm), gadolinium (Gd), and ytterbium (Yb) concentrations, as well as increased telomerase activity and a higher number of cells in S and G2/M phases, whereas total concentration of rare earth elements significantly correlated with telomerase activity in peripheral blood mononuclear cells [137].

Maternal environmental exposure to metal mixtures was also shown to affect telomere length in newborns and children. Specifically, maternal urinary barium (Ba), cadmium (Cd), and Pb levels were responsible for 35.4%, 24.5%, and 26.9% of the inverse association between maternal urinary metal (As, Ba, Cd, Ni, Pb) and cord blood telomere length, although, after adjustment for antioxidant intake, the observed association remained significant only in women with low antioxidant intake [138]. Maternal plasma As and Ba levels in the Guangxi Zhuang Birth Cohort were shown to contribute significantly to the inverse association between newborn telomere length and maternal plasma metal mixture levels. In turn, circulating Pb levels were characterized by an inverse association with telomere length only in males. An increase in each tertile of the metal mixture was shown to be associated with a 9.39% lower telomere length [139]. At the same time, analysis of both toxic and essential metals in mother–child pairs involved in Project Viva, a US pre-birth cohort, demonstrated a non-linear nearly U-shaped association between the first-trimester maternal blood Ba levels and cord blood telomere length, whereas selenium (Se) concentration was directly associated with longer telomeres. Despite a significant association between metal mixture or metals such as Pb with mtDNAcn, no significant relationship with telomere length was revealed for other metals studied [140].

Therefore, the existing data demonstrate that metal mixture exposure is associated with significant alteration of telomere length, mainly telomere shortening. In addition, certain metals as components of metal mixtures may be positively associated with telomere length, thus being indicative of the potential carcinogenic effect.

10.8 Conclusions

Existing data demonstrate that metal exposure interferes with both telomere length and telomerase activity. The potential mechanisms mediating the effect of metal overexposure on telomere shortening may involve oxidative stress, mitochondrial dysfunction, and inflammation [141]. The existing data, despite being rather heterogeneous, have shown specific patterns of telomere responsiveness to metal exposure. It appears that reduced telomere length may be considered as a potential biomarker of postnatal and prenatal exposure to Cd, as well as postnatal exposure to Pb and As. In turn, alterations in telomere length were shown to partially mediate the contribution of metal exposure to the development of diseases, including hypertension, kidney damage, and COPD. The effect of metals on telomere length and telomerase activity may also mediate the effects of metal exposure on cancer development as demonstrated for As when low doses of As promote cell proliferation and high-dose exposure reduces telomerase activity and possesses anticarcinogenic effect in cancer cell lines (Fig. 10.2).

Despite the lack of particular patterns of telomere length responsiveness upon exposure to other metals, existing data demonstrate that overexposure may interfere with telomere length and further studies are warranted. Telomere length was shown to be significantly affected by exposure to metal mixtures, resulting predominantly in telomere shortening. However, the particular effect of exposure strongly depends on mixture characteristics including its particular constituents and doses of specific metals.

Therefore, telomere length may be used as the potential biomarker of Cd, Pb, and As exposure, as well as a prognostic marker of the risk of metal-induced adverse health effects. At the same time, despite the rather high sensitivity of such biomarkers, their specificity is questionable, especially upon metal mixture exposure. Further studies are required to fill in existing gaps in the field by

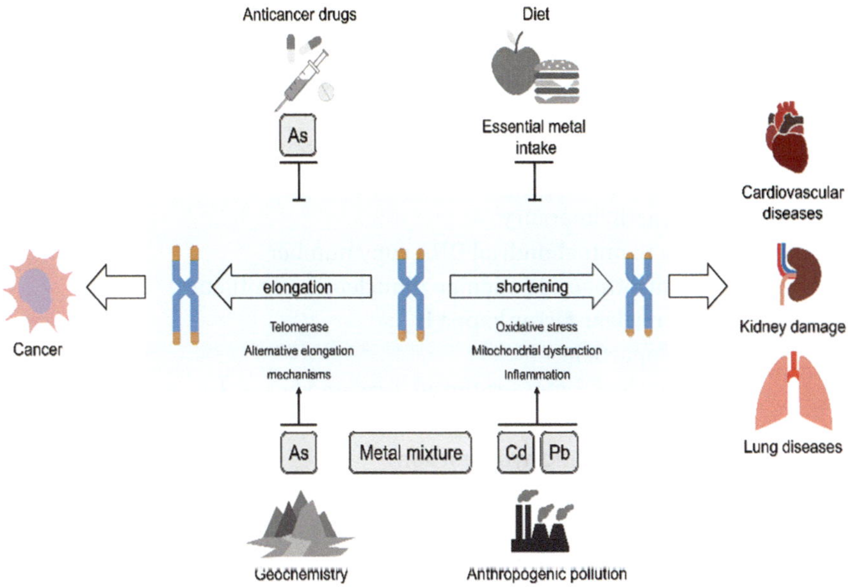

Figure 10.2 The potential effects of metal exposure on telomere length that may be involved in development of metal-induced diseases.

estimation of metal-specific responses, dose-dependence, as well as age and sex effects on the interaction between metal exposure and telomere length.

Acknowledgment

The study was performed with the support of the Russian Ministry of Science and Higher Education, Project No. FENZ-2023-0004.

Abbreviations

ALAD: δ-aminolevulinic acid dehydratase
APOE: apolipoprotein E
Bcl-2: B-cell lymphoma 2 protein
BMI: body mass index
CLPTM1L: cleft lip and palate transmembrane protein 1-like cluster on chromosome 5p15.33

COPD: chronic obstructive pulmonary disease
CVD: cardiovascular disease
DKC1: dyskerin pseudouridine synthase 1
Erα: estrogen receptor α
hTERT: human telomerase reverse transcriptase
JNK: c-Jun N-terminal kinase
MeHg: methylmercury
mtDNAcn: mitochondrial DNA copy number
NADS: nicotinamide adenine dinucleotide synthetase
NF-κB: nuclear factor kappa B
NP: nanoparticle
Nrf-2: nuclear factor erythroid 2-related factor 2
OBFC1: OB Fold-containing Protein 1
PAH: polyaromatic hydrocarbon
PCBs: polychlorinated biphenyls
POT1: protection of telomeres protein 1
Rb: retinoblastoma protein
RBC: red blood cells
ROS: reactive oxygen species
Sp1: specificity protein 1
TBARS: thiobarbituric acid-reactive species
TercKO: telomerase RNA component knockout
TERF2: telomeric repeat-binding factor 2
TERF2IP: TERF2 interacting protein
TERT: telomerase reverse transcriptase
TPP1: telomere-binding protein POT1-interacting protein 1
TRF-1/2: telomeric repeat-binding factor 1/2
USF2: upstream stimulatory factor 2

References

1. Smith, E. M., Pendlebury, D. F. and Nandakumar, J. (2020). Structural biology of telomeres and telomerase, *Cell. Mol. Life Sci.*, **77,** pp. 61–79.
2. Oeseburg, H., de Boer, R. A., van Gilst, W. H. and van der Harst, P. (2010). Telomere biology in healthy aging and disease, *Pflugers Arch.*, **459**, pp. 259–268.

3. Grill, S. and Nandakumar, J. (2021). Molecular mechanisms of telomere biology disorders, *J. Biol. Chem.*, **296**, pp. 100064.
4. Tsoukalas, D., Buga, A. M., Docea, A. O., Sarandi, E., Mitrut, R., Renieri, E., *et al.* (2021). Reversal of brain aging by targeting telomerase: a nutraceutical approach, *Int. J. Mol. Med.*, **48,** pp. 199.
5. Rossiello, F., Jurk, D., Passos, J. F. and d'Adda di Fagagna, F. (2022). Telomere dysfunction in ageing and age-related diseases, *Nat. Cell. Biol.*, **24**, pp. 135–147.
6. Haycock, P. C., Heydon, E. E., Kaptoge, S., Butterworth, A. S., Thompson, A. and Willeit, P. (2014). Leucocyte telomere length and risk of cardiovascular disease: systematic review and meta-analysis, *BMJ*, **349**, pp. g4227.
7. Xu, X., Hu, H., Lin, Y., Huang, F., Ji, H., Li, Y., *et al.* (2019). Differences in leukocyte telomere length between coronary heart disease and normal population: a multipopulation meta-analysis, *Biomed. Res. Int.*, **2019**, pp. 5046867.
8. Wang, J., Dong, X., Cao, L., Sun, Y., Qiu, Y., Zhang, Y., *et al.* (2016). Association between telomere length and diabetes mellitus: a meta-analysis, *J. Int. Med. Res.*, **44**, pp. 1156–1173.
9. Jin, X., Pan, B., Dang, X., Wu, H. and Xu, D. (2018). Relationship between short telomere length and stroke: a meta-analysis. *Medicine.*, **97**, pp. e12489.
10. Mundstock, E., Sarria, E. E., Zatti, H., Mattos Louzada, F., Kich Grun, L., *et al.* (2015). Effect of obesity on telomere length: systematic review and meta-analysis, *Obesity*, **23**, pp. 2165–2174.
11. Fu, J., Ji, X., Liu, J., Chen, X. and Shang, H. (2022). Meta-analysis of the connection between Alzheimer disease and telomeres, *Alzheimer Dis. Assoc. Disord.*, **36**, pp. 73–79.
12. Wang, T., Jia, Z., Li, S., Li, Y., Yu, T., Lu, T., *et al.* (2022). The association between leukocyte telomere length and chronic obstructive pulmonary disease is partially mediated by inflammation: a meta-analysis and population-based mediation study, *BMC Pulm. Med.*, **22,** pp. 320.
13. Smith, L., Luchini, C., Demurtas, J., Soysal, P., Stubbs, B., Hamer, M., *et al.* (2019). Telomere length and health outcomes: an umbrella review of systematic reviews and meta-analyses of observational studies, *Ageing Res. Rev.*, **51**, pp. 1–10.
14. Ma, H., Zhou, Z., Wei, S., Liu, Z., Pooley, K. A., Dunning, A. M., *et al.* (2011). Shortened telomere length is associated with increased risk of cancer: a meta-analysis, *PLoS One.*, **6**, pp. e20466.

15. Zhang, C., Chen, X., Li, L., Zhou, Y., Wang, C. and Hou, S. (2015). The association between telomere length and cancer prognosis: evidence from a meta-analysis, *PLoS One.*, **10**, pp. e0133174.
16. Wentzensen, I. M., Mirabello, L., Pfeiffer, R. M. and Savage, S. A. (2011). The association of telomere length and cancer: a meta-analysis, *Cancer Epidemiol. Biomarkers Prev.*, **20**, pp. 1238–1250.
17. Patel, C. J., Manrai, A. K., Corona, E. and Kohane, I. S. (2017). Systematic correlation of environmental exposure and physiological and self-reported behaviour factors with leukocyte telomere length, *Int. J. Epidemiol.*, **46**, pp. 44–56.
18. Assavanopakun, P., Sapbamrer, R., Kumfu, S., Chattipakorn, N. and Chattipakorn, S. C. (2022). Effects of air pollution on telomere length: evidence from in vitro to clinical studies, *Environ. Pollut.*, **312**, pp. 120096.
19. Miri, M., Nazarzadeh, M., Alahabadi, A., Ehrampoush, M. H., Rad, A., Lotfi, M. H., *et al.* (2019). Air pollution and telomere length in adults: a systematic review and meta-analysis of observational studies, *Environ. Pollut.*, **244**, pp. 636–647.
20. Louzon, M., Coeurdassier, M., Gimbert, F., Pauget, B. and de Vaufleury, A. (2019). Telomere dynamic in humans and animals: review and perspectives in environmental toxicology, *Environ. Int.*, **131**, pp. 105025.
21. Zhang, X., Lin, S., Funk, W. E. and Hou, L. (2013). Environmental and occupational exposure to chemicals and telomere length in human studies, *Occup. Environ. Med.*, **70**, pp. 743–749.
22. Rafati Rahimzadeh, M., Rafati Rahimzadeh, M., Kazemi, S. and Moghadamnia, A. A. (2017). Cadmium toxicity and treatment: an update, *Caspian J. Intern. Med.*, **8**, pp. 135–145.
23. Prozialeck, W.C. (2013). Biomarkers for Cadmium. In: Kretsinger, R.H., Uversky, V.N., Permyakov, E.A. (eds) *Encyclopedia of Metalloproteins*, Springer, New York, NY.
24. Zota, A. R., Needham, B. L., Blackburn, E. H., Lin, J., Park, S. K., Rehkopf, D. H., *et al.* (2015). Associations of cadmium and lead exposure with leukocyte telomere length: findings from National Health and Nutrition Examination Survey, 1999–2002, *Am. J. Epidemiol.*, **181**, pp. 127–136.
25. Nomura, S. J., Robien, K. and Zota, A. R. (2017). Serum Folate, Vitamin B-12, Vitamin A, γ-Tocopherol, α-Tocopherol, and Carotenoids do not modify associations between cadmium exposure and leukocyte telomere length in the General US Adult Population, *J. Nutr.*, **147**, pp. 538–548.

26. Grau-Perez, M., Zhao, J., Pierce, B., Francesconi, K. A., Goessler, W., Zhu, Y., *et al.* (2019). Urinary metals and leukocyte telomere length in American Indian communities: the strong heart and the strong heart family study, *Environ. Pollut.,* **246**, pp. 311–318.

27. Fillman, T., Shimizu-Furusawa, H., Ng, C. F. S., Parajuli, R. P. and Watanabe, C. (2016). Association of cadmium and arsenic exposure with salivary telomere length in adolescents in Terai, Nepal, *Environ. Res.*, **149**, pp. 8–14.

28. Mizuno, Y., Inaba, Y., Masuoka, H., Kibe, M., Kosaka, S., Natsuhara, K., *et al.* (2023). Determinants of oxidative stress among indigenous populations in Northern Laos: trace element exposures and dietary patterns, *Sci. Total Environ.*, **868**, pp. 161516.

29. Xia, F., Li, Q., Luo, X. and Wu, J. (2022). Association between urinary metals and leukocyte telomere length involving an artificial neural network prediction: findings based on NHANES 1999–2002, *Front. Public Health.*, **10**, pp. 963138.

30. Mizuno, Y., Konishi, S., Imai, H., Fujimori, E., Kojima, N. and Yoshinaga, J. (2019). Cadmium exposure and blood telomere length in Female University Students in Japan, *Biol. Trace Elem. Res.*, **192**, pp. 98–105.

31. Zhang, L., Song, L., Liu, B., Wu, M., Wang, L., Zhang, B., *et al.* (2019). Prenatal cadmium exposure is associated with shorter leukocyte telomere length in Chinese newborns, *BMC Med.*, **17**, pp. 27.

32. Wai, K. M., Umezaki, M., Kosaka, S., Mar, O., Umemura, M., Fillman, T., *et al.* (2018). Impact of prenatal heavy metal exposure on newborn leucocyte telomere length: a birth-cohort study, *Environ. Pollut.,* **243**, pp. 1414–1421.

33. Lin, S., Huo, X., Zhang, Q., Fan, X., Du, L., Xu, X., *et al.* (2013). Short placental telomere was associated with cadmium pollution in an electronic waste recycling town in China, *PloS one.*, **8**, pp. e60815.

34. Wai, K. M., Umezaki, M., Umemura, M., Mar, O. and Watanabe, C. (2020). Protective role of selenium in the shortening of telomere length in newborns induced by in utero heavy metal exposure, *Environ. Res.*, **183**, pp. 109202.

35. Yang, Q., Liu, R., Gao, Y., Kang, H., Zhang, Z., Han, Z., *et al.* (2022). Mediating effect of telomere length in a hypertension population exposed to cadmium: a case-control study, *J. Hum. Hypertens.*, 10.1038/s41371-022-00685-x. Advance online publication.

36. Wai, K. M., Umezaki, M., Mizuno, Y., Sawada, K., Shinya, O., Nakaji, S., *et al.* (2022, September). Effect of cadmium on the association

between blood pressures and telomere length: a population-based cross-sectional study in Japan, In *ISEE Conference Abstracts*, **2022**, No. 1.

37. Zhang, J. C., Li, S. J., Guo, J. Y., Zhang, G. Y., Kang, H., Shi, X. J., *et al.* (2022). Urinary cadmium and peripheral blood telomere length predict the risk of renal function impairment: a study of 547 community residents of Shanxi, China, *Environ. Sci. Pollut. Res. Int.*, **29**, pp. 71427–71438.
38. Lv, B. B., Yang, C. L., Tan, Z. X., Zheng, L., Li, M. D., Jiang, Y. L., *et al.* (2023). Association between cadmium exposure and pulmonary function reduction: potential mediating role of telomere attrition in chronic obstructive pulmonary disease patients, *Ecotoxicol. Environ. Saf.*, **251**, pp. 114548.
39. Chen, L., Zhao, Y., Liu, F., Chen, H., Tan, T., Yao, P., *et al.* (2022). Biological aging mediates the associations between urinary metals and osteoarthritis among U.S. adults, *BMC Med.*, **20**, pp. 207.
40. Huang, J., Okuka, M., Lu, W., Tsibris, J. C., McLean, M. P., Keefe, D. L., *et al.* (2013). Telomere shortening and DNA damage of embryonic stem cells induced by cigarette smoke, *Reprod. Toxicol.*, **35**, pp. 89–95.
41. Huang, J., Okuka, M., McLean, M., Keefe, D. L. and Liu, L. (2010). Telomere susceptibility to cigarette smoke-induced oxidative damage and chromosomal instability of mouse embryos in vitro, *Free Radic. Biol. Med.*, **48**, pp. 1663–1676.
42. Dai, W., Chen, H., Yu, R., He, L., Chen, B. and Chen, X. (2010). Effects of cadmium on telomerase activity, expressions of TERT, c-myc and P53, and apoptosis of rat hepatocytes, *J. Huazhong Univ. Sci. Technolog. Med. Sci.*, **30**, pp. 709–713.
43. Wang, M. and Lei, Y. X. (2015). Effects of tea polyphenols on proliferation and apoptosis of cadmium-transformed cells, *Int. J. Clin. Exp. Med.*, **8**, pp. 3054–3062.
44. Martínez-Campa, C. M., Alonso-González, C., Mediavilla, M. D., Cos, S., González, A. and Sanchez-Barcelo, E. J. (2008). Melatonin down-regulates hTERT expression induced by either natural estrogens (17beta-estradiol) or metalloestrogens (cadmium) in MCF-7 human breast cancer cells, *Cancer Lett.*, **268**, pp. 272–277.
45. Alfonso-De Matte, M. Y., Moses-Soto, H. and Kruk, P. A. (2002). Calcium-mediated telomerase activity in ovarian epithelial cells, *Arch. Biochem. Biophys.*, **399**, pp. 239–244.
46. Barbosa, F., Jr, Tanus-Santos, J. E., Gerlach, R. F. and Parsons, P. J. (2005). A critical review of biomarkers used for monitoring human exposure

to lead: advantages, limitations, and future needs, *Environ. Health Perspect.*, **113**, pp. 1669–1674.

47. Sakai, T. (2000). Biomarkers of lead exposure, *Ind. Health*, **38**, pp. 127–142.
48. Wang, T., Tu, Y., Wang, K., Gong, S., Zhang, G., Zhang, Y., *et al.* (2020). Associations of blood lead levels with multiple genotoxic biomarkers among workers in China: a population-based study, *Environ. Pollut.*, **273**, pp. 116181.
49. Wu, Y., Liu, Y., Ni, N., Bao, B., Zhang, C. and Lu, L. (2012). High lead exposure is associated with telomere length shortening in Chinese battery manufacturing plant workers, *Occup. Environ. Med.*, **69**, pp. 557–563.
50. Wang, T., Tu, Y., Zhang, G., Gong, S., Wang, K., Zhang, Y., *et al.* (2020). Development of a benchmark dose for lead-exposure based on its induction of micronuclei, telomere length changes and hematological toxicity, *Environ. Int.*, **145**, pp. 106129.
51. Pawlas, N., Płachetka, A., Kozłowska, A., Mikołajczyk, A., Kasperczyk, A., Dobrakowski, M., *et al.* (2016). Telomere length, telomerase expression, and oxidative stress in lead smelters, *Toxicol. Ind. Health.*, **32**, pp. 1961–1970.
52. Lu, Y., Liu, X., Zhao, Z., Ou, X., Yang, Y., Wei, Q., *et al.* (2021). Telomere length in peripheral leukocytes is a sensitive marker for assessing genetic damage among workers exposed to isopropanol, lead and noise: the case of an electronics manufacturer, *Genes. Environ.*, **43**, pp. 57.
53. Zhang, Y., Wang, T., Meng, Y., Zhang, G., Lei, C., Cui, S., *et al.* (2020). Changes of relative length of telomere and mRNA expression of telomere-binding protein POT1-interacting protein 1 in workers with occupational lead exposure, *China Occupational Medicine*, **6**, pp. 414–423.
54. Rohr, P., Campanelli Dos Santos, I., van Helvoort Lengert, A., Alves de Lima, M., Manuel Reis, R., Barbosa, F., Jr, *et al.* (2022). Absolute telomere length in peripheral blood lymphocytes of workers exposed to construction environment, *Int. J. Environ. Health Res.*, pp. 1–9. Advance online publication.
55. Pawlas, N., Płachetka, A., Kozłowska, A., Broberg, K. and Kasperczyk, S. (2015). Telomere length in children environmentally exposed to low-to-moderate levels of lead, *Toxicol. Appl. Pharmacol.*, **287**, pp. 111–118.

56. Alegría-Torres, J. A., Pérez-Rodríguez, R. Y., García-Torres, L., Costilla-Salazar, R. and Rocha-Amador, D. (2020). Exposure to arsenic and lead in children from Salamanca México, effects on telomeric lengthening and mitochondrial DNA, *Environ. Sci. Pollut. Res. Int.*, **27,** pp. 6420–6428.
57. Herrera-Moreno, J. F., Estrada-Gutierrez, G., Wu, H., Bloomquist, T. R., Rosa, M. J., Just, A. C., *et al.* (2022). Prenatal lead exposure, telomere length in cord blood, and DNA methylation age in the PROGRESS prenatal cohort, *Environ. Res.*, **205**, pp. 112577.
58. Wai, K. M., Umezaki, M., Umemura, M., Mar, O. and Watanabe, C. (2020). Protective role of selenium in the shortening of telomere length in newborns induced by in utero heavy metal exposure, *Environ. Res.*, **183**, pp. 109202.
59. Pottier, G., Viau, M., Ricoul, M., Shim, G., Bellamy, M., Cuceu, C., *et al.* (2013). Lead exposure induces telomere instability in human cells, *PloS one.*, **8,** pp. e67501.
60. Shah, A. J., Lakkad, B. C. and Rao, M. V. (2016). Genotoxicity in lead treated human lymphocytes evaluated by micronucleus and comet assays, *Indian J. Exp. Biol.*, **54**, pp. 502–508.
61. Liu, Q., Wang, H., Hu, D., Ding, C., Xu, H. and Tao, D. (2004). Effects of trace elements on the telomere lengths of hepatocytes L-02 and hepatoma cells SMMC-7721, *Biol. Trace Elem. Res.*, **100**, pp. 215–227.
62. Hughes M. F. (2006). Biomarkers of exposure: a case study with inorganic arsenic, *Environ. Health Perspect.*, **114**, pp. 1790–1796.
63. Marchiset-Ferlay, N., Savanovitch, C. and Sauvant-Rochat, M. P. (2012). What is the best biomarker to assess arsenic exposure via drinking water? *Environ. Int.*, **39**, pp. 150–171.
64. Gao, J., Roy, S., Tong, L., Argos, M., Jasmine, F., Rahaman, R., *et al.* (2015). Arsenic exposure, telomere length, and expression of telomere-related genes among Bangladeshi individuals, *Environ. Res.*, **136**, pp. 462–469.
65. Chatterjee, D., Adak, S., Banerjee, N., Bhattacharjee, P., Bandyopadhyay, A. K. and Giri, A. K. (2018). Evaluation of health effects, genetic damage and telomere length in children exposed to arsenic in West Bengal, İndia, *Mutat. Res. Genet. Toxicol. Environ. Mutagen.*, **836**, pp. 82–88.
66. Li, H., Engström, K., Vahter, M. and Broberg, K. (2012). Arsenic exposure through drinking water is associated with longer telomeres in peripheral blood, *Chem. Res. Toxicol.*, **25**, pp. 2333–2339.
67. De Loma, J., Krais, A. M., Lindh, C. H., Mamani, J., Tirado, N., Gardon, J., *et al.* (2022). Arsenic exposure and biomarkers for oxidative stress

and telomere length in indigenous populations in Bolivia, *Ecotoxicol. Environ. Saf.*, **231**, pp. 113194.

68. Jimenez Villarreal, J., Murillo Ortiz, B., Martinez Garza, S., Rivas Armendáriz, D. I., Boone Villa, V. D., Carranza Rosales, P., *et al.* (2018). Telomere length analysis in residents of a community exposed to arsenic, *J. Biochem. Mol. Toxicol.*, pp. e22230. Advance online publication.

69. Ameer, S. S., Xu, Y., Engström, K., Li, H., Tallving, P., Nermell, B., *et al.* (2016). Exposure to inorganic arsenic is associated with increased mitochondrial DNA copy number and longer telomere length in peripheral blood, *Front. Cell. Dev. Biol.*, **4**, pp. 87.

70. Farzan, S. F., Shahriar, M., Kibriya, M. G., Jasmine, F., Sarwar, G., Slavkovic, V., *et al.* (2021). Urinary arsenic and relative telomere length in 5–7 year old children in Bangladesh, *Environ. Int.*, **156**, pp. 106765.

71. Song, L., Liu, B., Zhang, L., Wu, M., Wang, L., Cao, Z., *et al.* (2019). Association of prenatal exposure to arsenic with newborn telomere length: Results from a birth cohort stud, *Environ. Res.*, **175**, pp. 442–448.

72. Herlin, M., Broberg, K., Igra, A. M., Li, H., Harari, F. and Vahter, M. (2019). Exploring telomere length in mother-newborn pairs in relation to exposure to multiple toxic metals and potential modifying effects by nutritional factors, *BMC Med.*, **17**, pp. 77.

73. Mannan, T., Ahmed, S., Akhtar, E., Ahsan, K. B., Haq, A., Kippler, M., *et al.* (2018). Associations of arsenic exposure with telomere length and naïve T cells in childhood: a birth cohort study, *Toxicol. Sci.*, **164**, pp. 539–549.

74. Yu, H. S., Liao, W. T. and Chai, C. Y. (2006). Arsenic carcinogenesis in the skin, *J. Biomed. Sci.*, **13**, pp. 657–666.

75. Chatterjee, D., Bhattacharjee, P., Sau, T. J., Das, J. K., Sarma, N., Bandyopadhyay, A. K., *et al.* (2015). Arsenic exposure through drinking water leads to senescence and alteration of telomere length in humans: a case-control study in West Bengal, India, *Mol. Carcinog.*, **54**, pp. 800–809.

76. Srinivas, N., Rachakonda, S., Hielscher, T., Calderazzo, S., Rudnai, P., Gurzau, E., *et al.* (2019). Telomere length, arsenic exposure and risk of basal cell carcinoma of skin, *Carcinogenesis.*, **40**, pp. 715–723.

77. Zhang, Y., Cao, E. H., Liang, X. Q. and Qin, J. F. (2003). Increasing sensitivity to arsenic trioxide-induced apoptosis by altered telomere state, *Eur. J. Pharmacol.*, **474**, pp. 141–147.

78. Liu, L., Trimarchi, J. R., Navarro, P., Blasco, M. A. and Keefe, D. L. (2003). Oxidative stress contributes to arsenic-induced telomere attrition, chromosome instability, and apoptosis, *J. Biol. Chem.*, **278**, pp. 31998–32004.
79. Phatak, P., Dai, F., Butler, M., Nandakumar, M. P., Gutierrez, P. L., Edelman, M. J., *et al.* (2008). KML001 cytotoxic activity is associated with its binding to telomeric sequences and telomere erosion in prostate cancer cells, *Clin. Cancer. Res.*, **14**, pp. 4593–4602.
80. Zhou, Q. and Xi, S. (2018). A review on arsenic carcinogenesis: epidemiology, metabolism, genotoxicity and epigenetic changes, *Regul. Toxicol. Pharmacol.*, **99**, pp. 78–88.
81. Khairul, I., Wang, Q. Q., Jiang, Y. H., Wang, C. and Naranmandura, H. (2017). Metabolism, toxicity and anticancer activities of arsenic compounds, *Oncotarget.*, **8**, pp. 23905–23926.
82. Mo, J., Xia, Y., Ning, Z., Wade, T. J. and Mumford, J. L. (2009). Elevated human telomerase reverse transcriptase gene expression in blood cells associated with chronic arsenic exposure in Inner Mongolia, China, *Environ. Health. Perspect.*, **117**, pp. 354–360.
83. Ferrario, D., Collotta, A., Carfi, M., Bowe, G., Vahter, M., Hartung, T., *et al.* (2009). Arsenic induces telomerase expression and maintains telomere length in human cord blood cells, *Toxicology.*, **260**, pp. 132–141.
84. Zhang, T. C., Schmitt, M. T. and Mumford, J. L. (2003). Effects of arsenic on telomerase and telomeres in relation to cell proliferation and apoptosis in human keratinocytes and leukemia cells in vitro, *Carcinogenesis.*, **24**, pp. 1811–1817.
85. Li, J. and Liu, S.X. (2003) Changes of telomerase activity and hTERT mRNA expression in the process of apoptosis of HL-60 cells induced by arsenic sulfide, *Xi Bao Yu Fen Zi Mian Yi Xue Za Zhi.*, **19,** pp. 595–597. (in Chinese).
86. Shi, Y., Hu, B., Guo, Y., Wang, H. and Xia, J. (2012). Inhibitory mechanism on growth of MA-891 cells by arsenic trioxide, *Zhongguo Zhong yao za zhi.*, **37**, pp. 637–642. (in Chinese).
87. Wang, Y., Fang, M. Y., Jiang, F. and Peng, H. J. (2004). Effects of arsenic trioxide, ginseng saponin and beta-elemene on telomere-telomerase system in K562 cell line, *Zhongguo shi yan xue ye xue za zhi.*, **12**, pp. 315–320. (in Chinese).
88. Wang, X. S., Wang, G. Y., Xu, H. T., Wang, K., Liu, M., Fu, S. B., *et al.* (2007). The effect of As2O3 on induction of apoptosis and inhibition

of telomerase activity in colon cancer LS-174T cells, *Zhonghua zhong liu za zhi.*, **29**, pp. 415–418. (in Chinese).

89. Chaudhary, A., Bhardwaj, S. K., Khan, A., Srivastava, A., Sinha, K. K., Ali, M., *et al.* (2022). Combinatorial effect of arsenic and herbal compounds in telomerase-mediated apoptosis induction in liver cancer, *Biol. Trace Elem. Res.*, 10.1007/s12011-022-03430-0.
90. Wang, X., Wang, G., Dong, D., Fu, S. and Yang, B. (2008). Inhibition on LS-174T cell growth and activity of telomerase in vitro and in vivo by arsenic trioxide, *Exp. Toxicol. Pathol.*, **60**, pp. 481–488.
91. Zhou, C., Boggess, J. F., Bae-Jump, V. and Gehrig, P. A. (2007). Induction of apoptosis and inhibition of telomerase activity by arsenic trioxide (As2O3) in endometrial carcinoma cells, *Gynecol. Oncol.*, **105**, pp. 218–222.
92. Guo, Z. X. and Jin, J. (2004). Effect of arsenic trioxide on telomerase and telomerase reverse transcriptase in KM3 cell line, *Zhongguo shi yan xue ye xue za zhi.*, **12**, pp. 346–349. (in Chinese).
93. Du, C., Li, D., Lin, Y. and Wu, M. (2001). Differentiation of human nasopharyngeal carcinoma xenografts and repression of telomerase activity induced by arsenic trioxide, *Natl. Med. J. India.*, **17**, pp. 67–70.
94. Zhang, Y., Sun, M., Shi, W., Yang, Q., Chen, C., Wang, Z., *et al.* (2015). Arsenic trioxide suppresses transcription of hTERT through down-regulation of multiple transcription factors in HL-60 leukemia cells, *Toxicol. Lett.*, **232**, pp. 481–489.
95. Chou, W. C., Hawkins, A. L., Barrett, J. F., Griffin, C. A. and Dang, C. V. (2001). Arsenic inhibition of telomerase transcription leads to genetic instability, *J. Clin. Invest.*, **108**, pp. 1541–1547.
96. Wang, Y. F., Sun, H. Y., Wang, Q. L. and Li, X. Q. (2003). Inhibiting effect of arsenic trioxide on telomerase activity of NB4 and Jurkat cell lines, *Zhongguo shi yan xue ye xue za zhi*, **11**, pp. 359–362. (in Chinese).
97. Chen, F., Xu, G., Li, Y. and Zhang, M. (2000). Regulation of telomerase activity in HL-60 and NB4 cells by arsenic trioxide, *Zhonghua xue ye xue za zhi.*, **21**, pp. 366–369. (in Chinese).
98. Caradonna, F. and Mauro, M. (2016). Role of the antioxidant defence system and telomerase in arsenic-induced genomic instability, *Mutagenesis.*, **31**, pp. 661–667.
99. Cheng, Y., Li, Y., Ma, C., Song, Y., Xu, H., Yu, H., Xu, S., Mu, Q., Li, H., Chen, Y. and Zhao, G. (2016). Arsenic trioxide inhibits glioma cell growth through induction of telomerase displacement and telomere dysfunction, *Oncotarget.*, **7**, pp. 12682–12692.

100. Shen, S. C., Yang, L. Y., Lin, H. Y., Wu, C. Y., Su, T. H. and Chen, Y. C. (2008). Reactive oxygen species-dependent HSP90 protein cleavage participates in arsenical As(+3)- and MMA(+3)-induced apoptosis through inhibition of telomerase activity via JNK activation, *Toxicol. Appl. Pharmacol.*, **229**, pp. 239–251. https://doi.org/10.1016/j.taap.2008.01.018
101. Ghaffari, S. H., Yousefi, M., Dizaji, M. Z., Momeny, M., Bashash, D., Zekri, A., *et al.* (2016). Arsenic trioxide induces apoptosis and incapacitates proliferation and invasive properties of U87MG glioblastoma cells through a possible NF-κB-mediated mechanism, *Asian Pac. J. Cancer. Prev.*, **17**, pp. 1553–1564. https://doi.org/10.7314/apjcp.2016.17.3.1553
102. Wai, K. M., Swe, T., Myar, M. T., Aisyah, C. R. and Hninn, T. S. S. (2023). Telomeres susceptibility to environmental arsenic exposure: shortening or lengthening? *Front. Public Health.*, **10**, pp. 1059248.
103. Perera, F., Lin, C. J., Qu, L. and Tang, D. (2018). Shorter telomere length in cord blood associated with prenatal air pollution exposure: benefits of intervention, *Environ. Int.*, **113**, pp. 335–340.
104. Yeates, A. J., Thurston, S. W., Li, H., Mulhern, M. S., McSorley, E. M., Watson, G. E., *et al.* (2017). PUFA status and methylmercury exposure are not associated with leukocyte telomere length in mothers or their children in the Seychelles child development study, *J. Nutr.*, **147**, pp. 2018–2024.
105. Crespo-López, M. E., Soares, E. S., Macchi, B. M., Santos-Sacramento, L., Takeda, P. Y., Lopes-Araújo, A., *et al.* (2019). Towards therapeutic alternatives for mercury neurotoxicity in the amazon: unraveling the pre-clinical effects of the superfruit açaí (Euterpe oleracea, Mart.) as juice for human consumption, *Nutrients.*, **11**, pp. 2585.
106. Roque, C. R., Sampaio, L. R., Ito, M. N., Pinto, D. V., Caminha, J. S. R., Nunes, P. I. G., *et al.* (2021). Methylmercury chronic exposure affects the expression of DNA single-strand break repair genes, induces oxidative stress, and chromosomal abnormalities in young dyslipidemic APOE knockout mice, *Toxicology.*, **464**, pp. 152992.
107. Liu, F. J., Barchowsky, A. and Opresko, P. L. (2010). The Werner syndrome protein suppresses telomeric instability caused by chromium (VI) induced DNA replication stress, *PloS one.*, **5**, pp. e11152.
108. Glaviano, A., Nayak, V., Cabuy, E., Baird, D. M., Yin, Z., Newson, R., *et al.* (2006). Effects of hTERT on metal ion-induced genomic instability, *Oncogene.*, **25**, pp. 3424–3435.

109. Jensen, D. M., Løhr, M., Sheykhzade, M., Lykkesfeldt, J., Wils, R. S., Loft, S., *et al.* (2019). Telomere length and genotoxicity in the lung of rats following intragastric exposure to food-grade titanium dioxide and vegetable carbon particles. *Mutagenesis.*, **34**, pp. 203–214.

110. Alswady-Hoff, M., Erdem, J. S., Phuyal, S., Knittelfelder, O., Sharma, A., Fonseca, D. M., *et al.* (2021). Long-term exposure to nanosized TiO2 triggers stress responses and cell death pathways in pulmonary epithelial cells, *Int. J. Mol. Sci.*, **22**, pp. 5349.

111. Wang, H., Ni, J., Guo, X., Zhou, T., Ma, X., Xue, J., *et al.* (2018). Shelterin differentially responds to oxidative stress induced by TiO2-NPs and regulates telomere length in human hepatocytes and hepatocarcinoma cells in vitro, *Biochem. Biophys. Res. Commun.*, **503**, pp. 697–702.

112. Wu, M., Wang, L., Song, L., Liu, B., Liu, Y., Bi, J., *et al.* (2021). The association between prenatal exposure to thallium and shortened telomere length of newborns, *Chemosphere*, **265**, pp. 129025.

113. Scinicariello, F. and Buser, M. C. (2016). Urinary antimony and leukocyte telomere length: an analysis of NHANES 1999–2002, *Environ. Res.*, **150**, pp. 513–518.

114. Mazidi, M., Kengne, A. P. and Banach, M. (2017). Mineral and vitamin consumption and telomere length among adults in the United States, *Pol. Arch. Intern. Med.*, **127**, pp. 87–90.

115. Mainous, A. G., 3rd, Wright, R. U., Hulihan, M. M., Twal, W. O., McLaren, C. E., Diaz, V. A., *et al.* (2013). Telomere length and elevated iron: the influence of phenotype and HFE genotype, *Am. J. Hematol.*, **88**, pp. 492–496.

116. Mainous, A. G., 3rd, Wright, R. U., Hulihan, M. M., Twal, W. O., McLaren, C. E., Diaz, V. A., *et al.* (2014). Elevated transferrin saturation, health-related quality of life and telomere length, *Biometals.*, **27**, pp. 135–141.

117. Shin, C. and Baik, I. (2017). Transferrin saturation concentrations associated with telomeric ageing: a population-based study, *Br J Nutr.*, **117**, pp. 1693–1701.

118. Martín, M., Millan, A., Ferraro, F., Tetzlaff, W. F., Lozano, C. E., Botta, E., *et al.* (2020). Leukocyte telomere length is associated with iron overload in male adults with hereditary hemochromatosis, *Biosci Rep.*, **40**, pp. BSR20201916.

119. Murillo-Ortiz, B., Ramírez Emiliano, J., Hernández Vázquez, W. I., Martínez-Garza, S., Solorio-Meza, S., Albarrán-Tamayo, F., *et al.* (2016).

Impact of oxidative stress in premature aging and iron overload in hemodialysis patients. *Oxid Med Cell Longev.*, **2016**, pp. 1578235.

120. Steele, S. L., Hsieh, A. Y. Y., Gadawski, I., Kroeun, H., Barr, S. I., Devlin, A. M., *et al.* (2021). Daily oral supplementation with 60 mg of elemental iron for 12 weeks alters blood mitochondrial DNA content, but not leukocyte telomere length in Cambodian women, *Nutrients.*, **13**, pp. 1877.
121. Brown, K. E., Meleah Mathahs, M., Broadhurst, K. A., Coleman, M. C., Ridnour, L. A., Schmidt, W. N., *et al.* (2007). Increased hepatic telomerase activity in a rat model of iron overload: a role for altered thiol redox state? *Free Radic Biol Med.*, **42**, pp. 228–235.
122. Lin, Z., Gao, H., Wang, B. and Wang, Y. (2018). Dietary copper intake and its association with telomere length: a population-based study, *Front Endocrinol (Lausanne)*, **9**, pp. 404.
123. Gong, H., Yu, Q., Yuan, M., Jiang, Y., Wang, J., Huang, P., *et al.* (2022). The relationship between dietary copper intake and telomere length in hypertension, *J Nutr Health Aging*, **26**, pp. 510–514.
124. Bar-Or, D., Thomas, G. W., Rael, L. T., Lau, E. P. and Winkler, J. V. (2001). Asp-Ala-His-Lys (DAHK) inhibits copper-induced oxidative DNA double strand breaks and telomere shortening, *Biochem Biophys Res Commun.*, **282**, pp. 356–360.
125. Bi, J., Wu, M., Liu, Y., Song, L., Wang, L., Liu, Q., *et al.* (2021). Association between maternal urinary manganese concentrations and newborn telomere length: results from a birth cohort study, *Ecotoxicol. Environ. Saf.*, **213**, pp. 112037.
126. Ijomone, O. M., Miah, M. R., Peres, T. V., Nwoha, P. U. and Aschner, M. (2016). Null allele mutants of trt-1, the catalytic subunit of telomerase in Caenorhabditis elegans, are less sensitive to Mn-induced toxicity and DAergic degeneration, *Neurotoxicology.*, **57**, pp. 54–60.
127. Rieuwerts, J. and Farago, M. (1996). Heavy metal pollution in the vicinity of a secondary lead smelter in the Czech Republic, *Appl Geochem.*, **11**, pp. 17–23.
128. Akber, M. A., Rahman, M. A., Islam, M. A. and Islam, M. A. (2019). Potential ecological risk of metal pollution in lead smelter-contaminated agricultural soils in Khulna, Bangladesh, *Environ Monit Assess.*, **191**, pp. 351.
129. Abdullahi, I. L. and Sani, A. (2020). Welding fumes composition and their effects on blood heavy metals in albino rats, *Toxicol Rep.*, **7**, pp. 1495–1501.

130. Meeker, J. D., Susi, P. and Flynn, M. R. (2007). Manganese and welding fume exposure and control in construction, *J Occup Environ Hyg.*, **4**, pp. 943–951.

131. Ko, J. L., Cheng, Y. J., Liu, G. C., Hsin, I. L. and Chen, H. L. (2017). The association of occupational metals exposure and oxidative damage, telomere shortening in fitness equipment manufacturing workers, *Ind Health.*, **55**, pp. 345–353.

132. Shoeb, M., Mustafa, G. M., Kodali, V. K., Smith, K., Roach, K. A., Boyce, G., *et al.* (2020). A possible relationship between telomere length and markers of neurodegeneration in rat brain after welding fume inhalation exposure, *Environ. Res.*, **180**, pp. 108900.

133. Shoeb, M., Kodali, V. K., Farris, B. Y., Bishop, L. M., Meighan, T. G., Salmen, R., *et al.* (2017). Oxidative stress, DNA methylation, and telomere length changes in peripheral blood mononuclear cells after pulmonary exposure to metal-rich welding nanoparticles, *NanoImpact.*, **5**, pp. 61–69.

134. Bai, Y., Fu, W., Guan, X., Wu, X., Li, G., Wei, W., *et al.* (2020). Co-exposure to multiple metals, TERT-CLPTM1L variants, and their joint influence on leukocyte telomere length, *Environ Int.*, **140**, pp. 105762.

135. Lai, X., Yuan, Y., Liu, M., Xiao, Y., Ma, L., Guo, W., *et al.* (2022). Individual and joint associations of co-exposure to multiple plasma metals with telomere length among middle-aged and older Chinese in the Dongfeng-Tongji cohort, *Environ. Res.*, **214**, pp. 114031.

136. Li, Z., Liu, H., Qian, Y., Li, X., Guo, C., Wang, Z., *et al.* (2020). Influence of metals from e-waste dismantling on telomere length and mitochondrial DNA copy number in people living near recycling sites, *Environ Int.*, **140**, pp. 105769.

137. Yu, L., Dai, Y., Yuan, Z. and Li, J. (2007). Effects of rare earth elements on telomerase activity and apoptosis of human peripheral blood mononuclear cells, *Biol. Trace Elem. Res.*, **116**, pp. 53–59.

138. Cowell, W., Colicino, E., Tanner, E., Amarasiriwardena, C., Andra, S. S., Bollati, V., *et al.* (2020). Prenatal toxic metal mixture exposure and newborn telomere length: modification by maternal antioxidant intake, *Environ. Res.*, **190**, pp. 110009.

139. Tang, P., He, W., Shao, Y., Liu, B., Huang, H., Liang, J., *et al.* (2022). Associations between prenatal multiple plasma metal exposure and newborn telomere length: effect modification by maternal age and infant sex, *Environ. Pollut.*, **315**, pp. 120451.

140. Smith, A. R., Lin, P. D., Rifas-Shiman, S. L., Rahman, M. L., Gold, D. R., Baccarelli, A. A., *et al.* (2021). Prospective associations of early pregnancy metal mixtures with mitochondria DNA copy number and telomere length in maternal and cord blood, *Environ Health Perspect.*, **129**, pp. 117007.

141. Lin, J. and Epel, E. (2022). Stress and telomere shortening: insights from cellular mechanisms, *Ageing Res Rev.*, **73**, pp. 101507.

Part IV

Diseases

Chapter 11

Telomere's Association with Diseases

Eleni Ntoumou
School of Medicine, University of Thessaly,
Viopolis, Larissa, Greece
eleni.ntoumou@idna.gr

11.1 Introduction

Telomeres, situated at the chromosomal ends, consist of noncoding repeats featuring the TTAGGG nucleotide sequence—a crucial element of genomic stability [1, 2]. As cells divide, these structures gradually shorten, triggering senescence and apoptosis upon reaching a critical length [2–4]. Disorders linked to genetic mutations that disrupt telomere homeostasis manifest as conditions associated with premature aging conditions. This spectrum includes bone marrow failure, pulmonary fibrosis, liver cirrhosis, and an increased susceptibility to cancer [5–9]. Collectively, these conditions are described by the term telomere biology disorders (TBD) [4].

Telomeres: Biomarkers of a Healthy Life and Successful Aging
Edited by Aristidis Tsatsakis

ISBN 978-981-5129-49-6 (Hardcover), 978-1-003-56809-4 (eBook)
www.jennystanford.com

11.2 Pathophysiology

Telomeres are crucial for maintaining the stability of chromosomes and protecting them from degradation during mitosis or inappropriate fusion with neighboring chromosomes [2, 4]. They specifically address the "end-replication" issue, which involves countering DNA loss and the gradual shortening of chromosomes with each cell division [3].

Linear DNA and damaged chromosomes are inherently unstable and have a propensity to fuse [10]. The result of significant telomere shortening, or broken chromosomes is abnormal recombination leading to end-to-end fusions and the initiation of "breakage-fusion-bridge" cycles collectively known as "crisis" [2, 4, 10]. The crisis is characterized by replicative senescence, chromosome end-to-end fusions, and extensive apoptosis. This process ultimately gives rise to abnormal derivative chromosomes contributing to genomic instability [10].

The structure of telomeres can trigger DNA damage responses as their ends are identified as double-stranded DNA breaks. Multiple mechanisms are in place to preserve the integrity of telomeres. The stabilizing configuration of telomeres is characterized by the "D-loop-T-loop" structure.

The T-loop is created by inserting the single-stranded G-strand terminus into the double-stranded telomere sequence. This process displaces the sequence strand of the duplex telomeric DNA and results in the formation of the D-loop at the insertion point [11]. Shelterin, a protein complex, shields telomeres by constructing and fortifying the "T-loop" structure. Furthermore, it facilitates and governs the elongation of telomeres [4, 12].

Telomeres consist of six subunits: telomere repeat-binding factors 1 and 2 (TRF1 and TRF2), repressor/activator protein 1 (RAP1), TRF1-interacting nuclear protein 2 (TIN2), TIN2-interacting protein 1 (TPP1), and protection of telomeres 1 (POT1). These subunits localize telomeric sequences and form complexes to distinguish telomeres from DNA damage sites. Telomerase, a ribonucleoprotein complex comprising telomerase reverse transcriptase (TERT) and an RNA component (TERC), maintains telomere length [1, 4, 12, 13]. Dyskerin stabilizes the telomerase complex, while RTEL1 regulates

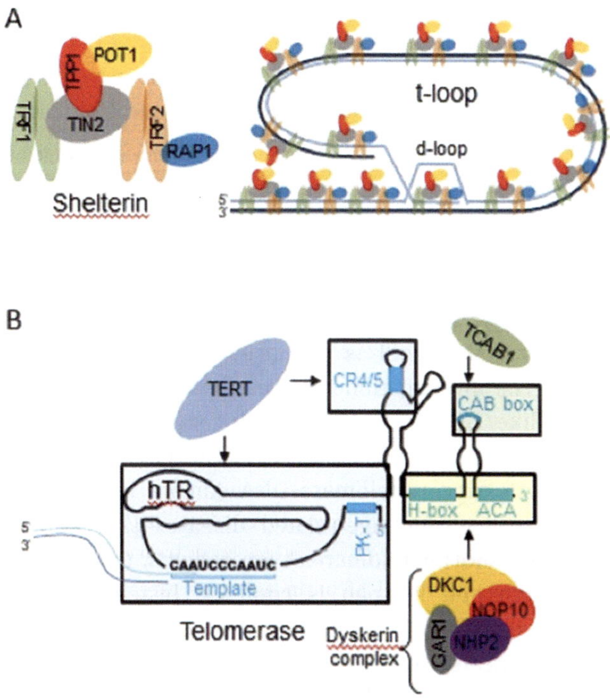

Figure 11.1 Telomerase and shelterin bind to telomeres. (A) Diagram showing the interaction between the six-subunit shelterin complex and telomeric DNA. (B) An illustration of the telomerase RNA component (hTR, indicated by the black line) and the several binding partners that comprise the telomerase complex [100].

telomere length during replication, and CST prevents telomeric DNA damage signaling by limiting telomerase action (Fig. 11.1) [4, 14–18]. Dysregulation of these components can lead to telomere biology disorders (TBD).

The Hayflick limit dictates a finite number of cell replications with telomere shortening triggering senescence and apoptosis [2, 3]. Leukocyte telomere length (LTL) at birth is approximately 10 kb with an attrition rate of 27–41 base pairs per year [19, 20]. Genetics play a crucial role in longer telomeres in individuals of African ancestry and accelerated LTL attrition in Down's syndrome [21]. Variable gene expression across cell lines leads to intra-individual telomere length variation. Extrinsic factors, such as obesity, smoking, and environmental exposures influence telomere dynamics contributing to accelerated cellular aging [21–24]. Short telomeres are implicated in aging-related degenerative defects and carcinogenesis, though precise mechanisms are not completely understood.

11.3 Telomeres in Aging

Replicative cellular senescence resulting from telomere shortening below a critical threshold is primarily explored in mouse and fish species. The investigation involves the deletion of telomerase components like TERC or TERT through genetic manipulation and successive inbreeding. In these models, the gradual reduction in telomere length triggers telomere DNA damage response (tDDR), cellular senescence, and age-related diseases [25, 26]. Despite humans having shorter telomeres than rodents, the link between telomere length and lifespan is complex. Instead, the pace of telomere shortening and the accumulation of short telomeres are suggested as indicators of lifespan [27].

Remarkably, even a small number of critically short telomeres can activate tDDR leading to cellular senescence in vivo [28]. This emphasizes the crucial role of individual telomeric DNA damage response events in determining cell fate and overall aging in organisms. Certainly, during aging, there is a noticeable elevation in the levels of DDR markers (DNA damage response) and TAFs (telomere-associated foci) across various mammalian tissues. Even mice, which possess elongated telomeres and exhibit elevated telomerase expression, show an age-dependent increase in dysfunctional telomeres. This phenomenon is observed in proliferating and non-proliferating tissues [29–33].

In skin melanocytes and CD8+ T cells, TAFs show an increase with age even when there is no concurrent telomere shortening. A recent investigation of telomere length in different tissues involving 952 individuals found that, across 24 tissues analyzed, 21 exhibited age-related telomeres shortening [21].

The detrimental effects of telomere shortening, a characteristic feature of aging, can be counteracted by the reverse-transcriptase activity of telomerase [34]. While most mammalian somatic cells lack telomerase expression leading to the gradual shortening of telomere sequences from chromosome ends over time, there are instances where telomere attrition limits the replicative lifespan of malignant cells, thereby attenuating carcinogenesis. In contrast to genomic instability, which promotes oncogenesis, telomere attrition is viewed as a distinctive hallmark of aging separately from genomic instability [35].

In humans, telomerase deficiency is associated with the premature onset of diseases, such as aplastic anemia, pulmonary fibrosis, and dyskeratosis congenita impairing the regenerative capacity of affected tissues [36]. Telomere attrition (shortening) is a natural occurrence during normal aging in various species influenced by factors, such as age, genetic variations, lifestyle, and social factors [27]. The rate of telomeric attrition depends on the proliferative activity of cells and it serves as a predictor of lifespan across different species. Deficiencies in shelterins, a group of proteins that regulate telomere length and inhibit the DNA damage at chromosome ends, can result in telomere uncapping. Loss-of-function models for the shelterin complex suggest a decrease in the regenerative capacity of tissues and an acceleration of the aging process, even when telomeres maintain their normal length.

Genetically modified animal models have provided insights into causal relationships between telomere attrition, cellular senescence, and organismal aging. Mice with shortened telomeres exhibit decreased lifespan, while those with lengthened telomeres show increased lifespan [37]. Remarkably, the premature aging phenotype of telomerase-deficient mice can be reversed when telomerase is reactivated [38]. Additionally, normal aging in mice can be delayed through pharmacological activation or employing systemic viral transduction of telomerase [39]. Mice with hyper-long telomeres demonstrate increased lifespan and improved metabolic health [40]. Modulating aging through telomerase activation has been shown in various contexts including maintaining physiological levels of telomerase in adult neurons to preserve cell survival and cognitive function in Alzheimer's disease models [41].

The leading hypothesis suggests that the process of aging and the development of age-related diseases are not primarily driven by telomere dysfunction alone. Instead, it is proposed that it is the activation of telomere dysfunction-induced tDDR (telomere DNA damage response) that triggers cellular senescence. This senescence, facilitated by SASP (senescence-associated secretory phenotype), contributes to the age-related decline in tissue functions [42]. It is important to note that senescence can occur independently of telomere dysfunction as observed during development. However, understanding the distinct roles of telomere-dependent and telomere-independent cellular senescence in the mechanisms of aging and age-related disorders is an area that still requires further investigation [43].

11.4 Human Telomere Diseases

11.4.1 Aplastic Anemia

Shortened telomeres have been observed in various human diseases, including aplastic anemia, initially attributed to "regenerative stress" or prolonged exposure to free oxygen radicals [44, 45]. The discovery of mutations in the DKC1 gene in individuals with dyskeratosis congenita, a constitutional marrow failure syndrome, provided a mechanism for these observations [14, 15]. Subsequent findings revealed mutations in the TERC [46] and other genes of the telomerase complex, such as NOP10 [47], NHP2 [48], and TINF2 [49] as well as mutations in the shelterin protein-encoding gene TINF250. DKC1 mutations typically result in early disease presentation in childhood characterized by mucocutaneous signs in severe cases and neurologic abnormalities in Hoyeraal-Hreidarsson syndrome [50]. On the other hand, TERT mutations were initially identified in adults with acquired aplastic anemia, often lacking distinctive physical features or a significant family history [6]. Approximately 10% of patients diagnosed with "idiopathic" aplastic anemia are found to have mutations in TERT or TERC.

All these mutations lead to markedly shortened telomeres allowing telomere length to serve as a screening test. The DKC1 gene is located on the X chromosome. The DKC1 gene encodes a protein called dyskerin, which is a component of the telomerase complex. The DKC1 gene mutation causes telomerase deficiency. While TERT and TERC mutations act dominantly, resulting in a dysfunctional telomere repair complex. NHP2 and NOP10 mutations follow a recessive pattern. TINF2 mutations lead to severe telomere shortening despite normal telomerase activity.

In some families with dyskeratosis congenita, there is anticipation of earlier and more severe symptoms in successive generations. While short telomeres can be inherited without apparent clinical effects in the presence of normal telomerase, most telomerase gene mutations exhibit variable penetrance [51] with family members showing a spectrum from overt disease to subtle laboratory or clinical manifestations. Some pedigrees may exhibit normal blood counts well into middle life despite underlying bone marrow abnormalities [52].

11.4.2 Telomeres and Respiratory Disorders

Idiopathic pulmonary fibrosis (IPF) represents the most prevalent manifestation among various types of interstitial lung diseases [53, 54]. It is characterized by progressive lung fibrosis leading to a deteriorating condition and a median survival of around three years [55]. The prevalence of IPF in Europe ranges from 1.25 to 23.4 cases per 100,000 individuals [56]. Typically affecting male smokers aged over 60, IPF is often identified by a usual interstitial pneumonia (UIP) pattern on chest high-resolution computed tomography (HRCT) or lung biopsy within the appropriate clinical context [55].

In at least 30% of patients with either sporadic or familial pulmonary fibrosis, genetic factors are implicated in elevating the risk of the condition [56, 58]. TERT and TERC mutations account for 8–15% of familial cases and 1–3% of sporadic cases of IPF [53, 57–62]. Other mutations related to telomeres, such as NAF1, PARN, RTEL1, DKC1, and TINF2, also play a role in the development of the condition.

Idiopathic pulmonary fibrosis (IPF) in familial cases typically presents at an earlier age and follows a more aggressive disease trajectory than its sporadic counterparts. This is accompanied by variations in both radiological and histological characteristics. Familial IPF tends to present earlier and exhibit a more aggressive disease course compared to sporadic cases displaying radiological and histological heterogeneity [54, 63]. Other interstitial lung diseases including non-specific interstitial pneumonia (NSIP), cryptogenic organizing pneumonia (COP), respiratory bronchiolitis-interstitial lung disease (RB-ILD), unclassifiable ILD, and combined pulmonary fibrosis and emphysema (CPFE), have also been observed in familial IPF [54, 59, 60, 63].

In both sporadic and familial IPF cases without telomere-related mutations, telomere length (TL) falls below the 10th percentile of age-matched controls [54]. Similarly, other sporadic forms of interstitial lung diseases have been associated with shorter telomeres and telomere-related mutations [64]. TL below the 10th percentile correlates with unfavorable outcomes in IPF patients undergoing immunosuppression leading to faster lung function deterioration, higher mortality rates, and poorer lung transplantation outcomes across various interstitial lung disease subtypes [54, 64, 65].

11.4.3 Telomeres and Hepatobiliary Conditions

Liver involvement occurs in up to 40% of patients with a TBD [9, 68] encompassing various manifestations, such as elevated liver enzyme levels (transaminitis), non-alcoholic steatohepatitis, nodular regenerative hyperplasia, cryptogenic liver cirrhosis, noncirrhotic portal hypertension, and hepatopulmonary syndrome (HPS). Biopsy results often reveal inflammatory and fibrotic components, hepatic nodular regeneration, cirrhosis, and idiopathic hemosiderosis [9, 66, 67].

HPS, a complication in TBD typically emerges in the first four decades of life occurring earlier than pulmonary fibrosis. Therefore, in younger TBD patients presenting with breathlessness, it is essential to consider evaluating for HPS, especially in the absence of pulmonary fibrosis. In non-alcoholic steatohepatitis, individuals with shorter telomeres are thought to be more susceptible to a second hit [67].

Beyond hereditary telomere-related mutations, chronic cellular injury, and exposure to hepatotoxic substances like drugs and alcohol can hasten telomere shortening contributing to the progression of liver fibrosis. Likewise, shorter telomeres and mutations in TERC and TERT promoters are associated with the development of various hepatobiliary tumors including hepatocellular carcinoma [66, 68].

11.4.4 Telomeres and Kidney Disorders

The aging process leads to adverse changes in the structure and function of kidneys. Several renal conditions, such as acute kidney injury, glomerulonephritis, diabetic nephropathy, polycystic kidney disease, and chronic kidney disease (CKD), are associated with cellular senescence and dysfunction in telomeres [69].

Chronic kidney disease, which is a debilitating and life-shortening disease whose prevalence is increasing globally, is a long-term condition that is characterized by a gradual loss of kidney function. Usually, other conditions that put a strain on the kidneys are responsible for the development of chronic kidney disease. In addition, it can often be the result of a combination of problems including hypertension, diabetes, elevated levels of cholesterol, and kidney infections, among many others [70–72].

Clinicians use a scale to define the severity of chronic kidney disease. This relies on the estimation of glomerular filtration rate and albuminuria [73–76]. According to this method, stage 1 chronic kidney disease patients demonstrate normal to high glomerular filtration rate, while stage 4 is associated with severely decreased glomerular filtration rate, and stage 5 corresponds to kidney [73].

Chronic kidney disease has also been defined as an independent risk factor for cardiovascular disease, cognitive dysfunction, hospitalization, and all-cause mortality. Interestingly, the risk of developing cardiovascular disease and all-cause mortality has been reported higher than the risk for progression to end-stage renal disease in older patients [77–79]. At the other end of the spectrum, when chronic kidney disease occurs at a much younger age and progresses to end-stage renal disease, the risk of cardiovascular mortality increases exponentially [77, 80]. Hence, this suggested that chronic kidney disease could be a clinical model of premature aging [81, 82].

Premature aging is a common feature of chronic kidney disease and other chronic diseases such as heart failure, chronic obstructive pulmonary disease, HIV infection, and rheumatoid arthritis [81, 83].

Progressive accumulation of deleterious changes over time, impairment of physiologic functions, and increased risk of disease and mortality are tightly associated with premature aging [82]. Indeed, clinical, and pathophysiological evidence suggest that premature aging is involved in the pathogenesis of systemic complications of many chronic organ diseases, which result in analogous phenotypes including premature vascular aging, osteoporosis, and muscle wasting [84]. Hence, improving the understanding of fundamental aging processes may be important in comprehending the complications associated with organ diseases such as chronic kidney disease.

Chronic kidney disease is responsible for promoting cellular senescence, and thus a premature aging phenotype, through toxic alterations in the internal milieu. Several mechanisms are accountable for these changes including DNA and mitochondria damage, increased reactive oxygen species generation, persistent inflammation, stem cell exhaustion, decreased klotho expression, telomere attrition, and altered nutrient sensing [82, 85].

11.4.5 Telomeres and Cancer

The development and progression of cancer are associated with biological processes, in which cells accumulate genomic instability, ultimately gaining the ability for indefinite replication—a hallmark of immortality [86]. Telomerase, the enzyme associated with immortality in cancer, is found in embryonic tissues and stays functional in germ cells. Nevertheless, it presents reduced expression in most body tissues to regulate cellular proliferation and prevent the initiation of carcinogenesis [87].

Telomerase reverse transcriptase (TERT), as the pivotal factor determining human telomerase activity, plays a crucial role in cancer initiation and progression [88].

Two crucial complexes, CST and shelterin, are involved in the regulation and maintenance of telomere length [89]. Genetic mutations in the genes governing these complexes can contribute to the pathogenesis of different types of cancer. Therefore, a comprehensive understanding of the molecular mechanisms that are involved in these proteins is indispensable, offering essential insights for devising therapeutic strategies to address such diseases.

When short telomeres were initially observed in colorectal cancer, it was hypothesized that telomere loss could contribute to the development of tumors and genetic instability [90]. In inflammatory bowel disease, a deficiency of telomerase has been identified in the histologically normal mucosa. In ulcerative colitis patients without dysplasia, chromosome losses were associated with telomere shortening, particularly in those progressing to cancer marked by the presence of anaphase bridges [91].

Chronic inflammation in Barrett's esophagus, resulting from prolonged exposure to gastroesophageal reflux, is a significant risk factor for esophageal cancer. The length of leukocyte telomeres at the initial presentation is inversely proportional to the later risk of esophageal cancer suggesting a potential genetic predisposition to repair with persistent oxidative stress [92]. Short leukocyte telomeres have been implicated as a risk factor or prognostic biomarker in various solid tumors. Accelerated telomere shortening is observed in recipients of human stem cell transplants with chronic graft-versus-host disease [93].

Hematologic malignancies offer advantages for telomere studies as telomere length can be easily measured in the cancer's cell of origin, and telomerase is typically active in hematopoietic stem cells. In dyskeratosis congenita, there is a significantly elevated risk of various tumors especially head and neck squamous cell carcinomas, skin, and anorectal cancers, and acute myeloid leukemia [90]. In acquired aplastic anemia, leukocyte telomere length is a major predictor of malignant clonal evolution with a substantial proportion of patients with short telomeres developing myelodysplastic syndrome and acute myeloid leukemia.

TERT hypomorphic variants are detected in around 8% of acute myeloid leukemia cases often linked to cytogenetic abnormalities resulting in decreased telomerase activity [66]. Telomerase mutations are found to be responsible for familial acute leukemia [94]. The presence of short telomeres is associated with the transformation to leukemia in myelodysplasia [95, 96], the development of secondary myelodysplasia and leukemia after chemotherapy and autologous hematopoietic cell transplantation [97, 98], and critically short telomeres in blast cells are correlated with chromosomal gains and losses [99].

11.5 Conclusions

Current research indicates that a multitude of factors, both genetic and non-genetic, may influence telomere length, and the complex interactions among these factors are not yet fully elucidated. While ongoing investigations are uncovering genetic mutations linked to telomere length maintenance, it is evident that additional studies are necessary. A significant challenge lies in deciphering how a combination of diverse factors—clinical, genetic, and disease-specific—along with telomere length, could contribute to identifying specific disease groups with distinct clinical behaviors, treatment responses, progression risk, and outcomes.

In conclusion, unraveling the intricate mechanisms of aging and cancer remains a formidable challenge. Nevertheless, insights into telomeres and telomerase activity motivated researchers to explore potential drugs targeting these mechanisms. The concept that inhibiting telomerase could serve as a promising therapeutic approach presents challenges, as several factors are under investigation.

References

1. Greider, C. W. & Blackburn, E. H. (1985). Identification of a specific telomere terminal transferase activity in tetrahymena extracts, *Cell*, **43**, pp. 405–413.
2. Greider, C. W. & Blackburn, E. H. A. (1989). Telomeric sequence in the RNA of Tetrahymena telomerase required for telomere repeat synthesis, *Nature*, **337**, pp. 331–337.
3. Levy, M. Z., Allsopp, R. C., Futcher, A. B., Greider, C. W. & Harley, C. B. (1992). Telomere end-replication problem and cell aging, *J. Mol. Biol.*, **225**, pp. 951–960.
4. Bertuch, A. A. (2016). The molecular genetics of telomere biology disorders, *RNA Biol.*, **13**, pp. 696–706.
5. Armanios, M. Y., Chen, J. J-L., Cogan, J. D., Alder, J. K., Ingersoll, R. G., Markin, C., *et al.* (2007). Telomerase mutations in families with idiopathic pulmonary fibrosis, *N. Engl. J. Med.*, **356**, pp. 1317–1326.
6. Yamaguchi, H., Calado, R.T., Ly, H., Kajigaya, S., Baerlocher, G. M., Chanock, S. G., *et al.* (2005). Mutations in TERT, the gene for telomerase

reverse transcriptase, in aplastic anemia, *N. Engl. J. Med.*, **352**, pp. 1413–1424.

7. Niewisch, M. R. & Savage, S. A. (2019). An update on the biology and management of dyskeratosis congenita and related telomere biology disorders, *Expert Rev. Hematol.*, **12**, pp. 1037–1052.
8. Schratz, K. E., Haley, L., Danoff, S. K., Blackford, A. L., DeZern, A. E., Gocke, C. D., *et al.* (2020). Cancer spectrum and outcomes in the Mendelian short telomere syndromes, *Blood*, **135**, pp. 1946–1956.
9. Feurstein, S., Adegunsoye, A., Mojsilovic, D., Vij, R., DePersia. A. H. W., Rajagopal, P. S., *et al.* (2020). Telomere biology disorder prevalence and phenotypes in adults with familial hematologic and/or pulmonary presentations, *Blood Adv.*, **13**, pp. 4873–4886.
10. McClintock, B. (1941). The Stability of Broken Ends of Chromosomes in Zea Mays. *Genetics*, **26**, pp. 234–282.
11. Griffith, J. D., Comeau, L., Rosenfield, S., Stansel, R. M., Bianchi, A., Moss, H., *et al.* (1999). Mammalian telomeres end in a large duplex loop, *Cell*, **97**, pp. 503–514.
12. De Lange, T. (2005). Shelterin: The protein complex that shapes and safeguards human telomeres, *Genes Dev.*, **19**, pp. 2100–2110.
13. Lemon, L. D., Morris, D. K. & Bertuch, A. A. (2019). Loss of Ku's DNA end binding activity affects telomere length via destabilizing telomere-bound Est1 rather than altering TLC1 homeostasis, *Sci. Rep.*, **9**, Article number: 10607.
14. Heiss, N. S., Knight, S. W., Vulliamy, T. J., Klauck, S. M., Wiemann, S., Mason, P. J., *et al.* (1998). X-linked dyskeratosis congenita is caused by mutations in a highly conserved gene with putative nucleolar functions, *Nat. Genet.*, **19**, pp. 32–38.
15. Mitchell, J. R., Wood, E. & Collins, K. (1999). A telomerase component is defective in the human disease dyskeratosis congenita, *Nature*, **402**, pp. 551–555.
16. Vannier, J. B., Pavicic-Kaltenbrunner, V., Petalcorin, M. I. R., Ding, H. & Boulton, S. J. (2012). RTEL1 dismantles T loops and counteracts telomeric G4-DNA to maintain telomere integrity, *Cell*, **149**, pp. 795–806.
17. Feng, X., Hsu, S. J., Bhattacharjee, A., Wang, Y., Diao, J., Price, C. M. (2018). CTC1-STN1 terminates telomerase while STN1-TEN1 enables C-strand synthesis during telomere replication in colon cancer cells, *Nat. Commun.*, **9**, Article number: 2827.

18. Keller, R. B., Gagne, K. E., Naheed Usmani, G., Asdourian, G. K., Williams, D. A., Hofmann, I., *et al.* (2012). CTC1 Mutations in a patient with dyskeratosis congenita, *Pediatr. Blood Cancer*, **59**, pp. 311–314.
19. Lubas, M., Christensen, M. S., Kristiansen, M. S., Domanski, M., Falkenby, L. G., Lykke-Andersen, S., *et al.* (2011). Interaction profiling identifies the human nuclear exosome targeting complex, *Mol. Cell.*, **43**, pp. 624–637.
20. Risom, L., Møller, P. & Loft, S. (2005). Oxidative stress-induced DNA damage by particulate air pollution, *Mutat. Res.*, **592**, pp. 119–137.
21. Demanelis, K., Jasmine, F., Chen, L. S., Chernoff, M., Tong, L., Delgado, D., *et al.* (2020). Determinants of telomere length across human tissues, *Science*, **369**, open access.
22. Vulliamy, T., Marrone, A., Szydlo, R., Walne, A., Mason, P. J., Dokal, I. (2004). Disease anticipation is associated with progressive telomere shortening in families with dyskeratosis congenita due to mutations in TERC, *Nat. Genet.*, **36**, pp. 447–449.
23. Slagboom, P. E., Droog, S. & Boomsma, D. I. (1994). Genetic determination of telomere size in humans: a twin study of three age groups, *Am. J. Hum. Genet.*, **55**, pp. 876.
24. Vaziri, H., Schächter, F., Uchida, I., Wei, L., Zhu, X., Effros, R., *et al.* (1993). Loss of telomeric DNA during aging of normal and trisomy 21 human lymphocytes, *Am. J. Hum. Genet.*, **52**, pp. 661–7.
25. Henriques, C. M., Carneiro, M. C., Tenente, I. M., Jacinto, A. & Ferreira, M. G. (2013). Telomerase is required for zebrafish lifespan, *PLoS Genet.*, **9**, pp. e1003214.
26. Blasco, M. A., Lee, H. W., Hande, M. P., Samper, E., Lansdorp, P. M., DePinho, R. A., *et al.* (1997). Telomere shortening and tumor formation by mouse cells lacking telomerase RNA, *Cell*, **91**, pp. 25–34.
27. Whittemore, K., Vera, E., Martínez-Nevado, E., Sanpera, C. & Blasco, M. A. (2019). Telomere shortening rate predicts species life span, *Proc. Natl. Acad. Sci. U. S. A.*, **116**, pp. 15122–15127.
28. Hemann, M. T., Strong, M. A., Hao, L. Y. & Greider, C. W. (2001). The shortest telomere, not average telomere length, is critical for cell viability and chromosome stability, *Cell*, **107**, pp. 67–77.
29. Hewitt, G., Jurk, D., Marques, F. D. M., Correia-Melo, C., Hardy, T., Gackowska, A., *et al.* (2012). Telomeres are favoured targets of a persistent DNA damage response in ageing and stress-induced senescence, *Nat. Commun.*, **3**, pp. 708.

30. Birch, J., Anderson, R. K., Correia-Melo, C., Jurk, D., Hewitt, G., Marques, F. D., *et al.* (2015). DNA damage response at telomeres contributes to lung aging and chronic obstructive pulmonary disease, *Am. J. Physiol. Lung Cell. Mol. Physiol.*, **309**, pp. L1124–L1137.
31. Farr, J. N., Fraser, D. G., Wang, H., Jaehn, K, Ogrodnik, M. B., Weivoda, M. M., *et al.* (2016). Identification of senescent cells in the bone microenvironment, *J. Bone Miner. Res.*, **31**, pp. 1920–1929.
32. Anderson, R., Lagnado, A., Maggiorani, D., Walaszczyk A., Dookun, E., Chapman, J., *et al.* (2019). Length-independent telomere damage drives post-mitotic cardiomyocyte senescence, *EMBO J.*, **38**, pp. e100492.
33. Ogrodnik, M., Zhu, Y., Langhi, L. G. P., Tchkonia, T., Krüger, P., Fielder, E., *et al.* (2019). Obesity-induced cellular senescence drives anxiety and impairs neurogenesis, *Cell Metab.*, **29**, pp. 1061–1077.
34. Chakravarti, D., LaBella, K. A. & DePinho, R. A. (2021). Telomeres: history, health, and hallmarks of aging, *Cell*, **184**, pp. 306–322.
35. López-Otín, C., Pietrocola, F., Roiz-Valle, D., Galluzzi, L. & Kroemer, G. (2023). Meta-hallmarks of aging and cancer, *Cell Metab.*, **35**, pp. 12–35.
36. Alder, J. K. & Armanios, M. (2022). Telomere-Mediated Lung Disease, *Physiol. Rev.*, **102**, pp. 1703–1720.
37. Tomás-Loba, A., Flores, I., Fernández-Marcos, P. J., Cayuela, M. L., Maraver, A., Tejera, A., *et al.* (2008). Telomerase reverse transcriptase delays aging in cancer-resistant mice, *Cell*, **135**, pp. 609–622.
38. Jaskelioff, M., Muller, F. L., Paik, J-H., Thomas, E., Jiang, S., Adams, A. C., Sahin, E., *et al.* (2011). Telomerase reactivation reverses tissue degeneration in aged telomerase-deficient mice, *Nature*, **469**, pp. 102–106.
39. Bernardes de Jesus, B., Vera, E., Schneeberger, K., Tejera, A. M., Ayuso, E., Bosch, F., *et al.* (2012). Telomerase gene therapy in adult and old mice delays aging and increases longevity without increasing cancer, *EMBO Mol. Med.*, **4**, pp. 691–704.
40. Muñoz-Lorente, M. A., Cano-Martin, A. C. & Blasco, M. A. (2019). Mice with hyper-long telomeres show less metabolic aging and longer lifespans, *Nat. Commun.*, **10**, pp. 4723.
41. Shim, H. S., Horner, J. W., Wu, C-J., Li, J., Lan, Z. D., Jiang, S., *et al.* (2021). Telomerase reverse transcriptase preserves neuron survival and cognition in Alzheimer's disease models, *Nat Aging*, **1**, pp. 1162–1174.

42. Gorgoulis, V., Adams, P. D., Alimonti, A., Bennett, D. C., Bischof, O., Bishop, C., *et al.* (2019). Cellular senescence: defining a path forward, *Cell*, **179**, pp. 813–827.
43. Di Micco, R., Krizhanovsky, V., Baker, D. & d'Adda di Fagagna, F. (2021). Cellular senescence in ageing: from mechanisms to therapeutic opportunities, *Nat. Rev. Mol. Cell Biol.*, **22**, pp. 75–95.
44. Ball, S. E., Gibson, F. M., Rizzo, S., Tooze, J. A., Marsh, J. C., Gordon-Smith, E. C. (1998). Progressive telomere shortening in aplastic anemia, *Blood*, **91**, pp. 3582–3592.
45. Brümmendorf, T. H., Maciejewski, J. P., Mak, J., Young, N. S. & Lansdorp, P. M. (2001). Telomere length in leukocyte subpopulations of patients with aplastic anemia, *Blood*, **97**, pp. 895–900.
46. Vulliamy, T., Marrone, A., Goldman, F., Dearlove, A., Bessler, M., Mason, P. J., *et al.* (2001). The RNA component of telomerase is mutated in autosomal dominant dyskeratosis congenita, *Nature*, **413**, pp. 432–435.
47. Walne, A. J., Vulliamy, T., Marrone, A., Beswick, R., Kirwan, M., Masunari, Y., *et al.* (2007). Genetic heterogeneity in autosomal recessive dyskeratosis congenita with one subtype due to mutations in the telomerase-associated protein NOP10, *Hum. Mol. Genet.*, **16**, pp. 1619–1629.
48. Vulliamy, T., Beswick, R., Kirwan, M., Marrone, A., Digweed, M., Walne, A., *et al.* (2008). Mutations in the telomerase component NHP2 cause the premature ageing syndrome dyskeratosis congenita, *Proc. Natl Acad. Sci. USA*, **105**, pp. 8073–8078.
49. Savage, S. A., Giri, N., Baerlocher, G. M., Orr, N., Lansdorp, P. M., Alter, B. P. (2008). TINF2, a component of the shelterin telomere protection complex, is mutated in dyskeratosis congenita, *Am. J. Hum. Genet.*, **82**, pp. 501–509.
50. Dokal, I. (2000). Dyskeratosis congenita in all its forms, *Br. J. Haematol.*, **110**, pp. 768–779.
51. Hodes, R. J., Hathcock, K. S., Weng, N-P. (2002). Telomeres in T and B cells, *Nat. New Biol.*, **2**, pp. 699–706.
52. Fogarty, P. F., Yamaguchi, H., Wiestner, A., Baerlocher, G. M., Sloand, E., Zeng, W. S., *et al.* (2003). Late presentation of dyskeratosis congenita as apparently acquired aplastic anaemia due to mutations in telomerase RNA, *Lancet*, **362**, pp. 1628–1630.
53. Armanios, M., Chen, J-L., Chang, Y-P. C., Brodsky, R. A., Hawkins, A., Griffin, C. A., *et al.* (2005). Haploinsufficiency of telomerase

reverse transcriptase leads to anticipation in autosomal dominant dyskeratosis congenita, *Proc. Natl. Acad. Sci. U.S.A.*, **102**, pp. 15960–15964.

54. Cronkhite, J. T., Xing, C., Raghu, G., Chin, K. M., Torres, F., Rosenblatt, R. L., *et al.* (2008). Telomere shortening in familial and sporadic pulmonary fibrosis, *Am. J. Respir. Crit. Care Med.*, **178**, pp. 729–737.
55. Raghu, G., Remy-Jardin, M., Myers, J. L., Richeldi, L., Ryerson, C. J., Lederer, D. J., *et al.* (2018). Diagnosis of idiopathic pulmonary fibrosis. An official ATS/ERS/JRS/ALAT clinical practice guideline, *Am. J. Respir. Crit. Care Med.*, **198**, pp. e44–e68.
56. Nalysnyk, L., Cid-Ruzafa, J., Rotella, P., & Esser, D. (2012). Incidence and prevalence of idiopathic pulmonary fibrosis: review of the literature, *Eur. Respir. Rev.*, **21**, pp. 355–361.
57. Allen, R. J., Porte, J., Braybrooke, R., Flores, C., Fingerlin, T. E., Oldham, J. M., *et al.* (2017). Genetic variants associated with susceptibility to idiopathic pulmonary fibrosis in people of European ancestry: a genome-wide association study, *Lancet Respir. Med.*, **5**, pp. 869–880.
58. Gable, D. L., Gaysinskaya, V., Atik, C. C., Conover Talbot Jr, C., Kang, B., Stanley, S. E., *et al.* (2019). ZCCHC8, the nuclear exosome targeting component, is mutated in familial pulmonary fibrosis and is required for telomerase RNA maturation, *Genes Dev.*, **33**, pp. 1381–1396.
59. Stuart, B. D., Choi, J., Zaidi, S., Xing, C., Holohan, B., Chen, R., *et al.* (2015). Exome sequencing links mutations in PARN and RTEL1 with familial pulmonary fibrosis and telomere shortening, *Nat. Genet.*, **47**, pp. 512–517.
60. Stanley, S. E., Gable, D. L., Wagner, C. L., Carlile, T. M., Hanumanthu, V. S., Podlevsky, J. D., *et al.* (2016). Loss-of-function mutations in the RNA biogenesis factor NAF1 predispose to pulmonary fibrosis-emphysema, *Sci. Transl. Med.*, **8**, pp. 351ra107.
61. Gaysinskaya, V., Stanley, S. E., Adam, S. & Armanios, M. (2020). Synonymous mutation in DKC1 causes telomerase RNA insufficiency manifesting as familial pulmonary fibrosis, *Chest*, **158**, pp. 2449–2457.
62. Alder, J. K., Stanley, S. E., Wagner, C. L., Hamilton, M., Hanumanthu, V. S., Armanios, M. (2015). Exome sequencing identifies mutant TINF2 in a family with pulmonary fibrosis, *Chest*, **147**, pp. 1361–1368.
63. Armanios, M. Y., Chen, J. J-L., Cogan, J. D., Alder, J. K., Ingersoll, R. G., Markin, C., *et al.* (2007). Telomerase mutations in families with idiopathic pulmonary fibrosis, *N. Engl. J. Med.*, **356**, pp. 1317–1326.

64. Newton, C. A., Zhang, D., Oldham, J. M., Kozlitina, J., Ma, S-F., Martinez, F. J., *et al.* (2019). Telomere length and use of immunosuppressive medications in idiopathic pulmonary fibrosis, *Am. J. Respir. Crit. Care Med.*, **200**, pp. 336–347.

65. Newton, C. A., Kozlitina, J., Lines, J. R., Kaza, V., Torres, F., Garcia, C. K. (2017). Telomere length in patients with pulmonary fibrosis associated with chronic lung allograft dysfunction and post–lung transplantation survival, *J. Hear. Lung Transplant.*, **36**, pp. 845–853.

66. Calado, R. T., Regal, J. A., Kleiner, D. E., Schrump, D. S., Peterson, N. R., Pons, V., *et al.* (2009). A spectrum of severe familial liver disorders associated with telomerase mutations, *PLoS One*, **4**, pp. e7926.

67. Gorgy, A. I., Jonassaint, N. L., Stanley, S. E., Koteish, A., DeZern, A. E., Walter, J. E., *et al.* (2015). Hepatopulmonary syndrome is a frequent cause of dyspnea in the short telomere disorders, *Chest*, **148**, pp. 1019–1026.

68. Kapuria, D., Ben-Yakov, G., Ortolano, R., Cho, M. H., Kalchiem-Dekel, O., Takyar, V., *et al.* (2019). The spectrum of hepatic involvement in patients with telomere disease, *Hepatology*, **69**, pp. 2579–2585.

69. Sturmlechner, I., Durik, M., Sieben, C. J., Baker, D. J. & van Deursen, J. M. (2017). Cellular senescence in renal ageing and disease, *Nat. Rev. Nephrol.*, **13**, pp. 77–89.

70. Krop, J. S., Coresh, J., Chambless, L. E., Shahar, E., Watson, R. L., Szklo, M., *et al.* (1999). A community-based study of explanatory factors for the excess risk for early renal function decline in blacks vs. whites with diabetes: the Atherosclerosis risk in communities study, *Arch. Intern. Med.*, **159**, pp. 1777–1783.

71. Levey, A. S., de Jong, P. E., Coresh, J., El Nahas, M., Astor, B. C., Matsushita, K., *et al.* (2011). The definition, classification, and prognosis of chronic kidney disease: a KDIGO controversies conference report, *Kidney Int.*, **80**, pp. 17–28.

72. Larson, M. G., Atwood, L. D., Benjamin, E. J., Cupples, L. A., D'Agostino, R. B., Sr., Fox, C. S., *et al.* (2007). Framingham Heart Study 100K project: genome-wide associations for cardiovascular disease outcomes, *BMC Med. Genet.*, **8**, pp. S5.

73. Drawz, P., & Rahman, M. (2015). Chronic kidney disease, *Ann. Intern. Med.*, **162**, ITC1.

74. Fink, H. A., Ishani, A., Taylor, B. C., Greer, N. L., MacDonald, R., Rossini, D., *et al.* (2012). AHRQ comparative effectiveness reviews. In *chronic*

kidney disease stages 1–3: screening, monitoring, and treatment, agency for healthcare research and quality (US), Report No.: **11**(12)-EHC075-EF.

75. Levey, A. S., Stevens, L. A., Schmid, C. H., Zhang, Y. L., Castro, A. F., III, Feldman, H. I., *et al.* (2009). A new equation to estimate glomerular filtration rate, *Ann Intern Med*, **150**, pp. 604–612.
76. Matsushita, K., Mahmoodi, B. K., Woodward, M., Emberson, J. R., Jafar, T. H., Jee, S. H., *et al.* (2012). Comparison of risk prediction using the CKD-EPI equation and the MDRD study equation for estimated glomerular filtration rate, *Jama*, **307**, pp. 1941–1951.
77. Go, A. S., Chertow, G. M., & Fan, D. (2005). Chronic kidney disease and the risks of death, cardiovascular events, and hospitalization, *Journal of Vascular Surgery*, **41**, pp. 177.
78. Hallan, S. I., Matsushita, K., Sang, Y., Mahmoodi, B. K., Black, C., Ishani, A., *et al.* (2012). Age and association of kidney measures with mortality and end-stage renal disease, *Jama*, **308**, pp. 2349–2360.
79. Rahman, M., Pressel, S., Davis, B. R., Nwachuku, C., Wright, J. T., Jr., Whelton, P. K., *et al.* (2006). Cardiovascular outcomes in high-risk hypertensive patients stratified by baseline glomerular filtration rate, *Ann. Intern. Med.*, **144**, pp. 172–180.
80. Foley, R. N. (2010). Clinical epidemiology of cardiovascular disease in chronic kidney disease, *J Ren Care*, **36**, pp. 4–8.
81. Shiels, P. G., & Ritzau-Reid, K. (2015). Biological ageing, inflammation and nutrition: how might they impact on systemic sclerosis? *Current Aging Science*, **8**, pp. 123–130.
82. Stenvinkel, P., & Larsson, T. E. (2013). Chronic kidney disease: a clinical model of premature aging [review], *American Journal of Kidney Diseases*, **62**, pp. 339–351.
83. Kooman, J. P., Kotanko, P., Schols, A., Shiels, P. G., & Stenvinkel, P. (2014). Chronic kidney disease and premature ageing [Article], *Nature Reviews Nephrology*, **10**, pp. 732–742.
84. Kooman, J. P., Shiels, P. G., & Stenvinkel, P. (2015). Premature aging in chronic kidney disease and chronic obstructive pulmonary disease: similarities and differences, *Curr. Opin. Clin. Nutr. Metab. Care*, **18**, pp. 528–534.
85. Shiels, P. G., McGuinness, D., Eriksson, M., Kooman, J. P., & Stenvinkel, P. (2017). The role of epigenetics in renal ageing, *Nat. Rev. Nephrol.*, **13**, pp. 471–482.

86. Vogelstein, B., Kinzler, K. W. (2015). The path to cancer — three strikes and you're out, *N. Engl. J. Med.*, **373**, pp. 1895–1898.
87. Krupp, G., Bonatz, G., Parwaresch, R. (2000). Telomerase, immortality, and cancer, *Biotechnol. Annu. Rev.*, **6**, pp. 103–140.
88. Yang, R., Han, Y., Guan, X. *et al.* (2023). Regulation and clinical potential of telomerase reverse transcriptase (TERT/hTERT) in breast cancer, *Cell Commun. Signal,* **21**, pp. 218.
89. Lim, C. J., Cech, T. R. (2021). Shaping human telomeres: from shelterin and CST complexes to telomeric chromatin organization, *Nat. Rev. Mol. Cell Biol.*, **22**, pp. 283–298.
90. Alter, B. P., Giri, N., Savage, S. A., Rosenberg, P. S. (2009). Cancer in dyskeratosis congenita, *Blood,* **113**, pp. 6549–6557.
91. O'Sullivan, J. N., Bronner, M. P., Brentnall, T. A., Finley, J. C., Shen, W-T., Emerson S. (2002). Chromosomal instability in ulcerative colitis is related to telomere shortening, *Nat. Genet.*, **32**, pp. 280–284.
92. Risques, R. A., Vaughan, T. L., Li, X., Odze, R. D., Blount, P. L., Ayub, K., *et al.* (2007). Leukocyte telomere length predicts cancer risk in Barrett's esophagus, *Cancer Epidemiol. Biomarkers Prev.*, **16**, pp. 2649–2655.
93. Baerlocher, G. M., Rovó, A., Müller, A., Matthey, S., Stern, M., Halter, J., *et al.* (2009). Cellular senescence of white blood cells in very long-term survivors after allogeneic hematopoietic stem cell transplantation: the role of chronic graft-versus-host disease and female donor sex, *Blood,* **114**, pp. 219–222.
94. Kirwan, M., Vulliamy, T., Marrone, A., Walne, A. J., Beswick, R., Hillmen, P., *et al.* (2009). Defining the pathogenic role of telomerase mutations in myelodysplastic syndrome and acute myeloid leukemia, *Hum. Mutat.*, **30**, pp. 1567–1573.
95. Ohyashiki, J. H., Ohyashiki, K., Fujimura, T., Kawakubo, K., Shimamoto, T., Iwabuchi, A., *et al.* (1994). Telomere shortening associated with disease evolution patterns in myelodysplastic syndromes, *Cancer Res.*, **54**, pp. 3557–3560.
96. Sieglová, Z., Zilovcová, S., Cermák, J., Ríhová, H., Brezinová, D., Dvoráková, R., *et al.* (2004). Dynamics of telomere erosion and its association with genome instability in myelodysplastic syndromes (MDS) and acute myelogenous leukemia arising from MDS: a marker of disease prognosis? *Leuk. Res.*, **28**, pp. 1013–1021.
97. Engelhardt, M., Ozkaynak, M. F., Drullinsky, P., Sandoval, C., Tugal, O., Jayabose, S., *et al.* (1998). Telomerase activity and telomere length

in pediatric patients with malignancies undergoing chemotherapy, *Leukemia*, **12**, pp. 13–24.

98. Chakraborty, S., Sun, C-L., Francisco, L., Sabado, M., Li, L., Chang, K. L., *et al.* (2009). Accelerated telomere shortening precedes development of therapy-related myelodysplasia or acute myelogenous leukemia after autologous transplantation for lymphoma, *J. Clin. Oncol.*, **27**, pp. 791–798.
99. Swiggers, S. J. J., Kuijpers, M. A., de Cort, M. J. M., Beverloo, H. B., Zijlmans, J. M. J. M. (2006). Critically short telomeres in acute myeloid leukemia with loss or gain of parts of chromosomes, *Genes Chromosomes Cancer*, **45**, pp. 247–256.
100. Batista, L. F. Z., Dokal, I., Parker, R. (2022). Telomere biology disorders: time for moving towards the clinic? *Trends Mol. Med.*, **28**, pp. 882–891.

Chapter 12

Telomere Length and Metabolomics in Autoimmune Diseases

Dimitris Tsoukalas,[a,b] Evangelia Sarandi,[b,c] Symeon Xenidis,[b,c] and Aristidis Tsatsakis[c]

[a] *EINUMM, European Institute of Molecular Medicine, Rome, Italy*
[b] *Metabolomic Medicine, Health Clinic for Autoimmune and Chronic Diseases, Athens, 10674, Greece*
[c] *Laboratory of Toxicology and Forensic Sciences, Medical School, University of Crete, Voutes, Heraklion, Greece*
research@metabolomicmedicine.com

12.1 Introduction: Background on Autoimmune Diseases

Autoimmune diseases (ADs) are a broad category of disorders caused by the immune system's loss of self-tolerance. Over 100 ADs are affecting 5–10% of the population. The most common ADs include type 1 diabetes (TD1), Hashimoto's thyroiditis (HT), rheumatoid arthritis (RA), systemic lupus erythematosus (SLE), psoriasis, multiple sclerosis (MS), and inflammatory bowel diseases (IBD) [1].

Telomeres: Biomarkers of a Healthy Life and Successful Aging
Edited by Aristidis Tsatsakis

ISBN 978-981-5129-49-6 (Hardcover), 978-1-003-56809-4 (eBook)
www.jennystanford.com

ADs are characterized by chronic, non-resolving, low-grade inflammation sharing common etiopathogenetic mechanisms that lead to self-tolerance loss [2]. They can be classified as organ-specific and systemic. In organ-specific ADs, autoimmune response targets a single organ, such as in the case of HT. In contrast, in systemic ADs, immunological dysfunction is reported in multiple organs, such as SLE [1].

Levels of comorbidity are very high in patients with ADs, especially in older individuals. Patients with rheumatoid arthritis often have two or more comorbid autoimmune diseases, with SLE and psoriatic arthritis being the most prevalent [3]. Even though different types of ADs and conditions with complex symptomatology and etiopathogenesis are being added, immune response dysregulation and oxidative stress are common hallmarks involving mononuclear phagocytes, autoreactive T cells, and the antibodies-producing plasma cells [4].

Autoimmunity is a multifactorial process where genetic and epigenetic factors contribute to the loss of self-tolerance, the dysregulation of immune response, and the disease's development. Autoreactive T cells are a dominant cell population in ADs through their interaction with antigen-presenting cells (APCs) as the early events of autoimmunity. The recognition of xenobiotics and autoantigens by APCs triggers the activation of innate immune response and, specifically, dendritic cells, macrophages, and natural killer cells. In addition, APCs present immunogenic peptides to T helper cells, activating the adaptive immune system. Activated T helper cells differentiate into various T cell types, such as Th1, Th2, Th17, and Tregs. Th2-cell signaling facilitates the activation of B cells that differentiate into plasma cells and produce tissue-damaging autoantibodies [5]. In many ADs, the loss of immunotolerance is promoted by negative regulation of the innate and adaptive immune response resulting in a decline in Tregs populations [1]. Th1-signaling facilitates the activation of autoreactive cytotoxic T cells, causing tissue damage through the secretion of cytotoxic agents and the Fas-Fas activation. Finally, Th-17 pathways have been associated with several ADs exerting a significant role in their progression.

12.2 Aging in Autoimmune Diseases

Aging is a complex biological process characterized by a gradual decline in the body's physiological functions over time. The relationship between aging and autoimmune diseases is multifaceted, and several factors contribute to the increased prevalence and severity of autoimmune conditions, especially in older individuals.

Aging is associated with changes in the immune system regarding the number and type of immune cells and their autoreactivity. In particular, the effectiveness of the immune response tends to decline reducing the ability to discriminate self from non-self-contributing to the development of autoimmune responses. It has been suggested that loss of self-tolerance may occur due to a mechanism that involves T-cell proliferation in response to lymphopenia. Lymphopenia can occur in normal physiological conditions or be associated with abnormal pathogenic status, such as autoimmune diseases. A possible mechanism includes the contribution of lymphopenia to the production of self-reactive T cells through lymphopenia-induced proliferation promoting autoimmunity. Homeostatic proliferation is responsible for regulating the generation of T cells and maintaining a significant number of naïve T cells. This process remains stable throughout adult life but increases in elderly individuals. Increased homeostatic proliferation is generally associated with healthy aging and is not linked to autoimmune diseases. Conversely, lymphopenia, or a low level of lymphocytes, has been associated with autoimmunity in animal models and human diseases. In patients with autoimmune diseases, lymphopenia may develop at an earlier age, and as a result, homeostatic proliferation increases to restore the number of lymphocytes. Excessive proliferation could lead to the selection of autoreactive T cells and the differentiation into memory-like cells. These cells have an altered phenotype, acquiring the hallmarks of effector cells promoting inflammation through rapid cytokine secretion. Therefore, peripheral tolerance mechanisms could be overcome causing the onset of autoimmune diseases [6].

Another contributor is the decline of the thymus function with age, leading to a decreased output of naïve T cells, potentially affecting immune surveillance and response. A reduced percentage of peripheral naive T cells can also lead to lymphopenia-induced proliferation, promoting autoimmunity. Following lymphopenia-induced proliferation, autoimmunity may occur through recognition of self with above-average affinity, recognition of neoantigens (e.g., produced by citrullination), lower T cell receptor activation thresholds, and hyperresponsiveness to growth factors. The ultimate results are differentiation into memory-like T cells, oligoclonal expansion, and increased autoreactive potential.

12.3 Telomere Shortening and Autoimmunity

Telomeres are protective structures at the ends of chromosomes, and their length decreases with each cell division. When telomeres become critically short after repeated divisions, cells acquire senescence phenotype or undergo apoptosis (programmed cell death) to avoid DNA damage. In cells with increased proliferation demands, such as activated T cells, telomerase elongates telomeres, increasing the replicative threshold of the cell. In patients with autoimmune diseases, telomere shortening may result from extrinsic factors, such as inflammation, mitochondrial dysfunction, and, ultimately, oxidative stress or dysfunctional telomerase activity. Data from different studies demonstrate a possible association between telomerase and inflammation [7, 8] and defective telomerase activities in ADs either increased [9, 10] or decreased [11–13]. Although telomerase may participate in the pathology of autoimmune diseases, it has been suggested as a potent therapeutic strategy. Telomerase overexpression in T cells [14] and small molecule telomerase activators [15] are two possible therapeutic strategies in Ads, and future studies will elucidate their potential clinical benefits. Ultimately, telomere shortening leads to immunosenescence, premature aging of immune cells, and dysfunctional immune responses, contributing to the exacerbation of autoimmune diseases through loss of self-tolerance and increased autoreactive cells (Fig. 12.1) [16]. Previous studies on common autoimmune diseases, such as rheumatoid arthritis, systemic lupus erythematosus, and multiple sclerosis have identified telomere shortening, telomerase dysfunction, and autoimmunity associations [17].

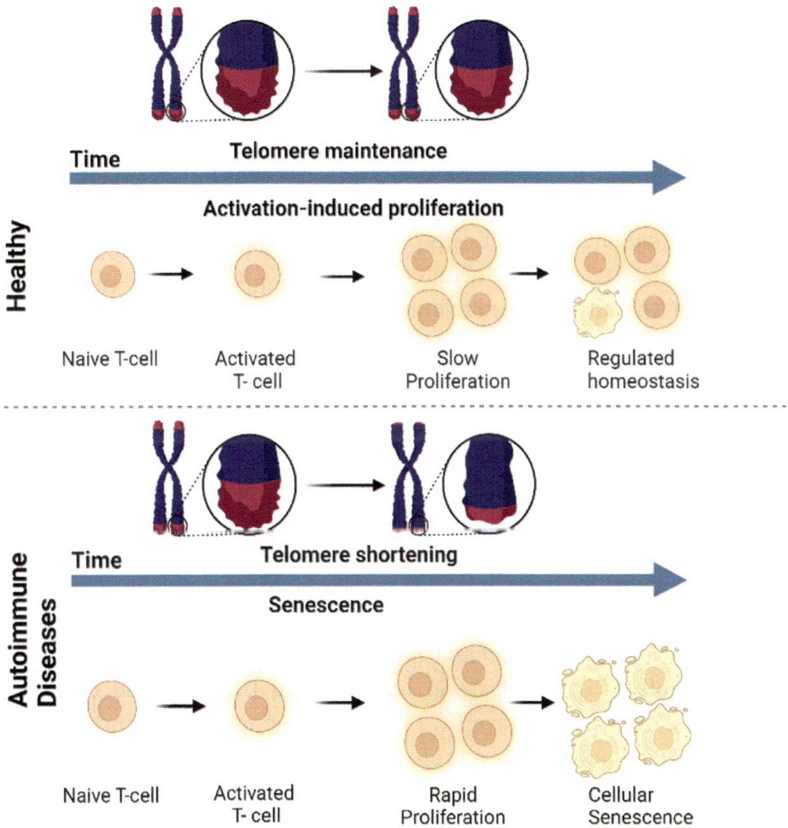

Figure 12.1 Telomere shortening in autoimmune diseases. (Top) Naïve T-cells proliferate upon stimulation by antigen-presenting cells and differentiation. The rate of activation-induced proliferation is a slow and well-regulated process. Telomerase activation facilitates telomere length maintenance and prolonged proliferation. (Bottom) In autoimmune diseases, dysfunctional telomerase and cellular stress (such as mitochondria and inflammatory signaling) lead to rapid cell proliferation and telomere shortening, ultimately leading to cellular senescence.

12.3.1 Rheumatoid Arthritis

Higher levels of telomeric erosion have been found in granulocytes, PBMCs, CD4 T cells, CD8 T cells, and hematopoietic progenitor cells of patients with RA [18–22]. The accelerated telomeric erosion is caused by various mechanisms, such as increased oxidative stress and homeostatic proliferation [10]. Dysfunction of the DNA break repair nuclease MRE11A is another mechanism responsible for telomeric impairment in CD4+ T cells of patients with RA [23]. Telomerase expression and activity have also been studied in patients with RA. However, the findings are contradictory, and the connection between telomerase and RA remains unclear. Fujii et al. showed that naive CD4+ T cells of RA patients have a reduced ability to upregulate telomerase activity [20]. Some studies indicate a link between RA and increased telomerase activity [6].

12.3.2 Intestinal Bowel Disease (IBD)

Short telomeres have been found in colon mucosa and leukocytes of IBD patients. Short telomeres may be involved in the etiology, pathology, and initiation of inflammation in IBDs. Increased telomere decay due to chronic inflammation, higher cell turnover, and adverse effects of lifestyle factors are possible mechanisms leading to abnormal telomere shortening in IBD patients [24]. Shorter telomere length is associated with severe clinical phenotypes in UC patients [25], dysplasia in longstanding UC [26], and tumor progression in progressive UC [27]. However, telomere shortening has not been found to play a role in anticipation of IBDs [28] and to be present in PBMCs of patients with UC and CD [29].

12.3.3 Psoriasis

Telomere dysfunction is suggested to be implicated in psoriasis. This hypothesis is explained by shorter telomeres and increased telomerase activity in patients with psoriasis T cells and PBMC [30, 31]. Telomerase activity in PBMCs has been linked to disease severity [30]. On the contrary, a recent study showed longer telomeres in the blood cells of patients with psoriasis [32].

12.3.4 SLE

The connection between telomeric dysfunction and the pathology of SLE remains controversial. Elevated telomeric erosion has been found in various cell types of patients with SLE [33–36]. However, other studies showed normal length [37, 38]. In this context, the contribution of telomeric attrition in disease activity is unclear since there are contradictory data [33, 35, 39]. Regarding telomerase activity, B cells have displayed higher levels indicating a possible link with disease activity [36, 40]. On the other hand, naïve T cells from patients with SLE had decreased telomerase activity [38]. Different expression patterns of specific telomeric proteins have also been demonstrated in patients with SLE [41].

12.4 Mitochondrial Dysfunction and Telomere Shortening

Mitochondrial dysfunction is one of the hallmarks of aging through its implication in cellular senescence, known as mitochondrial dysfunction-associated senescent response (MiDAS) [42]. Mitochondria are cellular organelles responsible for producing energy and metabolic substrates and for several other functions, from regulation of calcium and iron levels to cell fate and communication with different intra/extracellular compartments. Ingested carbohydrates, amino acids, fats, and their derivatives supply the tricarboxylic acid (TCA) cycle for energy production in the form of ATP in the mitochondria. Among the final steps of this metabolic cataract is oxidative phosphorylation, where NADH and FADH, produced in the TCA cycle, are the electron carriers of the electron chain transport, which ultimately provides protons to produce ATP through ATP synthase [43]. Reactive oxygen species (ROS) are generally produced through this process and removed by the cells' defensive mechanisms to prevent them from exerting their damaging effects on DNA, lipids, and proteins [44]. In senescent cells, accumulation of ROS caused by a leak in the electron transport chain or other endogenous (peroxisomes, endoplasmic reticulum, etc.) or exogenous (pollutants, xenobiotics, etc.) sources has several deleterious effects contributing to the senescent phenotype (SASP) [45]. In turn, mitochondrial dysfunction has been associated with telomere shortening, inflammation, and epigenetic alterations

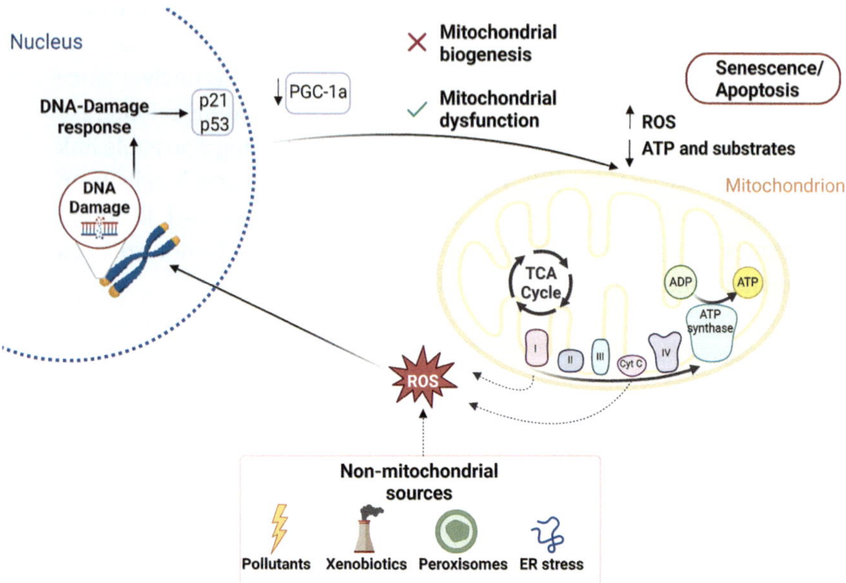

Figure 12.2 The crosstalk between mitochondria and telomeres contributing to cellular senescence.

through complex crosstalk in senescent cells leading to tissue aging and aging-related diseases (Fig. 12.2).

The association between telomere erosion and mitochondria emerged primarily through the observation that patients with genetic-driven mitochondrial diseases have shorter telomeres, but also through interventional studies demonstrating a beneficial effect of anti-oxidant substances on mitochondrial health, such as telomere length. In particular, mitochondrial encephalomyopathy with lactic acidosis and stroke-like episodes (MELAS) syndrome, and Leber hereditary optic neuropathy (LHON) syndrome are characterized by significant ablation of mitochondrial function and patients have significantly shorter telomeres [46]. In addition, several aging-related diseases, including neurodegenerative, cardiovascular, and autoimmune diseases, have been associated with mitochondrial dysfunction and telomere loss in separate studies. Further mechanistic studies would elucidate the contributing mechanisms. A plausible linking mechanism suggests that mitochondria-produced

ROS shuttle, in the nuclei cause telomere attrition and initiate the DNA damage response as early aging events. Damaged telomeres alter mitochondrial function and biosynthesis cascades, through complex molecular pathways, aggravating mitochondria-related aging [47]. The role of telomerase in this crosstalk has been studied in several experimental and human models shedding light on the underlying mechanisms. Briefly, telomerase's primary role is to lengthen telomeres and sustain cell survival. However, in cases of extensive oxidative stress, it has been shown that TERT (one of the protein telomerase subunits) translocates outside the nucleus in the cytoplasm and inside mitochondria, exerting protective and antioxidant effects, thereby, reducing ROS production and apoptosis [48].

Overall, the mitochondrial-telomere axis seems to present an aggravating cycle for aging, and several biomarkers have emerged [49]. Telomeres serve as biomarkers of accumulative damage, while mitochondria present an opportunity to analyze the ability to respond to stress and cells' functional capacity.

12.5 Metabolomics for the Analysis of Mitochondrial Function

Mitochondria are sensitive to environmental changes and their number and function are controlled through molecular mechanisms of mitochondrial biosynthesis and clearance, called mitophagy. Mitochondrial biosynthesis is promoted by the PGC-1 factor that is upregulated by the telomere-induced DNA damage response in a p-53-dependent manner (Fig. 12.2). Metabolomics, the study of small molecules that participate in metabolic networks within a biological system, effectively captures mitochondrial function and the impact of environmental cues. The TCA cycle constitutes a series of circular reactions leading to the conversion of one metabolite to another regulated by enzymes and their co-factors/co-enzymes (trace elements, vitamins, and amino acids). Capturing the mitochondrial metabolic profile under specific circumstances provides an overview of the mitochondrial state and possible factors causing the dysfunction (nutritional deficiencies, overnutrition, prolonged and unresolved stress, and exposure to toxicants). The advantage of metabolites is that due to their close association with the phenotype and their dynamic nature, they are sensitive biomarkers sensing external triggers and a detailed snapshot of the cell's reaction to the stimuli. In the case of mitochondrial dysfunctions, metabolites' absolute levels and their relative values as markers of enzymatic activity provide valuable information at early stages [50, 51]. Previous studies on the metabolomic profile of aging have identified changes in critical metabolic pathways associated with aging traits including dyslipidemia, hormonal imbalances, inflammation, oxidative stress, hormone metabolism, muscle changes, and nutritional requirements. Among the potent metabolic biomarkers, 2-ketoglutarate, 3-hydroxybutyrate, NAD, and NADPH have been proposed as key metabolites, given their central role in metabolic circuits associated with aging. These four metabolites play a significant role in the TCA cycle, and their association has been reported in human and animal studies of metabolomics-based aging, given the close relationship of metabolites with aging traits, efforts on constructing metabolomics-based biological age clocks, either alone or as part of a multi-omics platform [52, 53].

Findings on the association between metabolic changes and telomere length in humans are still scarce. The most studied type of cells are leukocytes, which are associated directly with ADs, implying a possible use of metabolomics and telomere length as biomarkers of ADs. A large study used data from six cohorts and found a positive association between certain metabolites involved in inflammation and oxidative stress with longer leukocyte telomere length (LTL). These metabolites are linked to homocysteine metabolism, a metabolic pathway met in several age-related and autoimmune diseases [54]. Other data showed a possible protective role of BCAAs on LTL, using targeted metabolomics, thus, implicating the potential cooperation of BCAAs and LTL in healthy aging [55]. Finally, a specific metabolic signature of leukocyte telomere length has been found in elite male soccer players [56]. In this study, sixty-seven metabolites and seven metabolic pathways showed significant associations with LTL including specific metabolites that can best predict LTL. Lipids, glutamine, xanthine, and beta-sitosterol, among other metabolites, may have a crucial impact on longevity in response to chronic exercise. More studies of these metabolites could clarify the metabolic pathways through which exercise decreases telomere erosion.

12.6 Mitochondrial-Targeted Interventions and Telomeres

Beyond their predictive and discriminative ability, metabolites are potent therapeutic targets against metabolic senescence and telomere-damaging oxidative stress.

Well-studied anti-aging interventions are calorie restriction and lifestyle habits improvement (smoking, physical exercise, and sleep) along with drug options, such as metformin, NMN, and resveratrol. Extensive research has also identified potent anti-aging agents focused on the involved mechanisms including senolytics, telomerase activators, anti-inflammatory and antioxidant mediators, and microbiome regulators [57–59]. As we deepen our knowledge of the mechanistic insights of aging and sequence of events, we require well-designed human studies to assess the applicability of metabolic biomarkers and telomeres and their response to known anti-aging interventions.

Several studies have examined the correlation of individuals' nutrient status with telomere length and nutrients, showing the most promising results commonly directly affect mitochondrial function as cofactors of the TCA cycle and oxidative phosphorylation. Senescent cells are characterized by dysfunctional mitochondria and increased ROS generation [60]. Therefore, cellular reprogramming to increase mitochondrial fitness has emerged as a novel therapeutic target [61].

B12 deficiency leads to accumulated methylmalonic acid, increasing oxidative stress [62] and disrupting normal succinic metabolism, negatively affecting complex II of oxidative phosphorylation. CoQ10 (ubiquinone) is a key cofactor and component of the mitochondrial electron transport chain and a strong antioxidant [63]. Selenium-dependent enzymes exhibit variable effects of mitochondrial function through increased biogenesis (Selenoprotein H), calcium homeostasis (Selenoprotein N and W), redox function (Selenoprotein O), and thyroid metabolism (deiodinases) [64]. B3 coenzymes are needed in more than 500 enzymes, which are required for energy metabolism [65]. It is metabolized to NAD+, which functions as an electron carrier in ATP production, or NADP+, which functions as a hydrogen donor and is vital in multiple metabolic pathways (PPP, TCA, glycolysis, β-oxidation, etc.) and possibly diseases [66]. Omega 3 fatty acids have been shown to help with chronic inflammation by decreasing oxidative stress, ROS production, and endoplasmic reticulum stress, which have a pivotal role in mitochondrial integrity [67]. The importance of vitamin D in physiological human metabolism is ubiquitous and its connection to mitochondrial function and biogenesis, oxidative stress, and chronic inflammation is thoroughly investigated [68, 69]. Other lipophilic antioxidant molecules (Vitamin A, E, etc.) are assumed to share biological mechanisms. Exercise as energy-demanding physiological stress exhibits great potential for mitochondrial dynamics, shape quantity, and functional quality [70].

The complex connection between mitochondria and telomeres is increasingly recognized among various study fields. Nutrients like B12, CoQ10, selenium, B3 coenzymes, and Omega 3 fatty acids as well as lifestyle factors like exercise, have shown significant impact on mitochondrial health, with the possibility to improve telomere length and slow cellular aging processes.

In Table 12.1, findings that demonstrate the beneficial effects of mitochondria-targeted nutraceuticals/interventions on telomeres and telomerase activity are presented:

Table 12.1 Mitochondrial targets and links with telomere length and telomerase activity

Nutrient/ intervention	Mitochondrial role	Effect on telomere length	Ref.
Vitamin B9–B12	Mitochondrial complex II	*Levels* Positive correlation with TL	[71, 72]
	Mitochondrial DNA	*Deficiency* Shorter TL	
Q10	Electron transport chain	*Supplementation* Less shortening	[73]
	Oxidative stress	Increased individual TL Telomerase activation	

Table 12.1 (*Continued*)

Selenium	Mitochondrial volume and biogenesis Selenoproteins Deiodinases	*Intake* Positive correlation with TL (especially in women)	[74, 75]
B3 (NMN)	NADH/NADPH precursor Oxidative stress	*Supplementation* Increased TL	[76]
Omega-3s	Oxidative stress Endoplasmic reticulum (ER) stress	*Supplementation* Increased TL Protection from attrition	[77, 78]
Vitamin D	Mitochondrial biogenesis	*Supplementation* Positive correlation with newborn TL	[79–81]
	Oxidative stress	Increased TL in chronic kidney disease patients Increased TL	
Lipophilic Antioxidants	Oxidative Stress	*Levels* Positive correlation with TL	[82]
Exercise	Mitochondrial Adaptation	Increased TL Telomerase activation	[83, 84]

References

1. Wang, L., Wang, F. S., Gershwin M. E. (2015). Human autoimmune diseases: a comprehensive update, *J. Intern. Med.*, **278**, pp. 369–95.
2. Cho, J. H., Feldman, M. (2015). Heterogeneity of autoimmune diseases: pathophysiologic insights from genetics and implications for new therapies, *Nat. Med.*, **21**, pp. 730–8.
3. Simon, T. A., Kawabata, H., Ray, N., Baheti, A., Suissa, S., Esdaile, J. M. (2017). Prevalence of co-existing autoimmune disease in rheumatoid arthritis: a cross-sectional study, *Adv. Ther.*, **34**, pp. 2481–90.
4. Fairweather, D., Root-Bernstein, R. (2015). *Autoimmune Disease: Mechanisms.* In: eLS. John Wiley & Sons Ltd., pp. 1–7.
5. Lou, Z., Casali, P., Xu, Z. (2015). Regulation of B cell differentiation by intracellular membrane-associated proteins and microRNAs: role in the antibody response, *Front Immunol.*, **6**, pp. 1–10.

6. Goronzy, J. J., Shao, L., Weyand, C. M. (2010). Immune aging and rheumatoid arthritis, *Rheum. Dis. Clin. North Am.*, **36**, pp. 297–310.
7. Dehbi, A. Z. A., Radstake, T. R. D. J., Broen, J. C. A. (2013). Accelerated telomere shortening in rheumatic diseases: cause or consequence? *Expert Rev. Clin. Immunol.*, **9**, pp. 1193–204.
8. Tamayo, M., Mosquera, A., Rego, J. I., Fernández-Sueiro, J. L., Blanco, F. J., Fernández, J. L. (2010). Differing patterns of peripheral blood leukocyte telomere length in rheumatologic diseases, *Mutat. Res.*, **683**, pp. 68–73.
9. Epel, E. S., Blackburn, E. H., Lin, J., Dhabhar, F. S., Adler, N. E., Morrow, J. D., *et al.* (2004). Accelerated telomere shortening in response to life stress. *Proc. Natl. Acad. Sci. U S A.*, **101**, pp. 17312–5.
10. Costenbader, K. H., Prescott, J., Zee, R. Y., De Vivo, I. (2011). Immunosenescence and rheumatoid arthritis: does telomere shortening predict impending disease? *Autoimmun Rev.*, **10**, pp. 569–73.
11. Artlett, C. M., Black, C. M., Briggs, D. C., Stevens, C. O., Welsh, K. I. (1996). Telomere reduction in scleroderma patients: a possible cause for chromosomal instability, *Br. J. Rheumatol.*, **35**, pp. 732–7.
12. Armanios, M. Y., Chen, J. J. L., Cogan, J. D., Alder, J. K., Ingersoll, R. G., Markin, C., *et al.* (2007). Telomerase mutations in families with idiopathic pulmonary fibrosis, *N. Engl. J. Med.*, **356**, pp. 1317–26.
13. Tsakiri, K. D., Cronkhite, J. T., Kuan, P. J., Xing, C., Raghu, G., Weissler, J. C., *et al.* Adult-onset pulmonary fibrosis caused by mutations in telomerase, *Proc. Natl. Acad. Sci. U S A.*, **104**, pp. 7552–7.
14. Weng, N-P. (2008). Telomere and adaptive immunity, *Mech. Ageing Dev.*, **129**, pp. 60–6.
15. Fauce, S. R., Jamieson, B. D., Chin, A. C., Mitsuyasu, R. T., Parish, S. T., Ng, H. L., *et al.* (2008). Telomerase-based pharmacologic enhancement of antiviral function of human CD8+ T lymphocytes, *The Journal of Immunology*, **181**, pp. 7400–6.
16. Liu, Z., Liang, Q., Ren, Y., Guo, C., Ge, X., Wang, L., *et al.* (2023). Immunosenescence: molecular mechanisms and diseases, *Signal Transduct. Target Ther.*, **8**, pp. 200.
17. Georgin-Lavialle, S., Aouba, A., Mouthon, L., Londono-Vallejo, J. A., Lepelletier, Y., Gabet, A. S., *et al.* (2010). The telomere/telomerase system in autoimmune and systemic immune-mediated diseases, *Autoimmun Rev.*, **9**, pp. 646–51.
18. Koetz, K., Bryl, E., Spickschen, K., O'Fallon, W. M., Goronzy, J. J., Weyand, C. M. (2000). T cell homeostasis in patients with rheumatoid arthritis, *Proceedings of the National Academy of Sciences*, **97**, pp. 9203–8.

19. Schönland, S. O., Lopez, C., Widmann, T., Zimmer, J., Bryl, E., Goronzy, J. J., *et al.* (2003). Premature telomeric loss in rheumatoid arthritis is genetically determined and involves both myeloid and lymphoid cell lineages, *Proceedings of the National Academy of Sciences*, **100**, pp. 13471–6.

20. Fujii, H., Shao, L., Colmegna, I., Goronzy, J. J., Weyand, C. M. (2009). Telomerase insufficiency in rheumatoid arthritis, *Proceedings of the National Academy of Sciences*, **106**, pp. 4360–5.

21. Colmegna, I., Diaz-Borjon, A., Fujii, H., Schaefer, L., Goronzy, J. J., Weyand, C. M. (2008). Defective proliferative capacity and accelerated telomeric loss of hematopoietic progenitor cells in rheumatoid arthritis, *Arthritis Rheum.*, **58**, pp. 990–1000.

22. Steer, S. E., Williams, F. M. K., Kato, B., Gardner, J. P., Norman, P. J., Hall, M. A., *et al.* (2007). Reduced telomere length in rheumatoid arthritis is independent of disease activity and duration, *Ann. Rheum. Dis.*, **66**, pp. 476–80.

23. Li, Y., Shen, Y., Hohensinner, P., Ju, J., Wen, Z., Goodman, S. B., *et al.* (2016). Deficient activity of the nuclease MRE11A induces T cell aging and promotes arthritogenic effector functions in patients with rheumatoid arthritis, *Immunity*, **45**, pp. 903–16.

24. Heba, A. C., Toupance, S., Arnone, D., Peyrin-Biroulet, L., Benetos, A., Ndiaye, N. C. (2021). Telomeres: new players in immune-mediated inflammatory diseases? *J. Autoimmun.*, **123**, pp. 102699.

25. Tahara, T., Shibata, T., Okubo, M., Kawamura, T., Sumi, K., Ishizuka, T., *et al.* (2015). Telomere length in non-neoplastic colonic mucosa in ulcerative colitis (UC) and its relationship to the severe clinical phenotypes, *Clin. Exp. Med.*, **15**, pp. 327–32.

26. Friis-Ottessen, M., Bendix, L., Kølvraa, S., Norheim-Andersen, S., De Angelis, P. M., Clausen, O. P. F. (2014). Telomere shortening correlates to dysplasia but not to DNA aneuploidy in longstanding ulcerative colitis, *BMC Gastroenterol.*, **14**, pp. 8.

27. Risques, R. A., Lai, L. A., Himmetoglu, C., Ebaee, A., Li, L., Feng, Z., *et al.* (2011). Ulcerative colitis-associated colorectal cancer arises in a field of short telomeres, senescence, and inflammation, *Cancer Res.*, **71**, pp. 1669–79.

28. Truta, B., Wohler, E., Sobreira, N., Datta, L. W., Brant, S. R. (2020). Role of telomere shortening in anticipation of inflammatory bowel disease, *World J. Gastrointest. Pharmacol. Ther.*, **11**, pp. 69–78.

29. Getliffe, K. M., Al Dulaimi, D., Martin-Ruiz, C., Holder, R. L., von Zglinicki, T., Morris, A., *et al.* (2005). Lymphocyte telomere dynamics and

telomerase activity in inflammatory bowel disease: effect of drugs and smoking, *Aliment. Pharmacol. Ther.*, **21**, pp. 121–31.

30. Liu, X., Lin, J., Wang, L., Zhang, Z., Hou, S., Yang, G. (2008). Telomerase activity in peripheral blood mononuclear cells of psoriatic patients correlates with disease severity, *The British Journal of Dermatology*, England, **158**, pp. 637–9.
31. Wu, K., Higashi, N., Hansen, E. R., Lund, M., Bang, K., Thestrup-Pedersen, K. (2000). Telomerase activity is increased and telomere length shortened in T cells from the blood of patients with atopic dermatitis and psoriasis, *J. Immunol.*, **165**, pp. 4742–7.
32. Beranek, M., Borsky, P., Fiala, Z., Andrys, C., Hamakova, K., Chmelarova, M., *et al.* (2023). Telomere length, oxidative and epigenetic changes in blood DNA of patients with exacerbated psoriasis vulgaris, *An. Bras. Dermatol.*, **98**, pp. 68–74.
33. Wu, C. H., Hsieh, S. C., Li, K. J., Lu, M. C., Yu, C. L. (2007). Premature telomere shortening in polymorphonuclear neutrophils from patients with systemic lupus erythematosus is related to the lupus disease activity, *Lupus*, **16**, pp. 265–72.
34. Montoya-Ortiz, G. (2013). Immunosenescence, aging, and systemic lupus erythematous, *Autoimmune Dis.*, **2013**, pp. 1–15.
35. Haque, S., Rakieh, C., Marriage, F., Ho, P., Gorodkin, R., The, L. S., *et al.* (2013). Shortened telomere length in patients with systemic lupus erythematosus, *Arthritis Rheum.*, **65**, pp. 1319–23.
36. Kurosaka, D., Yasuda, J., Yoshida, K., Yoneda, A., Yasuda, C., Kingetsu, I., *et al.* (2006). Abnormal telomerase activity and telomere length in T and B cells from patients with systemic lupus erythematosus, *J. Rheumatol.*, **33**, pp. 1102–7.
37. Beier, F., Balabanov, S., Amberger, C. C., Hartmann, U., Manger, K., Dietz, K., *et al.* (2007). Telomere length analysis in monocytes and lymphocytes from patients with systemic lupus erythematosus using multi-color flow-FISH, *Lupus*, **16**, pp. 955–62.
38. Fritsch, R. D., Shen, X., Illei, G. G., Yarboro, C. H., Prussin, C., Hathcock, K. S., *et al.* (2006). Abnormal differentiation of memory T cells in systemic lupus erythematosus, *Arthritis Rheum.*, **54**, pp. 2184–97.
39. Hoffecker, B. M., Raffield, L. M., Kamen, D. L., Nowling, T. K. (2013). Systemic lupus erythematosus and vitamin D deficiency are associated with shorter telomere length among African Americans: a case-control study, *PLoS One*, **8**, pp. e63725.
40. Klapper, W., Moosig, F., Sotnikova, A., Qian, W., Schröder, J. O., Parwaresch, R. (2004). Telomerase activity in B and T lymphocytes

of patients with systemic lupus erythematosus, *Ann. Rheum. Dis.*, **63**, pp. 1681–3.

41. Zhou, J. G., Qing, Y. F., Yang, Q. B., Xie, W. G., Zhao, M. C. (2011). Changes in the expression of telomere maintenance genes might play a role in the pathogenesis of systemic lupus erythematosus, *Lupus*, **20**, pp. 820–8.
42. Miwa, S., Kashyap, S., Chini, E., von Zglinicki, T. (2022). Mitochondrial dysfunction in cell senescence and aging, *Journal of Clinical Investigation*, **132**, pp. e158447.
43. Martínez-Reyes, I., Chandel, N. S. (2020). Mitochondrial TCA cycle metabolites control physiology and disease, *Nat Commun [Internet]*, **11**, pp. 1–11.
44. Cui, H., Kong, Y., Zhang, H. (2012). Oxidative stress, mitochondrial dysfunction, and aging, *J. Signal Transduct.*, **2012**, pp. 1–13.
45. de Almeida, A. J. P. O., de Oliveira, J. C. P. L., da Silva Pontes, L. V., de Souza Júnior, J. F., Gonçalves, T. A. F., Dantas, S. H., *et al.* (2022). ROS: basic concepts, sources, cellular signaling, and its implications in aging pathways, *Oxid. Med. Cell Longev.*, **2022**, pp. 1–23.
46. Oexle, K., Zwirner, A. (1997). Advanced telomere shortening in respiratory chain disorders, *Hum. Mol. Genet.*, **6**, pp. 905–8.
47. Zheng, Q., Huang, J., Wang, G. (2019). Mitochondria, telomeres and telomerase subunits, *Front Cell. Dev. Biol.*, **7**, pp. 1–10.
48. Gao, X., Yu, X., Zhang, C., Wang, Y., Sun, Y., Sun, H., *et al.* (2022). Telomeres and mitochondrial metabolism: implications for cellular senescence and age-related diseases, *Stem Cell Rev. Rep.*, **18**, pp. 2315–27.
49. Sahin, E., DePinho, R. A. (2012). Axis of ageing: telomeres, p53 and mitochondria, *Nat. Rev. Mol. Cell Biol.*, **13**, pp. 397–404.
50. Tsoukalas, D., Fragoulakis, V., Sarandi, E., Docea, A. O., Papakonstaninou, E., Tsilimidos, G. (2019). Targeted metabolomic analysis of serum fatty acids for the prediction of autoimmune diseases, *Front. Mol. Biosci.*, **6**, pp. 120.
51. Tsoukalas, D., Fragoulakis, V., Papakonstantinou, E., Antonaki, M., Vozikis, A., Tsatsakis, A., *et al.* (2020). Prediction of autoimmune diseases by targeted metabolomic assay of urinary organic acids, *Metabolites*, **10**, pp. 1–20.
52. Robinson, O., Lau, C. E. (2023). How do metabolic processes age: evidence from human metabolomic studies, *Curr. Opin. Chem. Biol.*, **76**, pp. 102360.
53. Panyard, D. J., Yu, B., Snyder, M. P. (2022). The metabolomics of human aging: advances, challenges, and opportunities, *Sci. Adv.*, **8**, pp. 1–13.

54. van der Spek, A., Broer, L., Draisma, H. H. M., Pool, R., Albrecht, E., Beekman, M., *et al.* (2019). Metabolomics reveals a link between homocysteine and lipid metabolism and leukocyte telomere length: the ENGAGE consortium, *Sci. Rep.*, **9**, pp. 11623.
55. Zhang, Y., Zhou, Q., Yang, R., Hu, C., Huang, Z., Zheng, C., *et al.* (2020). Serum branched-chain amino acids are associated with leukocyte telomere length and frailty based on residents from Guangxi longevity county, *Sci. Rep.*, **10**, pp. 10252.
56. Al-Muraikhy, S., Sellami, M., Domling, A. S., Rizwana, N., Agouni, A., Al-Khelaifi, F., *et al.* (2021). Metabolic rs, *Front. Mol. Biosci.*, **8**, pp. 727144.
57. Guo, J., Huang, X., Dou, L., Yan, M., Shen, T., Tang, W., *et al.* (2022). Aging and aging-related diseases: from molecular mechanisms to interventions and treatments, *Signal Transduct. Target Ther.*, **7**, pp. 391.
58. Tsoukalas, D., Buga, A. M., Docea, A. O., Sarandi, E., Mitrut, R., Renieri, E., *et al.* (2021). Reversal of brain aging by targeting telomerase: a nutraceutical approach, *Int. J. Mol. Med.*, **48**, pp. 1–11.
59. Tsatsakis, A., Renieri, E., Tsoukalas, D., Buga, A., Sarandi, E., Vakonaki, E., *et al.* (2023). A novel nutraceutical formulation increases telomere length and activates telomerase activity in middle aged rats, *Mol. Med. Rep.*, **28**, pp. 232.
60. Wiley, C. D., Velarde, M. C., Lecot, P., Liu, S., Sarnoski, E. A., Freund, A., *et al.* (2016). Mitochondrial dysfunction induces senescence with a distinct secretory phenotype, *Cell Metab.*, **23**, pp. 303–14.
61. Murphy, M. P., Hartley, R. C. (2018). Mitochondria as a therapeutic target for common pathologies, *Nat. Rev. Drug Discov.* **17**, pp. 865–86.
62. Okun, J. G., Hörster, F., Farkas, L. M., Feyh, P., Hinz, A., Sauer, S., *et al.* (2002). Neurodegeneration in methylmalonic aciduria involves inhibition of complex II and the tricarboxylic acid cycle, and synergistically acting excitotoxicity, *Journal of Biological Chemistry*, **277**, pp. 14674–80.
63. Littarru, G. P., Tiano, L. (2010). Clinical aspects of coenzyme Q10: an update, *Nutrition*, **26**, pp. 250–4.
64. Wesolowski, L. T., Semanchik, P. L., White-Springer, S. H. (2022). Beyond antioxidants: selenium and skeletal muscle mitochondria, *Front. Vet. Sci.*, **9**, pp. 1–12.
65. Depeint, F., Bruce, W. R., Shangari, N., Mehta, R., O'Brien, P. J. (2006). Mitochondrial function and toxicity: role of the B vitamin family on mitochondrial energy metabolism, *Chem. Biol. Interact.*, **163**, pp. 94–112.

66. Sun, C., Wang, K., Stock, A. J., Gong, Y., Demarest, T. G., Yang, B., *et al.* (2020). Re-equilibration of imbalanced NAD metabolism ameliorates the impact of telomere dysfunction, *EMBO J.*, **39**, pp. e103420.

67. Lepretti, M., Martucciello, S., Burgos Aceves, M., Putti, R., Lionetti, L. (2018). Omega-3 fatty acids and insulin resistance: focus on the regulation of mitochondria and endoplasmic reticulum stress, *Nutrients*, **10**, pp. 350.

68. Salles, J., Chanet, A., Guillet, C., Vaes, A. M. M., Brouwer-Brolsma, E. M., Rocher, C., *et al.* (2022). Vitamin D status modulates mitochondrial oxidative capacities in skeletal muscle: role in sarcopenia, *Commun. Biol.*, **5**, pp. 1288.

69. Phillips, E. A., Hendricks, N., Bucher, M., Maloyan, A. (2022). Vitamin D supplementation improves mitochondrial function and reduces inflammation in placentae of obese women, *Front. Endocrinol. (Lausanne)*, **13**, pp. 1–12.

70. Tanaka, T., Nishimura, A., Nishiyama, K., Goto, T., Numaga-Tomita, T., Nishida, M. (2020). Mitochondrial dynamics in exercise physiology, *Pflugers Arch.*, **472**, pp. 137–53.

71. Praveen, G., Sivaprasad, M., Reddy, G. B. (2022). Telomere length and vitamin B12, *Vitam. Horm.*, **119**, pp. 299–324.

72. Pusceddu, I., Herrmann, M., Kirsch, S. H., Werner, C., Hübner, U., Bodis, M., *et al.* (2016). Prospective study of telomere length and LINE-1 methylation in peripheral blood cells: the role of B vitamins supplementation, *Eur. J. Nutr.*, **55**, pp. 1863–73.

73. Opstad, T. B., Alexander, J., Aaseth, J. O., Larsson, A., Seljeflot, I., Alehagen, U. (2022). Selenium and coenzyme Q10 intervention prevents telomere attrition, with association to reduced cardiovascular mortality—sub-study of a randomized clinical trial, *Nutrients*, **14**, pp. 3346.

74. Shu, Y., Wu, M., Yang, S., Wang, Y., Li, H. (2020). Association of dietary selenium intake with telomere length in middle-aged and older adults, *Clinical Nutrition*, **39**, pp. 3086–91.

75. Gong, H., Yu, Q., Guo, D., Wang, Y., Duan, L., Huang, W., *et al.* (2023). The relationship between dietary selenium intake and telomere length among diabetes, *British Journal of Nutrition*, **129**, pp. 610–6.

76. Niu, K. M., Bao, T., Gao, L., Ru, M., Li, Y., Jiang, L., *et al.* (2021). The impacts of short-term NMN supplementation on serum metabolism, fecal microbiota, and telomere length in pre-aging phase, *Front. Nutr.*, **8**, pp. 1–12.

77. Ogłuszka, M., Lipiński, P., Starzyński, R. R. (2022). Effect of omega-3 fatty acids on telomeres—are they the elixir of youth? *Nutrients*, **14**, pp. 3723.
78. Barden, A. E., Moghaddami, M., Mas, E., Phillips, M., Cleland, L. G., Mori, T. A. (2016). Specialised pro-resolving mediators of inflammation in inflammatory arthritis, *Prostaglandins Leukot. Essent. Fatty Acids*, **107**, pp. 24–29.
79. Borras, M., Panizo, S., Sarró, F., Valdivielso, J. M., Fernandez, E. (2012). Assessment of the potential role of active vitamin D treatment in telomere length: a case–control study in hemodialysis patients, *Clin. Ther.*, **34**, pp. 849–56.
80. Daneels, L., Martens, D. S., Arredouani, S., Billen, J., Koppen, G., Devlieger, R., *et al.* (2021). Maternal vitamin D and newborn telomere length, *Nutrients*, **13**, pp. 2012.
81. Liu, J. J., Prescott, J., Giovannucci, E., Hankinson, S. E., Rosner, B., Han, J., *et al.* (2013). Plasma vitamin D biomarkers and leukocyte telomere length, *Am. J. Epidemiol.*, **177**, pp. 1411–1417.
82. Mazidi, M., Kengne, A. P., Cheskin, L. J., Banach, M. (2018). Serum lipophilic antioxidants levels are associated with leucocyte telomere length among US adults, *Lipids Health Dis.*, **17**, pp. 164.
83. Buttet, M., Bagheri, R., Ugbolue, U. C., Laporte, C., Trousselard, M., Benson, A., *et al.* (2022). Effect of a lifestyle intervention on telomere length: a systematic review and meta-analysis, *Mech. Ageing Dev.*, **206**, pp. 111694.
84. Semeraro, M. D., Smith, C., Kaiser, M., Levinger, I., Duque, G., Gruber, H. J., *et al.* (2020). Physical activity, a modulator of aging through effects on telomere biology, *Aging*, **12**, pp. 13803–23.

Chapter 13

Osteoarthritis

Lydia-Nefeli Thrapsanioti,[a] Aikaterini Berdiaki,[a] Fotios Kakridonis,[b] Aristidis Tsatsakis,[c,d] and Dragana Nikitovic[a]

[a] *Laboratory of Histology-Embryology, School of Medicine, University of Crete, Heraklion, Greece*
[b] *25th Department of Orthopaedics, KAT Attica General Hospital, Athens, Greece*
[c] *Laboratory of Toxicology, Medical School, University of Crete, Heraklion, Greece*
[d] *Lifeplus S.A., Science & Technological Park of Crete, Vassilika Vouton, Heraklion, Greece*
nikitovic@uoc.gr

13.1 Introduction

Osteoarthritis (OA) is a skeletal disease exhibiting abnormal reconstruction of the subchondral bone. OA is an age-related disease correlated to patient morbidity and mortality, and it presents a significant healthcare burden. Indeed, OA is a dynamic disease caused by the imbalance between restoration and destruction of joints, with complicated pathophysiology that affects the cartilage and neighboring tissues around it. Disease development is ordinarily gradual and causes pathological changes in the entire joint. These changes facilitate the breakdown of the articular cartilage

Telomeres: Biomarkers of a Healthy Life and Successful Aging
Edited by Aristidis Tsatsakis

ISBN 978-981-5129-49-6 (Hardcover), 978-1-003-56809-4 (eBook)
www.jennystanford.com

extracellular matrix (ECM), primarily type II collagen and aggrecan, and reduce the production of new cartilage ECM, ultimately resulting in joint dysfunction and disability [1]. The most severe symptoms of the affected individuals are evident in OA of the hips and knees, as pain and stiffness in these large weight-bearing joints frequently lead to considerable impairment needing surgical intervention. According to recent studies, it is estimated that OA incidence will continue to accelerate in the coming years due to the pandemic rise in obesity and the worldwide increase in life expectancy [2].

13.2 Role of Telomeres and Telomerase in Aging

Telomeres, the 5′-TTAGGG-3′ repetitive DNA sequence, are chromosomal end structures that safeguard DNA and guarantee genomic stability. Telomeres' size decreases in each mitotic cycle due to DNA polymerase's failure to maintain the length of the 3′ overhang [3]. Harley et al., in 1992, proposed the "telomere theory of cellular aging," and even continuing research has shown that telomere length (TL) and the start of age-related illnesses are correlated [4]. Indeed, telomere shortening (TS) or attrition has recently been characterized as one of the "hallmarks" of aging [5]. Telomeres are duplicated by a highly specialized ribonucleoprotein unit, known as telomerase, which consists of a protein component termed telomerase reverse transcriptase (TERT) and a crucial telomerase RNA component (TERC or RT) [6]. However, telomerase is absent in most mature human somatic cells and is only active in cells capable of reversing telomere shortening and supporting TL [7]. Other age-related diseases, such as cancer, cardiovascular disease, diabetes, rheumatoid arthritis, and psychiatric issues have all been linked to TL and telomerase activity [8]. Furthermore, Vakonaki et al. identified a link between TL and drug abuse, which results in accelerated biological aging. Therefore, the determination of TL and its maintenance through intervention might significantly contribute to the postponement of the aging process and the treatment of a variety of age-related disorders, ultimately leading to longevity [9]. The "BIOTEL" database was recently built to calculate a wide variety of TL statistics, biological age, and applications of telomere biology research [9].

13.3 Critical Components of OA Pathology

The characteristics of OA include subchondral sclerosis, osteophyte development, and progressive loss of hyaline cartilage. Due to the pathogenesis's complexity, it is currently illusive and characterized as complicated and multimodal [10]. Weight-bearing joints' cartilage experiences fibrillations, loses resiliency, and experiences localized ECM loss. As knowledge grows, OA is becoming more and more recognized as a condition affecting the entire joint, with pathological changes occurring in all of the joint's tissues, including the cartilage, synovium, subchondral bone, and connected musculature. Indeed, the other two major OA events—oxidative stress and cartilage degeneration—strongly correlate with chronic synovitis, an infection of the joint membrane [11]. ROS and mitochondrial dysfunction are linked processes in the pathogenesis of OA. Most ROS production occurs in mitochondria, making them a vulnerable target for ROS destructive effects [12, 13]. Adenosine triphosphate (ATP) loss, mtDNA alteration, and mitochondrial respiratory chain suppression are all results of excessive ROS. Therefore, the inflammation brought on by these processes promotes cell mortality and functional failure. In addition to speeding up the aging process, mtDNA mutation and loss also attenuate mitochondrial respiratory failure and fasten excessive ROS generation [14]. Tumor necrosis factor (TNF) and interleukin 1β (IL-1β) are pro-inflammatory proteins that increase the generation of ROS and NO in mitochondria. Human chondrocyte cultures from OA patients showed decreased membrane potential in OA cartilage as well as respiratory dysfunction of mitochondria as a consequence of the entire signaling event.

13.4 Role of Aging in OA: Correlation with Telomeres and Telomerase

Aging is an irrevocable and inevitable biological process that contributes to the etiology of numerous illnesses, including diabetes, osteoarthritis, Alzheimer's disease, cardiovascular disease, cancer, obesity, and other metabolic abnormalities. Nowadays, as the human life span and the percentage of older adults rise, the worldwide financial impact of aging-related illnesses increases, and effective preventive and therapeutic techniques are desperately required. Furthermore, due to aging, the bone deteriorates in composition, structure, and function, predisposing it to osteoporosis [15, 16]. Notably, in a recent meta-analysis of case-control designed studies TL of peripheral blood leukocytes (PBLs) was found to be shorter In OA compared to healthy controls. These data suggest that the TL of PBLs may be immediately correlated with the pathogenesis of OA [17]. Moreover, in a cohort of patients, the TS in PBLs exhibited faster attrition in patients with knee OA [18]. Furthermore, low relative TL in PBLs in keen OA is associated with poorer physical performance in these patients [19]. Another critical point is that PBLs TL was found to be a persistent risk factor for knee OA, independent of other health parameters [20]. Likewise, incident hand OA was bound to be robustly correlated with decreased PBLs TL [21].

13.5 Parameters Correlated to TS and Telomerase Activity Loss in OA

The signature of cellular aging needs to be more adequately understood. The events of aging result in a well-established state of terminal growth-arrest-denominated senescence [22]. Senescence is caused by multifaceted factors that induce progressive damage to essential cellular structures. One of the most prominent factors is inflammation. Indeed, inflammatory stress causes chondrocytes in OA joints to behave differently than they would in healthy joints. Importantly it has been shown that the release of radical oxygen species (ROS) causes genomic instability and parallel telomere instability, which results in senescence and impairment in the function of human chondrocytes [23]. The metabolic shift research by Arra et al. revealed that OA chondrocytes have higher amounts of lactate dehydrogenase A (LDHA) and are more dependent on glycolysis. Since LDHA knockout lowers ROS production and delays

OA progression, targeting LDHA-mediated ROS generation in OA chondrocytes may help develop new therapies [24, 25].

13.5.1 Chondrocyte Metabolic Status

The complicated interaction between chondrocytes' anabolic and catabolic intracellular signaling regulates the homeostasis of the cartilage. By increasing the expression of Sox9 and the production of type II collagen and aggrecan, anabolic signaling helps maintain the chondrogenic profile [26]. Notably, cloned chondroprogenitors maintained similar Sox9 expression but exhibited longer telomeres in comparison to non-clonal dedifferentiated chondrocytes [27]. Nevertheless, in pathological conditions, catabolic signaling induces chondrocytes to synthesize proteases like MMP-13 and a disintegrin and ADAM metallopeptidase with thrombospondin type 1 motif 5 (ADAMTS5), which ultimately causes atrophy or death of chondrocytes. Chondrocyte catabolism occurs in a low-grade inflammatory environment and is regulated by damage-associated molecular patterns (DAMPs), which are the breakdown products of proteins, proteoglycans, and cellular materials like uric acids, cause a sterile inflammatory response by interacting with particle recognition receptors (PRRs), such as Toll-like receptors (TLRs) on the surface of immune cells, TLR signaling, and its downstream canonical nuclear factor kappa B (NF-B) signaling [28]. DAMPs exert location-dependent roles outside and inside the cell and have been correlated to aberrant telomeres [29]. Furthermore, through significant production of ROS and oxidative stress, selenium deficiency also speeds up the chondrocyte's catabolic process [30]. Mitochondrial function has also been implicated in cell senescence [31]. Moreover, OA has been suggested to be a mitochondrial disease [32]. Indeed, chondrocyte mitochondrial dysfunction correlated to oxidative stress and decreased autophagy facilitates cell catabolism and cell death [33]. Moreover, in a recent study, an enhanced rate of TS in PBLs seems to be facilitated by disrupted mitochondrial function and increased knee OA initiation [34]. Interestingly, derivative embryonic stem cells (ntESCs) with elongated telomeres support correct chondrocyte differentiation and maintenance, suggesting that the TL of surrounding cells and consequent metabolic profile affect chondrocyte wellbeing [35].

13.5.2 MMPs' Activity and Expression

OA is characterized by irreversible and non-linear deterioration of joint cartilage facilitated by MMP action (Table 13.1). The primary cause of cartilage ECM loss is excessive MMP synthesis, triggered by IL-1 and TNF-a, which are characterized as key OA cytokines [36]. MMP-1 and MMP-13 are known to be critical players in ECM breakdown. Notably, TS has been correlated with increased MMP expression [37]. Moreover, mean TL was found to be shorter in chondrocytes near the OA lesion compared to cells positioned at distal sites in the same joint, indirectly correlating TL with ECM breakdown [38]. Thus, MMP-1, secreted by synovial lining cells, and MMP-13, produced by chondrocytes, are implicated in the breakdown of type II collagen. MMP-13 can break down aggrecan, in addition to type II collagen, and thus plays a dual function in ECM degradation [39]. MMP-2, MMP-3, and MMP-9, in addition to MMP-1 and 13 expressions, are increased and linked with the breakdown of non-collagen matrix components of the joints. It is essential to note that each collagenase subfamily member can cleave the collagen triple helix. While MMP-13 and MMP-1 preferably break type II and type III collagen, MMP-8 selectively cleaves type I collagen. Interestingly, MMP-13 has 5–10 times more effect on type-II collagen; however, the higher expression of MMP-1 surpasses its comparative efficacy to degrade type-II collagen, as corroborated by MMP-1's several-fold higher expression compared to MMP-13.

13.5.3 Cytokines

Among the most prominent mediators in OA pathogenesis is IL-1β (Table 13.1). Indeed, this interleukin is directly associated with the induction of chondrocyte senescence and OA [40]. IL-1β, one of the 11 members of the IL-1 family, activates various catabolic pathways by triggering the transcription factor NF-B and several other signaling cascades. To cause pro-inflammatory effects, IL-1β has a dual function (autocrine and paracrine). The fundamental

Table 13.1 A summary of key mediators correlated with telomere/ telomerase status in the onset of OA

Molecules	Role in OA	Ref.
MMP-1 and MMP-13	Breakdown of type II collagen and MMP-3 can also cause aggrecan degradation.	[39]
MMP-2, MMP-3, and MMP-9	They are linked with the breakdown of non-collagen matrix components of the joints.	[39]
MMP-8	Selectively cleaves type I collagen.	[39]
IL-1	Inhibits the production of type II collagen and aggrecan.	[41]
	It also increases the synthesis of MMPs (especially MMP-1, 3, and 13), which are detrimental to articular cartilage.	
	It influences chondrocytes' synthesis of disintegrin and Metalloproteinase with Thrombospondin motif 4 (ADAMTS4). Multiple effects on cartilage, firstly by reducing its restoration capability and then by activating proteases and having a direct negative impact on chondrocytes.	[44]
IL-6	IL-6 gene expression and protein secretion under telomerase inhibition were investigated in several studies and showed that gene levels and protein secretion were decreased by TERT inhibition in cells under inflammatory stimulus actions.	[46]
	IL-6-mediated increases in telomerase activity are associated with reduced cellular senescence.	[47]
	IL-6 also reduces senescence and enhances telomerase activity.	
Wnt/β-catenin pathway	Wnt activity has been linked to the degradation of the cartilage matrix by related ECM-degrading proteases.	[8]
	The DNA damage responses (DDRs) are activated as telomeres shorten and start to uncap, resulting in the downregulation of Wnt pathway components and target genes (TRF1, TRF2, TIN2, and POT1).	[49]

(*Continued*)

Table 13.1 (*Continued*)

Molecules	Role in OA	Ref.
	The Wnt-to-telomere capping portion of the feedback loop showed the significance of TERF2 regulation by β-catenin in cancer cells.	[50]
MAPK-p38	The release of MMP-1 and MMP-13, which break down collagen and raise IL-1 and TNF levels, was caused by the induction of MAPK-p38.	[8]
	In several animal models, MMP-3 expression was reduced by inhibiting the MAPK-p38 pathway.	

cells of the joint, such as chondrocytes, synoviocytes, macrophages, and osteoblasts, regulate its production. The most critical impact of IL-1 is to decrease ECM synthesis and metabolism. It is well established that IL-1β inhibits the production of type II collagen and aggrecan, two crucial structural ECM proteins [41]. It also increases the synthesis of MMPs (especially MMP-1, 3, and 13), which are detrimental to articular cartilage. IL-1β also influences chondrocytes' synthesis of disintegrin and metalloproteinase with thrombospondin motif 4 (ADAMTS4). IL-1β was shown to decrease telomerase activity in chondrocytes, which was attenuated by treating these cells with a non-steroidal anti-inflammatory drug and a cyclooxygenase inhibitor, feprazone [42]. Furthermore, blocking IL-1β normalized telomerase expression in chondrocytes isolated from cartilage-subchondral bone explants from OA patients [43]. In conclusion, IL-1β has multiple effects on cartilage, first by reducing its restoration capability and then by activating proteases and having a direct negative impact on chondrocytes [44]. Interleukin-6 (IL-6) is a multi-functional cytokine, and its increase in circulation with age is considered an important aging biomarker [45]. The age-associated changes in telomere attrition increase circulating inflammatory cytokines like IL-6. The pro-inflammatory IL-6 is a cytokine with pleiotropic effects, which is involved in both pro – and anti-inflammatory actions and is associated with structural changes in joints that characterize OA. TERT, the telomerase reverse transcriptase catalytic subunit, is required to induce IL6, IL1-β, and TNF genes by the NF-kB factor. As telomerase participates in the induction of cytokine expression, IL-6 gene expression and protein secretion under telomerase inhibition were investigated in several models. In glial cells, gene levels and protein secretion were decreased by TERT inhibition under inflammatory stimulus actions. On the other hand, TERT inhibition interrupted the protective effects of tibolone on cell death [46, 47]. The observation that IL-6 also reduces senescence and enhances telomerase activity raises the hypothesis that cell proliferation and telomerase activity are regulated by common intracellular signaling pathways [46, 47]. Furthermore, IL-6-mediated increases in telomerase activity are associated with reduced cellular senescence. Butorphanol, an anti-inflammatory agent, attenuates TNF-α induced IL-6 elevation and telomerase downregulation in human chondrocyte-articular cells [48].

13.5.4 Wnt/β-Catenin Signaling

An additional signaling pathway that is enhanced in OA is Wnt/β-catenin (Table 13.1). The Wnt peptides are localized to the intercellular space, and when they bind to their particular receptor, frizzle protein, and low-density lipoprotein receptor-associated protein, complex formation is triggered. The complexing of these proteins prevents β-catenin phosphorylation and degradation, enabling it to translocate to the nucleus and exert its transcriptional activities. Baseline Wnt activity is critical for maintaining the metabolic balance of chondrocytes; however, elevated Wnt activity, as seen in OA, has been linked to the degradation of the cartilage matrix by related ECM-degrading proteases [8]. MMP-13, ADAMTS4, and ADAMTS5 expressions were significantly elevated in β-catenin overexpressing animals, whereas cartilage thickness was reduced, and ECM degradation was increased. Inhibiting Wnt/β-Catenin diminished the intensity of OA illness and decreased cartilage catabolism in a mouse model [8]. Telomere capping and Wnt are connected via a positive feedback loop. Telomeres in healthy, normal cells are long enough and occupied by shelterin to maintain the capped state, promoting the regular production of Wnt pathway constituents. The DNA damage responses (DDRs) are activated as telomeres shorten and start to uncap, resulting in the downregulation of Wnt pathway components and target genes, including those that express the shelterins TRF1, TRF2, TIN2, and POT1 [49]. As a result, the mutual support that Wnt signaling and telomere capping usually share is lost. The positive feedback is restored by reactivating the Wnt pathway using agonists such as GSK-3 inhibitors, which upregulate shelterins and induce telomere capping. Other studies have also suggested a relationship between Wnt and telomeres. For example, Diala et al. described the Wnt-to-telomere capping portion of the feedback loop and showed the significance of TERF2 regulation by β-catenin in cancer cells [50]. A family of serine-threonine protein kinases called MAPK, which can be triggered by various variables, such as physical stress, infection, inflammation, and extracellular cues, is also one of these critical signaling networks contributing to OA. For example, the release of MMP-1 and MMP-13, which break down collagen and raise IL-1 and TNF levels, was caused by the induction of MAPK-p38. In several animal models, MMP-3 expression was reduced by inhibiting the MAPK-p38 pathway [8]. Notably, IL-1β induces downstream p38 MAPK activation and enhances caveolin 1 expression correlated to chondrocyte senescent phenotype and TS. Moreover, caveolin 1 overexpression and p38 MAPK triggering attenuated chondrocyte ability to synthesize type II collagen and aggrecan [51].

The same OA risk factors that apply to older adult populations, such as obesity, joint damage, genetics, and bone abnormalities, also apply to younger communities. Some evidence indicates that older adults will develop OA faster than younger adults following an acute joint injury, such as an anterior cruciate ligament tear. Some risk factors for the development of OA, such as calcification of joint tissues, increased bone turnover, and degenerative changes in the meniscus and joint ligaments, seem to be more prevalent in older adult groups [52].

Injuries to the anterior cruciate ligament (ACL) also increase the risk of developing knee OA. In addition, they frequently result in post-traumatic OA in young people who have sustained sports-related injuries. Although the exact changes that take place in aging ligaments are unknown, decreasing fibril diameter and rising stiffness from collagen crosslinking may raise the risk for ACL.

Although it is evident that changes in the bone can affect how OA develops or progresses, the exact process by which this occurs is unclear. Aging has recently been found to increase the chance of developing bone marrow lesions in asymptomatic people [52].

Oxidative stress and decreased levels of growth factors have been found to lead to increased susceptibility to cell death, reduced matrix synthesis, and repair. Furthermore, a rise in the number of cells with aged secretory characteristics stimulates matrix degradation and increased cytokine and MMP production [52].

A summary of the main signaling pathways/ mechanisms correlated to TS contribution to OA pathogenesis is schematically depicted in Fig. 13.1.

13.6 Therapeutic Implications

In OA cases, chondrocyte cellular senescence and apoptosis are believed to be primarily caused by oxidative stress and persistent inflammation. With targeted antioxidant treatment, chondrocytes and MSCs may be shielded from oxidative stress-related harm and inflammation. In this regard, Hudita et al. showed that an acetylated fatty acid mixture from celadrin decreased the secretion of inflammatory mediators and facilitated the chondrogenic differentiation process of human adipose-derived stem cells using an in vitro scaffold-free 3D MSC culture model of chondrogenesis. A possible diagnostic tool for the identification and prognosis of OA is the evaluation of TL in chondrocytes and/or peripheral blood leukocytes (PBL). Along these lines, the effects of etomidate, an intravenous anesthetic exhibiting antioxidant and anti-inflammatory effects, were examined in OA. Indeed, etomidate exerted a protective effect in an IL-1β- induced chondrocytes, OA model. This therapeutic, among others, induced enhanced telomerase activity [53].

Additionally, MSCs are currently being researched as a possible OA treatment since they have great potential in promoting chondrocytes' regeneration and differentiation into cartilage. The necessary characteristics of MSCs as cell-based therapeutic agents are their ability to stimulate cartilage formation, vascularization, anti-inflammation, and immunoregulation. Phase I/II clinical studies

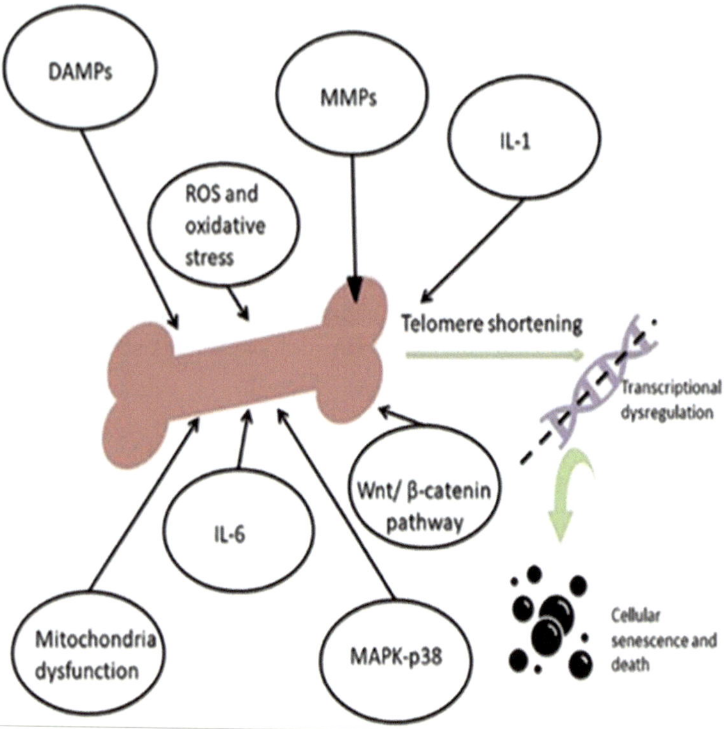

Figure 13.1 Factors affecting chondrocyte cellular senescence and death in OA. Excessive ROS production and the resulting oxidative stress, mitochondrial dysfunction, altered metabolism, and specific extra- and intracellular mediators are correlated with telomere shortening, transcriptional dysregulation, and subsequent cellular senescence and death leading to OA.

have shown signs of pain alleviation and functional improvement. However, there are risks and limitations in the use of MSCs that should be realized and treated carefully, such as the inadequate understanding of MSCs, regarding their physiological properties and cellular functions in vitro and in vivo and the fact that the therapeutic efficacy of MSCs in preclinical and clinical studies is influenced by many factors, such as the cell culture conditions, the cell density, the time and location for MSC transplantation [24]. Notably, applying adipogenic stromal-vascular fraction cells with retained TL in a prospective study resulted in patient pain relief and better physical performance [54]. In an in vivo study, the systemic transplantation of adult multipotent muscle-derived stem/progenitor cells resulted in telomere protection of normally aged mice [55]. Due to the avascular nature of cartilage and/or the injured vasculature of significant defects, healing from bone and osteochondral diseases has proven to be challenging. This lack of nourishment and cells has made recovery difficult for patients. Since it is challenging to guarantee cell viability and a high probability of tissue deterioration, traditional therapies like microfractures and cell-based treatment are not always effective [56]. Alternative therapies, including TL protection and telomerase activity enhancement, are important therapy targets.

13.7 Conclusions

Osteoarthritis is one of the most prevalent chronic diseases impacting the aging population, with high morbidity and mortality rates. According to accumulating data, TS may serve as an epigenetic factor in the development of this disease. As a result, the assessment of the progression of OA may benefit from the measurement of chondrocyte TL and/or PBL. Finding the causes of this pathology and age-related changes is crucial for further investigation. More research involving larger cohorts is necessary to get unbiased findings and improve our comprehension of the connection between TL, inflammation, and aging. Further understanding of the pathophysiology of degenerative joint disorders could arise from this.

References

1. Ashruf, O. S. & Ansari, M. Y. (2022). Natural compounds: potential therapeutics for the inhibition of cartilage matrix degradation in osteoarthritis, *Life (Basel)*, **13**, pp. 102.
2. Sowers, M. R. & Karvonen-Gutierrez, C. A. (2010). The evolving role of obesity in knee osteoarthritis, *Curr Opin Rheumatol*, **22**, pp. 533–537.

3. Aubert, G. & Lansdorp, P. M. (2008). Telomeres and aging, *Physiol Rev,* **88**, pp. 557–579.
4. Harley, C. B., Vaziri, H., Counter, C. M. & Allsopp, R. C. (1992). The telomere hypothesis of cellular aging, *Exp Gerontol,* **27**, pp. 375–382.
5. Lopez-Otin, C., Blasco, M. A., Partridge, L., Serrano, M. & Kroemer, G. (2023). Hallmarks of aging: an expanding universe, *Cell,* **186**, pp. 243–278.
6. Masutomi, K., Possemato, R., Wong, J. M., Currier, J. L., Tothova, Z., Manola, J. B., *et al.* (2005). The telomerase reverse transcriptase regulates chromatin state and DNA damage responses, *Proc Natl Acad Sci U S A,* **102,** pp. 8222–8227.
7. Cong, Y. S., Wright, W. E. & Shay, J. W. (2002). Human telomerase and its regulation, *Microbiol Mol Biol Rev,* **66**, pp. 407–425.
8. Li, Z., Dai, A., Yang, M., Chen, S., Deng, Z. & Li, L. (2022). p38MAPK Signaling pathway in osteoarthritis: pathological and therapeutic aspects, *J Inflamm Res,* **15**, pp. 723–734.
9. Vakonaki E, Tzatzarakis M, Tsiminikaki K, *et al.* (2019). Effect of chronic and heavy drug abuse on biological aging, *World Academy of Sciences Journal,* **1**, pp. 67–73.
10. Holden, M. A., Nicolson, P. J. A., Thomas, M. J., Corp, N., Hinman, R. S. & Bennell, K. L. (2023). Osteoarthritis year in review 2022: rehabilitation, *Osteoarthritis Cartilage,* **31**, pp. 177–186.
11. Fragkiadaki, P., Nikitovic, D., Kalliantasi, K., Sarandi, E., Thanasoula, M., Stivaktakis, P. D., *et al.* (2020). Telomere length and telomerase activity in osteoporosis and osteoarthritis, *Exp Ther Med,* **19**, pp. 1626–1632.
12. Valko, M., Leibfritz, D., Moncol, J., Cronin, M. T., Mazur, M. & Telser, J. (2007). Free radicals and antioxidants in normal physiological functions and human disease, *Int J Biochem Cell Biol,* **39**, pp. 44–84.
13. Henrotin, Y. E., Bruckner, P. & Pujol, J. P. (2003). The role of reactive oxygen species in homeostasis and degradation of cartilage, *Osteoarthritis Cartilage,* **11**, pp. 747–755.
14. Liu JT, Guo X, Ma WJ, *et al.* (2010). Mitochondrial function is altered in articular chondrocytes of an endemic osteoarthritis, Kashin–Beck disease, *Osteoarthritis and Cartilage* **18**, pp. 1218–1226.
15. Franceschi, C., Garagnani, P., Morsiani, C., Conte, M., Santoro, A., Grignolio, A., *et al.* (2018). The continuum of aging and age-related diseases: common mechanisms but different rates, *Front Med (Lausanne),* **5**, pp. 61.

16. Chen, S., Gan, D., Lin, S., Zhong, Y., Chen, M., Zou, X., *et al.* (2022). Metformin in aging and aging-related diseases: clinical applications and relevant mechanisms, *Theranostics,* **12**, pp. 2722–2740.
17. Xie, H., Ma, Y., Shao, M., Kong, J., Zhou, T., Wang, F., *et al.* (2022). Telomere length in patients with osteoarthritis: a systematic review and meta-analysis, *Aging Clin Exp Res,* **34**, pp. 495–503.
18. Guillen, R., Otero, F., Mosquera, A., Vazquez-Mosquera, M., Rego-Perez, I., Blanco, F. J., *et al.* (2021). Association of accelerated dynamics of telomere sequence loss in peripheral blood leukocytes with incident knee osteoarthritis in osteoarthritis initiative cohort, *Sci Rep,* **11**, pp. 15914.
19. Manoy P, Yuktanandana P, Tanavalee A, *et al.* (2020). Telomere shortening is associated with poor physical performance in knee osteoarthritis, *Biomedical Reports,* **13**, pp. 27.
20. Mosquera, A., Rego-Perez, I., Blanco, F. J. & Fernandez, J. L. (2019). Leukocyte telomere length in patients with radiographic knee osteoarthritis, *Environ Mol. Mutagen.,* **60**, pp. 298–301.
21. McAlindon, T., Roberts, M., Driban, J., Schaefer, L., Haugen, I. K., Smith, S. E., *et al.* (2018). Incident hand OA is strongly associated with reduced peripheral blood leukocyte telomere length, *Osteoarthritis Cartilage,* **26**, pp. 1651–1657.
22. Mollano, A. V., Martin, J. A. & Buckwalter, J. A. (2002). Chondrocyte senescence and telomere regulation: implications in cartilage aging and cancer (a brief review), *Iowa Orthop J,* **22**, pp. 1–7.
23. Yudoh, K., Nguyen v, T., Nakamura, H., Hongo-Masuko, K., Kato, T. & Nishioka, K. (2005). Potential involvement of oxidative stress in cartilage senescence and development of osteoarthritis: oxidative stress induces chondrocyte telomere instability and downregulation of chondrocyte function, *Arthritis Res Ther,* **7**, pp. R380–391.
24. Jiang, Y. (2022). Osteoarthritis year in review 2021: biology, *Osteoarthritis Cartilage,* **30**, pp. 207–215.
25. Arra, M., Swarnkar, G., Ke, K., Otero, J. E., Ying, J., Duan, X., *et al.* (2020). LDHA-mediated ROS generation in chondrocytes is a potential therapeutic target for osteoarthritis, *Nat Commun,* **11**, pp. 3427.
26. Hardingham, T. E., Oldershaw, R. A. & Tew, S. R. (2006). Cartilage, SOX9 and notch signals in chondrogenesis, *J Anat,* **209**, pp. 469–480.
27. Khan, I. M., Bishop, J. C., Gilbert, S. & Archer, C. W. (2009). Clonal chondroprogenitors maintain telomerase activity and Sox9 expression

during extended monolayer culture and retain chondrogenic potential, *Osteoarthritis Cartilage,* **17**, pp. 518–528.

28. Liu-Bryan, R. (2013). Synovium and the innate inflammatory network in osteoarthritis progression, *Curr Rheumatol Rep,* **15**, pp. 323.
29. Huang, J., Xie, Y., Sun, X., Zeh, H. J., 3rd, Kang, R., Lotze, M. T., *et al.* (2015). DAMPs, ageing, and cancer: The 'DAMP Hypothesis', *Ageing Res Rev,* **24**, pp. 3–16.
30. Lei, L., Mu, J., Zheng, Y. & Liu, Y. (2023). Selenium deficiency-induced oxidative stress causes myocardial injury in calves by activating inflammation, apoptosis, and necroptosis, *Antioxidants (Basel),* **12**, pp. 229.
31. Miwa, S., Kashyap, S., Chini, E. & von Zglinicki, T. (2022). Mitochondrial dysfunction in cell senescence and aging, *J Clin Invest,* **132**, pp. e158447.
32. Fernandez-Moreno, M., Rego-Perez, I. & Blanco, F. J. (2022). Is osteoarthritis a mitochondrial disease? What is the evidence, *Curr Opin Rheumatol,* **34**, pp. 46–53.
33. Loeser, R. F., Collins, J. A. & Diekman, B. O. (2016). Ageing and the pathogenesis of osteoarthritis, *Nat Rev Rheumatol,* **12**, pp. 412–420.
34. Fajardo, R. G., Farina, F. O., Rey, A. M., Rego-Perez, I., Blanco, F. J. & Garcia, J. L. F. (2021). Relationship between the dynamics of telomere loss in peripheral blood leukocytes from knee osteoarthritis patients and mitochondrial DNA haplogroups, *J Rheumatol,* **48**, pp. 1603–1607.
35. Tsai, L. K., Ou-Yang, H., Xu, J., Chen, C. M., Chang, W. F. & Sung, L. Y. (2022). Effects of recloning on the telomere lengths of mouse terc(+/−) nuclear transfer-derived embryonic stem cells, *Stem Cells Dev,* **31**, pp. 720–729.
36. Bondeson, J., Blom, A. B., Wainwright, S., Hughes, C., Caterson, B. & van den Berg, W. B. (2010). The role of synovial macrophages and macrophage-produced mediators in driving inflammatory and destructive responses in osteoarthritis, *Arthritis Rheum,* **62**, pp. 647–657.
37. Fukuda, K. (2009). [Progress of research in osteoarthritis. Involvement of reactive oxygen species in the pathogenesis of osteoarthritis], *Clin Calcium,* **19**, pp. 1602–1606.
38. Price, J. S., Waters, J. G., Darrah, C., Pennington, C., Edwards, D. R., Donell, S. T., *et al.* (2002). The role of chondrocyte senescence in osteoarthritis, *Aging Cell,* **1**, pp. 57–65.
39. Elliott, S., Hays, E., Mayor, M., Sporn, M. & Vincenti, M. (2003). The triterpenoid CDDO inhibits expression of matrix metalloproteinase-1,

matrix metalloproteinase-13 and Bcl-3 in primary human chondrocytes, *Arthritis Res Ther,* **5**, pp. R285–291.

40. Ashraf, S., Cha, B. H., Kim, J. S., Ahn, J., Han, I., Park, H., *et al.* (2016). Regulation of senescence associated signaling mechanisms in chondrocytes for cartilage tissue regeneration, *Osteoarthritis Cartilage,* **24**, pp. 196–205.
41. Kulkarni, P., Martson, A., Vidya, R., Chitnavis, S. & Harsulkar, A. (2021). Pathophysiological landscape of osteoarthritis, *Adv Clin Chem,* **100**, pp. 37–90.
42. Huang, Z., Lan, J. & Gao, X. (2021). Feprazone mitigates IL-1beta-induced cellular senescence in chondrocytes, *ACS Omega,* **6**, pp. 9442–9448.
43. Clerigues, V., Guillen, M. I., Gomar, F. & Alcaraz, M. J. (2012). Haem oxygenase-1 counteracts the effects of interleukin-1beta on inflammatory and senescence markers in cartilage-subchondral bone explants from osteoarthritic patients, *Clin Sci (Lond),* **122**, pp. 239–250.
44. Vincent, T. L. (2019). IL-1 in osteoarthritis: time for a critical review of the literature, *F1000Res,* **8**, pp. 1–8.
45. Dockrell, H. M. & Smith, S. G. (2017). What have we learnt about BCG vaccination in the last 20 years? *Front Immunol,* **8**, pp. 1134.
46. Gonzalez-Giraldo, Y., Garzon-Benitez, A. V., Forero, D. A. & Barreto, G. E. (2019). TERT inhibition leads to reduction of IL-6 expression induced by palmitic acid and interferes with the protective effects of tibolone in an astrocytic cell model, *J Neuroendocrinol,* **31**, pp. e12768.
47. Liao, Y., Ren, Y., Luo, X., Mirando, A. J., Long, J. T., Leinroth, A., *et al.* (2022). Interleukin-6 signaling mediates cartilage degradation and pain in posttraumatic osteoarthritis in a sex-specific manner, *Sci Signal,* **15**, pp. eabn7082.
48. Zhang, C., Jiang, S., Lu, Y. & Yuan, F. (2022). Butorphanol tartrate mitigates cellular senescence against tumor necrosis factor-alpha (TNF-alpha) in human HC-A chondrocytes, *Bioengineered,* **13**, pp. 5434–5442.
49. Fernandez, R. J., 3rd & Johnson, F. B. (2018). A regulatory loop connecting WNT signaling and telomere capping: possible therapeutic implications for dyskeratosis congenita, *Ann N Y Acad Sci,* **1418**, pp. 56–68.
50. Diala, I., Wagner, N., Magdinier, F., *et al.* (2013). Telomere protection and TRF2 expression are enhanced by the canonical Wnt signalling pathway, *EMBO Rep,* **14**, pp. 356–363.
51. Dai, S. M., Shan, Z. Z., Nakamura, H., Masuko-Hongo, K., Kato, T., Nishioka, K. & Yudoh, K. (2006). Catabolic stress induces features of chondrocyte

senescence through overexpression of caveolin 1: possible involvement of caveolin 1-induced down-regulation of articular chondrocytes in the pathogenesis of osteoarthritis, *Arthritis Rheum,* **54**, pp. 818–831.

52. Shane Anderson, A. & Loeser, R. F. (2010). Why is osteoarthritis an age-related disease? *Best Pract Res Clin Rheumatol,* **24**, pp. 15–26.
53. Yin, M. & Xu, Y. (2022). The protective effects of etomidate against interleukin-1beta (IL-1beta)-induced oxidative stress, extracellular matrix alteration and cellular senescence in chondrocytes, *Bioengineered,* **13**, pp. 985–994.
54. Labarre, K. W. & Zimmermann, G. (2022). Infiltration of the Hoffa's fat pad with stromal vascular fraction in patients with osteoarthritis of the knee: results after one year of follow-up, *Bone Rep,* **16**, pp. 101168.
55. Thompson, S. D., Pichika, R., Lieber, R. L., Budinger, G. R. S. & Lavasani, M. (2021). Systemic transplantation of adult multipotent stem cells functionally rejuvenates aged articular cartilage, *Aging Dis,* **12**, pp. 726–731.
56. Hudita, A., Galateanu, B., Dinescu, S., Costache, M., Dinischiotu, A., Negrei, C., *et al.* (2020). In vitro effects of cetylated fatty acids mixture from celadrin on chondrogenesis and inflammation with impact on osteoarthritis, *Cartilage,* **11**, pp. 88–97.

Chapter 14

Microbiome

George Pantazidis
Personal Wellness Health, Kalamaria, Greece
george.panta@personalwellness.health

14.1 Introduction

The microscopic universe of microorganisms, spanning bacteria to viruses, is extensively explored revealing their profound impact on the intricate fabric of life. The evolutionary journey, marked by endosymbiosis and the emergence of mitochondria and chloroplasts, uncovers the pivotal shift from anaerobic to aerobic life.

The microbiome is central to maintaining ecological equilibrium, particularly in its profound influence on the health of multicellular organisms notably within the human context. Navigating the interdisciplinary landscape of microbiome research, the focus lies on the dynamic symbiosis between microorganisms and human cells emphasizing the profound impact on health and well-being specifically centered around the gut microbiota.

Various facets of the relationship between the gut microbiota and health conditions are explored offering valuable insights into the impact of dysbiosis on diseases, genetic variations influencing

Telomeres: Biomarkers of a Healthy Life and Successful Aging
Edited by Aristidis Tsatsakis

ISBN 978-981-5129-49-6 (Hardcover), 978-1-003-56809-4 (eBook)
www.jennystanford.com

the gut microbiota, and the involvement of intestinal bacteria in metabolic defects and disease development. Finally, the role of the gut microbiota in metabolic syndrome, neurological disorders, allergies, oxidative stress, diet, and longevity is probed providing a holistic perspective on potential personalized therapeutic approaches.

14.2 Microbiome: the Emergence and Evolution of Life

When exploring the biosphere, the largest potential ecosystem, which encompasses the solid surface of the Earth and the atmosphere where the phenomenon of life develops, we encounter microorganisms everywhere. These small life forms, imperceptible to the naked eye, have contributed to the emergence of life and continue to play a pivotal role in its evolution. These microorganisms include bacteria, archaea, protozoa, fungi, and viruses.

Following the formation of the initial primordial cell through the assembly of biological macromolecules, according to the Endosymbiotic theory, we witness the emergence of prokaryotic cells and subsequently eukaryotic cells, the origin of which is the product of endosymbiosis between aerobic and anaerobic bacteria. Aerobic bacteria evolved into mitochondria, organelles that provide the necessary energy for the survival of anaerobic bacteria and led to their transformation into the first eukaryotic cells. In some other anaerobic environments, endosymbiosis resulted in the creation of plant eukaryotic cells. These eukaryotic cells, with the help of cyanobacteria, which served as chloroplasts, performed photosynthesis, and produced oxygen, both in aquatic environments and on land. This condition aided the evolution of life and the appearance of the first multicellular organisms. Mitochondria and chloroplasts are semi-autonomous organelles with their own genetic material and protein synthesis systems. Their appearance substantially contributed to the transition of the cell from anaerobic to aerobic life and the development of complexity and biodiversity on the planet [1].

Microorganisms participate in biological cycles, carry out reactions, ensure the bioavailability of essential chemicals, and meet the energy needs at both the cellular level of an organism and the balance of ecosystems. They even contribute to the generation of deposits of various energy sources for the development beyond the life and economy of the planet.

The totality of microorganisms and genes that exist in their genetic material is called the microbiome. It constitutes a distinct world, the balance of which is an essential requirement for protecting the planet from ecological disruptions and safeguarding the health of all multicellular organisms, particularly humans. The microbiome contributes to better living conditions for all organisms, improves their quality of life, and achieves longevity.

14.3 Analysis and Identification of the Microbiome

The analysis of the microbiome is an interdisciplinary approach that involves microbiology, genetics, ecology, biochemistry, molecular biology, and evolutionary biology.

The development of biological sciences has made it possible to apply omics technologies, which form the basis of metagenomics. To decrypt the identity of microorganisms, present on the planet, samples are initially collected from biotic and abiotic factors of ecosystems. Subsequently, there is a sequencing of the DNA bases of specific segments of their genetic material followed by the introduction of data into bioinformatics analysis systems.

In the last 15 years, the advent of next-generation sequencing (NGS) technology has brought about tremendous changes in microbiological research. After the application of Sanger sequencing, which could be used for the genetic analysis of microorganisms from cultures, cutting-edge NGS technology enabled the genetic analysis of non-cultivable microorganisms, which represent more than 99% of microorganisms today.

Specifically, the 16S rRNA gene can be used as a phylogenetic marker for bacterial classification, and the fungal genetic regions

ITS (internal transcribed spacer) for fungi. In bacteria, the 16S rRNA gene with a length of 1500 base pairs includes nine variable regions (V1–V9) scattered among strongly conserved sequences. The use of these nine variable regions is a significant tool for distinguishing bacterial strains. However, difficulties in their discrimination arise due to the similarity of the sequence of some of these variable regions. The problem of potential misclassification of bacteria at the genus and species level is resolved by the continuous development of science for the creation of a more comprehensive metagenomic analysis platform and the parallel application of the quantitative real-time polymerase chain reaction (qRT-PCR) method. This method allows rapid detection and quantification of target genes. qRT-PCR is highly sensitive and is considered the gold standard, especially in the fields of microbial diagnostics and the application of therapeutic schemes with probiotics.

Today, for both human gut and endometrial microbiota, as well as the microbiota mapped by detecting and quantifying bacteria in the human oral and nasal cavities, we have acquired data that can explain the emergence and assist in the treatment of chronic diseases, such as metabolic syndrome and obesity, inflammatory bowel diseases, autoimmune diseases, neurological and dermatological disorders, and human fertility.

14.4 Human Microbiome

Definition of the microbiome: The human microbiome is the essential microflora that resides on or within human tissues, bodily fluids, and anatomical sites as well as the genes present in these microorganisms [1]. Microorganisms in the human body colonize the skin, respiratory tissues, the urogenital and gastrointestinal tracts, and nearly any surface or cavity in the human body. They form a complex ecosystem composed of approximately 10^{14} bacterial cells, a substantial number relative to the total number of cells in the human body, of which a high percentage (20–40%) cannot be cultured.

Modern perspectives on the human microbiome primarily emerged from two major research programs that began in 2007: The

Human Microbiome Project funded by the U.S. National Institutes of Health (NIH), and a similar program funded by the European Union (MetaHIT Consortium) focusing on the gut microbiota. Both programs aimed to correlate the biodiversity of the human microbiome with differences in metabolic function and diseases of various individuals as well as to identify prospects for improving human health by monitoring or modifying the human microbiome. The human microbiome constitutes a dynamic functional system that develops in space and time in parallel with the normal development of the organism.

Human health is affected by both the interactions between microorganisms as well as between these microorganisms and human cells. The composition of the human microbiome is related to age. From the early stages of human life, the microbiome composition significantly affects the development of the immune system. Many exogenous and endogenous factors, such as diet, antimicrobial defense strategies, and immunity, affect human microbiota, particularly the gut microbiota, which hosts the largest number and variety of microbial populations. In turn, the microbiome's bioactive products shape human cells functioning locally and remotely. For example, bacteria break down dietary fiber into short-chain fatty acids (SCFAs) through fermentation. These SCFAs, such as acetate, propionate, and butyrate, serve as bioactive products with profound effects:

- **Locally: Gut Epithelial Cells**: SCFAs act as a primary energy source for the cells lining the intestinal walls (enterocytes). Butyrate, in particular, is known to enhance the health and integrity of the gut epithelial barrier influencing local cell function.
- **Remotely: Immune Modulation**: SCFAs can modulate immune responses systemically affecting immune cells in distant locations. For instance, butyrate has been shown to regulate immune cell activity in the spleen and peripheral blood.

Microbiota develops in various parts of the body from birth following ecological succession principles (Fig. 14.1). In fact, the microbiome of a 4-year-old neonate is related to the microbial

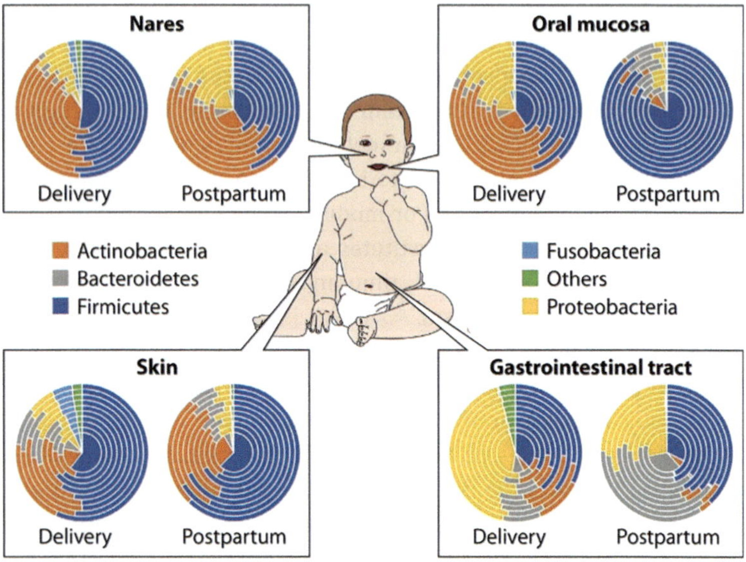

Figure 14.1 Microbial composition at various sites of the infant body at early stages of development with concentric circles indicating variability in different individuals [3].

composition of the same child at 120 days of age and even at 34 years of age indicating the importance of initial founding microorganisms in the microbial successional trajectories that follow [2]. The types of microorganisms acquired in early infancy play a crucial role in shaping the ongoing development of the microbiome emphasizing the enduring influence of early-life microbial colonization on an individual's microbiome into adulthood. Therefore, recent literature findings suggest that early-life microbiota can provide information about disease origin and the ability to identify those individuals at higher risk of developing the disease. Thus, the potential for timely, targeted intervention to prevent disease development might be possible. For example, the gut microbiome and metabolic dysfunction in infancy are characteristics of a higher risk of developing atopy and asthma in childhood. Furthermore, specific metabolites originating from microorganisms found at elevated concentrations in the feces of infants with asthma promote key features of established disease [3].

Today, study data indicates that the number of microorganisms in the human microbiome is in the order of tens of trillions, with 90% of them residing in the gut. They outnumber human cells by a factor of 10, and, to put it simply, the human entity consists of 90% microbes and 10% human cells. More than 10,000 different microbial species have been identified in the human body. Their genes are at least 100 times more numerous than human genes, and while individual humans share 99.9% genetic similarity with each other, their microbiomes can differ by 80–90% (individual microbial fingerprint).

People are colonized by microbes at birth, and this colonization process evolves with a remarkable degree of variability depending on factors, such as the type of delivery (natural delivery or cesarean section), feeding practices (breastfeeding or formula feeding), antibiotic use, and necessary infant care (Fig. 14.2). In the early years of life, the human microbiome is highly variable and is continuously

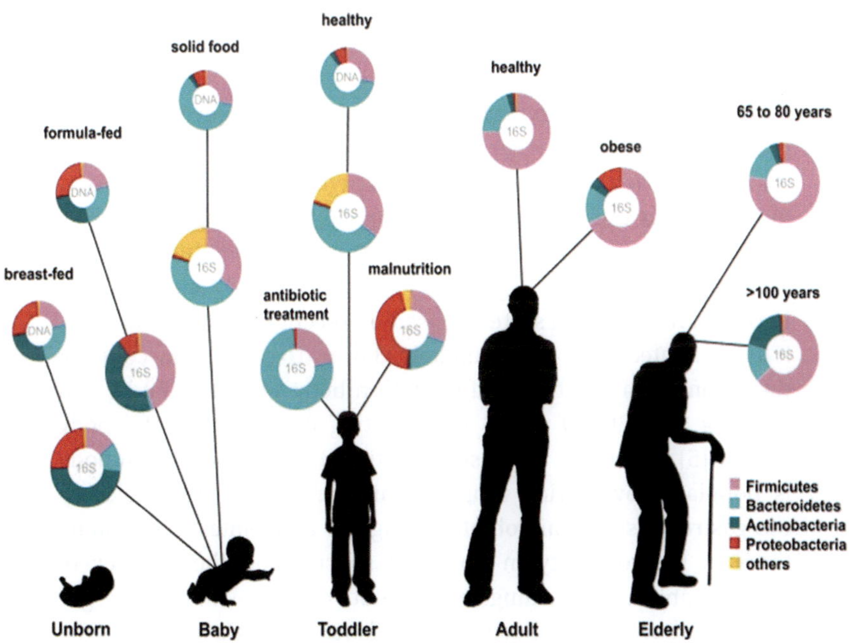

Figure 14.2 Relative abundance of important microbe genera in the composition of the human microbiota in various life stages [4].

enriched until adulthood, when it stabilizes. The adult microbiome is unique, although it can change to a lesser extent than in childhood and is influenced by dietary habits, hormonal disturbances as well as factors, such as travel, illnesses, and treatments. Lastly, in old age, the microbiome differentiates compared to younger ages and is affected by dietary changes, medication use, susceptibility to infections, and inflammatory conditions [4].

The post-genomic analysis will contribute to our understanding of microbial function, productivity, and interactions with the human host in space and time under various environmental influences. Comprehensive high-resolution studies applied to samples collected from different regions of the human body documenting the microbiome's function, productivity, and the host's response will lead to a broader understanding of our coevolution with microorganisms. Knowledge of our microbiome will be the most significant tool for shaping a balanced life full of health, energy, and well-being.

14.5 Human Intestinal Microbiota

The human body hosts many microorganisms. However, there are certain organs in which there are significantly more microorganisms than others, as they come into contact with the external environment, such as the oral cavity, skin, intestines, and vagina. In these areas, the types of microorganisms that are abundant differ.

The growth of microorganisms in the human body mainly occurs in the gastrointestinal system. Based on recent computational data, it is estimated that approximately 3.8×10^{13} bacteria colonize the colon of an adult individual with a body weight of 70 kg and a young age (20–30 years) representing 0.3% of the total body weight [5]. Generally, the gastrointestinal tract of the human body is populated by a wide range of microorganisms that make up the gastrointestinal microbiota. Along the gastrointestinal system, there is heterogeneity in both the species and the number of microorganisms. Regarding the qualitative composition of the gut flora, lactobacilli, helicobacter, and *Veillonella* bacteria develop in the stomach, while bacilli, streptococci, actinobacteria, actinomycetes, and corynebacteria develop in the small intestine (duodenum, jejunum, and ileum). Bacteria of the *Lachnospiraceae* family develop in the large intestine (colon). Regarding the quantitative composition of the gastrointestinal microbiota, the number of microorganisms is equal to 10 bacteria/g in the stomach, 10^3 bacteria/g in the regions of the small intestine and specifically in the duodenum, 10^5 bacteria/g in the jejunum, and it is 10^7 bacteria/g in the ileum. Finally, the majority of microorganisms, specifically 10^{12} bacteria/g found in feces, are located in the colon (large intestine). Consequently, along the gastrointestinal tract from the stomach to the small and large intestines, there is an increase in both the variety and abundance of microorganisms [6].

Today, due to the increased presence of microorganisms in the colon, when we refer to the microorganisms of the gastrointestinal system, we use the terms "gut microbiota" and "gut microbiome," respectively. The term "gut microbiota" refers to the total number of the microorganisms that inhabit the gastrointestinal system of humans and consists of bacteria, viruses, and eukaryotic microorganisms, while the term "gut microbiome" is the total of the genes of the microorganisms of the intestinal microflora of a person, which primarily live in the area of the colon [6].

The first catalog of microbial genes in the human gut was developed through metagenomic analysis of 124 European individuals by Qin et al. [7]. It includes 3.3 million genes with over 99% of them being of bacterial origin and the rest involving viral or eukaryotic genes. According to a more comprehensive reference gene catalog of the human gut microbiome announced by Li et al. [8], the gut microbiome contains approximately 9.9 million genes.

The bacterial phyla with their representative genera that make up the gut microbiota are as follows:

- **Bacteroidetes**: Gram-negative bacteria, including genera, such as *Bacteroides*, *Prevotella*, and *Corynebacterium*.
- **Firmicutes**: Gram-positive bacteria, including genera, such as *Bacillus*, *Clostridium*, *Mycoplasma*, *Faecalibacterium*, *Ruminococcus*, *Eubacterium*, *Streptococcus*, *Staphylococcus*, *Lactococcus*, *Lactobacillus*, *Enterococcus*, and *Roseburia*.
- **Actinobacteria**: Gram-positive bacteria, including genera, such as *Bifidobacterium*, *Eggerthella*, *Collinsella*, and *Propionibacterium*.

- **Proteobacteria**: Gram-negative bacteria, including genera, such as *Escherichia*, *Salmonella*, *Shigella*, *Klebsiella*, *Citrobacter*, *Helicobacter*, and *Serratia*.
- **Fusobacteria**: Gram-negative bacteria, including the genus *Fusobacterium*.
- **Verrucomicrobia**: Gram-negative bacteria, including the genus *Akkermansia*.

The gut microbiota is influenced by various factors, such as lifestyle, age, environment, health, medication, genetic material, metabolites, hormones, immunity, and diet.

Each person's gut microbiota is unique and changes throughout their life, from birth to old age. Among these factors, diet appears to have a particularly significant impact on the composition of the gut microbiota.

Bacteria in the gut interact with each other and with the host. There is a mutual relationship between the host and the bacteria that coexist with it. The host serves as a growth and nutrition space for symbiotic intestinal bacteria. In turn, the bacteria favor the host by facilitating the absorption of digested foods, ensuring the bioavailability of micronutrients, meeting the energy needs of the organism, and strengthening its resistance to various infections.

Specifically, the gut microbiota contributes to:

- Protecting the intestine from pathogenic microorganisms
- Maintaining the structural integrity of the intestinal mucosa
- Regulating intestinal motility
- Developing a healthy immune system
- Producing anti-inflammatory substances
- Producing 80% of antibodies (IgA)
- Host metabolism
- Drug metabolism
- Plant fibers, mucus, and fatty acids digestion
- Vitamins synthesis (mainly K and B complex vitamins)

According to Hollister et al. [9], enterotypes described in healthy adults can be classified into three types: enterotype 1 (abundant in *Bacteroides*), enterotype 2 (abundant in *Prevotella*), and enterotype 3 (abundant in *Ruminococcus*). Enterotype 1 bacteria exhibit a broad saccharolytic potential with the ability to produce energy from dietary carbohydrates and proteins, while enterotype 2 degrades glycoproteins in the gut mucus layer. Enterotype 3 is associated with mucin degradation and membrane sugar transport. These enterotypes also play significant metabolic roles with enterotype 1 being associated with the synthesis of biotin (B7), riboflavin (B2), pantothenic acid (B5), and ascorbic acid (C). Enterotype 2 is dominant in the synthesis of thiamine (B1) and folic acid (B9).

Today, an increasing number of studies highlight bidirectional interactions between the gastrointestinal tract, the enteric nervous system, and the central nervous system, discussing the gut-brain axis, which positions the gut microbiota as our "second brain" [10]. This axis is formed by a vast number of beneficial microorganisms and neural fibers that continuously interact and, through specific signaling molecules such as neurotransmitters, enhance mood and ensure mental health. Gut bacteria stimulate the enteric nervous system, which, in turn, controls functions like immune responses, digestion, heart rate, and mood. Some gut bacteria also trigger the release of serotonin, a neurotransmitter that stabilizes mood, while others participate in the synthesis of gamma-aminobutyric acid (GABA), another neurotransmitter with inhibitory roles. On the other hand, changes in the gut microbiota composition have been associated with the pathogenesis of various neurological disorders, including stress, autism, depression, Parkinson's disease, and Alzheimer's disease. Moreover, essential neurotransmitters, such as norepinephrine (NA), dopamine (DA), and acetylcholine (ACh) are produced by intestinal bacteria, influencing both neurological diseases and gastrointestinal disorders as well as fat metabolism [11].

It is clear that diet plays an exceptionally important role in shaping the composition of the gut microbiota. Research findings indicate that dietary changes can lead to significant, temporary changes in gut microbiota within 24 hours [12]. In pathological conditions, as previously mentioned, there is a disruption in the balance of microorganisms. Adopting the right dietary pattern results in the composition of a balanced gut microbial community. Maintaining gut health and avoiding dietary inflammation contribute significantly to the prevention of chronic pathological conditions while ensuring maximum energy and well-being.

14.6 Dysbiosis

Dysbiosis is the disorder or imbalance of microbial populations, both in terms of their numbers and diversity, which is associated with damage or leakage in the intestine. This condition increases the risk of bacterial translocation, which is the movement of bacterial antigens or substances from the gut mucosa into the bloodstream, leading to a range of phenomena such as the development of chronic systemic inflammation and damage to various human organs.

Dysbiosis results in the abnormal functioning of the human immune system and has a negative impact on health, contributing to various pathological conditions. Specifically, disruptions in the composition of the gut microbiota are linked to complex and multifactorial diseases. These include autoimmune diseases, idiopathic inflammatory bowel diseases (such as Crohn's disease), colorectal cancer, obesity, neurological disorders, acne, and various types of allergies that manifest as atopic dermatitis.

However, dysbiosis is not a well-defined condition. Various indicators have been proposed and applied to characterize it. Such indicators can help in diagnosing diseases and adverse conditions, predicting treatment outcomes, and providing information beyond assessments of gut microbial diversity. It is worth noting that some researchers have even applied the term dysbiosis in situations related to improved health conditions; for example, type 2 diabetes treatment with metformin. Given that the prefix "dys-" means "bad," "difficult," or "disordered," we consider the term to imply an adverse condition that may result from the loss of beneficial microorganisms, excessive growth of potentially harmful organisms, and a loss of overall microbial diversity.

The recognized markers of dysbiosis can be categorized into five groups based on the following methodology. Specifically, the gut microbiota (GA) dysbiosis test, developed by genetic analysis AS in Oslo, Norway, represents a large-scale analysis of bacterial markers that determine dysbiosis in the gut microbiota. It uses a set of 54 detectors targeting the 16S rRNA gene (V3–V7 region) covering more than 300 bacterial markers related to the phyla *Firmicutes*, *Bacteroidetes*, *Proteobacteria*, *Actinobacteria*, and *Verrucomicrobia*,

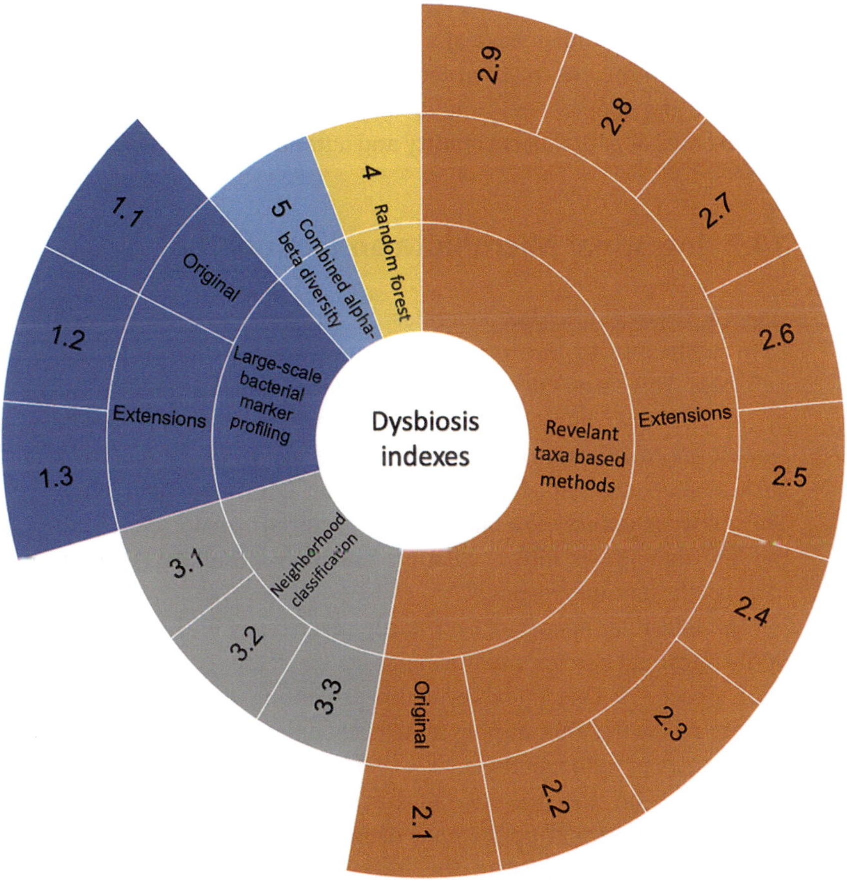

Figure 14.3 Diagram illustrating the appearance of different indices used to characterize the dysbiosis of microbial communities. The numbers presented at the outermost level refer to various indices [13].

encompassing 10 bacterial classes, 36 genera, and more than 300 species.

The GA dysbiosis test assigns a score of 1–5 to each sample (Fig. 14.3). A score greater than 2 indicates that the microbial profile differs from a selected reference population, thus characterizing it as "dysbiosis." A score of 2 or lower is defined as "eubiosis" indicating a healthy state. The GA dysbiosis test, as described above, was initially developed, and validated for the diagnosis and prediction of inflammatory bowel diseases (IBD) and irritable bowel syndrome (IBS). However, studies have also applied the test to assess its correlation with the effects of various interventions, both therapeutic (invasive and non-invasive) and dietary, in gastrointestinal diseases and in cases of pathological obesity and autoimmune diseases [13].

14.7 Intestinal Microbiota and Immunity

One of the most important roles of the intestinal microbiota is to contribute to the formation of an antimicrobial protection network. This protection network includes the microorganisms of the intestinal microbiota themselves, which act competitively against the colonization of pathogenic bacteria as well as substances such as mucus, antimicrobial proteins, and IgA immunoglobulins. This network reduces the likelihood of bacterial translocation from the intestinal lumen into circulation, thus preventing the initiation of a specific immune response.

The intestinal microbiota primarily contributes to the integrity of the intestinal barrier and the maintenance of the gastrointestinal tract structure. This is achieved by promoting the synthesis of protein molecules that inhibit cellular shedding or by maintaining the integrity of tight junctions.

In the colon, the presence of mucus produced by the Goblet cells of the intestinal epithelium, composed of mucin molecules, is continuous and dense in the lower layers, with outer layers containing nutrients like glycans for the growth of microorganisms [14]. This mucus layer forms a protective barrier for epithelial cells, making it difficult for pathogenic factors to access cell receptors. In contrast, in the small intestine where mucus is absent, antimicrobial function is achieved through the participation of proteins such as cytokines and lysozyme produced and secreted by Paneth cells [15].

The PTPN2 gene in intestinal epithelial cells acts as a negative regulator of signaling induced by the proinflammatory cytokine IFN-γ, which plays a significant role in the pathogenesis of Crohn's disease (CD) and increases the permeability of the intestinal epithelial barrier. PTPN2 protects the function of the epithelial barrier by limiting IFN-γ's ability to increase epithelial permeability, preventing the induction of a protein that forms pores (claudin-2). Loss of PTPN2 function also leads to significant changes in the gut microbiota, specifically increasing E. coli, exacerbating inflammation in IBD conditions [16].

Additionally, the overgrowth of pathogenic bacteria is controlled by the presence of IgA immunoglobulins produced by plasma cells of the intestinal *lamina propria* following activation by resident dendritic cells. IgA plays a fundamental role in the defense of the mucosa by coating and trapping microorganisms. The production of IgA is influenced significantly by the protein expressed by the My-D88 gene. This molecule acts as a mediator of intracellular signaling from cell surface receptors like TLR and IL-1 to the interior of cells involved in IgA secretion, promoting the synthesis of nuclear transcription factors, which, in turn, regulate genes involved in the control of immune responses and inflammatory reactions in the body.

Our bodies host beneficial bacteria, while also coming into contact with pathogens from the environment. The immune system can recognize commensal bacteria, while simultaneously having the capability for antimicrobial action. The microflora in the intestine contributes to the host's resistance to various infections but also facilitates the absorption of nutrients derived from food digestion. The ability to distinguish between potential pathogens and harmless microorganisms is accomplished by pattern-recognition receptors (PRRs) found in the epithelial and immune cells of the gut. These receptors include toll-like receptors, NOD-like receptors, RIG-I-like receptors, and cell-surface C-type lectin-like receptors [17]. When PRRs recognize molecular patterns (pathogen-associated molecular patterns-PAMP) related to pathogenic bacteria or other microorganisms (such as lipopolysaccharides LPS, peptidoglycans, glycans, proteins, and nucleic acids), they activate cellular responses to neutralize the pathogenic microorganism including the activation of the transcription factor NF-κB, which, in turn, can regulate inflammation.

NF-κB targets inflammation not only by directly increasing the production of inflammatory cytokines, chemokines, and adhesion molecules but also by regulating cell proliferation, apoptosis, morphogenesis, and differentiation. The inflammatory response is triggered by proinflammatory cytokines like tumor necrosis factor (TNF), interleukin-1 (IL-1), and interleukin-6 (IL-6). These cytokines are pleiotropic[a] proteins that regulate cell death in inflammatory tissues, modify vascular endothelial permeability, recruit blood cells to inflamed tissues, and induce the production of acute-phase proteins [18]. Therefore, initially, the innate defense mechanisms of the organism are activated to combat pathogens. If an effective neutralization does not occur, the organism's adaptive immune defense is activated.

Specifically, macrophages characterized by the production of proinflammatory cytokines like IL-1, IL-6, interleukin-12 (IL-12), TNF-α, and chemokines, promote the differentiation of Th1[b] and Th17[c] T-cells, which, in turn, mediate inflammation. Conversely, macrophages that produce anti-inflammatory cytokines like interleukin-10 (IL-10) and interleukin-13 (IL-13) have predominantly anti-inflammatory effects and contribute to tissue healing.

CD4+ T-cells differentiate into various subsets of effector T-cells including Th1, Th2, Th17, follicular helper T-cells (Tfh), and regulatory T (Treg) cells. Th1 and Th17 cells are generally considered proinflammatory T-lymphocytes because they mediate inflammatory responses against infections and autoimmune conditions. Th1 cells are characterized by the secretion of IFN-γ, a cytokine that promotes cellular immunity and participates in inflammatory processes. NF-κB promotes the differentiation of Th1 cells by regulating T-cell receptor (TCR) signaling and inducing cytokines like IL-12 that drive Th1 differentiation. Th17 cells, on the other hand, are known for producing interleukin-17 (IL-17), a proinflammatory cytokine that activates monocytes and neutrophils at the site of inflammation in response to pathogen invasion or autoantigens. The differentiation of CD4+ T-cells is also regulated by cytokines secreted by antigen-presenting cells and other immune cells as well as innate factors of T-cells. Th2 cells

[a]Pleitropic gene is the gene that influences more than one characteristic, which is not related to each other.

[b]Th1 T-cells, or T-helper type 1 cells, are a subset of T-helper cells that primarily produce interferon-gamma and play a key role in cell-mediated immunity.

[c]Th17 T-cells, or T-helper type 17 cells, produce interleukin-17 and are involved in immune responses against extracellular bacteria and fungi.

promote humoral immune responses in which specific antibodies are generated against extracellular pathogens through the secretion of interleukin-4 (IL-4) and other cytokines. Regulatory T (Treg) cells formed by the differentiation of CD4+ T-cells, play a crucial role in controlling immune responses to prevent autoimmunity and chronic inflammation. Another subset of T-cells known as follicular helper T (Tfh) cells contributes to the maturation of B-cells ultimately producing antibodies through the production of interleukin-22 (IL-22).

The education of the human immune system by the gut microbiota is essential both for establishing tolerance to the beneficial microorganisms that help sustain the body in various ways and for developing the immune defense of the human organism, both innate and adaptive, against the invasion of pathogens, thus ensuring health. Disruption of such a complex mechanism like the immune system would lead to the development of inflammation, which could be the cause of many chronic diseases.

14.8 Intestinal Microbiota and Diseases

14.8.1 Gastrointestinal Diseases

14.8.1.1 Irritable bowel syndrome (IBS)

It is a chronic gastrointestinal disorder characterized by recurring symptoms such as abdominal pain and abnormal bowel habits in the absence of an obvious organic cause. It is one of the most common diseases observed in patients visiting gastroenterology clinics. Based on the Rome IV criteria, widely used for diagnosing IBS and classifying its subtypes based on stool characteristics and bowel movements, the following conditions are recognized [19]:

- IBS-D with predominant diarrhea
- IBS-C with predominant constipation
- IBS-M mixed subtype
- IBS-U unclassified

Current treatments for IBS chosen in medical practice are generally symptomatic with limited effectiveness. The use of antibiotics, modified diets, lifestyle changes, and exposure to pathogens can disrupt the gut microbiota balance and lead to exacerbation. Small intestinal bacterial overgrowth (SIBO), characterized by an overgrowth of bacteria similar to those in the colon, such as *Klebsiella*, *Enterococcus*, and *Escherichia*, is often observed in the small intestine of IBS patients [20, 21]. SIBO can potentially cause increased intestinal permeability, low-grade inflammation, altered motility, and reduced absorption of bile salts as well as affect the activity of the enteric nervous system (ENS). In addition to the bacteria mentioned above, overgrowth of ancient gut species has also been associated with IBS symptoms. For instance, *Methanobrevibacter smithii* produces abundant methane gas in the small intestine, influencing intestinal motility and delaying transit potentially relating to IBS-C [22]. Furthermore, microbial diversity in stool samples from IBS patients is lower than in healthy individuals. Reduced levels of *Faecalibacterium prausnitzii*, *Bifidobacterium*, and *Lactobacillus* have been observed in IBS cases, especially in IBS-D [23]. Bacteria, such as *Escherichia coli*, *Campylobacter jejuni*, and *Salmonella spp*., as well as viruses like cytomegalovirus, and parasites (*Blastocystis*, *Cryptosporidium*, *Giardia*), are often identified as causative microorganisms in cases of post-infectious IBS [11]. In IBS-related dysbiosis, both the quality and quantity of microbial metabolites (bile acids [Bas], short-chain fatty acids [SCFAs], vitamin D, vitamin B6, and tryptophan [Trp]), neurotransmitters (histamine [His], serotonin [5HT], glutamic acid [Glu], γ-aminobutyric acid [GABA], norepinephrine [NA], dopamine [DA], and acetylcholine [Ach]), compounds related to TLR receptors, neuroendocrine factors (GLP-1, PYY), and proteins are significantly altered compared to those in healthy conditions (Fig. 14.4) [11].

Dysfunction of the gut barrier and increased epithelial permeability, visceral hypersensitivity, pain, changes in bowel motility, immune cell activation, and the development of inflammation are key features in the pathogenesis of IBS.

14.8.1.2 Inflammatory bowel diseases (IBDs)

These include Crohn's disease (CD) and ulcerative colitis (UC), which affect 0.3–0.5% of the global population [24]. The onset and devel-

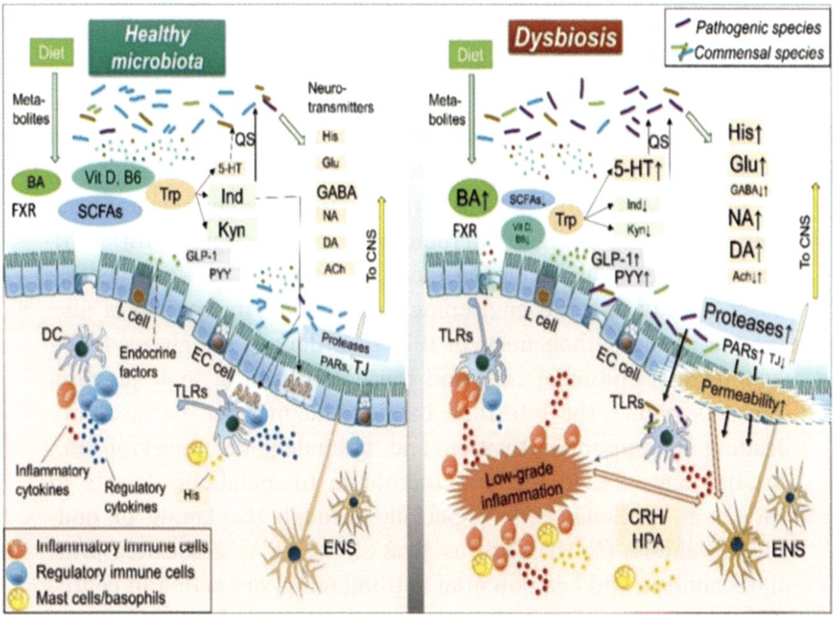

Figure 14.4 Mechanisms of intestinal dysfunction caused by dysbiosis in irritable bowel syndrome (IBS) [11].

opment of IBD, a type of idiopathic inflammatory gastrointestinal disease (IIGD), are influenced by multiple factors, such as genetic susceptibility, immune factors, and gut microbiota [25, 26].

Several studies have confirmed that the gut microbiota composition in IIGD patients is significantly different from that of healthy individuals [27, 28]. Compared to healthy individuals, levels of *Bifidobacterium longum* in UC, as well as *Eubacterium rectale, Faecalibacterium prausnitzii, Roseburia intestinalis*, and other beneficial bacteria in CD and UC, are significantly reduced. Meanwhile, bacteria from the *Ruminococcus* genus and *Bacteroides fragilis* are increased in both CD and UC [29]. In CD patients, *Clostridium leptum* is decreased, while *Actinomyces spp., Veillonella spp.*, and *Escherichia coli* are increased. In UC patients, *E. coli* and *Eubacterium rectum* are increased, while *Akkermansia muciniphila* is decreased [30].

Klebsiella pneumoniae invades the intestinal epithelial cells and interacts with macrophages to induce the release of interleukin IL-1β and tumor necrosis factor (TNF) [31]. *Fusobacterium nucleatum* activates caspase 3 (CARD3) through NOD2 in the colonic epithelial cells, thereby inducing the IL-17F, NF-κB signaling pathway and promoting the development of intestinal inflammation [32].

Genetic variations that affect the immune system play a crucial role in shaping the gut microbiota in the etiology of IBD [33]. There is increasing evidence that the interplay between genetic susceptibility and the environment in the gut microbiota is also related to the pathogenesis of IBD. Disorders in the glycosylation of intestinal epithelial cells and the destruction of their junction proteins reduce the intestinal barrier and increase permeability leading to immune activation and ultimately the onset of IBD. Studies have linked the gut microbiota to metabolic defects in intestinal epithelial cells, especially through the family of nod-like receptors (NLR), such as NLRX1, which is associated with mitochondria and has potential anti-inflammatory action in colitis. The NLRX1 receptor is essential for maintaining barrier function in the intestinal epithelial cells and contributes to glutamine metabolism that alleviates inflammation.

Faecalibacterium prausnitzii produces butyrate, which belongs to short-chain fatty acids (SCFAs) and has anti-inflammatory effects. SCFAs regulate the immunity of the mucosa, promoting the growth of B-cells and the differentiation and expansion of regulatory T-cells (Treg), and may activate the production of pro-inflammatory cytokines. Butyric acid can act on the immune cells in the intestinal mucosa and increase the quantity and activity of Treg while inhibiting the activity of neutrophils, macrophages, and dendritic cells. Dysbiosis and the increase of inflammatory cells in the intestine of IBD patients are associated with the reduction of SCFAs [34].

On the other hand, intestinal bacteria control the transformation of bile acids to regulate host immunity [35]. Modified bile acids can activate two types of immune cells, Tregs, and Th17, which regulate the immune response by suppressing or promoting inflammation.

Immunoglobulin A (IgA) is the most common subtype of antibodies in the intestine. It is transported by polymeric IgA receptors (pIgR) to host epithelial cells and is then released into the intestinal lumen as secretory IgA (sIgA). In a stable environment, sIgA is essential for the dynamic balance within the gut microbiota.

The interaction between T-cells and the gut microbiota can influence the onset of IBD. The response triggered by Th cells protects the host from harmful pathogens, but the overactivation of Th cells is associated with the initiation and development of intestinal inflammation. It is generally believed that the development of Crohn's disease (CD) is mainly associated with Th1 cells and the activation of Th17 cells, while the onset of ulcerative colitis (UC) is a result of the interaction between Th1 and Th2 cells [36, 37]. Studies have shown that the frequency of IBD is more correlated with the activity of Th17 cells. The cytokines produced by Th17 cells are mainly IL-17 and IL-22, which play a vital role in mediating immune damage and autoimmune diseases. IL-22 is considered to have a protective role when acute colitis occurs.

Treg cells are primarily used to maintain the balance of T cells. According to data for humans, the development of IBD is associated with the reduction or abnormal function of Treg cells. Due to the lack of immune suppression regulation of Treg cells, Th cells (Th1, Th2, and Th17) can trigger an excessive immune response in the intestine ultimately leading to damage to the intestinal mucosa [38]. Th17 and Treg cells are in balance under normal conditions. Excessive increases in Th17 and decreases in Treg cells lead to an imbalance in the Th17/Treg ratio. The disruption of this balance can lead to damage to the intestinal mucosa. IL-6 and low levels of TGF-β can stimulate T cells to differentiate into Th17. High levels of TGF-β can suppress the production of Th17 cells and promote the production of Treg cells. Th17 cells can also inhibit the proliferation of Treg cells. Th17 cells increase, and Treg cells decrease in the peripheral blood of patients with IBD indicating that the Th17/Treg imbalance plays a significant role in the development and maintenance of IBD. The gut microbiota can induce the differentiation of T-cells into Th17 or Treg cells by shaping the intestinal microenvironment [39]. Conversely, other intestinal bacteria can also promote the increase of Treg cells with anti-inflammatory action.

Therefore, dysbiosis, cytokine imbalance, and disruption of the mucosal barrier contribute to the induction of mucosal inflammation and the development of IBD. Today, therapeutic protocols based on monoclonal antibodies, mainly targeting TNF, in combination with specialized dietary protocols supported by specific probiotics and nanomedicines (HABN), can lead to effective remission of IBD. Along with cutting-edge technology for analyzing the gut microbiota, metabolic analysis, and immune response analysis, we can predict the personalized response of patients to specific drugs.

14.8.2 Colorectal Cancer

Colorectal cancer is a particularly common cancer. The transition from dysplastic adenoma to adenocarcinoma is due to mutations that include oncogenes, such as the adenomatous polyposis coli (APC) gene, P53 (TP53), and the beta-catenin gene (CTNNB1) as well as oncogenes such as KRAS. Environmental factors such as diet and lifestyle also seem to influence the development of this cancer since its incidence is much lower in developing countries than in developed ones. Inflammation in the intestine is associated with the development of polyps and adenocarcinomas in the colon. The gut microbiota can affect the carcinogenesis mechanism either through diet or its anti-inflammatory action on intestinal mucus. Increased levels of *Bacteroides, Clostridium spp*, and *Bifidobacterium spp* are associated with colorectal cancer development, while conversely, the gut microbiota of individuals with a low risk of cancer is abundant in bacteria that produce lactic acid, such as *Lactobacillus spp.*, and *Eubacterium aerofaciens*. Additionally, bacteria with polyketide synthase genes produce colibactin, a toxin that causes severe DNA damage in infected cells. Other bacteria are likely to be involved in the evolution of colorectal cancer through products that activate TLR and induce the cytokine IL-17 synthesis by helper T lymphocytes, which activates the STAT3 transcription factor in epithelial cells, increasing their survival and proliferation, leading to additional mutations, resulting in dysplasia and possibly cancer. Other studies report that *Fusobacterium nucleatum* as well as bacteria like *Peptostreptococcus, Parvimonas*, and *Porphyromonas*, which are components of the oral microbiome, may be related to cancer development [40].

Fusobacterium nucleatum is a common element of the oral cavity, but if it is abundant in the colon, it is associated with regional lymph node metastasis [41] and, eventually, colon cancer formation [42]. *Fusobacterium nucleatum* promotes colorectal cancer through multiple mechanisms. *Fusobacterium nucleatum* has a direct interaction with epithelial cells, invading them after binding to specific adhesion molecules (FadA) and activating genes that promote inflammation [43]. Also, *Fusobacterium nucleatum*, with another protein, Fap2, binds to a receptor on T cells and natural killer cells, eventually blocking cytotoxic activity against cancer cells [44]. On the other hand, several post-genomic studies have identified significant enrichment of bacteria that produce short-chain fatty acids (SCFAs), particularly butyric acid (*Lachnospiraceae* and *Faecalibacterium*), in healthy controls compared to those suffering from colorectal cancer as well as in patients with a decreased presence of common bacteria (*Bifidobacteria, Lactobacillus, Ruminococcus*) that generally produce SCFAs. SCFAs strengthen barrier functions, have anti-inflammatory effects, and regulate the immune response by mechanisms such as reducing oxygen levels in mucus cells [45]. In this way, SCFAs have strong anti-inflammatory and anticancer effects [46]. Butyric acid suppresses carcinogenesis through multiple mechanisms by regulating cell proliferation and apoptosis, inducing Treg cells, and maintaining epithelial barrier function by increasing tight junction expression, which is essential for preventing inflammation. Diet can prevent or increase gastrointestinal cancers by regulating the gut microbiota [47]. The Mediterranean diet pattern is one of the healthiest and most sustainable dietary models, based mainly on vegetables, fruits, legumes, nuts, cereals, fish, and unsaturated fats such as olive oil. Compliance with the MedDiet model has been reported to positively affect the gut microbiota and the function of the immune system as well as the metabolic balance of the human body [48]. Adopting the Mediterranean dietary pattern is based on the regular consumption of monounsaturated fatty acids (MUFAs) and polyunsaturated fatty acids (PUFAs), polyphenols and other antioxidants, high intake of prebiotic fibers and low glycemic index carbohydrates and consuming more plant proteins than animal proteins [49]. Recent data indicate that as compliance with the MedDiet pattern increases, mortality is lower, and the frequency of gastrointestinal diseases decreases [48, 50]. Moreover, according to the European Prospective Investigation into Cancer and Nutrition

(EPIC), adherence to the MedDiet pattern delayed the onset of colorectal cancer.

14.8.3 Metabolic Syndrome

Metabolic syndrome (MS), as defined by the World Health Organization (WHO), is a complex group of metabolic disorders characterized by abdominal obesity, hypertension, insulin resistance, and hyperlipidemia [51]. MS is a phenotype created by the complex interaction of host intrinsic factors, such as genetics, the endocrine system, the immune system, oxidative stress, and the gut microbiome, as well as external factors like diet, medication, and lifestyle. Recent evidence indicates the role of gut microbiota as a significant factor affecting the host's normal metabolism.

Individuals with MS often have alterations in their gut microbiota composition and may exhibit dysbiosis, which can lead to metabolic imbalance in the host. This is caused by a low-grade inflammatory response in the body, which weakens the gut barrier and results in insulin resistance, setting off a chain of events that promotes the progression of MS. Consuming a typical Western diet high in fat and sugars fuels the evolution and development of MS.

Sugars and processed foods lead to gut dysbiosis and metabolic endotoxemia, resulting in low-grade inflammation, insulin resistance, dyslipidemia, obesity, and metabolic disorders. Conversely, dietary fiber is a critical nutritional component that maintains gut health by regulating macronutrients and the host's physiology. Dietary fiber enhances insulin sensitivity, helps with weight management, and reduces inflammation by increasing short-chain fatty acids (SCFAs) produced by gut microbiota, which can reinforce the gut barrier and reduce the risk of inflammation and metabolic diseases [52].

Obesity is characterized by an altered *Firmicutes/Bacteroides* ratio, with a higher relative abundance of *Firmicutes*. This occurs because *Firmicutes* bacteria more efficiently metabolize energy sources compared to *Bacteroidetes*, also promoting the efficient absorption of calories and, consequently, weight gain. Additionally, the risk of atherosclerosis has been linked to the gut microbiota, especially due to enhanced choline and phosphatidylcholine metabolism that generates the pro-atherogenic compound trimethylamine-N-oxide (TMAO). Specifically, anaerobic bacteria, such as *Bacteroides, Alistipes,* and *Bilophila* have been found to increase with the consumption of animal protein from red meat and are associated with elevated levels of trimethylamine-N-oxide (TMAO), which increases the risk of cardiovascular diseases. Overall, higher consumption of animal protein leads to a decrease in the total number of bacteria and, more specifically, beneficial species such as *Bifidobacterium* and *Eubacterium*. Additionally, *Lactobacillus spp.* has been shown to alleviate metabolic complications associated with obesity. Obese individuals, with a high initial relative abundance of *Akkermansia muciniphila*, tend to have greater improvements in metabolic parameters related to obesity (insulin tolerance, plasma triglycerides, and body fat distribution) following dietary intervention [12].

Disorders of liver enzymes, such as increased gamma-glutamyl transpeptidase (GGT), are closely related to atherosclerosis, cardiovascular disease, and decreased glucose tolerance [53]. They can predict the risk of diabetes, hypertension, plaque sclerosis, and independent cardiovascular disease [54]. The likely reason is that GGT is involved not only in extracellular glutathione hydrolysis but also serves as an indicator of oxidative stress and subclinical inflammation [55], which are considered important mechanisms in atherosclerosis.

Gut microbiota in individuals with hyperlipidemia is characterized by low microbial diversity, high abundance of *Actinobacteria*, and a lower abundance of the phyla *Proteobacteria* and *Bacteroidetes*. Furthermore, hypertensive patients also display a dysbiosis pattern due to the lack of diversity in their gut microbiota. Studies have shown that, as compared to healthy controls, pre-hypertensive and hypertensive populations exhibited a significant reduction in microbial abundance and increased prevalence of harmful bacteria, such as *Prevotella* and *Klebsiella*.

Depending on the pathological condition identified within the metabolic syndrome, both individualized dietary intervention and the application of specific enhancement protocols will improve the microbial balance and pathological indicators.

14.8.4 Neurological Disorders

In the human body, the communication between the nerve cells of the gut and the brain through the gut-brain axis highlights the crucial role of the gut microbiota. The regulation of neuroinflammation and gastrointestinal symptoms through the gut-brain axis has a significant impact on the neurological function of the body not only through the secretion of neurotransmitters but also through synapses and the immune system. Studies have shown that patients with inflammatory bowel disease (IBD) often suffer from anxiety and depression which may be related to changes in the gut microbiota.

Brain activity can regulate the gut microbiota through the hypothalamic-pituitary-adrenal (HPA) axis. The brain can control gut functions, such as peripheral motility, gastric acid and mucus secretion, antimicrobial peptides, and other peptides, intestinal permeability, and the immune response, through sympathetic and parasympathetic nerve fibers directly or by stimulating the enteric nervous system. Consequently, these changes in gut physiology can influence the composition and activity of the microbiota. Furthermore, the host's neuroendocrine system can communicate with the gut microbiota directly through the release of signaling molecules of the host including catecholamines, serotonin (5HT), dynorphin, and cytokines, released by neurons, immune cells, and enteroendocrine cells. The gut microbiota can influence the central nervous system (CNS) through molecules such as peptide-1 resembling glucagon and peptide YY released by enteroendocrine cells (EECs) of the intestinal epithelium as well as neuroactive molecules (γ-aminobutyric acid, 5HT, norepinephrine, and dopamine), short-chain fatty acids (SCFAs), and secondary bile acids that could enter the systemic circulation and travel to the brain to regulate neuronal function [56].

Specifically, in patients with schizophrenia (SCZ), disturbances in the *Lactobacillales* family were observed. In patients with major depressive disorder (MDD), changes were observed in various families, including *Bifidobacteriales*, *Flavobacteriales*, and *Sphingobacteriales*. In patients with multiple sclerosis (MS), increased levels of *Pseudomonas*, *Mycoplasma*, *Haemophilus*, *Blautia*,

Methanobrevibacter, Akkermansia, and *Dorea* and reduced levels of *Parabacteroides, Adlercreutzia*, and *Prevotella* were found. Disturbances in the presence of *Veionella parvula, Bacteroides caccae, Bacteroides coprocola, Bacteroides ovatus, Bacteroides uniformis* as well as bacteria of the *Collinsela, Gemmiger, Streptococcus, Uribacter,* and *Lachnospiraceae* families were observed in patients with attention deficit hyperactivity disorder (ADHD). In patients on the autism spectrum (ASD), disruptions were observed in the genera *Bacteroidetes, Desulfovibrio, Devosia, and Dialister.*

At the gender level, the most common disorder observed in conditions, such as ADHD, anorexia nervosa (AN), and bipolar disorder (BD) was an increase in *Actinobacteria*. Similarly, in conditions like Alzheimer's disease (AD), amyotrophic lateral sclerosis (ALS), generalized anxiety disorder (GAD), ADHD, and MDD, a decrease in *Firmicutes* was observed. At the genus level, the most frequent change in ALS and MS was an increase in the bacterium *Akkermansia* and an increase in the bacteria of the *Bacteroides* genus in patients with ADHD, AN, GAD, and MS [57].

Finally, studies have shown that patients with Parkinson's disease (PD) had increased levels of *Akkermansia* in their feces, while bacteria of the *Clostridium, Faecalibacterium*, and *Prevotella genera*, as well as the content of short-chain fatty acids (SCFA), were significantly lower than in healthy individuals indicating that the gut ecological imbalance of PD patients was related to the reduction of SCFA levels [58, 59].

The regulation of the gut microbiota and the maintenance of health through dietary improvements and reinforcement with specific probiotics, such as *Lactobacillus rhamnosus,* which has been found to function as a therapeutic supplement and may reduce the risk of neuropsychiatric disorders in infants with autism spectrum disorders, as well as the administration of prebiotics or fecal microbiota transplantation (FMT), could lead to new insights for the treatment of neurological and psychological disorders.

14.8.5 Allergies

From birth, microorganisms from the environment begin to colonize various parts of the human body. Vaginal birth, as opposed to cesarean section, and breastfeeding have been shown to increase the diversity of a baby's microbiota, providing protection from allergies later in life. Breastfeeding directly provides beneficial bacteria of the genera *Lactobacillus* and *Bifidobacterium* to the infant and is rich in sugars known as oligosaccharides that nourish these microbes, which, in turn, aid in the development of the baby's immune system through molecular signals.

Through the gut microbiota-immune system axis, food allergy (FA) pathogenesis can be directly neutralized with microbial components or indirectly through the action of metabolites such as short-chain fatty acids (SCFAs). These molecules promote epithelial integrity, gut permeability, mucus production, tolerogenic dendritic cells (DCs), regulatory T-cell (Treg) differentiation, cytokine production, and the release of secretory IgA by plasma cells. The gut microbiota also regulates immunity through Th2 T-cells, influences tolerance, and the presence of basophils. As a result of dysbiosis, the immune response via Th2 and B cells is worsened, and IgE levels produced by B cells increase. Food allergy essentially arises from a breakdown of immunological tolerance to dietary antigens that the body encounters [60].

Moreover, many forms of FA may be associated with the subsequent development of other allergic manifestations, such as asthma, rhinitis, atopic dermatitis, and urticaria, as well as other conditions, such as functional gastrointestinal disorders (FGIDs), inflammatory bowel diseases (IBD), and psychiatric disorders like autism spectrum disorders (ASD), attention-deficit/hyperactivity disorder (ADHD), and obsessive-compulsive disorder (OCD).

Studies of the gut microbiota in children with food allergy, as well as in experimental animal models, reveal conflicting evidence regarding microbial population disruptions with the most common being an increase in *Bacteroides* and *Ruminococcus* and a decrease in *Lactobacillus* and *Bifidobacterium* [61]. Finally, asthma and atopy are complex diseases that affect and are influenced by the microbial communities that inhabit the gut and the respiratory tract, which, in turn, are affected by various environmental factors, from diet and antibiotic administration to early local microbial exposure.

14.9 Oxidative Stress – Diet – Longevity

Oxidative stress corresponds to the disruption of the redox signaling pathway in cells due to an increase in the level of reactive oxygen species (ROS) beyond the level of antioxidant mechanisms. Neurodegenerative diseases (NDDs), primarily Alzheimer's disease (AD) and Parkinson's disease (PD), are mainly caused by oxidative damage, increased ROS production, neuroinflammation, and disrupted energy metabolism, which also affects the gut microbiota.

Dysbiosis in the gut and neuroinflammation are the main causes of the pathophysiology of various neurological disorders (Fig. 14.5). Oxidative stress leads to cellular damage through lipid peroxidation, protein oxidation, and nucleic acid damage. In fact, oxidative stress is considered a part of the normal aging process, but it is known to be involved in chronic brain disorders, such as AD, PD, and depression. Additionally, it plays a significant role in metabolic disorders related

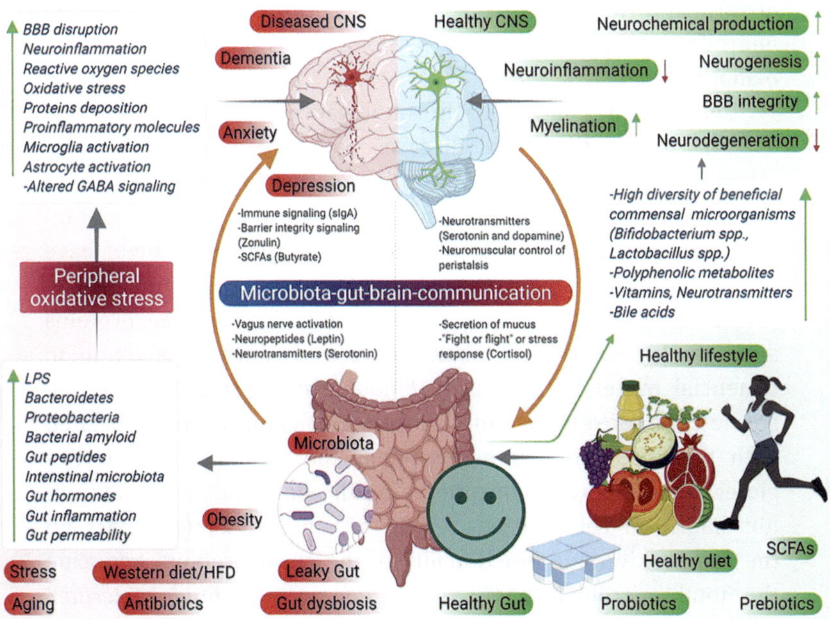

Figure 14.5 Microbiota–gut–brain axis and the effect of oxidative stress in neurodegeneration [62].

to lifestyle, such as type 2 diabetes, non-alcoholic fatty liver disease, non-alcoholic steatohepatitis, obesity, cardiovascular diseases, and cancer.

Antioxidants, whether enzymatic or non-enzymatic, endogenous, or exogenous, protect the brain from oxidative stress by preventing the generation of ROS, scavenging free radicals, or inactivating the products of free radical reactions. The first line of the antioxidant defense mechanism includes the use of endogenous enzymes, such as superoxide dismutase (SOD), glutathione peroxidase (GPx), glutathione reductase, and catalase. The second line of antioxidant defense includes the use of endogenous non-enzymatic molecules, such as thioredoxin, ferritin, transferrin, ceruloplasmin, leukotrienes, and metallothionein. Moreover, other enzymatic cofactors like coenzyme Q10 and alpha-lipoic acid, as well as metabolites like bilirubin, melatonin, and uric acid, play a significant role in the antioxidant defense mechanism. Similarly, vitamins A, E, and C, flavonoids, phenolic acids, and carotenoids are also known to have strong potential antioxidant defense against neurodegeneration and other pathological conditions caused by oxidative stress.

Today, studies highlight the importance of diet in regulating the risk of many chronic diseases by shaping a balanced gut microbiota, regulating metabolism, and controlling immune system function. Popular dietary patterns, including the Western, gluten-free, omnivorous, vegetarian, vegan, and Mediterranean diets, have been studied for their ability to regulate the gut microbiota (Fig. 14.6). In several studies, a Western diet high in animal proteins and fats, low in dietary fiber, led to a significant reduction in beneficial bacteria, specifically *Bifidobacterium* and *Eubacterium* species. The consumption of a Western diet has also been associated with the production of nitrosamines that promote cancer. The gluten-free diet (GFD), despite being the only effective treatment for diagnosed celiac disease (CD), has an inevitable impact on the composition and functionality of the gut microbiota, reducing the total microbial mass with a decrease in *Bifidobacterium*, *Lactobacillus*, *Prevotella*, *Eubacterium*, and *Roseburia* species, while only increasing *Enterobacterium*. Vegan and vegetarian diets are enriched with fermentable plant foods; however, they led to a

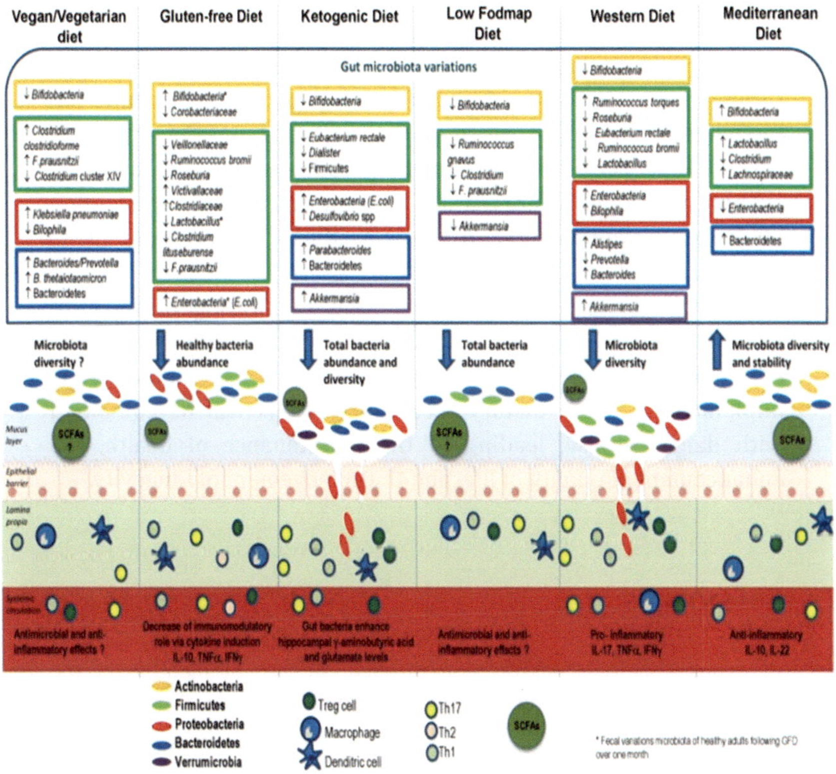

Figure 14.6 Effect of dietary pattern on the gut microbiota and immune function in the intestine [63].

reduction in *Bifidobacterium* species and, in general, microbial diversity, although the studies conducted did not provide precise details on the composition of the microbiota [6]. The Mediterranean diet is considered a balanced diet characterized by a beneficial fatty acid profile rich in monounsaturated and polyunsaturated fatty acids, high levels of polyphenols and other antioxidants, a high intake of dietary fiber and other carbohydrates with a low glycemic index, and a relatively greater intake of plant proteins than animal proteins. Specifically, it includes olive oil, various fruits, vegetables, grains, legumes, and nuts, moderate consumption of fish, poultry, and red wine, and reduced intake of dairy products, red meat, and processed meat.

Precision medicine, based on an increasing amount of data derived from cutting-edge technology, both in the analysis of the microbiome and in investigating each individual's phenotype through metabolomic analysis, is leading to new therapeutic approaches for many diseases that have strong genetic and epigenetic correlations. These new treatment paradigms will rely not only on pharmacological intervention but primarily on the prevention of disease development and the subsequent management of its progression.

Through systematic assessment and monitoring of each individual's specific needs, personalized dietary recommendations enriched with special enhancement protocols will ultimately be implemented. These dietary recommendations will be combined with daily exercise, leading to the maintenance of health, the enhancement of quality of life, and the achievement of longevity.

References

1. Scouras, Z. (2019). Traveling through the age of man-life in the anthropocaine, *Germanos Publications*, pp. 167–170.
2. Rackaityte, E., Lynch, S. V. (2020). The human microbiome in the 21st century, *Nature Communications,* **11**, pp. 1–3.
3. Milani, C., Duranti, S., Bottacini, F., Casey, F., Turroni, F., Mahony, J., *et al.* (2017). The first microbial colonizers of the human gut: composition, activities, and health implications of the infant gut microbiota, *ASM Journals Microbiology and Molecular Biology Reviews*, **81**, pp. 1–67.
4. Ottman, N., Smidt, H., de Vos, W. M., Belzer, C. (2012). The function of our microbiota: who is out there and what do they do? *Front Cell Infect Microbiol.*, **2,** pp. 1–11.
5. Sender, R., Fuchs, S., Milo, R. (2016). Revised estimates for the number of human and bacteria cells in the body, *PLoS Biol.,* pp. 1–14.
6. Mentis, A-F. A, Gypas, F., Mentis, A. (2013). Human enteric microbiome: Its role in health and disease, *Archives of Hellenic Medicine*, **30**, pp. 272–288.
7. Qin, J., Li, R., Raes, J., Arumugam, M., Burgdor, K. S., Manichanh, C., *et al.* (2010). Human gut microbial gene catalogue established by metagenomic sequencing, *Nature*, **4**, pp. 59–65.

8. Li, J., Jia, H., Cai, X., Zhong, H., Feng, Q., Sunagawa, S., *et al.* (2014). An integrated catalog of reference genes in the human gut microbiome, *Nature Biotechnology*, **32**, pp. 834–41.
9. Hollister, E. B., Gao, C., Versalovic, J. (2014). Compositional and functional features of the gastrointestinal microbiome and their effects on human health, *Gastroenterology*, **146**, pp. 1449–1458.
10. Kim, N., Yun, M., Oh, Y. J., Choi, H. J. (2018). Mind-altering with the gut: modulation of the gut-brain axis with probiotics, *Journal of Microbiology*, **56**, pp. 172–182.
11. Mishima, Y., Ishihara, S. (2020). Molecular mechanisms of microbiota-mediated pathology in irritable bowel syndrome, *International Journal of Molecular Science*, **21**, pp. 8664.
12. Singh, R. K., Chang, H. W., Yan D., Lee, K. M., Ucmak, D., Kirsten Wong, K., *et al.* (2017). Influence of diet on the gut microbiome and implications for human health, *Journal of Translational Medicine*, **15**, pp. 73.
13. Wei, S., Bahl, M. I., Baunwall, S. M. D., Hvas, C. D., Licht, T. R. (2021). Determining gut microbial dysbiosis: a review of applied indexes for assessment of intestinal microbiota imbalances, *Appl. Environ. Microbiol.*, **87**, pp. e00395–21.
14. Johansson, M. E. V., Holmen-Larsson, J. M., Hansson, G. C. (2011). The two mucus layers of colon are organized by the MUC2 mucin, whereas the outer layer is a legislator of host-microbial interactions, *Proc. Natl. Acad. Sci. U S A*, **108**, pp. 4659–65.
15. Salzman, N. H., Underwood, M. A., $\kappa\alpha\iota$ Bevins, C. L. (2007). Paneth cells, defensins and the commensal microbiota: a hypothesis on intimate interplay at the intestinal mucosa, *Semin. Immunol.*, **19**, pp. 70–83.
16. McCole, D. F. (2012). Regulation of epithelial barrier function by the inflammatory bowel disease candidate gene, PTPN2, *Ann. N Y Acad Sci*, **1257**, pp. 108–114.
17. Takeuchi, O., Akira, S. (2010). Pattern recognition receptors and inflammation, *Cell*, **140**, pp. 805–20.
18. Liu, T., Zhang, L., Joo, D., Sun, S. C. (2017). NF-κB signaling in inflammation, *Signal Transduct. Target Ther.*, **2**, pp. 17023.
19. Schmulson, M. J., Drossman, D. A. (2017). What Is New in Rome IV, *J. Neurogastroenterol. Motil.*, **23**, pp. 151–163.
20. Takakura, W., Pimentel, M. (2020). Small intestinal bacterial overgrowth and irritable bowel syndrome: an update, *Front. Psychiatry*, **11**, pp. 664.
21. Shah, A., Talley, N. J., Jones, M., Kendall, B. J., Koloski, N., Walker, M. M., *et al.* (2020). Small intestinal bacterial overgrowth in irritable

bowel syndrome: a systematic review and meta-analysis of case-control studies, *Am. J. Gastroenterol.*, **115**, pp. 190–201.

22. Ghoshal, U., Shukla, R., Srivastava, D., Ghoshal, U. C. (2016). Irritable bowel syndrome, particularly the constipation-predominant form, involves an increase in *Methanobrevibacter smithii*, which is associated with higher methane production, *Gut Liver*, **10**, pp. 932–938.
23. Liu H. N., Wu, H., Chen, Y. Z., Chen, Y. J., Shen, X. Z., Liu, T. T. (2017). Altered molecular signature of intestinal microbiota in irritable bowel syndrome patients compared with healthy controls: a systematic review and meta-analysis, *Dig. Liver Dis.*, **49**, pp. 331–337.
24. Ng, S. C., Kamm, M. A., Yeoh, Y. K., Chan, P. K. S., Zuo, T., Tang, W., *et al.* (2020). Scientific frontiers in faecal microbiota transplantation: joint document of Asia-Pacific Association of Gastroenterology (APAGE) and Asia-Pacific Society for Digestive Endoscopy (APSDE), *Gut*, **69**, pp. 83–91.
25. Manichanh, C., Borruel, N., Casellas, F., and Guarner, F. (2012). The gut microbiota in IBD, *Nat Rev Gastroenterol. Hepatol.*, **9**, pp. 599–608.
26. Schaubeck, M., Clavel, T., Calasan, J., Lagkouvardos, I., Haange, S. B., Jehmlich, N., *et al.* (2016). Dysbiotic gut microbiota causes transmissible Crohn's disease like ileitis independent of failure in antimicrobial defence, *Gut*, **65**, pp. 225–37.
27. Mosca, A., Leclerc, M., and Hugot, J. P. (2016). Gut microbiota diversity and human diseases: should we reintroduce key predators in our ecosystem? *Front. Microbiol.*, **7**, pp. 1–22.
28. Oligschlaeger, Y., Yadati, T., Houben, T., Condello Oliván, C. M., Shiri-Sverdlov, R. (2019). Inflammatory bowel disease: a stressed "gut/feeling", *Cells*, **8**, pp. 659.
29. Vich Vila, A., Imhann, F., Collij, V., Jankipersadsing, S. A., Gurry, T., Mujagicet, Z., *et al.* (2018). Gut microbiota composition and functional changes in inflammatory bowel disease and irritable bowel syndrome, *Sci. Transl. Med.*, **10**, pp. eaap8914.
30. Pittayanon, R., Lau, J. T., Leontiadis, G. I., Tse, F., Yuan, Y., Surette, M., *et al.* (2020). Differences in gut microbiota in patients with vs without inflammatory bowel diseases: a systematic review, *Gastroenterology*, **158**, pp. 930–946.
31. Read, E., Curtis, M. A., Neves, J. F. (2021). The role of oral bacteria in inflammatory bowel disease, *Nat. Rev. Gastroenterol. Hepatol.*, **18**, pp. 731–742.

32. Chen, Y., Chen, Y., Cao, P., Su, W., Zhan, N., Dong, W. (2020). *Fusobacterium nucleatum* facilitates ulcerative colitis through activating IL-17F signaling to NF-κB via the upregulation of CARD3 expression, *J. Pathol.*, **250**, pp. 170–182.

33. Hu, S., Vich Vila, A., Gacesa, R., Collij, V., Stevens, C., Fu, J. M., *et al.* (2021). Whole exome sequencing analyses reveal gene-microbiota interactions in the context of IBD, *Gut*, **70**, pp. 285–296.

34. Goncalves, P., Araujo, J. R., Di Santo, J. P. (2018). A cross-talk between microbiota-derived short-chain fatty acids and the host mucosal immune system regulates intestinal homeostasis and inflammatory bowel disease, *Inflamm. Bowel Dis.*, **24**, pp. 558–572.

35. Campbell, C., McKenney, P. T., Konstantinovsky, D., Isaeva, O. I., Schizas, M., Verter, J., *et al.* (2020). Bacterial metabolism of bile acids promotes generation of peripheral regulatory T cells, *Nature*, **581**, pp. 475–479.

36. Chao, K., Zhang, S., Yao, J., He, Y., Chen, B., Zeng, Z., *et al.* (2014). Imbalances of CD4(+) T-cell subgroups in Crohn's disease and their relationship with disease activity and prognosis, *J. Gastroenterol. Hepatol.*, **29**, pp. 1808–14.

37. Lopetuso, L. R., Napoli, M., Rizzatti, G., Gasbarrini, A. (2018). The intriguing role of rifaximin in gut barrier chronic inflammation and in the treatment of Crohn's disease, *Expert. Opin. Investig. Drugs*, **27**, pp. 543–551.

38. Sun, X., He, S., Lv, C., Sun, X., Wang, J., Zheng, W., *et al.* (2017). Analysis of murine and human Treg subsets in inflammatory bowel disease, *Mol. Med. Rep.*, **16**, pp. 2893–2898.

39. Lin, L., Zhang, J. (2017). Role of intestinal microbiota and metabolites on gut homeostasis and human diseases, *BMC Immunology*, **18**, pp. 1–25.

40. Ağagündüz, D., Cocozza, E., Cemali, Ö., Bayazıt, A. D., Nanì, M. F., Cerqua, I., *et al.* (2023). Understanding the role of the gut microbiome in gastrointestinal cancer: a review, *Front. Pharmacol.*, **14**, pp. 1–17.

41. Warnakulasuriya, S. (2009). Global epidemiology of oral and oropharyngeal cancer, *Oral Oncol.*, **45**, pp. 309–16.

42. Mima, K., Nishihara, R., Qian, Z. R., Cao, Y., Sukawa, Y., Nowak, J. A., *et al.* (2016). *Fusobacterium nucleatum* in colorectal carcinoma tissue and patient prognosis, *Gut*, **65**, pp. 1973–1980.

43. Rubinstein, M. R., Wang, X., Liu, W., Hao, Y., Cai, G., Han, Y. W. (2013). *Fusobacterium nucleatum* promotes colorectal carcinogenesis by modulating E-cadherin/β-catenin signaling via its FadA adhesin, *Cell Host Microbe*, **14**, pp. 195–206.

44. Mima, K., Sukawa, Y., Nishihara, R., Qian, Z. R., Yamauchi, M., Inamura, K., *et al.* (2015). *Fusobacterium nucleatum* and T cells in colorectal carcinoma, *JAMA Oncology*, **1**, pp. 653–61.

45. Tilg, H., Adolph, T. E., Gerner, R. R., Moschen, A. R. (2018). The intestinal microbiota in colorectal cancer, *Cancer Cell*, **33**, pp. 954–964.

46. Bultman, S. J. (2014). Emerging roles of the microbiome in cancer, *Carcinogenesis*, **35**, pp. 249–55.

47. Ploger, S., Stumpff, F., Penner, G. B., Schulzke, J. D., Gabel, G., Martens, H. *et al.* (2012). Microbial butyrate and its role for barrier function in the gastrointestinal tract, *Ann. N. Y. Acad. Sci*, **1258**, pp. 52–9.

48. Tsigalou, C., Paraschaki, A., Karvelas, A., Kantartzi, K., Gagali, K., Tsairidis, D. *et al.* (2021). Gut microbiome and Mediterranean diet in the context of obesity: current knowledge, perspectives and potential therapeutic targets, *Metabol. Open*, **9**, pp. 100081.

49. Garcia-Mantrana, I., Selma-Royo, M., Alcantara, C., Collado, M. C. (2018). Shifts on gut microbiota associated to Mediterranean diet adherence and specific dietary intakes on general adult population, *Front. Microbiol.*, **9**, pp. 890.

50. Khalili, H., Håkansson, N., Chan, S. S., Chen, Y., Lochhead, P., Ludvigsson, J. F. *et al.* (2020). Adherence to a Mediterranean diet is associated with a lower risk of later-onset Crohn's disease: results from two large prospective cohort studies, *Gut*, **69**, pp. 1637–1644.

51. Saklayen, M. G. (2018). The global epidemic of the metabolic syndrome, *Curr. Hypertens. Rep.*, **20**, pp. 12.

52. Thomas, M. S., Blesso, C. N., Calle, M. C., Chun, O. K., Puglisi, M., Fernandez, M. L. (2022). Dietary influences on gut microbiota with a focus on metabolic syndrome, *Metab. Syndr. Relat. Disord.*, **20**, pp. 429–439.

53. Krishnamurthy, H.A. (2013). The serum gamma glutamyl transpeptidase: a noninvasive diagnostic bio marker of chronic anicteric non-alcoholic liver diseases, *J. Clin. Diagn. Res.*, **7**, pp. 691–694.

54. Shiraishi, M., Tanaka, M., Okada, H., Hashimoto, Y., Nakagawa, S., Kumagai, M., *et al.* (2019). Potential impact of the joint association of total bilirubin and gamma-glutamyltransferase with metabolic syndrome, *Diabetol. Metab. Syndr.*, **11**, pp. 12.

55. Alissa, E. M. (2019). Relationship between serum gamma-glutamyltransferase activity and cardiometabolic risk factors in metabolic syndrome, *J. Family Med. Prim. Care*, **7**, pp. 430–434.

56. Wang, X., Liang, Z., Wang, S., Ma, D., Zhu, M Feng, J. (2022). Role of gut microbiota in multiple sclerosis and potential therapeutic implications, *Curr. Neuropharmacol.*, **20**, pp. 1413–1426.
57. Zang, Y., Lai, X., Li, C., Ding, D., Wang, Y, Zhu, Y. (2023). The role of gut microbiota in various neurological and psychiatric disorders: an evidence mapping based on quantified evidence, *Mediators Inflamm.*, **2023**, pp. 5127157.
58. Zhu, M., Liu, X., Ye, Y., Yan, X., Cheng, Y., Zhao, L., Chen, F., Ling, Z. (2023). Gut microbiota: a novel therapeutic target for Parkinson's disease, *Front. Immunol.*, **13**, pp. 937555.
59. Unger, M. M., Spiegel, J., Dillmann, K. U., Grundmann, D., Philippeit, H., Burmann, J., *et al.* (2016). Short chain fatty acids and gut microbiota differ between patients with Parkinson's disease and age-matched controls, *Parkinsonism Relat. Disord.*, **32**, pp. 66–72.
60. Zhao, W., Ho, H. E., Bunyavanich, S. (2018). The gut microbiome in food allergy, *Ann. Allergy Asthma Immunol.*, **122**, pp. 276–282.
61. Canani, R. B., Paparo, L., Nocerino, R., Di Scala, C., Della Gatta, G. D., Maddalena, Y., *et al.* (2019). Gut microbiome as target for innovative strategies against food allergy, *Front. Immunol.*, **10**, pp. 191.
62. Shandilya, S., Kumar, S., Jha, N. K., Kesari, K. K., Ruokolainen, J. (2022). Interplay of gut microbiota and oxidative stress: perspective on neurodegeneration and neuroprotection, *J. Adv. Res.*, **38**, pp. 223–244.
63. Rinninella, E., Cintoni, M., Raoul, P., Lopetuso, L. R., Scaldaferri, F, Pulcini, G., *et al.* (2019). Food components and dietary habits: keys for a healthy gut microbiota composition, *Nutrients*, **11**, pp. 2393.

Chapter 15

Intestinal Microbiota and Human Telomere Length: A Dynamic Crosstalk between Two Worlds

Taxiarchis Konstantinos Nikolouzakis,[a] Michael Koukakis,[b] Aristidis Tsatsakis,[b,c] and John Tsiaoussis[a]

[a]*Department of Anatomy, Medical School, University of Crete, Crete, Greece*
[b]*Laboratory of Toxicology, Medical School, University of Crete, Heraklion, Greece*
[c]*Lifeplus S.A., Science & Technological Park of Crete, Vassilika Vouton, Heraklion, Greece*
tknikolouzakis@gmail.com

15.1 Introduction

Aging is a progressive and dynamic degenerative process, often accompanied by tissue stem cell depletion, tissue inflammation, cellular senescence, and metabolic dysfunction [1].

Popular aging theories agree that the aging phenotype is caused by an imbalance between stressors and stress-buffering mechanisms [2]. The loss of compensatory reserves leads to the accumulation of unrepaired DNA damage [3].

Telomeres: Biomarkers of a Healthy Life and Successful Aging
Edited by Aristidis Tsatsakis

ISBN 978-981-5129-49-6 (Hardcover), 978-1-003-56809-4 (eBook)
www.jennystanford.com

Telomeres can be used as a typical marker of aging because their length reflects the replication potential of cells. Furthermore, telomeres are particularly vulnerable to oxidative damage [2].

Persistent DNA damage can activate the tumor suppressor genes p53 and p21, and cause cell senescence [4]. Inflammation is also considered one of the biological characteristics of aging [5]. Nuclear factor-kappa B (NF-κB) is the central component of cellular responses to damage, stress, and inflammation, and it is considered the most relevant transcription factor in mammalian aging [6]. Chronic activation of the NF-κB-cyclooxygenase-2 (COX-2)-reactive oxygen species (ROS) axis results in accelerated aging in multiple tissues by the levels of oxidative stress and inflammation [7]. Therefore, the inhibition of NF-κB and COX-2 activation can delay many aging-related symptoms and rescue cell senescence. Humans and animals are constantly exposed to various stresses that may accelerate their aging processes [8].

Many external factors may influence aging processes, such as ionizing radiation [9], high temperature [10], and poor living environment [11]. High-density crowding is an important social stress factor in animals [12], which may accelerate the aging processes in humans and animals.

In modern society, high-density stress could lead to increased social stress as reflected by a subsequent increase in corticosterone (CORT) levels, leading to the appearance of premature aging features, for example, gray hair [8] or hair loss [13]. People living in crowded urban areas usually have a higher probability of developing mental illnesses than those living in countryside areas [14]. Repeated exposure to environmental stressors has been shown to shorten the lifespan of *Caenorhabditis elegans* [8]. An increase in population density can reduce the lifespan of Drosophila melanogaster (*D. melanogaster*) [15].

In nature, the variation in the population density of animals is largely driven by external (climate, food, and predators) and intrinsic (crowding and competing) factors. Density dependence is an important mechanism in regulating the population dynamics of animals. High density can increase social stress [13,15] and induce negative effects on immune function [15], which may eventually contribute to the low survival rate of animals and a decline in their population [16]. High-density crowding stress could decrease the fitness of animals through various regulatory mechanisms, such as the regulation of physiological, behavioral, genetic, senescence, neurology, and gut microbes [17,18].

All these mechanisms are closely related to high-density crowding stress. However, the density-dependent aging processes of animals have not yet been fully evaluated in mammals.

15.2 Microbiota

The microorganisms living in our body are collectively referred to as microbiota and include bacteria, fungi, and protozoa. The microbiota serves multiple physiological functions, although its overall importance has not been fully grasped yet. A state of balance between "good" bacteria and "harmful" bacteria (called "eubiosis") is therefore paramount to maintain the homeostasis of its hosting organism. In contrast, the perturbation of this balance (called "dysbiosis") is related to the development of several pathological conditions. For example, the microbiota works synergistically with the immune system to avoid colonization from pathogenic bacteria and viruses.

The microbiota also plays a role in metabolism, participating in digestion by aiding micronutrient absorption (amino acids and short-chain fatty acids) and part of their further degradation as well.

Although dysbiosis has been clearly associated with numerous ailments, it is not clear whether a causal relationship exists between these two phenomena or, instead, if anomalies in the microbiota composition represent an epiphenomenon of the underlying pathological processes. Similarly, the eventual pre-emptive or even therapeutic effects deriving from microbiota manipulation remain unclear.

However, there is now evidence that the microbiota, particularly gut microbiota, exerts a modulatory function on the brain, possibly even modulating behavior [19]. Indeed, experimental data in animal models show that central nervous system neurotransmission can be profoundly disturbed by the absence of a normal gut microbiota [20] and that alterations of eubiosis with induced acute bacterial infection might induce cognitive alterations [21]. In humans, data have correlated alterations of microbiota to the manifestation of autism spectrum disorder (ASD) [22].

Interestingly, a recent translational study operated transplants of gut microbiota from human donors with ASD controls into germ-free mice revealing that colonization with ASD microbiota was sufficient to induce hallmark autistic behaviors [23].

Other severe psychiatric disorders, such as SCZ and MDD [24], show substantial microbiota imbalances. Relevant to this study protocol is the evidence that a proportion of this altered gut–brain communication in severe mental disorders, determined by a pathological microbiota, is determined through an immunomodulatory action, which includes a rise in the activity of inflammatory pathways [25].

15.2.1 Possible Crosstalk Between Gut Microbiota and Telomere Length

Initially, progressive chromosome shortening occurs during cell replication and is observed with the aging process. Senescent cells accumulate with age, secrete inflammatory cytokines, and have well-established roles in promoting degenerative diseases and pathology with aging [26].

In addition, many of the environmental exposures (sedentary lifestyle, unhealthy diet, drugs, and smoking) that lead to ROS elevation, are also associated with shortened telomeres [27]. Importantly, because dysfunctional mitochondria during aging generate more ROS, this sets up a vicious cycle in which telomeres may suffer further insult from oxidative damage. Accumulating evidence from human and animal models suggests that oxidative damage to telomeric DNA is responsible for accelerated telomere shortening under oxidative stress [26]. These injuries include damaged single-strand breaks, purines, pyrimidines, and a basic site [26].

Guanine is the most susceptible of the natural bases to oxidation, commonly generating 8-Oxoguanine, which is even more sensitive to oxidation. Furthermore, there is data that shows the antioxidant peroxiredoxin 1, which scavenges H_2O_2, is enriched at telomeres, and PRDX1 loss inherent to the aging process starts with telomeres damage [27].

Finally, the habitual genomic DNA damage repair mechanisms (base excision, nucleotide excision repair, mismatch repair, homologous recombination, and non-homologous end joining) are not efficient during aging. In addition, several species of GM in pathological contexts are related to increased oxidative stress and inflammation [28].

Increased abundance of several bacteria species, such as *Enterotoxigenic B. fragilis, Fusobacterium varium, Adherent-invasive Escherichia coli, Campylobacter concisus,* and *Fusobacterium nucleatum* is linked with inflammatory diseases, such as inflammatory bowel disease (IBD) and metabolic-associated fat liver disease (MAFLD), respectively [29].

Oxidative stress mediated by the human microbiome occurs through its ability to alter the cellular ROS by modulating mitochondrial activity [30,31]. It has been hypothesized that GM may be related to telomere shortening. Some bacterial species synthesize enzymes capable of fermenting non-digestible polysaccharides into digestible compounds, known as short-chain fatty acids (SCFAs) [32]. It is known that *Bifidobacteria longum* and *Eubacterium rectale* degrade indigestible oligosaccharides into acetate and butyrate, two of the three most common SCFAs [32]. These gut-derived metabolites are linked to the regulation of skeletal muscle function and metabolism [33]. Thus, the process of SCFAs in old age is multifaceted, and its potential role in the prevention of sarcopenia is currently being discussed [34].

Furthermore, SCFAs have been linked to reduced oxidative stress and inflammation. Huang et al. pointed out that SCFAs, mainly acetate, butyrate, and the GPR43 agonist, could attenuate oxidative stress and inflammation of glomerular mesangial cells (GMCs) induced by high glucose and LPS circulation. In addition, they reduced the generation of ROS and pro-inflammatory cytokines (MCP-1, IL-1, and ICAM-1) [35].

Thus, although further studies are needed to define better the mechanisms by which the microbiota can reduce oxidative stress and inflammation, it is already possible to consider the existence of this crosstalk [35]. The intestinal microbiota can also be modulated by antioxidant metabolism. For example, antioxidant substrates from fermented foods can play significantly essential roles in reducing oxidative stress by hindering lipid peroxidation [36].

The *Lachnospiraceae* and *Ruminococcaceae* families can produce reactive sulfur species (RSS) and enhance the antioxidant capacity of the host [37]. Aging is commonly characterized by low anti-oxidative defense systems, specifically in glutathione peroxidase levels, the most potent biological anti-oxidative reductant [38]. In agreement, excessive ROS production (H_2O_2, singlet oxygen, and others) has been observed in aging [39].

Thus, it seems that the gut microbiota may also influence the telomere-shortening process by participating in the balance of the antioxidant profile and ROS levels in cells.

15.3 Gut Microbiota and Immunity in Eubiosis

Gut-associated lymphoid tissues (GALTs) consist of crypt patches, Peyer's patches, and isolated lymphoid follicles (ILFs). Antigen-presenting cells in GALTs can take up and present antigens and this could stimulate lymphocytes and lead to inflammation or tolerance [40]. In the fetus, the development of Peyer's patches is encouraged by lymphoid tissue inducer (LTi) cells in the nonexistence of inhabiting bacteria. However, Peyer's patch size in specific-pathogen-free mice is larger than those in germ-free mice [41]. In contrast to Peyer's patches, the maturation of the crypt patches and the ILFs needs gut microbiota stimulation [42].

The maturation of the immune system requires commensal microorganisms; therefore, it "learns" to differentiate between pathogenic bacteria and commensal microbes (that are analogous to quasi-self-antigens and tolerated antigens) [43]. Pattern recognition receptors (PRRs), such as toll-like receptors (TLRs), in the membrane of epithelial cells and lymphoid cells of the small intestine, have been implicated in this differential recognition and are responsible for the development of a normal mucosal immune system of the intestine [22].

In addition, TLRs inhibit the inflammatory response and promote immunological tolerance to normal microbial flora. TLRs identify various microbe-associated molecular patterns (MAMPs) including different bacterial antigens (e.g., lipopolysaccharides, capsular polysaccharides, muramic acid, peptidoglycan, unmethylated bacterial DNA CpG motifs, and flagellin) and activate the innate intestinal immune response [43].

After TLR stimulation, a signaling cascade is triggered, resulting in the release of nuclear factor kappa-light-chain-enhancer of activated B cells (NF-kB), that activates genes encoding cytokines, acute phase proteins, chemokines, and other mediators of the humoral immune response [44]. TLR activity declines during the first weeks of life to permit the expansion of the gut microbiota community in a steady state. Additionally, TLR stimulation by normal intestinal microbiota antigens signals the inhibition of inflammatory reactions which is important to maintain intestinal homeostasis [45].

15.4 Microbiota and Dysbiosis

Our current knowledge of the architecture of healthy microbiota comes from multiple studies in individuals with no overt signs of disease [46]. This structure includes *Bacteroidetes* and *Firmicutes* as the dominant bacterial phyla present in stool samples and Proteobacteria and Actinobacteria being a small but consistent presence in most people. Broadly defined, dysbiosis is any change to the composition of the resident commensal communities relative to the community found in healthy individuals.

In the last decade, several studies have documented significant changes in the structure of microbial communities in patients and mouse models of inflammatory bowel diseases (IBD) such as Crohn's and ulcerative colitis (UC) [47], diabetes [48], asthma [49], and allergies and even autism [48]. Given the emerging importance of the microbiota to host development, it is speculated that these observed changes in microbial composition are contributing factors to the initiation and/or persistence of many of these diseases.

There are multiple ways that the structure of the microbial community can be influenced. This includes the genetics of the host, diet, infection, or medical interventions (such as antibiotics). The hygiene hypothesis originally proposed that antibiotic usage and lifestyle alterations that limit microbial exposure were predisposing populations of people in developed countries to autoimmune disease [50]. Therefore, it was suggested that, due to the inability to differentiate between pathogen and commensal, antibiotics disturb microbiota structure and, subsequently, the co-evolutionary relationship between our immune system and the symbionts we host. Since then, a significant amount of research has gone into exploring the functional importance of microbiota and the influence antibiotic treatment has on its architecture [9]. Interestingly, antibiotics commonly used in the clinic have significant impacts on our microbial residents. Importantly, many antibiotics have long-lasting effects on the microbiota, leading to the permanent loss of some organisms, while others outgrow and persist.

While these studies have documented dysbiosis in the context of disease or antibiotic use, recent investigations have begun to identify the causality between dysbiosis and disease progression. Collectively, these studies now allow us to better understand what dysbiosis is and begin to categorize it into three types that will be discussed in depth here. These include (i) loss of beneficial microbial organisms, (ii) expansion of pathobionts or potentially harmful microorganisms, and (iii) loss of overall microbial diversity. These three types of dysbiosis are not mutually exclusive and may all occur concurrently.

This review is intended to help synthesize the current data to allow a more defined understanding of what dysbiosis is and how it influences health, immune system development, and disease.

15.5 Microbiota-Immunity Interaction in Dysbiosis

Metabolic disorders, such as diabetes mellitus, obesity, and atherosclerosis are hallmarks of chronic low-grade inflammation. Immune cells-parenchymal cells crosstalk have a decisive role in the pathogenesis of metabolic disorders in metabolically highly active organs like the adipose tissue [51]. Increasing evidence suggests that gut microbiota-derived metabolites can enter systemic circulation through the gut barrier and stimulate metabolic inflammation [18].

It has been indicated that interactions between the host immune system and gut microbiota are implicated in type I diabetes. For instance, germ-free non-obese diabetic mice with MyD88 deficient signaling vigorously develop type I diabetes, although the disease could be attenuated by microbial colonization. *Akkermansia muciniphila* depletion translocated endotoxin-activated CCR2+ monocytes to systemic circulation. This, in turn, triggers innate pancreatic B1a cells, followed by decreased insulin sensitivity [52].

Additionally, the crosstalk between microbiota and immunity plays an important role in obesity. In obesity, microbiota-derived tryptophan metabolites induce white adipose tissue inflammation, via the miR-181 family of micro RNAs [53]. Recently, high-fat diet-induced murine obesity has been reported to be decreased by NLRP12 through SCFA derived from members of the *Lachnospiraceae* family [54].

15.6 Dysbiosis of Gut Microbiota and Cancer

The interaction between gut microbiota and the immune system is assumed to affect cancer immune surveillance. The existence of *Fusobacterium nucleatum* in the colon cancer microenvironment directly inhibits the killing of tumors by NK cells. This is partially due to the binding of bacterial Fap2 protein to the human TIGIT (T cell immune receptor with Ig and ITIM domains) receptor [55].

Furthermore, an abundance of *F. nucleatum* in the human colorectal carcinoma microenvironment could decrease CD3+ T cells, which are associated with a better clinical prognosis [56]. In primary or metastatic liver tumors, gut commensal *Clostridium* species consume bile acids as messengers to boost the antitumor response of hepatic CXCR6+ NKT cells [57]. The anticancer immunotherapeutic response is reported to be modulated by microbiota. For example, large numbers of commensals *Enterococcus faecium, Bifidobacterium longum*, and *Collinsella aerofaciens* fuel T cell-promoted responses to anti-PD-1 therapy in either preclinical model or cases have metastasized melanoma [58].

Another study revealed an association between excess of fecal *Akkermansia muciniphila* and PD-1 blockade effectiveness in epithelial tumors patients, due to CCR9+CXCR3+CD4+ T lymphocyte influx and IL-12 expression [59]. Immune response to other anticancer therapy, such as CTLA-4 blockade [60] or cyclophosphamide [60, 61] was also associated with different gut microbiota patterns. Interestingly, unfolding the gut microbiota role regarding anticancer immune surveillance and immunotherapy may show promise in enhancement of treatment response in cancer patients, and needs to be extensively studied [62].

Besides gut microbiota, a recent study discovered that cancer immunity could be regulated by intra-tumor tissue microbiome. For example, intra-pancreatic adenocarcinoma microbiota in mice and humans stimulates carcinogenesis by inducing a tolerogenic immune pathway, including suppression of monocyte differentiation through selective TLRs and T cell energy (inactive T cell) [63].

Additionally, the existence of Gammaproteobacteria in colon cancer of mice or human pancreatic adenocarcinoma results in resistance to anticancer gemcitabine [64]. Interestingly, in long-term pancreatic adenocarcinoma surviving patients, intra-tumor microbiota shows high microbial heterogeneity, that can stimulate robust immune infiltration and antitumor immune response [65]. These studies highlight the therapeutic role of intra-tumor tissue microbiota calling for further mechanistic studies (Fig 15.1).

15.7 Conclusions

It is quite suggestive that the mechanisms of aging and longevity are distinct paths that modulate the lifespan of all beings. However, biological aging is a multi-factorial and complex process where the physiological systems intertwine. Thus, more detailed research into how the crosstalk between the microbiome and telomere integrity influences cellular senescence and understanding which exercise characteristics enhance this process can be essential for overall health and longevity. Defining the mechanisms that mediate this interaction is essential in developing optimized lifestyle interventions to reduce chronic disease risk during aging. We hope

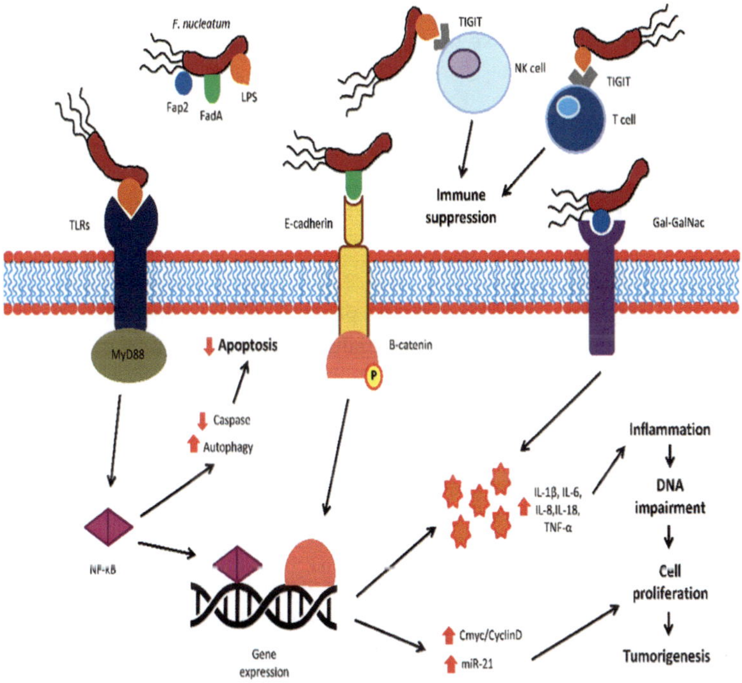

Figure 15.1 Schematic summary of the molecular pathways of *F. nucleatum* in CRC tumorigenesis. *F. nucleatum* mediates its oncogenic properties through three major components: The Fap2 and FadA molecules along with the LPS. LPS can interact with TLRs (namely TLR2 or TLR4), activating the MyD88 and NF-κB pathway. This interaction leads to reduced caspase activity and increased autophagy resulting in reduced apoptosis. Furthermore, FadA binds to E-cadherin causing dephosphorylation and activation of β-catenin. NF-κB and β-catenin alter the gene expression, increasing the synthesis of pro-inflammatory cytokines (IL-1β, IL-6, IL-8, IL-18, and TNF-α) and upregulating oncogenic pathways of Cmyc/CyclinD and miR-21. The pro-inflammatory state is further enhanced by the binding of Fap2 to Gal-GalNAc. Additionally, the interaction of LPS with the TIGIT receptor of NK and T cells leads to the suppression of antitumor immunity. Eventually, these events create inflammation, which impairs DNA, promotes cell proliferation, and results in CRC tumorigenesis. CRC: colorectal cancer; Gal-GalNAc: D-galactose-β (1–3)-N-acetyl-D-galactosamine; IL: interleukin, LPS: lipopolysaccharide; miR: microRNA; NF-κB: nuclear factor kappa-beta; NK: natural-killer; TIGIT: T-cell immunoglobulin and immunoreceptor tyrosine-based inhibitory motif domain; TLR: toll-like receptor; TNF-α: tumor necrosis factor-alpha; Upward red arrows: enhancement/stimulation; Downward red arrows: reduction. Adapted from Koliarakis et al. [16], under Creative Commons CC BY 4.0.

our insights stimulate future research and more open debate about the relevance of exercise on the gut microbiota and telomere in the aging context.

References

1. Liu, J., Huang, S., Zhang, X., *et al.* (2022). Gut microbiota reflect the crowding stress of space shortage, physical and non-physical contact in Brandt's voles (Lasiopodomys brandtii), *Microbiol Res*, **255**, pp. 1–10.
2. Casella, G., Munk, R., Kim, K.M., Piao, Y., De, S., Abdelmohsen, K. *et al.* (2019). Transcriptome signature of cellular senescence, *Nucleic Acids Res,* **47**, pp. 7294–7305.
3. Karlsson, F.H., Tremaroli, V., Nookaew, I., *et al.* (2013). Gut metagenome in European women with normal, impaired and diabetic glucose control, *Nature*, **498**, pp. 99–103.
4. Abbas, H.A., MacCio, D.R., Coskun, S., *et al. (*2010). Mdm2 is required for survival of hematopoietic stem cells/progenitors via dampening of ROS-induced p53 activity, Cell Stem Cell, **7**, pp. 606–617.
5. Frampton, J., Murphy, K.G., Frost, G., Chambers, E.S. (2020). Short-chain fatty acids as potential regulators of skeletal muscle metabolism and function, *Nat Metab*, **2**, pp. 840–848.
6. Gur, C., Ibrahim, Y., Isaacson, B., *et al.* (2015). Binding of the Fap2 protein of fusobacterium nucleatum to human inhibitory receptor TIGIT protects tumors from immune cell attack, *Immunity*, **42**, pp. 344–355.
7. Huttenhower, C., Gevers, D., Knight, R., *et al.* (2012). Structure, function and diversity of the healthy human microbiome, *Nature*, **486**, pp. 207–214.
8. Virtue, A.T., McCright, S.J., Wright, J.M., *et al.* (2019). The gut microbiota regulates white adipose tissue inflammation and obesity via a family of microRNAs, *Sci Transl Med*, **11**, pp. 1–26.
9. Buffie, C.G., Jarchum, I., Equinda, M., *et al.* (2012). Profound alterations of intestinal microbiota following a single dose of clindamycin results in sustained susceptibility to Clostridium difficile-induced colitis, *Infect Immun*, **80**, pp. 62–73.
10. Cryan, J.F. and Dinan, T.G. (2012). Mind-altering microorganisms: the impact of the gut microbiota on brain and behaviour, *Nat Rev Neurosci*, **13**, pp. 701–712.

11. Routy, B., Le Chatelier, E., Derosa, L., *et al.* (2018). Gut microbiome influences efficacy of PD-1-based immunotherapy against epithelial tumors, *Science*, **359**, pp. 91-97 .
12. Hotamisligil, G.S. (2017). Inflammation, metaflammation and immunometabolic disorders, *Nature*, **542**, pp. 177–185.
13. Charbonnel, N., Chaval, Y., Berthier, K., Deter, J., Morand, S., Palme, R. *et al.* (2008). Stress and demographic decline: a potential effect mediated by impairment of reproduction and immune function in cyclic vole populations, *Physiol Biochem Zool*, **81**, pp. 63–73.
14. Gopalakrishnan, V., Spencer, C.N., Nezi, L., *et al.* (2018). Gut microbiome modulates response to anti-PD-1 immunotherapy in melanoma patients, *Science*, **359**, pp. 97–103.
15. Cattan, V., Mercier, N., Gardner, J.P., *et al.* (2008). Chronic oxidative stress induces a tissue-specific reduction in telomere length in CAST/Ei mice, *Free Radic Biol Med*, **44**, pp. 1592–1598.
16. Koliarakis, I., Messaritakis, I., Nikolouzakis, TK, Hamilos, G., Souglakos, J., Tsiaoussis, J. (2019). Oral Bacteria and Intestinal Dysbiosis in Colorectal Cancer, *Int J Mol Sci*, **20**, pp. 4146.
17. Ma, C., Han, M., Heinrich, B., *et al.* (2018). Gut microbiome-mediated bile acid metabolism regulates liver cancer via NKT cells, *Science*, **360**.
18. Thomas, C.M., Versalovic, J. (2010). Probiotics-host communication modulation of signaling pathways in the intestine, *Gut Microbes*, **1**, pp. 1–16.
19. Coretti, L., Paparo, L., Riccio, M.P., *et al.* (2018). Gut microbiota features in young children with autism spectrum disorders, *Front Microbiol*, **9**, 2018.
20. Choi, S., Zhang, B., Ma, S., *et al.* (2021). Corticosterone inhibits GAS6 to govern hair follicle stem-cell quiescence, *Nature*, **592**, pp. 428–432.
21. Frank, D.N., St. Amand, A.L., Feldman, R.A., Boedeker, E.C., Harpaz, N., Pace, N.R. (2007). Molecular-phylogenetic characterization of microbial community imbalances in human inflammatory bowel diseases, *Proc Natl Acad Sci U S A*, **104**, pp. 13780–13785.
22. Clarke, G., Grenham, S., Scully, P., *et al.* (2013). The microbiome-gut-brain axis during early life regulates the hippocampal serotonergic system in a sex-dependent manner, *Mol Psychiatry*, **18**, pp. 666–673.
23. Shanahan, F. (2005). Physiological basis for novel drug therapies used to treat the inflammatory bowel diseases, I. Pathophysiological basis and prospects for probiotic therapy in inflammatory bowel disease, *Am J Physiol - Gastrointest Liver Physiol*, **288**, pp. G417–G421.

24. Espinoza, S.E., Guo, H., Fedarko, N., *et al.* (2008). Glutathione peroxidase enzyme activity in aging, *Journals Gerontol - Ser A Biol Sci Med Sci*, **63**, pp. 505–509.
25. Ebi, K.L., Capon, A., Berry, P., *et al.* (2021). Hot weather and heat extremes: health risks, *Lancet (London, England)*, **398**, pp. 698–708.
26. Barnes, R.P., Fouquerel, E., Opresko, P.L. (2019). The impact of oxidative DNA damage and stress on telomere homeostasis, *Mech Ageing Dev*, **177**, pp. 37–45.
27. Aeby, E., Ahmed, W., Redon, S., Simanis, V. Lingner, J. (2016). Peroxiredoxin 1 Protects Telomeres from Oxidative Damage and Preserves Telomeric DNA for Extension by Telomerase, *Cell Rep*, **17**, pp. 3107–3114.
28. Bander, Z. Al, Nitert, M.D., Mousa, A., Naderpoor, N. (2020). The gut microbiota and inflammation: An overview, *Int J Environ Res Public Health*, **17**, pp. 1–22.
29. Zhang, J., Zhao, X., Jiang, Y., *et al.* (2017). Antioxidant status and gut microbiota change in an aging mouse model as influenced by exopolysaccharide produced by Lactobacillus plantarum YW11 isolated from Tibetan kefir, *J Dairy Sci*, **100**, pp. 6025–6041.
30. Zitvogel, L., Ayyoub, M., Routy, B., Kroemer, G. (2016). Microbiome and Anticancer Immunosurveillance, *Cell*, **165**, pp. 276–287.
31. Zorov, D.B., Plotnikov, E.Y., Silachev, D.N., *et al.* (2014). Microbiota and mitobiota. Putting an equal sign between mitochondria and bacteria, *Biochem*, **79**, pp. 1017–1031.
32. Riquelme, E., Zhang, Y., Zhang, L., *et al.* (2019). Tumor Microbiome Diversity and Composition Influence Pancreatic Cancer Outcomes, *Cell*, **178**, pp. 795-806.
33. Forsythe, P., Bienenstock, J. (2010). Immunomodulation by commensal and probiotic bacteria, *Immunol Invest*, **39**, pp. 429–448.
34. López-Otín, C., Blasco, M.A., Partridge, L., Serrano, M., Kroemer, G. (2023). Hallmarks of aging: An expanding universe, *Cell*, **186**, pp. 243–278.
35. Huang, S., Guoliang, L.I., Pan, Y., *et al.* (2021). Density-induced social stress alters oxytocin and vasopressin activities in the brain of a small rodent species, *Integr Zool*, **16**, pp. 149–159.
36. Zhang, B., Ma, S., Rachmin, I., *et al.* (2020). Hyperactivation of sympathetic nerves drives depletion of melanocyte stem cells, *Nature*, **577**, pp. 676–681.

37. Truax, A.D., Chen, L., Tam, J.W., *et al.* (2018). The Inhibitory Innate Immune Sensor NLRP12 Maintains a Threshold against Obesity by Regulating Gut Microbiota Homeostasis, *Cell Host Microbe*, **24**, pp. 364-378.
38. Regier, D.A., Kuhl, E.A., Kupfer, D.J. (2013). The DSM-5: Classification and criteria changes, *World Psychiatry*, **12**, pp. 92–98.
39. Strachan, D.P. (2000). Family size, infection and atopy: the first decade of the "hygiene hypothesis.", *Thorax*, **55** (Suppl 1), pp. S2–S10.
40. Bouskra, D., Brézillon, C., Bérard, M., Werts, C., Varona, R., Boneca, I.G. *et al.* (2008). Lymphoid tissue genesis induced by commensals through NOD1 regulates intestinal homeostasis, *Nature*, **456**, pp. 507–510.
41. Jurk, D., Wilson, C., Passos, J.F., *et al.* (2014). Chronic inflammation induces telomere dysfunction and accelerates ageing in mice, *Nat Commun*, **2**, pp. 1–14.
42. Nakanishi, Y., Sato, T., Ohteki, T. (2015). Commensal Gram-positive bacteria initiates colitis by inducing monocyte/macrophage mobilization, *Mucosal Immunol*, **8**, pp. 152–160.
43. Roux, A.V.D., Merkin, S.S., Arnett, D., *et al.* (2001). Neighborhood of Residence and Incidence of Coronary Heart Disease, *N Engl J Med*, **345**, pp. 99–106.
44. Tan, B.L., Norhaizan, M.E., Liew, W.P.P., Rahman, H.S. (2018). Antioxidant and oxidative stress: A mutual interplay in age-related diseases, *Front Pharmacol*, **9**, pp. 1–28.
45. Pushalkar, S., Hundeyin, M., Daley, D., *et al.*: The pancreatic cancer microbiome promotes oncogenesis by induction of innate and adaptive immune suppression, *Cancer Discov*, **8**, pp. 403–416.
46. Huang, W., Guo, H.L., Deng, X., Zhu, T.T., Xiong, J.F., Xu, Y.H., Xu, Y. (2017). Short-Chain Fatty Acids Inhibit Oxidative Stress and Inflammation in Mesangial Cells Induced by High Glucose and Lipopolysaccharide, *Exp Clin Endocrinol Diabetes*, **125**, pp. 98–105.
47. Francino, M.P. (2014). Early development of the gut microbiota and immune health, *Pathogens*, **3**, pp. 769–790.
48. Abrahamsson, T.R., Jakobsson, H.E., Andersson, A.F., Björkstén, B., Engstrand, L., Jenmalm, M.C. (2014). Low gut microbiota diversity in early infancy precedes asthma at school age, *Clin Exp Allergy*, **44**, pp. 842–850.
49. Kamada, N., Seo, S.U., Chen, G.Y., Núñez, G. (2013). Role of the gut microbiota in immunity and inflammatory disease, *Nat Rev Immunol*, **13**, pp. 321–335.

50. Shen, Y., Xu, J., Li, Z., *et al.* (2018). Analysis of gut microbiota diversity and auxiliary diagnosis as a biomarker in patients with schizophrenia: A cross-sectional study, *Schizophr Res*, **197**, pp. 470–477.
51. Hayden, M.S., Ghosh, S. (2008). Shared principles in NF-kappaB signaling, *Cell*, **132**, pp. 344–362.
52. Viaud, S., Saccheri, F., Mignot, G., *et al.* (2013). The intestinal microbiota modulates the anticancer immune effects of cyclophosphamide, *Science*, **342**, pp. 971–976.
53. Bodogai, M., O'Connell, J., Kim, K., *et al.* (2018). Commensal bacteria contribute to insulin resistance in aging by activating innate B1a cells, *Sci Transl Med*, **10**, pp. 1–26.
54. Tilg, H., Zmora, N., Adolph, T.E., Elinav, E. (2020). The intestinal microbiota fuelling metabolic inflammation, *Nat Rev Immunol*, **20**, pp. 40–54.
55. Graves, J.L., Mueller, L.D. (1993). Population density effects on longevity, *Genetica*, **91**, pp. 99–109.
56. Manchia, M., Paribello, P., Arzedi, C., *et al.* (2020). A multidisciplinary approach to mental illness: do inflammation, telomere length and microbiota form a loop? A protocol for a cross-sectional study on the complex relationship between inflammation, telomere length, gut microbiota and psychiatric disorders, *BMJ Open*, **10**, pp. 1–7.
57. Lustgarten, M.S. (2019). The Role of the Gut Microbiome on Skeletal Muscle Mass and Physical Function: 2019 Update, *Front Physiol*, **10**, pp. 1–4.
58. Geller, L.T., Barzily-Rokni, M., Danino, T., *et al.* (2017). Potential role of intratumor bacteria in mediating tumor resistance to the chemotherapeutic drug gemcitabine, *Science*, **357**, pp. 1156–1160.
59. Rivière, A., Gagnon, M., Weckx, S., Roy, D., De Vuyst, L. (2015). Mutual cross-feeding interactions between Bifidobacterium longum subsp. longum NCC2705 and Eubacterium rectale ATCC 33656 explain the bifidogenic and butyrogenic effects of arabinoxylan oligosaccharides, *Appl Environ Microbiol*, **81**, pp. 7767–7781.
60. Uchiyama, J., Akiyama, M., Hase, K., Kumagai, Y., Kim, Y.G. (2022). Gut microbiota reinforce host antioxidant capacity via the generation of reactive sulfur species, *Cell Rep*, **38**, pp. 1–15.
61. Vétizou, M., Pitt, J.M., Daillère, R., *et al.* (2015). Anticancer immunotherapy by CTLA-4 blockade relies on the gut microbiota, *Science*, **350**, pp. 1079–1084.

62. Zhu, L., Baker, S.S., Gill, C., Liu, W., Alkhouri, R., Baker, R.D., Gill, S.R. (2013). Characterization of gut microbiomes in nonalcoholic steatohepatitis (NASH) patients: a connection between endogenous alcohol and NASH, *Hepatology*, **57**, pp. 601–609.
63. Parracho, H.M.R.T., Bingham, M.O., Gibson, G.R., McCartney, A.L. (2005). Differences between the gut microflora of children with autistic spectrum disorders and that of healthy children, *J Med Microbiol*, **54**, pp. 987–991.
64. Gareau, M.G., Wine, E., Rodrigues, D.M., *et al.* (2011). Bacterial infection causes stress-induced memory dysfunction in mice, *Gut*, **60**, pp. 307–317.
65. Rakoff-Nahoum, S., Paglino, J., Eslami-Varzaneh, F., Edberg, S., Medzhitov, R. Recognition of commensal microflora by toll-like receptors is required for intestinal homeostasis, *Cell*, **118**, pp, 229–241.

Chapter 16

Cardiovascular Diseases and Telomeres

Sergey Savko,[a] Christina Tsitsimpikou,[b] Emmanouel Papadakis,[c] Demetrios Spandidos,[d] Aristidis Tsatsakis,[e,f] and Konstantinos Tsarouhas[g]

[a] *Department of Medical Elementology, University Department, Peoples' Friendship University of Russia (RUDN University), Moscow, Russia*
[b] *General Chemical State Laboratory, Greece*
[c] *Onassis Cardiac Surgery Centre, Athens, Greece*
[d] *Laboratory of Clinical Virology, Medical School, University of Crete, Heraklion, Greece*
[e] *Laboratory of Toxicology, Medical School, University of Crete, Heraklion, Greece*
[f] *Lifeplus S.A., Science & Technological Park of Crete, Vassilika Vouton, Heraklion, Greece*
[g] *University Hospital of Larissa, Larissa, Greece*
d.t.d.savko@gmail.com

16.1 Introduction

Aging is a well-established factor that increases the risk of developing cardiovascular diseases (CVDs), including hypertension, myocardial infarction (MI), stroke, chronic heart failure (HF), atherosclerosis [1], and other numerous pathophysiological conditions, the accumulation of endothelial damage over time, hypertrophy, altered

Telomeres: Biomarkers of a Healthy Life and Successful Aging
Edited by Aristidis Tsatsakis

ISBN 978-981-5129-49-6 (Hardcover), 978-1-003-56809-4 (eBook)
www.jennystanford.com

ventricular diastolic function, diminished systolic reverse, and increased arterial stiffness [2]. It is believed that many pathophysiological processes either occur due to cellular or subcellular damage leading to a progressive age-related accumulation of biological "garbage" materials such as lipofuscin, an undegradable lysosomal pigment and aberrant proteins [3], or due to disruption of signaling pathways and modification of chromatin structure. A phenomenon called STASIS: stress or aberrant signaling-induced senescence [4, 5]. STASIS is associated with exposure to increased production of reactive oxygen species (ROS) and reduced extracellular proteolytic activity [6]. However, the primary regulators of STASIS involve the dysfunction of p53, p38MAPK, and cyclin-dependent kinase inhibitors p16INK4a (p16) and p21CIP1 (p21) which prevent the G1 phase of the cell cycle [7, 8]. Several studies have described increased p16INK4a expression in kidneys, myocardium, ventricles, and cardiac arteries [9, 10], thereby senescence-associated cell cycle inhibitor p16INK4a is associated with developing cardiovascular diseases and a decrease in their regenerative capacity [11].

Another cellular senescence mechanism involves telomere depletion, also known as replicative senescence. This process leads to chromosomal instability and ultimately results in cell cycle arrest and senescence [12]. Telomeres are specialized DNA-protein complexes located at the ends of linear chromosomes, protecting the chromosome's ends from degradation during replication and preventing the triggering of the DNA damage repair machinery [13]. Therefore, in the scientific consensus, telomeres were suggested as a systemic indicator of biological aging and a putative biomarker of cardiovascular disease [14]. Several epidemiological studies have shown an association between short telomere length (TL) and cardiovascular disease (CVD) [15–17].

16.2 Cardiovascular Risk Factors Associated with Telomeres

Cardiovascular disease is a leading cause of morbidity and mortality worldwide. CVD and its risk factors have been associated with

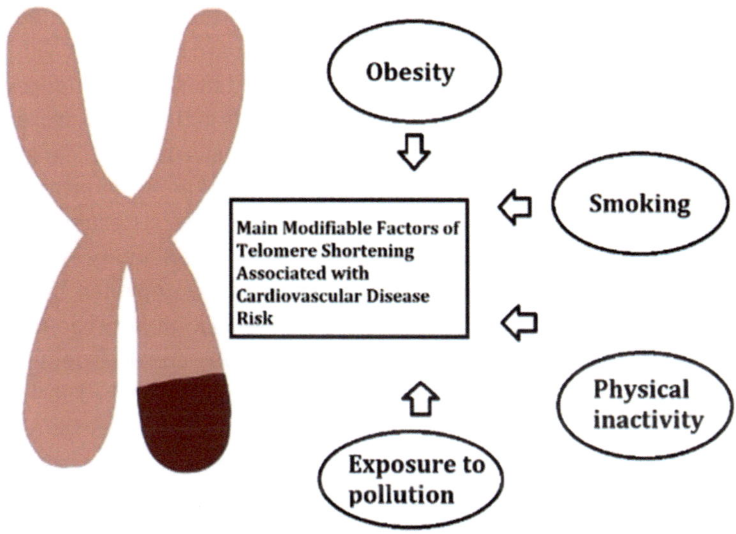

Figure 16.1 Major modifiable factors leading to telomere shortening.

cellular aging and telomere shortening. Studies have shown a correlation between telomere length and cardiovascular risk factors, such as smoking, alcohol, obesity, hypercholesterolemia, and diabetes mellitus (Fig. 16.1) [18].

Obesity, a risk factor for CVD and metabolic disorders, has also been linked to telomere shortening [19]. Thus, a study by Valdes et al. concluded that telomeres in obese women were found to be 240 bp shorter than those in lean women ($p = 0.026$) [20]. Furthermore, some studies have confirmed the relationship between the length of leukocyte telomeres and low physical activity [21, 22]. A high-fat diet may also be a trigger for shortening telomeres [23]. A study by Bloom SI et al. revealed that obesity induced by a high-fat diet and aging modify the expression of genes that are involved in the control of telomeres, specifically telomeric repeat-binding factor 2 (Terf2), protection of telomeres 1B (Pot1b), and the mouse telomerase reverse transcriptase (mTert) [24]. A meta-analysis by Müezzinler et al. including 16 eligible studies confirmed a plausible inverse association between body mass index and leukocyte telomere length regardless of gender [25]. Similar findings, that obesity was associated with shorter telomere length, are shown in a meta-analysis by Khosravaniardakani et al. [26]. There are several hypotheses regarding body mass index-induced alterations in C-reactive protein (CRP) levels. CRP levels are an important mediator for the association of leukocyte telomere length (LTL) and obesity since obesity is known to continuously increase the cumulative burden of chronic inflammation [27]. Other studies have shown that a cumulative load of high interleukin-6 (IL-6) and high tumor necrosis factor-α (TNF-α) is accompanied by an increased risk of short LTL but found no association between CRP and LTL [28]. Data on the association of CRP and LTL require clarification because there are conflicting results described in the literature [29], and some authors admit a genetically determined relationship between CRP and telomere length [30]. Increased inflammatory activity may stimulate the production of reactive oxygen species, resulting in damage to telomeric DNA [31]. In particular, TNF-α can modulate telomerase activity [32, 33]. This may explain the effect of obesity on telomere length.

Smoking, another major risk factor for CVD, has also been associated with telomere shortening. A previously mentioned study by Valdes et al. concluded that telomere length was significantly shorter in current and former smokers compared to non-smokers. For each pack-year smoked, there was an additional loss of 5 bp telomere length (18%) compared to the overall cohort [19]. In a systematic review of Barragán et al., 27 observational studies were analyzed, and most of them showed an association between tobacco smoking and reduced telomere length [34]. In addition, the authors observed that two studies have reported no correlation between tobacco smoking and TL [35, 36]. These results should be refined in the future but the consensus of the studies carried out rather supports the hypothesis of a correlation between smoking and telomere length. The mechanism of telomere shortening may be the result of epigenetic effects, due to increased oxidative stress, inflammation, and DNA methylation [37, 38]. In addition, an interesting study was conducted comparing the content of cotinine in pregnant smokers, secondhand smokers, and non-smokers. Thus, maternal levels of cotinine, a marker of secondhand smoke exposure during pregnancy, were found to be associated with a 3.90% reduction in telomere length in children, compared with non-smoking [39]. The mechanism of telomere shortening due to smoking is unclear; however, this may cause pathogenetic changes in the cardiovascular system, including endothelial dysfunction, altering of the lipidemic profile, exacerbation of hypertension, and diabetes or damage to cardiomyocytes and smooth muscle cells at a cellular level [8, 40].

Telomere shortening is also associated with other cardiovascular risk factors, such as hypercholesterolemia [41], homocysteinemia [42], and physical inactivity [43]. The precise findings of telomere shortening and its relationship with various pathologies remain unclear but most studies on telomere depletion have shown a relation with an increase in oxidative stress in tissue [44, 45]. In addition, it has been shown that a change in nutritional status is reflected in telomere shortening, so Xu et al. proved that multivitamin intake is associated with telomere length in women (aged 35–74 years) [46]. This is a preliminary suggestion of the influence of nutritional status on telomere shortening and association with cardiovascular risk. Thus, this direction is very promising for further scientific research.

16.3 Hypertension (High Blood Pressure)

High blood pressure, or hypertension, is a pervasive health concern that poses a substantial challenge in the field of medicine. This chronic condition affects millions of individuals worldwide and significantly increases the risk of cardiovascular diseases, strokes, and other related complications [47]. Emerging research has shed light on a fascinating connection between this condition and telomere shortening, offering new insights into its underlying mechanisms and potential avenues for intervention. Epidemiological studies have shown that hypertension is more prevalent in certain demographic groups. Age is a significant risk factor, as the prevalence of hypertension tends to increase with advancing age. Additionally, gender variations can be observed, with men having a higher incidence of hypertension at a younger age, while women surpass men in prevalence during later stages of life.

In particular, among the numerous factors that lead to the development of hypertension, the most important pathogenetic contribution is endothelial cell dysfunction, which is associated with telomere depletion as the bioavailability of NO is reduced [48], whose dysfunction directly leads to the development of vascular hypertension [49]. Additionally, it has been shown that endothelial dysfunction is present in metabolic syndrome and dyslipidemia, and can be associated with obesity, hyperhomocysteinemia, and a sedentary lifestyle [50].

Several studies have shown that the length of telomeres is associated with the replicative potential of endothelial cells [51, 52]. Aviv et al. hypothesized that essential hypertension, commonly considered a genetically predisposed disease, could also be caused by the shortening of telomeres on specific chromosomes depending on age [53]. Recent findings confirm that changes in telomerase activity and the length of telomeres may be implicated in the development of essential hypertension [54]. However, telomerase activity can be reversibly upregulated by fibroblast growth factor-2 (FGF-2) and nitric oxide [55], which allows consideration of therapeutic modulation of essential hypertension and cardiovascular decompensation associated with telomere depletion. Nevertheless, it is necessary to note the very important finding by Morgan et al. that arterial telomere uncapping is a significant predictor of hypertension, while arterial mean telomere length is not associated with telomere uncapping or p53/cyclin-dependent kinase inhibitor 1A (P21)-induced senescence and hypertension [56]. Therefore, the conclusion about the association between telomere length and arterial hypertension should be clarified in the future.

Regarding the replication potential of endothelial cells, there is evidence that estrogen activates the PI3K/Akt pathway in endothelial cells by increasing telomerase activity [57]. This may explain the role of telomeres in mediating the protective effects of estradiol on the cardiovascular system [58]. This is consistent with the findings of several studies that higher telomerase activity and longer telomeres are more common in women than in men [59, 60]. Meanwhile, mitogens, cell cycle regulation proteins, and hormonal drugs acting on telomeres may be potential new therapeutic agents in the treatment of cardiovascular disorders.

In addition to the integrity of endothelial tissue, telomeres are described in the literature as a factor influencing systemic arterial pressure and vascular stiffness. There is a positive correlation between leukocyte telomere length and diastolic blood pressure [60]. Benetos et al. showed that systolic and pulsed blood pressure are also inversely related to the length of leukocyte telomeres [61], so it is worth postulating a relationship between telomere length and the pathophysiology of hypertension.

16.4 Ischemic Heart Diseases

Atherosclerosis, the underlying cause of many cardiovascular diseases, has long been a subject of intense research and investigation. Over the years, scientists have unearthed various factors contributing to the development of this disease. Among them, previously described telomeres have emerged as intriguing players with the potential to influence atherosclerosis development. Atherosclerosis is a multifocal immunoinflammatory disease characterized by lipid accumulation and transformation, inflammation of smooth muscle cells, and necrotic cellular debris in the intimal space [62].

Several epidemiological studies have investigated the association between telomere length and atherosclerotic plaque formation. Some studies report an inverse correlation, indicating that individuals with shorter telomeres are more susceptible to plaque development [63]. Others present conflicting results, suggesting a lack of a definitive relationship [64]. However, a study by Sobenin et al. showed that telomere length may be directly proportional to the progression of atherosclerosis. The positive association between telomere length and atherosclerosis progression can be attributed to several factors. Firstly, it may be explained by the migration of smooth muscle and pericyte-like cells, as well as macrophages, into the developing atherosclerotic lesions. This migration leads to alterations in the cellular composition of the intima, contributing to disease progression. Additionally, in advanced atherosclerotic lesions, the functional activity of cells may be inhibited, further influencing the relationship between telomere length and atherosclerosis [65].

Nevertheless, most studies do support a relationship between telomere shortening and the development of atherosclerotic complications. Thus, recent observational data obtained in large populations have further confirmed the association between short leukocyte telomeres and coronary disease. This is fundamentally important because atherosclerosis is a major underlying process leading to the development of coronary heart disease. In a study involving 66,618 subjects, 17,235 of whom were diagnosed with ischemic heart disease, researchers used polymerase chain reaction (PCR) assessment to measure leukocyte telomere length. The results revealed that individuals with a telomere length that was 200 base pairs shorter had a multivariable-adjusted hazard ratio of 1.02 for developing ischemic heart disease [66].

Also worth noting is the study of Codd et al. that conducted a genome-wide association analysis, leading to the identification of seven genomic regions that impact the average telomere length. Additionally, a weighted genetic risk score analysis, involving 22,233 subjects from the CARDIoGRAM cohort (refers to a large-scale genetic study that aimed to investigate the genetic factors associated with coronary artery disease), demonstrated that the collective effects of these variants were associated with an elevated risk of coronary disease. The study's findings shed light on the potential interplay between telomere biology and coronary disease development, providing valuable insights into the genetic factors contributing to cardiovascular health [67]. At the same time, atherosclerosis is a complex and multifactorial condition. Therefore, in the discussion about the impact of telomere length on the development of atherosclerosis, it is important to examine all the pathogenetic components of the condition and their associations with telomere shortening.

First, from what has been written above, we know that endothelial dysfunction characterized by impaired nitric oxide production, increased inflammation, and oxidative stress, is an early event in atherosclerosis development. Shortened telomeres in endothelial cells have been implicated in the initiation of endothelial dysfunction creating a microenvironment conducive to plaque formation. For example, VanderLaan et al. have shown that atherosclerosis tends to develop more prominently in areas of blood vessels that experience low and fluctuating wall shear stress (WSS) rather than high and steady laminar WSS. Endothelial cells exposed to oscillatory WSS exhibit increased cell turnover and adopt a pro-oxidant, pro-inflammatory phenotype similar to the canonical senescence-associated secretory phenotype [68]. This heightened cell turnover has been linked to telomere attrition, which is associated with the development of atherosclerosis. Besides, endothelial cells are most susceptible to DNA damage and telomere dysfunction precisely at sites associated with the development of atherosclerosis [69].

Vascular smooth muscle cells (VSMCs) are also crucial participants in the pathogenesis of atherosclerosis. As telomeres shorten, VSMCs may undergo cellular senescence, which impairs their functionality and promotes the formation of unstable atherosclerotic plaques [70]. While endothelial dysfunction initiates atherosclerosis by allowing the infiltration of lipoproteins into the arterial wall, VSMCs actively participate in the subsequent stages of the disease. Their role involves migration, proliferation, and phenotypic changes, which contribute to plaque formation and progression [71]. Vascular smooth muscle cells possess the ability to adapt and respond to vascular injury by undergoing phenotypic and functional changes. When the blood vessel sustains damage, VSMCs can transition from their quiescent contractile phenotype to a proinflammatory phenotype. In chronic inflammation that occurs in atherosclerosis cells acquire a pro-atherosclerotic phenotype, leading to increased VSMC dedifferentiation and the formation of extracellular matrix within plaque areas [72]. The attrition of telomeres may result from the increased rates of VSMC proliferation during the early development of atherosclerotic lesions. Matthews et al. concluded that advanced plaque VSMCs barely show any telomere presence indicating an inverse correlation between telomere length and the severity of atherosclerosis [73]. Also, analysis of human atherosclerotic plaques showed decreased expression of telomeric repeat binding factor 2 (TRF2) in VSMCs within the plaques [74]. In summary, the differences observed in VSMCs between atherosclerotic plaques and healthy vessels suggest that plaque VSMCs undergo premature senescence. The upregulation of telomere proteins shortened telomeres and decreased proliferation collectively indicate the involvement of VSMC senescence in the progression of atherosclerosis.

One cannot overlook such a factor in the development of ischemic insufficiency and atherosclerosis as dyslipidemia. Novau-Ferré et al. drew some noteworthy findings: total and medium high-density lipoprotein (HDL) particles were linked to shorter telomeres, as well as lower expression levels of telomerase reverse transcriptase (TERT). On the other hand, large HDL particles were associated with longer telomeres and higher expression of TERT [75]. Therefore, one can postulate a certain association between telomere length and the development of ischemic insufficiency associated with atherosclerosis, which should be further elucidated in subsequent studies.

16.5 Heart Failure and Cardiomyopathies

Heart failure encompasses a spectrum of cardiovascular diseases characterized by impaired cardiac function resulting in reduced blood flow and decreased tissue oxygenation. Despite significant research efforts to understand the causes and treatment of these conditions, the influence of telomere length on their development remains a captivating and unexplored subject of study. Emerging research indicates that individuals suffering from chronic heart failure exhibit a diminished average leukocyte telomere length [76]. Several studies have shown that telomere length has been associated with various factors that contribute to the predisposition of congestive heart failure, premature myocardial infarction, and activation of the renin-angiotensin-aldosterone system (RAAS) [77]. The literature describes that, in elderly individuals, a shorter leukocyte telomere length has been found to be associated with a decrease in left ventricular ejection fraction (LVEF), which is a measure of the heart's pumping efficiency [78]. Additionally, the findings of Leri et al. revealed that late-generation Terc−/− mice (refer to mice that have been genetically engineered to lack the gene for telomerase RNA component), characterized by telomerase deficiency and telomere shortening, experience impaired regeneration of cardiomyocytes and increased cardiomyocyte death. These cellular changes contribute to the development of pathological cardiac remodeling and severe ventricular dysfunction in these mice [79]. Also, research by Aung et al. demonstrated that the application of Mendelian randomization analysis revealed a potential causal genetic link between leukocyte telomere length and left ventricular mass, ventricular size, and left ventricular stroke volume. Moreover, it was observed that individuals with longer telomere length had a reduced risk of developing heart failure, even after accounting for potential confounding factors [80]. At the same time, associations between other heart diseases and telomere length are not always found. Thus, in groups of black African ancestry, there is no significant association between the average relative leucocyte telomere length and idiopathic dilated cardiomyopathy (IDC) or its severity [81]. Furthermore, telomere shortening, which is influenced by oxidative stress, has been associated with cellular senescence and reduced regenerative capacity. In the context of heart failure, this could lead to a decreased ability of the heart to repair and regenerate damaged tissue, exacerbating the condition.

Bernhard et al. explored the impact of the UCP2 gene status on circulating leukocyte telomere length. A significant association was observed between the presence of a functional promoter UCP2 variant, leading to increased oxidative stress through the downregulation of gene expression, and shorter telomere length compared to individuals lacking the variant. This finding provides compelling evidence for a direct link between mitochondrial ROS production, mediated by the UCP2 gene, and the accelerated erosion of telomeres [82]. Also, the process of telomere shortening was found to occur concurrently with several cellular changes, including elevated superoxide production, increased expression of NOX2 (NADPH oxidase 2), heightened activity of HDAC6 (histone deacetylase 6), reduction in the telomere-specific antioxidant PRDX1 (peroxiredoxin 1), and an increase in oxidative DNA damage [83]. Accumulation of oxidative damage has been observed over the lifespan of a cell, leading to cellular senescence. This is because of the abundance of guanines in the telomeres structure which renders them highly susceptible to damage induced by oxidative stress [84].

Myocardial remodeling occurs with aging, and it accompanies diseases such as valvular diseases. While there is substantial

Table 16.1 Mechanisms of interaction between cellular alterations in cardiomyopathy and heart failure and telomere dysfunction

	Described mechanisms	Ref.
Myocardial cells	Telomere shortening, defective expression of TRF2, increased expression of p53, Chk2, increased apoptosis, and cardiac myocyte hypertrophy	[79, 88]
Endothelial cells	Telomere shortening, hTER expression alters the regenerative capacity of endothelial progenitor cells	[51, 89]
Circulating leukocytes	Telomere shortening, dysfunction of telomerase reverse transcriptase (TERT), a marker of oxidative stress and inflammation	[90, 91]

research on telomere length and various cardiovascular conditions, valvular diseases have not been extensively explored in the context of telomeres. Increased hemodynamic stress on the aortic valve (AV) can lead to higher rates of endothelial cell (EC) turnover, resulting in telomere loss and focal areas of EC senescence [85]. This impaired regeneration of valvular EC may contribute to the progression of aortic valve diseases. This process of cell senescence has been found to be significant in patients with valvular diseases. A recent study by Wang et al. showed that patients with valvular diseases had shorter telomere length, which may be a factor in the development of CAVS in a European population [86]. Further research in this area will lead to a better understanding of the mechanisms underlying these associations and explore potential therapeutic implications.

Therefore, assessment of telomere length might be a useful biomarker of disease progression, such as heart failure, cardiomyopathies, and valvular diseases (Table 16.1). However, the main inquiry regarding the link between telomere length and heart failure pertains to its causality. Is short telomere length, a direct contributor to the onset and advancement of heart failure, or is it a consequence of heart failure itself, or its underlying causes, leading to accelerated telomere shortening? Perhaps the truth lies somewhere in the middle. Assessing telomere length could potentially serve as a valuable biomarker for monitoring disease progression, including heart failure. On the other hand, heart failure is a complex condition influenced by various factors. It is possible that heart failure or its underlying causes, such as oxidative stress, inflammation, and cellular damage, may lead to accelerated telomere shortening as a secondary effect [87].

16.6 Cerebrovascular Diseases

Cerebrovascular diseases refer to a group of medical conditions that impact the blood vessels supplying the brain. These conditions include ischemic stroke, hemorrhagic stroke, and transient ischemic attacks (TIAs). An ischemic stroke occurs when there is a blockage or reduction of blood flow to the brain, while hemorrhagic stroke results from a burst blood vessel in or around the brain. TIAs are brief episodes of reduced blood flow to the brain, often considered warning signs of potential stroke [92].

Cerebrovascular diseases can have severe consequences, including high mortality rates and long-term disability. Mortality rates from stroke vary globally with higher rates observed in low- and middle-income countries. Understanding the relationship between telomere length dynamics and the development and progression of cerebrovascular diseases could provide valuable insights into potential therapeutic interventions. By targeting and modulating telomere length, it might be possible to slow down or even reverse the cellular aging process, mitigate the damage caused by cerebrovascular events, and enhance the recovery and rehabilitation of stroke survivors. Such interventions could potentially reduce disability rates, improve the quality of life for stroke survivors, and alleviate the burden on healthcare systems.

Previously, the available observational data showed a consistent negative association between telomere length and the risk of coronary heart disease, independent of conventional vascular risk factors. In other words, individuals with longer telomeres tend to have a lower likelihood of developing coronary heart disease, even after accounting for traditional risk factors, such as high blood pressure, high cholesterol, and smoking. On the other hand, the relationship between telomere length and cerebrovascular disease, which includes conditions such as stroke, is less well-established and remains uncertain [93]. Fyhrquist et al. reported an association between telomeres and cerebrovascular diseases including stroke and vascular dementia [94]. We mentioned earlier that telomere depletion is associated with endothelial dysfunction, inflammation, and atherosclerotic processes. All the factors described above play an important role in the pathogenesis of stroke and transient ischemic attack. Thus, shortening telomere length is closely related to early-onset and delayed carotid atherosclerosis, which is associated with cerebrovascular diseases [95]. Studies involving diverse population cohorts of Chinese and Europeans have reported that a shortened telomere length serves as an independent risk biomarker for stroke [96, 97]. These findings support a meta-analysis from 2018 consisting of 12 studies and including 25,340 participants that shortened telomere length is associated with stroke risk [98].

Despite the positive relationship between short LTL and stroke, the underlying mechanisms behind this correlation are not yet fully understood. Several signaling pathways have been proposed as potential contributors to this positive association. Thus, the apelin-apelin receptor-mediated signaling pathway and histone deacetylases-mediated epigenetic regulation are among the pathways that might play a role [99]. In the context of stroke and telomere length, it may contribute to the association between short telomeres and an increased risk of stroke. These changes could influence the expression of genes involved in various biological processes, including inflammation, oxidative stress, and cell survival, which are all relevant to stroke pathogenesis [100]. As of today, we have insufficient information to explain the mechanisms of telomere shortening in cerebrovascular diseases, but this needs to be clarified in the future.

16.7 Arrhythmias

Arrhythmias, or abnormal heart rhythms, have also been a subject of interest in the context of telomere shortening. Arrhythmia refers to an irregular heart rhythm, where the only normal rhythm is known as normal sinus rhythm. In this rhythm, an electrical impulse originates in the sinoatrial (SA) node and travels through the atrioventricular (AV) node, bundle of His, bundle branches, and Purkinje fibers. Any deviation from this pathway leads to arrhythmia [101]. As people age, the electrical system of the heart undergoes natural changes. The heart's conduction system, which regulates the rate and rhythm of heartbeats, can become less efficient and more susceptible to interruptions or abnormalities. These changes can lead to the development of arrhythmias in older individuals. The prevalence of arrhythmias varies across different populations and is influenced by various factors, such as age, gender, and underlying medical conditions. It is estimated that approximately 2% of the general population experience arrhythmias at some point in their lives. However, the prevalence increases significantly with age, particularly after the age of 60. This rise in prevalence is due to the increased presence of risk factors such as heart disease and hypertension, which are commonly associated with arrhythmias.

The increase in the prevalence of arrhythmias is mainly due to factors such as an aging population. While conditions like rheumatic heart disease and hypertension have experienced a decline in their prevalence over the past years, new factors like obesity and possibly metabolic syndrome, or even the shortening of telomeres, have emerged as potential contributors that could amplify the occurrence of arrhythmias. This highlights the evolving landscape of arrhythmia risk factors and emphasizes the need for continued monitoring and intervention to address these changing dynamics [102]. In particular, Sawhney et al. showed that in patients with ischemic cardiomyopathy, there is an observed association between the occurrence of ventricular arrhythmias (VAs) and specific telomere-related factors, including leucocyte telomere length, load-of-short telomeres, and/or telomerase activity. These telomere-related parameters may play a role in the development or progression of VAs in individuals with ischemic cardiomyopathy [103].

Genotyping studies have also shown the relationship between telomerase activity, a particular genetic variant (SNP) situated within the TERC locus, and the occurrence of ventricular arrhythmias (VA) among individuals with ischemic cardiomyopathy. Notably, individuals with homozygosity for the C-allele display a significant influence on telomerase expression, which is connected to an elevated likelihood of encountering ventricular arrhythmias within this specific group of patients [104]. Other studies support the hypothesis that shortened telomeres may be a potential biomarker for predicting atrial fibrillation recurrence [105].

Furthermore, Gao et al. showed that activation of the Smad-dependent TGF-β signaling pathway (TGF-β/Smad) was found to be significantly increased in the lungs of G3 Terc−/− mice, a type of mice with shortened telomeres. This activation suggests that the process of shortening telomeres can potentially exacerbate tissue fibrosis, a condition characterized by excessive buildup of fibrous tissue. The activation of TGF-β/Smad signaling is not only relevant in promoting tissue fibrosis in the lungs but is also a crucial pathway in cardiac fibrosis and the persistence of atrial fibrillation. This indicates that the mechanism by which telomere shortening contributes to fibrosis might be similar across various organ systems [106]. There is a large number of studies on telomere length and the associated increased risk of ventricular and supraventricular arrhythmias, but the mechanisms explaining this relationship remain unclear.

16.8 Congenital and Acquired Heart Defects

Research on the relationship between telomere length and congenital heart defects (CHD) has been relatively limited and more focused on acquired heart defects. However, there have been a few studies that have investigated the association between telomere length and CHD. Congenital heart diseases are a group of structural abnormalities present at birth that affect the heart's form and function. Research in 2019 suggests that telomere length may be a contributing factor in the pathogenesis of CHD. Studies have identified associations between altered telomere dynamics and specific types of CHDs, such as atrial septal defects, tetralogy of Fallot, and ventricular septal defects. These findings hint at the potential influence of telomere length on the development and severity of CHDs [107].

Note the research by Vecoli et al. from 2016. The authors studied the magnitude of health risks of low-dose radiation exposure among patients with surgically repaired congenital heart disease. The study intended to investigate whether telomeres are shorter in patients with grown-up congenital heart disease (GUCH) and whether specific genes may influence how radiation affects their genetic stability. It has been found that individuals with grown-up congenital heart disease have noticeably shorter telomere length compared to those without the condition. There is a significant negative link between LTL and cumulative radiation exposure. Interestingly, patients with specific genetic variations in DNA repair genes XRCC3 or XRCC1 were shown to have even shorter LTL. These significant findings indicate that GUCH patients might undergo early biological aging and that certain genetic variations could influence the impact of radiation on the development of degenerative diseases related to telomeres. Further research is required to delve deeper into these mechanisms and explore potential interventions to mitigate these effects [108].

Valvulopathy, also known as acquired heart defects, refers to conditions that affect the valves of the heart. The heart has four valves — the mitral valve, tricuspid valve, aortic valve, and pulmonary valve — which help regulate the flow of blood throughout the heart. Valvular diseases occur when there is a malfunction or damage to one or more of these valves. Common examples of valvular diseases include valvular stenosis, valvular regurgitation, infective endocarditis, and mitral valve prolapse [109]. Valvular diseases are caused by the infiltration of lipids, the presence of chronic inflammation, and the development of calcification. We previously described the relationship between lipid imbalance and chronic inflammation at the focus of telomere length shortening, but we did not consider the progression of calcification as a factor. A study by Saraieva et al. showed that telomeres length (TL) was shorter in calcified areas of aortic valves in patients with calcific aortic valve disease (CAVD), and shorter in both calcified and non-calcified areas of valves from patients with aortic stenosis (AS) compared to individuals without AS. These findings indicate that TL may play a role in the development of clinically significant AS and that TL may undergo local changes during the calcification process [110].

In other studies, it has been observed that atherosclerotic lesions, which share similarities in terms of oxidative stress and inflammation with stenotic aortic valves, have shorter telomeres compared to healthy blood vessels [111]. Quite similar results were obtained by Kurz et al. in a prospective study of 193 patients with planned surgery for calcific aortic valve stenosis. The results of the study suggest that calcifying aortic stenosis in the elderly is associated with shorter leukocyte telomere length [112]. Among other things, the authors also suggest that chronic inflammation, high cholesterol, and increased oxidative stress could potentially contribute to the development of calcific aortic valve stenosis, as well as accelerate leukocyte telomere erosion on their own.

However, it is important to note that longer telomere length does not always have a positive effect on the surgical treatment of valve heart defects, as indicated in other research studies. In fact, an increase in mortality after transcatheter aortic valve replacement has been associated with longer leukocyte telomere length. This may be due to the increased proliferative capacity of cells, which can result in myeloid and systemic inflammation. On the other hand, decreased TRF-2 expression at telomeres may lead to a decrease in the number of circulating endothelial progenitor cells (EPCs) and accumulation of senescent valve endothelial cells, which is associated with enhanced cell death and senescence in patients with aortic stenosis [113]. Therefore, no conclusions regarding medical use can be drawn yet. Now, despite the abundance of studies, it is worth acknowledging that we still know too little.

16.9 Conclusions

Almost every cardiovascular condition has been shown by both in vivo and in vitro studies to be associated with telomere length. However, data up to now do not answer the question of the pathogenesis of these relationships. Since heart failure, arrhythmias, and ischemic heart disease are primarily diseases of the elderly, it is not surprising to find a decrease in replicative potential in cells of affected organs. Preserving the replicative potential of cells on the other hand has not yet been proven to be an effective therapeutic strategy to prevent the onset of cardiovascular disease.

References

1. North, B. J., & Sinclair, D. A. (2012). The intersection between aging and cardiovascular disease, *Circulation Research*, **110**, pp. 1097–1108.
2. Lakatta, E. G., & Levy, D. (2003). Arterial and cardiac aging: major shareholders in cardiovascular disease enterprises: Part I: aging arteries: a "set up" for vascular disease, *Circulation*, **107**, pp. 139–146.
3. Terman, A., Gustafsson, B., & Brunk, U. T. (2006). Mitochondrial damage and intralysosomal degradation in cellular aging, *Molecular Aspects of Medicine*, **27**, pp. 471–482.
4. Drayton, S., & Peters, G. (2002). Immortalisation and transformation revisited, *Current Opinion in Genetics & Development*, **12**, pp. 98–104.
5. Gire, V. (2005). Senescence: a telomeric limit to immortality or a cellular response to physiologic stresses? *Medecine Sciences: M/S*, **21**, pp. 491–497.
6. Bertram, C., & Hass, R. (2008). Matrix metalloproteinase-7 and the 20 S proteasome contribute to cellular senescence, *Science Signaling*, **1**, pt1.
7. Kiyono, T. (2007). Molecular mechanisms of cellular senescence and immortalization of human cells, *Expert Opinion on Therapeutic Targets*, **11**, pp. 1623–1637.
8. Serrano, M., Hannon, G. J., & Beach, D. (1993). A new regulatory motif in cell-cycle control causing specific inhibition of cyclin D/CDK4, *Nature*, **366**, pp. 704–707.
9. Stenvinkel, P., Luttropp, K., McGuinness, D., Witasp, A., Qureshi, A. R., Wernerson, A., *et al.* (2017). CDKN2A/p16INK4a expression is associated with vascular progeria in chronic kidney disease, *Aging (Albany NY)*, **9**, pp. 494.
10. Melk, A., Schmidt, B. M., Vongwiwatana, A., Rayner, D. C., & Halloran, P. F. (2005). Increased expression of senescence-associated cell cycle inhibitor p16INK4a in deteriorating renal transplants and diseased native kidney, *American Journal of Transplantation*, **5**, pp. 1375–1382.
11. Westhoff, J. H., Hilgers, K. F., Steinbach, M. P., Hartner, A., Klanke, B., Amann, K., *et al.* (2008). Hypertension induces somatic cellular senescence in rats and humans by induction of cell cycle inhibitor p16 INK4a, *Hypertension*, **52**, pp. 123–129.
12. Van Deursen, J. M. (2014). The role of senescent cells in ageing, *Nature*, **509**, pp. 439–446.
13. Verdun, R. E., & Karlseder, J. (2007). Replication and protection of telomeres, *Nature*, **447**, pp. 924–931.

14. Bekaert, S., De Meyer, T., Rietzschel, E. R., De Buyzere, M. L., De Bacquer, D., Langlois, M., *et al.* (2007). Telomere length and cardiovascular risk factors in a middle-aged population free of overt cardiovascular disease, *Aging Cell*, **6**, pp. 639–647.
15. Fitzpatrick, A. L., Kronmal, R. A., Gardner, J. P., Psaty, B. M., Jenny, N. S., Tracy, R. P., *et al.* (2007). Leukocyte telomere length and cardiovascular disease in the cardiovascular health study, *American Journal of Epidemiology*, **165**, pp. 14–21.
16. D'Mello, M. J., Ross, S. A., Briel, M., Anand, S. S., Gerstein, H., & Paré, G. (2015). Association between shortened leukocyte telomere length and cardiometabolic outcomes: systematic review and meta-analysis, *Circulation: Cardiovascular Genetics*, **8**, pp. 82–90.
17. O'Donnell, C. J., Demissie, S., Kimura, M., Levy, D., Gardner, J. P., White, C., *et al.* (2008). Leukocyte telomere length and carotid artery intimal medial thickness: the Framingham heart study, *Arteriosclerosis, Thrombosis, and Vascular Biology*, **28**, pp. 1165–1171.
18. Yeh, J. K., & Wang, C. Y. (2016). Telomeres and telomerase in cardiovascular diseases, *Genes*, **7**, pp. 58.
19. Dankel, S. J., Loenneke, J. P., & Loprinzi, P. D. (2017). The impact of overweight/obesity duration and physical activity on telomere length: an application of the WATCH paradigm, *Obesity Research & Clinical Practice*, **11**, pp. 247–252.
20. Valdes, A. M., Andrew, T., Gardner, J. P., Kimura, M., Oelsner, E., Cherkas, L. F., *et al.* (2005). Obesity, cigarette smoking, and telomere length in women, *The Lancet*, **366**, pp. 662–664.
21. Cherkas, L. F., Hunkin, J. L., Kato, B. S., Richards, J. B., Gardner, J. P., Surdulescu, G. L., *et al.* (2008). The association between physical activity in leisure time and leukocyte telomere length, *Archives of Internal Medicine*, **168**, pp. 154–158.
22. Shadyab, A. H., LaMonte, M. J., Kooperberg, C., Reiner, A. P., Carty, C. L., Manini, T. M., *et al.* (2017). Association of accelerometer-measured physical activity with leukocyte telomere length among older women, *Journals of Gerontology Series A: Biomedical Sciences and Medical Sciences*, **72**, pp. 1532–1537.
23. Ng, S. F., Lin, R. C., Maloney, C. A., Youngson, N. A., Owens, J. A., & Morris, M. J. (2014). Paternal high-fat diet consumption induces common changes in the transcriptomes of retroperitoneal adipose and pancreatic islet tissues in female rat offspring, *The FASEB Journal*, **28**, pp. 1830–1841.

24. Bloom, S. I., Tuluca, A., Ives, S. J., & Reynolds, T. H. (2020). High-fat diet induced obesity and age influence the telomere shelterin complex and telomerase gene expression in mouse adipose tissue, *Physiological Reports*, **8**, pp. e14461.
25. Müezzinler, A., Zaineddin, A. K., & Brenner, H. (2014). Body mass index and leukocyte telomere length in adults: a systematic review and meta-analysis, *Obesity Reviews*, **15**, pp. 192–201.
26. Khosravaniardakani, S., Bokov, D. O., Mahmudiono, T., Hashemi, S. S., Nikrad, N., Rabieemotmaen, S., *et al.* (2022). Obesity accelerates leukocyte telomere length shortening in apparently healthy adults: a meta-analysis, *Frontiers in Nutrition*, **9**, pp. 812846.
27. Gao X., Li, S., Dong, S., Li, J., Yan, Y., Zhang, T., *et al.* (2021). Association between body weight and telomere length is predominantly mediated through C-reactive protein, *The Journal of Clinical Endocrinology & Metabolism*, **106**, pp. e4634–e4640.
28. O'Donovan, A., Pantell, M. S., Puterman, E., Dhabhar, F. S., Blackburn, E. H., Yaffe, K., *et al.* (2011). Cumulative inflammatory load is associated with short leukocyte telomere length in the health, aging and body composition study, *PloS One*, **6**, pp. e19687.
29. Shin, D., Shin, J., & Lee, K. W. (2019). Effects of inflammation and depression on telomere length in young adults in the United States, *Journal of Clinical Medicine*, **8**, pp. 711.
30. Rode, L., Nordestgaard, B. G., Weischer, M., & Bojesen, S. E. (2014). Increased body mass index, elevated C-reactive protein, and short telomere length, *The Journal of Clinical Endocrinology & Metabolism*, **99**, pp. E1671–E1675.
31. Jaiswal, M., LaRusso, N. F., Burgart, L. J., & Gores, G. J. (2000). Inflammatory cytokines induce DNA damage and inhibit DNA repair in cholangiocarcinoma cells by a nitric oxide-dependent mechanism, *Cancer Research*, **60**, pp. 184–190.
32. Parish, S. T., Wu, J. E., & Effros, R. B. (2009). Modulation of T lymphocyte replicative senescence via TNF-α inhibition: role of caspase-3, *The Journal of Immunology*, **182**, pp. 4237–4243.
33. Akiyama, M., Yamada, O., Hideshima, T., Yanagisawa, T., Yokoi, K., Fujisawa, K., *et al.* (2004). TNFalpha induces rapid activation and nuclear translocation of telomerase in human lymphocytes, *Biochemical and Biophysical Research Communications*, **316**, pp. 528–532.
34. Barragán R, Ortega-Azorín C, Sorlí JV, et al. (2021). Effect of physical activity, smoking, and sleep on telomere length: a systematic review of observational and intervention studies, *J. Clin. Med.*, **11**, pp. 76.

35. Cassidy, A., De Vivo, I., Liu, Y., Han, J., Prescott, J., Hunter, D. J., *et al.* (2010). Associations between diet, lifestyle factors, and telomere length in women, *The American Journal of Clinical Nutrition*, **91**, pp. 1273–1280.

36. Flannagan, K. S., Jansen, E. C., Rozek, L. S., Rentschler, K. M., Roman, A. V., Ramirez-Zea, M., et al. (2017). Sociodemographic correlates and family aggregation of leukocyte telomere length in adults and children from Mesoamerica, *American Journal of Human Biology: the Official Journal of the Human Biology Council*, **29**, 10.1002/ajhb.22942.

37. Lei, M. K., Gibbons, F. X., Simons, R. L., Philibert, R. A., Beach, S. R. H. (2020). The effect of tobacco smoking differs across indices of DNA methylation-based aging in an African American sample: DNA methylation-based indices of smoking capture these effects, *Genes (Basel)*, **11**, pp. 311.

38. Marcon, F., Siniscalchi, E., Andreoli, C., Allione, A., Fiorito, G., Medda, E., Guarrera, S., Matullo, G., & Crebelli, R. (2017). Telomerase activity, telomere length and hTERT DNA methylation in peripheral blood mononuclear cells from monozygotic twins with discordant smoking habits, *Environmental and Molecular Mutagenesis*, **58**, pp. 551–559.

39. Osorio-Yáñez, C., Clemente, D. B. P., Maitre, L., Vives-Usano, M., Bustamante, M., Martinez, D., *et al.* (2020). Early life tobacco exposure and children's telomere length: the HELIX project, *The Science of the Total Environment*, **711**, pp. 135028.

40. Bernhard, D., & Laufer, G. (2008). The aging cardiomyocyte: a mini-review, *Gerontology*, **54**, pp. 24–31.

41. Strandberg, T. E., Saijonmaa, O., Fyhrquist, F., Tilvis, R. S., Strandberg, A. Y., Miettinen, T. A., *et al.* (2011). Telomere length in old age and cholesterol across the life course, *Journal of the American Geriatrics Society*, **59**, pp. 1979–1981.

42. Ma, F., Lv, X., Du, Y., Chen, H., Liu, S., Zhao, J., *et al.* (2019). Association of leukocyte telomere length with mild cognitive impairment and Alzheimer's disease: role of folate and homocysteine, *Dementia and Geriatric Cognitive Disorders*, **48**, pp. 56–67.

43. Shadyab, A. H., LaMonte, M. J., Kooperberg, C., Reiner, A. P., Carty, C. L., Manini, T. M., *et al.* (2017). Leisure-time physical activity and leukocyte telomere length among older women, *Experimental Gerontology*, **95**, pp. 141–147.

44. Wolkowitz, O. M., Mellon, S. H., Epel, E. S., Lin, J., Dhabhar, F. S., Su, Y., *et al.* (2011). Leukocyte telomere length in major depression:

correlations with chronicity, inflammation and oxidative stress: preliminary findings, *PloS One*, **6**, pp. e17837.

45. Comporti, M., Signorini, C., Leoncini, S., et al. Ethanol-induced oxidative stress: basic knowledge, *Genes Nutr.*, **5**, pp. 101–109.

46. Xu, Q., Parks, C. G., DeRoo, L. A., Cawthon, R. M., Sandler, D. P., & Chen, H. (2009). Multivitamin use and telomere length in women, *The American Journal of Clinical Nutrition*, **89**, pp. 1857–1863.

47. Hall, J. E., Granger, J. P., do Carmo, J. M., da Silva, A. A., Dubinion, J., George, E., *et al.* (2012). Hypertension: physiology and pathophysiology, *Comprehensive Physiology*, **2**, pp. 2393–2442.

48. Higashi, Y., Kihara, Y., & Noma, K. (2012). Endothelial dysfunction and hypertension in aging, *Hypertension Research: Official Journal of the Japanese Society of Hypertension*, **35**, pp. 1039–1047.

49. Widlansky, M. E., Gokce, N., Keaney, J. F., Jr, & Vita, J. A. (2003). The clinical implications of endothelial dysfunction, *Journal of the American College of Cardiology*, **42**, pp. 1149–1160.

50. Endemann, D. H., & Schiffrin, E. L. (2004). Endothelial dysfunction, *Journal of the American Society of Nephrology: JASN*, **15**, pp. 1983–1992.

51. Chang, E., Harley, C. B. (1995). Telomere length and replicative aging in human vascular tissues, *Proc Natl Acad Sci U S A.*, **92**, pp. 11190–11194.

52. Harley, C. B., Futcher, A. B., & Greider, C. W. (1990). Telomeres shorten during ageing of human fibroblasts, *Nature*, **345**, pp. 458–460.

53. Aviv, A., & Aviv, H. (1999). Telomeres and essential hypertension, *American Journal of Hypertension*, **12**, pp. 427–432.

54. Ma, L., Li, Y., & Wang, J. (2015). Telomeres and essential hypertension, *Clinical Biochemistry*, **48**, pp. 1195–1199.

55. Vasa, M., Breitschopf, K., Zeiher, A. M., & Dimmeler, S. (2000). Nitric oxide activates telomerase and delays endothelial cell senescence, *Circulation Research*, **87**, pp. 540–542.

56. Morgan RG, Ives SJ, Walker AE, et al. (2014). Role of arterial telomere dysfunction in hypertension: relative contributions of telomere shortening and telomere uncapping, *J. Hypertens.*, **32**, pp. 1293–1299.

57. Simoncini, T., Hafezi-Moghadam, A., Brazil, D. P., Ley, K., Chin, W. W., & Liao, J. K. (2000). Interaction of oestrogen receptor with the regulatory subunit of phosphatidylinositol-3-OH kinase, *Nature*, **407**, pp. 538–541.

58. Dubey, R. K., & Jackson, E. K. (2001). Estrogen-induced cardiorenal protection: potential cellular, biochemical, and molecular mechanisms,

American Journal of Physiology, Renal Physiology, **280**, pp. F365–F388.

59. Nawrot, T. S., Staessen, J. A., Gardner, J. P., & Aviv, A. (2004). Telomere length and possible link to X chromosome, *Lancet (London, England)*, **363**, pp. 507–510.
60. Jeanclos, E., Schork, N. J., Kyvik, K. O., Kimura, M., Skurnick, J. H., & Aviv, A. (2000). Telomere length inversely correlates with pulse pressure and is highly familial, *Hypertension (Dallas, Tex.: 1979)*, **36**, pp. 195–200.
61. Benetos, A., Okuda, K., Lajemi, M., Kimura, M., Thomas, F., Skurnick, J., *et al.* (2001). Telomere length as an indicator of biological aging: the gender effect and relation with pulse pressure and pulse wave velocity, *Hypertension (Dallas, Tex.: 1979)*, **37**, pp. 381–385.
62. Björkegren, J. L. M., & Lusis, A. J. (2022). Atherosclerosis: recent developments, *Cell*, **185**, pp. 1630–1645.
63. Samani, N. J., Boultby, R., Butler, R., Thompson, J. R., & Goodall, A. H. (2001). Telomere shortening in atherosclerosis, *Lancet (London, England)*, **358**, pp. 472–473.
64. De Meyer, T., Rietzschel, E. R., De Buyzere, M. L., Langlois, M. R., De Bacquer, D., Segers, P., *et al.* (2009). Systemic telomere length and preclinical atherosclerosis: the Asklepios Study, *European Heart Journal*, **30**, pp. 3074–3081.
65. Sobenin, I. A., Khasanova, Z. B., Tolstik, T. V., Zotova, U. S., Markin, A. M., & Doroshchuk, N. A. (2022). Telomere length in atherosclerotic lesions of human aortic intima, *Atherosclerosis*, **355**, pp. 32.
66. Scheller Madrid, A., Rode, L., Nordestgaard, B. G., & Bojesen, S. E. (2016). Short telomere length and ischemic heart disease: observational and genetic studies in 290 022 individuals, *Clinical Chemistry*, **62**, pp. 1140–1149.
67. Codd, V., Nelson, C. P., Albrecht, E., Mangino, M., Deelen, J., Buxton, J. L., *et al.* (2013). Identification of seven loci affecting mean telomere length and their association with disease, *Nature Genetics*, **45**, pp. 422–427e4272.
68. VanderLaan, P. A., Reardon, C. A., & Getz, G. S. (2004). Site specificity of atherosclerosis: site-selective responses to atherosclerotic modulators, *Arteriosclerosis, Thrombosis, and Vascular Biology*, **24**, pp. 12–22.
69. Bloom, S. I., Tucker, J. R., Lim, J., Thomas, T. G., Stoddard, G. J., Lesniewski, L. A., *et al.* (2022). Aging results in DNA damage and telomere dysfunction that is greater in endothelial versus vascular

smooth muscle cells and is exacerbated in atheroprone regions, *GeroScience*, **44**, pp. 2741–2755.

70. Gorenne, I., Kavurma, M., Scott, S., & Bennett, M. (2006). Vascular smooth muscle cell senescence in atherosclerosis, *Cardiovascular Research*, **72**, pp. 9–17.
71. Rudijanto A. (2007). The role of vascular smooth muscle cells on the pathogenesis of atherosclerosis, *Acta medica Indonesiana*, **39**, pp. 86–93.
72. Chistiakov, D. A., Orekhov, A. N., & Bobryshev, Y. V. (2015). Vascular smooth muscle cell in atherosclerosis, *Acta physiologica (Oxford, England)*, **214**, pp. 33–50.
73. Matthews, C., Gorenne, I., Scott, S., Figg, N., Kirkpatrick, P., Ritchie, A., *et al.* (2006). Vascular smooth muscle cells undergo telomere-based senescence in human atherosclerosis: effects of telomerase and oxidative stress, *Circulation Research*, **99**, pp. 156–164.
74. Wang, J., Uryga, A. K., Reinhold, J., Figg, N., Baker, L., Finigan, A., *et al.* (2015). Vascular smooth muscle cell senescence promotes atherosclerosis and features of plaque vulnerability, *Circulation*, **132**, pp. 1909–1919.
75. Novau-Ferré, N., Rojas, M., Gutierrez-Tordera, L., Arcelin, P., Folch, J., Papandreou, C., *et al.* (2023). Lipoprotein particle profiles associated with telomere length and telomerase complex components, *Nutrients*, **15**, pp. 2624.
76. van der Harst, P., van der Steege, G., de Boer, R. A., Voors, A. A., Hall, A. S., Mulder, M. J., et al. (2007). Telomere length of circulating leukocytes is decreased in patients with chronic heart failure, *Journal of the American College of Cardiology*, **49**, pp. 1459–1464.
77. Vasan RS, Demissie S, Kimura M, *et al.* (2008). Association of leukocyte telomere length with circulating biomarkers of the renin-angiotensin-aldosterone system: the Framingham Heart Study, *Circulation*, **117**, pp. 1138–1144.
78. Collerton, J., Martin-Ruiz, C., Kenny, A., Barrass, K., von Zglinicki, T., Kirkwood, T., *et al.* (2007). Telomere length is associated with left ventricular function in the oldest old: the Newcastle 85+ study, *European Heart Journal*, **28**, pp. 172–176.
79. Leri, A., Franco, S., Zacheo, A., Barlucchi, L., Chimenti, S., Limana, F., *et al.* (2003). Ablation of telomerase and telomere loss leads to cardiac dilatation and heart failure associated with p53 upregulation, *The EMBO Journal*, **22**, pp. 131–139.

80. Aung, N., Wang, Q., van Duijvenboden, S., Burns, R., Stoma, S., Raisi-Estabragh, Z., *et al.* (2023). Association of longer leukocyte telomere length with cardiac size, function, and heart failure, *JAMA Cardiology,* **8**, pp. 808–815.
81. Raymond, A. R., Norton, G. R., Sareli, P., Woodiwiss, A. J., & Brooksbank, R. L. (2013). Relationship between average leucocyte telomere length and the presence or severity of idiopathic dilated cardiomyopathy in black Africans, *European Journal of Heart Failure,* **15**, pp. 54–60.
82. Bernhard, D., Laufer, G. (2008) The aging cardiomyocyte: a mini-review, *Gerontology,* **54**, pp. 24–31
83. Brandt, M., Dörschmann, H., Khraisat, S., Knopp, T., Ringen, J., Kalinovic, S., *et al.* (2022). Telomere shortening in hypertensive heart disease depends on oxidative DNA damage and predicts impaired recovery of cardiac function in heart failure, *Hypertension (Dallas, Tex.: 1979),* **79**, pp. 2173–2184.
84. Houben, J. M., Moonen, H. J., van Schooten, F. J., & Hageman, G. J. (2008). Telomere length assessment: biomarker of chronic oxidative stress? *Free Radical Biology and Medicine,* **44**, pp. 235–246.
85. Matsumoto, Y., Adams, V., Walther, C., Kleinecke, C., Brugger, P., Linke, A., *et al.* (2009). Reduced number and function of endothelial progenitor cells in patients with aortic valve stenosis: a novel concept for valvular endothelial cell repair, *European Heart Journal,* **30**, pp. 346–355.
86. Wang, J., Hao, Y., Zhu, Z., Liu, B., Zhang, X., Wei, N., *et al.* (2022). Causality of telomere length associated with calcific aortic valvular stenosis: a Mendelian randomization study, *Frontiers in Medicine,* **9**, pp. 1077686.
87. Grahame, T. J., & Schlesinger, R. B. (2012). Oxidative stress-induced telomeric erosion as a mechanism underlying airborne particulate matter-related cardiovascular disease, *Particle and Fibre Toxicology,* **9**, pp. 1–19.
88. Oh, H., Wang, S. C., Prahash, A., Sano, M., Moravec, C. S., Taffet, G. E., *et al.* (2003). Telomere attrition and Chk2 activation in human heart failure, *Proceedings of the National Academy of Sciences of the United States of America,* **100**, pp. 5378–5383.
89. Murasawa, S., Llevadot, P., Silver, M., Isner, J.M., Losordo, D.W., Asahara, T. (2002). Constitutive human telomerase reverse transcriptase expression enhances regenerative properties of endothelial progenitor cells, *Circulation,* **106**, pp. 1133–1139.

90. Romaine, S. P. R., Denniff, M., Codd, V., Nath, M., Koekemoer, A., Anker, S. D., *et al.* (2022). Telomere length is independently associated with all-cause mortality in chronic heart failure, *Heart (British Cardiac Society)*, **108**, pp. 124–129.
91. Oh, H., Taffet, G. E., Youker, K. A., Entman, M. L., Overbeek, P. A., Michael, L. H., *et al.* (2001). Telomerase reverse transcriptase promotes cardiac muscle cell proliferation, hypertrophy, and survival, *Proceedings of the National Academy of Sciences of the United States of America*, **98**, pp. 10308–10313.
92. Levi, F., Lucchini, F., Negri, E., & La Vecchia, C. (2002). Trends in mortality from cardiovascular and cerebrovascular diseases in Europe and other areas of the world, *Heart (British Cardiac Society)*, **88**, pp. 119–124.
93. Haycock, P. C., Heydon, E. E., Kaptoge, S., Butterworth, A. S., Thompson, A., & Willeit, P. (2014). Leucocyte telomere length and risk of cardiovascular disease: systematic review and meta-analysis, *Bmj*, **349**, pp. g4227.
94. Fyhrquist, F., Saijonmaa, O., & Strandberg, T. (2013). The roles of senescence and telomere shortening in cardiovascular disease, *Nature Reviews Cardiology*, **10**, pp. 274–283.
95. Toupance, S., Labat, C., Temmar, M., *et al.* (2017). Short telomeres, but not telomere attrition rates, are associated with carotid atherosclerosis, *Hypertension*, **70**, pp. 420–425.
96. Ellehoj, H., Bendix, L., & Osler, M. (2016). Leucocyte telomere length and risk of cardiovascular disease in a cohort of 1,397 Danish men and women, *Cardiology*, **133**, pp. 173–177.
97. Ding, H., Chen, C., Shaffer, J. R., Liu, L., Xu, Y., Wang, X., *et al.* (2012). Telomere length and risk of stroke in Chinese, *Stroke*, **43**, pp. 658–663.
98. Jin X, Pan B, Dang X, Wu H, Xu D. (2018). Relationship between short telomere length and stroke: a meta-analysis, *Medicine (Baltimore)*, **97**, pp. e12489.
99. Wu, Y., Wang, X., Zhou, X., Cheng, B., Li, G., Bai, B. (2017). Temporal expression of apelin/apelin receptor in ischemic stroke and its therapeutic potential., *Front. Mol. Neurosci.*, **10**, pp. 1.
100. Tian, Y., Wang, S., Jiao, F., Kong, Q., Liu, C., Wu, Y. (2019). Telomere length: a potential biomarker for the risk and prognosis of stroke, *Front. Neurol.*, **10**, pp. 624.

101. Desai, D. S., & Hajouli, S. (2022). *Arrhythmias*. In StatPearls. StatPearls Publishing.

102. Lakshminarayan, K., Anderson, D. C., Herzog, C. A., Qureshi, A. I. (2008). Clinical epidemiology of atrial fibrillation and related cerebrovascular events in the United States, *Neurologist*, **14**, pp. 143–150.

103. Sawhney, V., Campbell, N. G., Brouilette, S. W., Coppen, S. R., Harbo, M., Baker, V., *et al.* (2016). Telomere shortening and telomerase activity in ischemic cardiomyopathy patients: potential markers of ventricular arrhythmia, *International Journal of Cardiology*, **207**, pp. 157–163.

104. Sawhney, V., Brouilette, S., Campbell, N., Coppen, S., Baker, V., Hunter, R., *et al.* (2018). Association of genetic variation in telomere-related SNP and telomerase with ventricular arrhythmias in ischemic cardiomyopathy, *Pacing and Clinical Electrophysiology: PACE*, **41**, pp. 261–266.

105. Su, C., Liu, Z., Gao, Y., Liu, Y., Hu, R. M., Liu, J., *et al.* (2019). Study on the relationship between telomere length changes and recurrence of atrial fibrillation after radiofrequency catheter ablation, *Journal of Cardiovascular Electrophysiology*, **30**, pp. 1117–1124.

106. Gao, Y., Liu, Y., Fu, Y., Wang, Q., Liu, Z., Hu, R., *et al.* (2021). The potential regulatory role of hsa_circ_0004104 in the persistency of atrial fibrillation by promoting cardiac fibrosis via TGF-β pathway, *BMC Cardiovascular Disorders*, **21**, pp. 25.

107. Shealy, C. N. (2015). Telomere rejuvenation for health & longevity, *Anti-Aging Therapeutics*, **XVI**, pp. 187–198.

108. Vecoli, C., Borghini, A., Foffa, I., Ait-Ali, L., Picano, E., & Andreassi, M. G. (2016). Leukocyte telomere shortening in grown-up patients with congenital heart disease, *International Journal of Cardiology*, **204**, pp. 17–22.

109. Iung, B., & Vahanian, A. (2014). Epidemiology of acquired valvular heart disease, *The Canadian Journal of Cardiology*, **30**(9), pp. 962–970.

110. Saraieva, I., Benetos, A., Labat, C., Franco-Cereceda, A., Bäck, M., Toupance, S. (2021). Telomere length in valve tissue is shorter in individuals with aortic stenosis and in calcified valve areas, *Front. Cell Dev. Biol.*, **9**, pp. 618335.

111. Okuda, K., Khan, M. Y., Skurnick, J., Kimura, M., Aviv, H., & Aviv, A. (2000). Telomere attrition of the human abdominal aorta: relationships with age and atherosclerosis, *Atherosclerosis*, **152**, pp. 391–398.

112. Kurz, D. J., Kloeckener-Gruissem, B., Akhmedov, A., Eberli, F. R., Bühler, I., Berger, W., *et al.* (2006). Degenerative aortic valve stenosis, but

not coronary disease, is associated with shorter telomere length in the elderly, *Arteriosclerosis, Thrombosis, and Vascular Biology*, **26**, pp. e114–e117.

113. Hoffmann, J., Tabata, N., Mas-Peiro, S., Spyridopoulos, I., Sinning, J. M., Berkowitsch, A., *et al.* (2022). Longer leukocyte telomere length is associated with myeloid inflammation and increased mortality after transcatheter aortic valve replacement, *European Heart Journal Open*, **2**, pp. oeac045.

Chapter 17

Decelerating Cardiovascular Aging: Diet, Exercise, and Medication

Konstantinos Tsarouhas,[a] Christina Tsitsimpikou,[b] and Emmanouel Papadakis[c]

[a] *University Hospital of Larissa, Larissa, Greece*
[b] *General Chemical State Laboratory, Greece*
[c] *Onassis Cardiac Surgery Centre, Athens, Greece*
ktsarouhas14@yahoo.gr

17.1 Effect of Diet, Exercise, and Medication on Cardiovascular Aging

Structural and functional decline of the myocardium and the aorta is associated with the phenomenon of cardiovascular aging. Regarding myocardium, there are several hallmarks of cardiovascular aging namely myocardial diastolic dysfunction, myocardial fibrosis, and hypertrophy. Oxidative stress, mitochondrial dysfunction, inflammation, and apoptosis are the main culprit pathogenic processes involved in these pathologies. Lipofuscin accumulation has also been reported in the aging heart. On the other hand, the aorta in the elderly presents an enlarged lumen and thickened wall and is

Telomeres: Biomarkers of a Healthy Life and Successful Aging
Edited by Aristidis Tsatsakis

ISBN 978-981-5129-49-6 (Hardcover), 978-1-003-56809-4 (eBook)
www.jennystanford.com

characterized by arterial dysfunction. Collagen deposition, increased apoptosis, and inflammation are very common in the aging aorta. Reduced nitric oxide bioavailability and endothelial dysfunction lead to aortic stiffness [1].

Senescence of the main cell components of the aortic wall is observed in aging, evident by specific staining in the pathologic laboratory as beta-galactosidase staining. The main senescent cells in the aging aorta are endothelial and smooth muscle cells. Their cell death leads to aortic extracellular matrix degradation. Impaired angiogenesis in the aging aorta leads further to microvascular rarefaction, a reduction in the density of aortic micro-vessels. Along with the senescent cells, the cells adopt a senescence-associated secretory phenotype (SASP) that makes them pro-inflammatory and spreads the inflammation to the surrounding tissue cells, via what it is called a paracrine action. Inflammatory factors circulate downstream, while the endothelial cell barrier is disrupted. Tissue microenvironment changes and inflammation are the main contributors of cellular senescence to vascular aging [2].

In cardiovascular aging, autophagy, a salvatory mechanism of tissue function, is significantly suppressed, while a considerable rise in reactive oxygen species occurs. It is thought that in cardiovascular aging the mTOR signaling is overactivated, while AMPK activity is reduced. Also, an activation of the PI3K/Akt signaling pathway was reported. In response to these changes, the initiation of autophagy is attenuated as a result of suppression of the function of the autophagy ULK1 initiation complex. At the same time, negative transcriptional regulation of autophagy occurs as both the FOXO (a subgroup of the Forkhead family of transcription factors) and the TFEB (transcription factor EB) action is attenuated, which is considered pro-autophagic [1].

Chromosome telomere length role in cardiovascular disease is nowadays increasingly recognized as reduced telomere length is linked to several cardiovascular diseases, e.g., atherosclerosis, coronary artery disease, heart failure, and peripheral artery disease (Fig. 17.1). Telomerase activation and thus increased telomere length is associated with a healthy lifestyle, and exercise and is found to be augmented through the action of several drugs, such

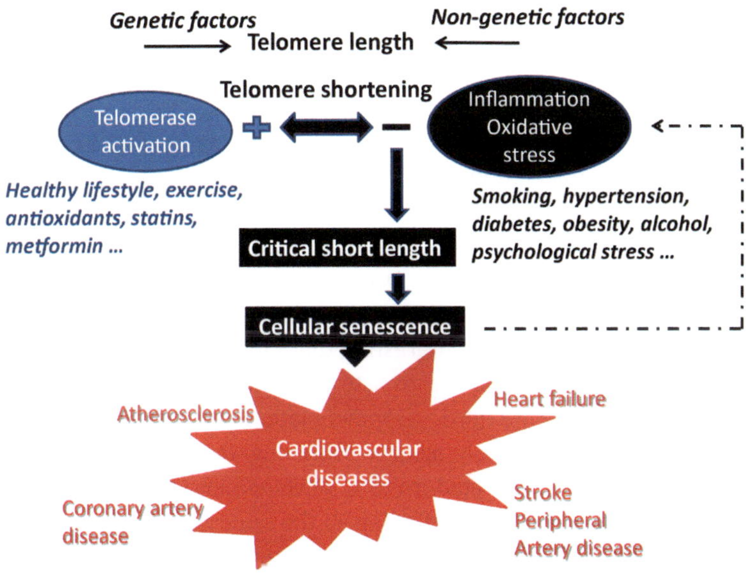

Figure 17.1 Schematic overview of telomere length and cardiovascular disease.

as statins, pioglitazone, and antioxidants. There is an equilibrium between telomerase activation and non-genetic factors that provoke inflammation and oxidative stress which result in telomere shortening. Unhealthy habits like smoking and alcohol abuse and several diseases, such as hypertension, diabetes, obesity, and psychological stress result in telomere shortening and, in the end, cellular senescence, the hallmark of cardiovascular aging [3].

Regarding endothelial and vascular smooth muscle senescence, several triggers were identified with the main representatives being telomere and DNA damage, epigenetic stress, oncogene activation, loss of tumor suppression factors, and increased levels of angiotensin II. In this process, the presence of aged collagen, disturbed blood flow in the aorta and the coronary vessels, and the reduced availability of nitric oxide (NO), all lead to endothelial and smooth muscle cell senescence, and arterial stiffness, primary features of vascular aging. In this regard, high glucose values are associated with an increased presence of glycated collagen which further confers to the vicious cycle of vascular inflammation stiffening and degeneration [4]. Replicative incompetence is observed in the respective cells, impaired angiogenesis ensues, and ultimately arterial stiffening.

Arterial stiffening as a function of vascular aging is well characterized and is connected with factors affecting cardiovascular health, such as smoking, diabetes, hyperlipidemia, and hypertension, and is more prominent in women. Less-known cardiovascular influences such as oxidative stress and DNA damage can be the culprit of arterial stiffening as well as low-grade chronic inflammation and telomere shortening. It is interesting that low birth weight and fetal programming are connected to arterial stiffening, thus connecting early life features with the development later in life of characteristics of vascular aging, namely arterial stiffening. It is known that low birth weight is connected to the development later in life of hypertension and arterial stiffening. At the same time, the influences in fetal life which cause growth retardation and impaired growth, it is thought that induce epigenetic changes which can affect the offspring (the next generation). Fetal programming in this aspect can involve changes to sympathetic nervous system activation and renin-angiotensin system balance in response to fetal life stressors. Indices of arterial stiffening as the pulse wave velocity of the blood flow in the aorta can integrate all the major changes occurring in the vessel wall with aging. Carotid stiffness is also an excellent marker of vascular aging.

Mechanisms of vascular aging range from diverse sources and pathways and give birth to several different cardiovascular pathologies. Identifying those mechanisms offers new possibilities to deter these detrimental vascular influences and potentially slow down the course of vascular aging. Apart from the mechanisms already mentioned, namely endothelial and vascular smooth muscle senescence, aortic stiffening, and chromosome telomere length attrition, impaired nuclear factor erythroid 2–related factor (NRF-2) signaling, has also been described as a factor of vascular aging, leading to dysfunctional mechanisms of oxidative stress resistance, induction of nitrative stress, NAD+ depletion, and NF-kB activation. The molecular target of rapamycin (mTOR) dysregulation, along with dysregulation of sirtuins and AMPK has also been implicated in the process. Involvement of miRNAs has been recorded and impaired DNA methylation whose role in epigenetic modification in protein synthesis is well known. Genomic instability was also reported in the mechanisms of vascular aging. mTOR is an autophagy repressor. AMPK (AMP-activated protein kinase) acts on mTOR suppressing its action. It should be noted that AMPK is very sensitive to changes in the cell energy status. On the other hand, sirtuins are enzymes involved in protein acetylation (deacetylases) which in turn are major determinants of autophagy induction in cell homeostasis [2].

It is evident from the above-mentioned mechanisms that in vascular aging, inflammation ensues in the vascular tree, extracellular matrix (ECM) remodeling occurs and there is an impaired mechanism of vascular healing. At the same time, atherosclerosis is augmented. Cellular energetics of the vascular wall, focusing on the production, distribution, and use of energy typically via the production of ATP (adenosine triphosphate) through cellular respiration, are impaired. The presence of inflammation in vascular aging is fundamental and is associated with the paracrine effect in surrounding cells at the tissue level. As a result, regarding the vascular system, the term "inflammaging" was used to describe the combined action of inflammation with the other features of vascular aging. For each of these mechanisms of vascular aging, potential interventions and medications were suggested to inhibit the causal features of the pathology with the first ever tested being diet.

The trigger to study specific diets to contemplate vascular aging and aging, in general, came from the observation of the extended lifespan of residents of the Japanese city of Okinawa. Regarding cardiovascular mortality, the Okinawans presented striking differences in mortality from coronary artery disease compared to Americans but also significantly lower from other Japanese. Also, mortality for different cancer types, such as breast and prostate cancer, was considerably reduced. At the same time, the traditional Okinawan diet is known for its low caloric content, and it is mainly comprised of carbohydrates with a low content of fat and protein [5]. Okinawans usually present low weight and have a low body surface area (BMI). This phenomenon led to active research regarding the potential of caloric restriction to contribute to an increased lifespan, healthy aging, and healthy cardiovascular aging.

What was found was that across all living organisms and especially mammals, caloric restriction inhibits the action of mTOR and suppresses the levels of insulin growth factor 1 (IGF-1). This, in turn, leads to the activation of the PI3K/Akt pathway with favorable effects on the FOXO transcription factors. It is thought that IGF-1 actions are central to the nutrient-sensing pathways and that its inhibition suppresses in part the main pathways of aging [6]. The final steps of the aging pathways are not clearly understood at the moment.

In human skeletal muscle, it is found that **caloric restriction** suppresses inflammation and augments mitochondrial biogenesis. Also, autophagy is increased, and DNA repair is activated. In terms of metabolic adaptations, diet improves lipidemic profile and reduces insulin and glucose levels, reduces leptin levels, increases adiponectin levels, and reduces angiotensin I levels. As a result of caloric restriction, the physiological adaptations involve improved endothelial function, lowering of arterial blood pressure, improved diastolic myocardial function, and an improvement of the autonomic system regulation of heart rhythm shown by an improved heart rate variability. All these favorable changes are translated to a reduced risk of coronary artery disease and cardiac arrhythmias and a low risk of stroke. Why does diet in terms of caloric restriction drive the antiaging effects? Probably because at times of significant deprivation of food, organisms, and cells reduce their function and reproduction to divert energy for the cell-sustaining systems [7]. Thus, in organism evolution starvation periods trigger antiaging modifications.

Apart from caloric restriction, protein restriction seems to increase the levels of stress-resistance genes both in laboratory experiments and in clinical settings. This occurs as a result of activation of mTOR signaling and augmented levels of general control nonderepressible 2 (GCN2) protein kinase. In humans, it was found that both low-calorie diet and low protein diet reduced IGF-1 concentrations, a main molecular determinant of aging. Several methods tried to reproduce the positive anti-aging effects of low-calorie diets as intermittent fasting programs in many of which the caloric restriction is minimal, and the positive effects are induced by alternate day feeding or fasting 5 days a week and 2 days free diet or time restricting feeding namely fasting for several hours per day with no caloric restriction. It is believed that the same effects on IGF-1 could be induced in part by intermittent fasting. Caloric restriction and intermittent fasting are believed to alleviate vascular dysfunction linked to aging [8]. An alternate way to reproduce these favorable effects is through caloric restriction mimetics medication, with the main representatives of this class being rapamycin, resveratrol, and metformin. Flavonoids and carotenoids are also studied. The theoretical background of these attempts is also based on the hormesis phenomenon, as described below, to induce the stress resistance phenotype typical of antiaging favorable cellular modifications.

Hormesis represents the favorable cell reaction to low-level exposure to cell stressors such as caloric restriction. A similar effect could be replicated using different types of food/diet, which can initially act as stressors or even present a negative action to cells such as flavonoids, but in the long run, they stimulate favorable surviving and anti-aging compensation mechanisms acting as preconditioning factors. In this regard, the Mediterranean diet contains low doses of cell stressors that are capable of suppressing inflammaging. The Mediterranean diet includes the consumption of vegetables and fruits, whole grain cereals, fish, large quantities of monounsaturated fat such as olive oil, and low consumption of meat and moderate alcohol. Nutritional hormetins in the Mediterranean diet are considered phytochemicals, namely carotenoids and phenolic compounds found in olives and legumes which have the potential to activate the nuclear erythroid factor 2 (Nrf2). Also, resveratrol found in red wine can activate the Nrf2 pathway and induce sirtuin action while it can block the NF-kB action [9].

At the molecular level, for the antiaging compounds, rapamycin is known to inactivate its molecular target mTOR, and metformin acts to suppress AMPK activity. Spermidine directly increases autophagy and reduces the activity of histone acetyltransferase (HAT) limiting epigenetic modifications and active transcription in the nucleus.

In humans, there is accumulating evidence that several compounds impact arterial aging. Omega-3 fish oils improve endothelial function and reduce arterial stiffening. Lycopene and quercetin increase SIRT signaling and reduce arterial dysfunction. Also, curcumin was found able to increase the Nrf-2 activity and improve endothelial function. **Exercise, caloric restriction, and caloric restriction (CR) mimetic drugs induce autophagy, and thus, have the potential to slow down cardiovascular aging**. This occurs by ultimately reducing myocardial hypertrophy and fibrosis and attenuating diastolic myocardial dysfunction and arterial stiffening. Endothelial function is enhanced, and vascular wall thickening is attenuated [10]. We have previously shown in a publication of our group, that resveratrol administration in rats augmented Akt expression in rats' hearts [11]. Also, interestingly it is found that vascular function can be improved in adults involved in strenuous exercise marathons such as marathon running. Tomato juice supplementation, a high source of lycopene, improved endothelial function and oxidative stress markers after 2 months of use in marathon runners [12]. In this sport, cardiovascular adaptations to marathon running seem to go hand in hand with markers of inflammation which at least have a predictive ability of the specific patterns of myocardial hypertrophy if not partially implicated in this process [13].

Simple interventions such as **dietary sodium restriction** can improve healthy vascular aging evidenced by a reduction of systolic blood pressure and carotid-femoral pulse wave velocity. A 5.2 gr reduction of salt daily intake can significantly reduce pulse wave velocity independently of blood pressure values [14]. In terms of the reduction of **carotid augmentation index** values and of **aortic pulse wave velocity, central markers of cardiovascular aging**, it is reported that sodium restriction can achieve a significantly greater reduction compared to exercise in postmenopausal women with systolic hypertension. However, the role of exercise in restoring healthy cardiovascular aging and in reducing cardiovascular mortality should not be underestimated.

In major observational studies, such as the Aerobics Center Longitudinal study, a prospective cohort study that involved 55.000 persons, was found that exercise, specifically running, reduced cardiovascular mortality in runners compared to non-exercising individuals. A recent study has also shown that increased physical activity can lead to healthy microvascular aging by suppressing p66, a mitochondrial adaptor and source of ROS. Retinal arterial to venular diameter was significantly higher in exercising individuals compared to healthy sedentary and sedentary at-risk persons. P66 expression was significantly attenuated in exercising persons along with reduced 3-nitrotyrosine levels, indicative of reduced oxidative stress levels. It was found that exercise induces epigenetic modifications, and DNA methylation is one of them. Exercise augmented p66 gene methylation thus suppressing its activity [15]. Acute bouts of aerobic exercise also have the potential to increase telomerase activity in mononuclear cells in humans compared to resistance exercise. The acute effect was studied after a session of 45 minutes of walking or running. Chronic aerobic exercise training was also able to increase telomere length in peripheral blood mononuclear cells in previously inactive persons. Interval aerobic training had an analogous effect.

A very interesting study followed previously inactive people trained to compete in the London Marathon. In persons older than 37 years, exercise significantly reduced central aortic blood pressure and improved aortic distensibility. Running also improved all aortic stiffness indices. Exercise led to a reduction of 4 mmHg of central aortic systolic pressure in participants of the 6-month training program. When aortic biological age was calculated from the relationship between chronological age and arterial stiffness, it was found that the 6-month exercise program reduced the estimated aortic age by 4 years. This effect was more pronounced in older, male participants, with higher blood pressure, and in the slower runners. It should be noted that first-time marathon runners usually are half an hour slower than the average runner [16]. Exercise training is thought to reduce aortic stiffness, a hallmark of vascular aging, by both reducing blood pressure and also inducing structural changes in the aortic wall, thus presenting a load-independent effect.

Exercise training decreases inflammation and ECM remodeling; the latter by a reduction in proteolytic mechanisms activity. At the same time, it increases wall shear stress which in turn increases NO availability in the arterial wall. A reduction in sympathetic tone and the activity of the renin-angiotensin system contributes to an improvement in the vascular smooth muscle cells' function in the aortic wall and at the end in the aortic elastic properties [17].

Data from the Cooper Center Longitudinal study show that **the most active individuals presented the lowest prevalence of myocardial hypertrophy** in the form of concentric hypertrophy which is closely linked to diastolic dysfunction. Biomarkers of myocardial stress and injury as the NT-proBNP and troponin were found in a separate analysis of the Cardiovascular Health Study to be minimally increased in the most active persons among 2,900 older adults over an observation period of 2–3 years. However, exercise should be accompanied by a healthy diet to maximize its positive effects in preventing vascular aging and cardiometabolic disease. Especially in the prevention of diabetes, which in many cases is a major triggering factor of accelerated vascular aging, it was found from meta-analysis that maintaining normal weight is of the greatest value in the prevention of diabetes and that even high levels of physical activity when they are combined with obesity present several times higher risk for diabetes development compared to cases of low physical activity but with normal weight [18].

Countering arterial stiffness and thus vascular aging can be facilitated with the simplest forms of exercise. The stretching exercise was able to reduce arterial stiffness in middle-aged and older men compared to non-exercising people. Vascular endothelial function was improved with stretching exercise and the resting heart rate and diastolic blood pressure were reduced. Vascular endothelial function can be assessed in the clinical setting with the measurement of flow-mediated dilatation (FMD) of the brachial artery. In older men, it was found that exercise, specifically 8 weeks of aerobic exercise, could significantly improve FMD and that the FMD values achieved in older individuals with exercise were comparable to FMD values in younger non-exercising persons. **Carotid compliance is another sensitive marker of arterial stiffness.** In later middle age and older adults, it was found that aerobic exercise in the form of running, rowing, and swimming had a positive effect in improving carotid compliance compared to healthy untrained controls while resistance training increased carotid compliance.

Very interesting data on the role of exercise on vascular aging came from the EXAMIN Age study, in which the effects of 12 weeks of high-intensity interval training of Nordic walking were studied in older individuals with a mean age of 59 years. Even though Nordic walking did not reduce aortic pulse wave velocity (PWV), a commonly used index of arterial stiffness, in sedentary adults at risk for cardiovascular disease, it was evident that healthy active older adults presented the lowest PWV values compared to sedentary, healthy and at-risk persons. Taking in mind the results of the cardiorespiratory exercise test, with every 10 ml/min/kg increase in maximal oxygen uptake (VO2max), PWV dropped by 0.8 m/s, and a linear association of the two indices was found [19].

To decelerate vascular aging, apart from the already-mentioned strategies of exercise, caloric restriction, low sodium intake, adhering to a healthy diet (Mediterranean highly recommended), smoking cessation, and avoiding excess drinking should also be implemented. **Pharmacological interventions** were also studied in animal models with research mainly focusing on rapamycin, metformin, and resveratrol and secondly on the role of statins, antihypertensive drugs, and NAD+ precursors.

Antihypertensive treatment was effective in reducing PWV in patients with mild and moderate essential hypertension, irrespective of the blood pressure lowering achieved. In the short-term studies, angiotensin-converting enzyme inhibitors (ACEI) significantly reduced PWV compared to placebo and calcium channel antagonists. In long-term studies, all the major classes of antihypertension medication, namely diuretics, ACEI, Calcium Channel Blockers, and beta-blockers, effectively reduced arterial stiffness. In a meta-analysis of the Sprint clinical trial, it was found that the intensive antihypertensive treatment reduced all-cause mortality compared to the standard one only when arterial stiffness was reduced, thus linking a determinant of vascular aging with all-cause death. In the standard treatment, PWV reduction responders had an impressive 42% mortality risk reduction [20]. Very effective in reducing central aortic systolic and pulse pressure was the combination of sacubitril/valsartan compared to olmesartan in the Parameter study, an effect achieved already in the 12th week of treatment and maintained to the 52nd week of treatment.

Statins also showed their ability to reduce arterial stiffness indices such as aortic PWV and augmentation index in hypertensive and hypercholesterolemic patients. Statin pleiotropic effects, favorable action on vascular endothelial function, and inflammation suppression are the possible mechanisms involved. Statins were found capable of increasing telomerase activity in blood mononuclear cells and increasing telomere length in older adults. Statin treatment also reduced the rate of telomere shortening which naturally occurs each year (effect of aging).

Telomerase activity is usually reduced by obesity and diabetes while lifestyle changes such as diet and exercise increase telomerase activity through inflammation reduction and epigenetic changes. Bariatric surgery and anti-diabetic medication as dipeptidyl peptidase IV (DPP IV) inhibitors and peroxisome proliferator-activated receptors (PPARs) improve insulin sensitivity and increase telomerase activity. Regarding telomerase activity opposite actions were reported depending on which pathway of telomerase action is activated. Reduced telomere length of inflammatory cells is associated with delaying coronary artery disease (CAD) appearance (in this case the canonical pathway of telomerase function is involved). On the other hand, when non-canonical pathways of telomerase action are activated, reduced telomerase activity is connected to senescence and DNA damage which in turn accelerates CAD. In a previous study in patients with metabolic syndrome, it was found that telomerase activity was increased in peripheral blood mononuclear cells along with markers of inflammation and endothelial dysfunction. The increased telomerase activity was inversely correlated with high-density lipoprotein levels and positively with a marker of endothelial dysfunction, namely Asymmetric Dimethylarginine (ADMA) [12].

Other pharmacological interventions to achieve healthy vascular aging are AMPK activators with the main representative being metformin, and sirtuin activators with resveratrol being the most well-known, anti-cytokine therapy with anti-TNF-a medications to stand out, and peroxisome proliferator-activated receptor gamma (PPAR-gamma) agents for example pioglitazone. Rapamycin, the main mTOR inhibitor, apart from protecting from in-stent restenosis and cardiac allograft vasculopathy, reduces arterial stiffness. In experiments in mice, rapamycin increased survival when administered later in life. This effect was considered a result of aging deceleration or a retardation of death from cancer. On the other hand, resveratrol was able to improve endothelial function in overweight patients with mild hypertension as resveratrol supplementation improved flow-mediated dilatation of the brachial artery.

Metformin's action on vascular aging is more complex. Metformin suppresses IGF-1 and insulin and inhibits PAI-1 and TNF-a. It also inhibits NF-Kb and activates the PI3/Akt pathway. Thus, it reduces oxidative stress and cell senescence. Metformin acts on AMPK and mTOR and in turn, favors cellular survival and increases autophagy [21, 22].

Cardiovascular aging research recently focuses on senolytic drugs, which could have the ability to suppress senescence. Myocardial cell senescence in aging hearts leads to compensatory myocardial hypertrophy which in cases of additional stress as ischemia or hypertension could lead to the spread of senescence to neighboring myocardial cells and potentially to decompensation overriding myocardial adaptive mechanisms [23]. Senolytic drugs can act directly on senescent cells and in laboratory experiments on mice, it is found that they can help in the clearance of senescent cells and improve vascular relaxation. A reduction of vascular calcification was also noted. The main representatives are dasatinib and quercetin. Quercetin is a plant flavonol and is found in many fruits and vegetables. Dasatinib is an anti-cancer drug, a tyrosine kinase inhibitor, used to treat different types of leukemia. Fisetin another flavonol and naticlovax, another anti-cancer drug, are thought to be senolytic. Senolytics were found capable of increasing survival in experiments in mice. Dasatinib and quercetin administration also reduced inflammation and cytokine secretion in human adipose tissue.

As the adult population ages, the deceleration of aging features as vascular aging whose consequences span to major cardiovascular problems such as coronary artery disease and heart failure, becomes a significant quest. Healthy diet interventions and exercise can help in this direction. Active research is also conducted on new drugs that can become game-changers or new ways of using already-known medical compounds to slow down the main components of vascular aging.

References

1. Abdellatif, M., Sedej, S., Carmona-Gutierrez, D., Madeo, F., Kroemer, G. (2018). Autophagy in cardiovascular aging, *Circ Res*, **123,** pp. 803–24.
2. Ungvari, Z., Tarantini, S., Donato, A. J., Galvan, V., Csiszar, A. (2018). Mechanisms of vascular aging, *Circ Res,* **123**, pp. 849–67.
3. Yeh, J. K., Wang, C. Y. (2016). Telomeres and telomerase in cardiovascular diseases, *Genes (Basel)*, **7**, pp. 58.
4. Yin, H., Pickering, J. G. (2016). Cellular senescence and vascular disease: novel routes to better understanding and therapy, *Can J Cardiol,* **32**, pp. 612–23.
5. Le Couteur, D. G., Solon-Biet, S., Wahl, D., Cogger, V. C., Willcox, B. J., Willcox, D. C., *et al.* (2016). New horizons: dietary protein, ageing and the Okinawan ratio, *Age Ageing*, **45**, pp. 443–7.
6. Fontana, L., Partridge, L., Longo, V. D. (2010). Extending healthy life span–from yeast to humans, *Science*, **328**, pp. 321–6.
7. Fontana, L. (2018). Interventions to promote cardiometabolic health and slow cardiovascular ageing, *Nat Rev Cardiol*, **15**, pp. 566–77.
8. Mirzaei, H., Suarez, J. A., Longo, V. D. (2014). Protein and amino acid restriction, aging and disease: from yeast to humans, *Trends Endocrinol Metab*, **25**, pp. 558–66.
9. Martucci, M., Ostan, R., Biondi, F., Bellavista, E., Fabbri, C., Bertarelli, C., *et al.* (2017). Mediterranean diet and inflammaging within the hormesis paradigm, *Nutr Rev.*, **75**, pp. 442–55.
10. LaRocca, T. J., Martens, C. R., Seals, D. R. (2017). Nutrition and other lifestyle influence on arterial aging, *Ageing Res Rev.*, **39**, pp. 106–19.
11. Hashemzaei, M., Barani, A. K., Iranshahi, M., Rezaee, R., Tsarouhas, K., Tsatsakis, A. M., *et al.* (2016). Effects of resveratrol on carbon monoxide-induced cardiotoxicity in rats, *Environ Toxicol Pharmacol*, **46**, pp. 110–5.

12. Samaras, A., Tsarouhas, K., Paschalidis, E., Giamouzis, G., Triposkiadis, F., Tsitsimpikou, C., *et al.* (2014). Effect of a special carbohydrate-protein bar and tomato juice supplementation on oxidative stress markers and vascular endothelial dynamics in ultra-marathon runners, *Food Chem Toxicol*, **69**, pp. 231–6.
13. Tsarouhas, K., Tsitsimpikou, C., Samaras, A., Saravanis, C., Kolovou, G., Bacopoulou, F., *et al.* (2022). Cardiovascular adaptations and inflammation in marathon runners, *Exp Ther Med*, **24**, pp. 699.
14. D'Elia, L., Galletti, F., La Fata, E., Sabino, P., Strazzullo, P. (2018). Effect of dietary sodium restriction on arterial stiffness: systematic review and meta-analysis of the randomized controlled trials, *J Hypertens*, **36**, pp. 734–43.
15. Streese, L., Khan, A. W., Deiseroth, A., Hussain, S., Suades, R., Tiaden, A., *et al.* (2020). Physical activity may drive healthy microvascular ageing via downregulation of p66 (Shc), *Eur J Prev Cardiol*, **27**, pp. 168–76.
16. Bhuva, A. N., D'Silva, A., Torlasco, C., Jones, S., Nadarajan, N., Van Zalen, J., *et al.* (2020). Training for a first-time marathon reverses age-related aortic stiffening, *J Am Coll Cardiol*, **75**, pp. 60–71.
17. Chirinos, J. A. (2020). The run against arterial aging, *J Am Coll Cardiol*, **75**, pp. 72–5.
18. Cloostermans, L., Wendel-Vos, W., Doornbos, G., Howard, B., Craig, C. L., Kivimaki, M., *et al.* (2015). Independent and combined effects of physical activity and body mass index on the development of type 2 diabetes: a meta-analysis of 9 prospective cohort studies, *Int J Behav Nutr Phys Act*, **12**, pp. 147.
19. Deiseroth, A., Streese, L., Kochli, S., Wust, R. S., Infanger, D., Schmidt-Trucksass, A., *et al.* (2019). Exercise and arterial stiffness in the elderly: a combined cross-sectional and randomized controlled trial (EXAMIN AGE), *Front Physiol*, **10**, pp. 1119.
20. Vlachopoulos, C., Terentes-Printzios, D., Laurent, S., Nilsson, P. M., Protogerou, A. D., Aznaouridis, K., *et al.* (2019). Association of estimated pulse wave velocity with survival: a secondary analysis of SPRINT, *JAMA Netw Open*, **2**, pp. e1912831.
21. Nowak, K. L., Rossman, M. J., Chonchol, M., Seals, D. R. (2018). Strategies for achieving healthy vascular aging, *Hypertension*, **71**, pp. 389–402.
22. Barzilai, N., Crandall, J. P., Kritchevsky, S. B., Espeland, M. A. (2016). Metformin as a tool to target aging, *Cell Metab*, **23**, pp. 1060–5.
23. Childs, B. G., Li, H., van Deursen J. M. (2018). Senescent cells: a therapeutic target for cardiovascular disease, *J Clin Invest*, **128**, pp. 1217–28.

Chapter 18

Male and Female Infertility

Elisavet Kouvidi,[a] Elisavet Renieri,[b,c] and Aristidis Tsatsakis[b,c]
[a] *Phenotypos Lab, Athens, Greece*
[b] *Laboratory of Toxicology, Medical School, University of Crete, Heraklion, Greece*
[c] *Lifeplus S.A., Science & Technological Park of Crete,*
Vassilika Vouton, Heraklion, Greece
ekouvidi@gmail.com, medp2011622@med.uoc.gr, tsatsaka@uoc.gr

18.1 Introduction

Telomeres are specific, highly conserved, non-coding DNA structures located at the ends of eukaryotic chromosomes, which protect them from degradation, recombination, or end-to-end fusion, and thus are essential for maintaining genomic integrity and stability. Human telomeres consist of a 5–20-kb double-stranded (ds) 5′-TTAGGG-3′ tandem repeat region and a 50–300-nucleotide single-stranded (ss) G-rich overhang at the 3′ end, which folds back onto duplex telomeric DNA forming a "T-loop" structure [1, 2]. The regulation of telomere function is accomplished through associations between telomeric DNA and numerous directly or indirectly binding proteins [3]. Shelterin is a six-protein complex consisting of TRF1 (telomere repeat factor), TRF2, TIN2 (TRF1-interacting nuclear factor), RAP1 (repressor activator protein), TPP1 (telomere protection protein),

Telomeres: Biomarkers of a Healthy Life and Successful Aging
Edited by Aristidis Tsatsakis

ISBN 978-981-5129-49-6 (Hardcover), 978-1-003-56809-4 (eBook)
www.jennystanford.com

and POT1 (protection of telomeres) subunits, which implicated in the formation of "T-loops" and safeguards telomeres from degradation and DNA damage responses [4–6].

Most normal human somatic cells (e.g., fibroblasts, skin epidermal cells, peripheral blood leukocytes, etc.) lose about 50–150 bp of their telomeric repeats per cell cycle during aging and have a limited replicative capacity of about 40–60 passages in culture [7, 8]. Telomere loss is caused by the "end replication problem" in which there is unidirectional 5′–3′ DNA replication and incomplete replication of the 3′ DNA strand ends [9–11]. When a minimum critical number of 1–2 kb telomeric repeats or telomere length (TL) is reached, it acts as a "mitotic clock" and it triggers a DNA damage response, which signals cell cycle exit and leads to replicative senescence of cells [10–12].

Certain cells that continuously divide, such as germline cells, basal epidermal cells, proliferative granulosa cells, hematopoietic stem cells, uterine endometrial cells, activated lymphocytes, and various cancers, overcome their telomere attrition by telomerase, ribonucleoprotein enzyme complex which binds to the 3′ G–overhang and elongates the telomeric 3′ end repeat sequence [10, 13–15] (Fig. 18.1). Telomerase consists of two subunits: telomerase reverse transcriptase (TERT), which is a catalytic protein with reverse transcriptase activity and consists of four functional domains; and telomerase RNA component (TERC), which serves as the template for telomeric DNA synthesis. Numerous proteins, such as dyskerin (DKC1), nucleolar protein 10 (NOP10), non-histone protein 2 (NHP2), glycine-arginine rich 1 (GAR1), and ATPases (pontin, reptin), are associated with telomerase complex and regulate telomerase structure, function, biogenesis, and localization [16, 17]. Some somatic and germ cells and certain types of cancer (10–15%) maintain their telomere length through a telomerase-independent mechanism termed alternative lengthening of telomeres (ALT), which relies on telomere sister chromatid exchanges (T-SCE) and homologous recombination [14, 18, 19]. ALT appears to lead to the formation of longer telomeres compared to the lengths obtained after telomerase activity. However, it is a mechanism not yet fully elucidated [20].

Telomerase is activated during embryogenesis at the blastocyst stage, at which the longest telomeres are found, localizing to

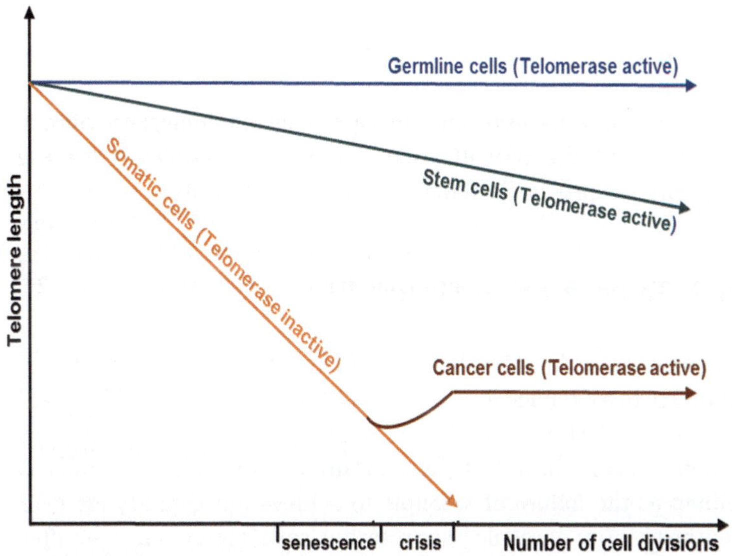

Figure 18.1 Telomere length in different cells in relation to the number of cell divisions.

inner cell mass [21, 22]. TL has been shown to be synchronized among tissues of the human fetus and newborn and no TL difference between male and female newborns has been observed [23, 24]. However, in adults, telomerase is inactivated, and TL varies between chromosomes, between cell types, across tissues, and among individuals [23, 25, 26]. Interestingly, telomeres in females have shown to be slightly longer (176 bp) than in males of similar age, a difference associated with a protective effect due to female hormones [19, 23, 25, 26]. This great variability in TL among adults is due to influences of several genetic, epigenetic, and environmental factors (e.g., oxidative stress, inflammation, lifestyle factors, physiological stress, and exposure to carcinogens) occurring in extra-uterine life [17, 21, 23, 27].

TL has been suggested to be a biomarker of cellular senescence and of biological aging and a risk factor for age-related diseases, such as cardiovascular disease, type 2 diabetes mellitus, neurodegenerative diseases, osteoporosis, aplastic anemia, dyskeratosis, etc. [8, 10, 15]. Aging also has a negative effect on reproductive aging and capacity. Due to the strong association between aging and telomeres, several studies have investigated the relationship between telomere length and the development of male and female infertility.

This chapter discusses the emerging role of telomeres in human infertility and the potential use of TL as a biomarker for the diagnosis and prognosis of male and female infertility.

18.2 Telomeres and Infertility

In recent years, there has been a tendency for couples to postpone childbirth to a later age due to social and economic factors. Biological age causes dysfunction of both male and female reproductive systems, decline in fertility, and eventually infertility. Infertility is defined as the failure of a couple to achieve a pregnancy after 12 months or more of regular, unprotected, sexual intercourse, or after 6 months for women aged 35 and older [28]. Approximately 1 in 6 couples face infertility problems worldwide; estimates suggest that between 48 million couples and 186 million individuals live with infertility globally [28]. The male factor is solely responsible for about 30% of infertility cases, the female factor alone for another 30%, and the remaining 30–40% is due to both partners or for unknown reasons (idiopathic infertility) [29].

Age-related infertility is a multifactorial process involving genetic, epigenetic, molecular, and cellular factors, such as increased aneuploidy, mitochondrial dysfunction, oxidative stress, dysfunctional DNA damage response, autophagy, and inflammation [30–32]. Although both men and women face an age-related decline in fertility, there are differences concerning the time of onset, duration, and outcome of age-dependent fertility due to differences between male and female gametogenesis, spermatogenesis, and oogenesis respectively (Table 18.1) [33]. Gametogenesis is the process by which undifferentiated primordial germ cells (PGCs), arising during embryonic development, undergo several mitotic divisions (~34 in males and 22 in females) and meiosis, a cell division characterized by one round of DNA replication followed by

Table 18.1 Differences between spermatogenesis in males and oogenesis in females

Spermatogenesis	Oogenesis
1. The production of spermatozoa from spermatogonia	1. The production of oocytes from oogonia
2. A continuous process begins at puberty throughout old age	2. A discontinuous process begins during fetal development, pauses in prophase I/prophase II/metaphase II, and ends at menopause
3. Millions of spermatozoa are produced per day	3. One oocyte is produced per month
4. All stages occur in testes	4. Occurs mostly in ovaries. The last stages occur in the oviduct
5. All spermatogonia give rise to spermatids	5. Only a few oogonia give rise to oocytes
6. Spermatids undergo metamorphosis into differentiated spermatozoa	6. No metamorphosis process
7. Four small, motile gametes/meiosis	7. One large, non-motile gamete/meiosis

two successive cell divisions, meiosis I (MI) and meiosis II (MII), and produce differentiated haploid gametes [34, 35]. Male gametes or spermatozoa and female gametes or oocytes (eggs) are the specialized cells responsible for the reproductive potential, thus, any alteration in their quantity and quality can lead to infertility [36, 37].

Telomeres have been demonstrated to play a critical role in meiosis. During prophase I, which is subdivided into leptotene, zygotene, pachytene, and diplotene, telomeres attach to the nuclear envelope and cluster to form the meiotic bouquet configuration, which is essential for successful homologous chromosome pairing, synapsis, recombination, and segregation [38–40]. Recently accumulated evidence has shown that dysfunction of germ cell telomeres may contribute to abnormal fertilization of gametes, leading to abnormal embryo cleavage and further development, suggesting their important role in gametogenesis and fertility [37, 39, 41]. Germ cell telomeres are longer (13–20 kb) than those of somatic cells (4 kb) with spermatozoa telomeres being longer than those of oocytes because they maintain their telomerase activity to avoid telomere erosion and chromosome segregation, and to ensure the delivery of full-length chromosomes to the progeny [10, 11, 19, 22]. Significant differences have been observed in telomere dynamics between spermatogenesis and oogenesis. Thus, we will present separately the relationship between telomere length and the development of male and female infertility.

18.3 Telomeres and Male Infertility

The male factor is responsible for up to 50% of infertility cases, being solely responsible for 20–30% of infertility cases and contributing along with a female factor in another 20–30% of cases [29, 42]. Male infertility affects around 7% of the male population and can be caused by several factors including genetic, environmental, anatomical, physiological, endocrine, and immunological [29, 42]. Evaluation of male infertility should include a complete medical and reproductive history, a physical examination, and semen analysis. Semen analysis is the fundamental test for assessing male infertility, as it measures sperm parameters including concentration, motility, morphology, volume, etc., which are important for sperm fertilization capacity. Abnormal semen parameters have predictive value in the determination of male infertility. However, in almost 40% of infertile men, the etiology is still unknown (idiopathic male infertility), and it has been suggested that an underlying genetic/epigenetic factor not yet identified may be involved [42]. Thus, the identification of a new diagnostic and prognostic biomarker for the evaluation of semen and male infertility is of major interest.

Although in men there is no critical age at which sperm production or function and fertility cease, the increasing trend of delayed childbearing in advanced Western countries has also effects on male fertility. Many studies have shown that men aged $>$ 50 years experience significant changes in their reproductive organs and their endocrine system leading to defective spermatogenesis, deterioration of sperm quality, and decrease of sperm parameters [36, 43, 44]. Consequently, advanced paternal age has been associated with lower pregnancy rates, increased time to pregnancy, male infertility, poor embryo quality, low birth weight, short life expectancy, and unhealthy childhood outcomes, such as congenital birth defects and achondroplasia, autism, schizophrenia, and certain types of cancer [36, 45].

Accumulating research has been focused on male germ cell telomere dynamics. Male germ cells have an average TL of 10–20 kb [19]. Unlike somatic cells, sperm telomere length (STL) is increased with advancing age in the same individual, possibly due to over-representation/selection of a subset of sperm with longer telomeres in older men [10, 46]. Depending on the methodology used, sperm telomere length (STL) has been shown to become longer/year by 17 bp, 70 bp, 135 bp, and 57 bp [10, 36, 47, 48]. It has generally been thought that with age, sperm telomere elongation results from the continued effects of telomerase. However, the ALT pathway has also been proposed because of the high STL heterogeneity with age [36, 49]. Studies have shown variation in telomere length between sperm subpopulations in the same man as telomeres of different lengths are found in a single ejaculation [14, 50]. In addition, a positive correlation has been observed between STL and leukocyte TL (LTL) within the individual; the longer the LTL, the longer the STL [48, 51]. Moreover, advanced paternal age at conception has been positively correlated with longer LTL and STL in the offspring of older fathers, thus confirming the telomere length heritability [33, 46, 51, 52]. However, there are also studies showing contrasting results due to differences in techniques, sample storage, study settings, and severity of the diagnosis [50, 53].

It is well-established that sperm telomeres play a significant role in meiosis. Extensive research has been dedicated to investigating TL changes during spermatogenesis (Fig. 18.2). In brief, spermatogenesis in humans is a continuous, complex process, which occurs in the seminiferous tubules of the testes from puberty throughout life [34]. The duration of the human spermatogenic cycle takes approximately 64–72 days [54, 55]. Spermatogenesis begins with mitotic proliferation and differentiation of diploid male PGCs, called spermatogonia. There are two spermatogonia subtypes: undifferentiated type A (Adark and Apale) and differentiated type B. Type A spermatogonia proliferate either to renew themselves or to differentiate into intermediate and type B spermatogonia, which

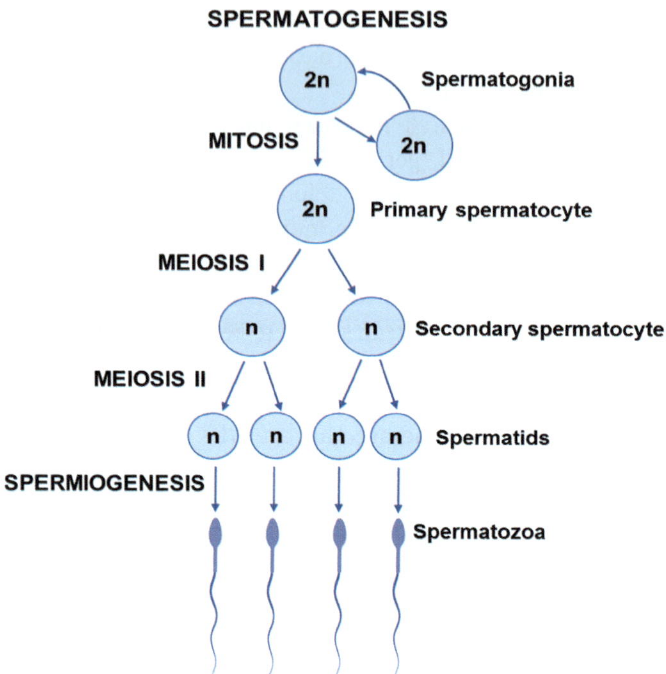

Figure 18.2 Schematic representation of spermatogenesis.

undergo mitotic proliferation and form preleptotene spermatocytes. Preleptotene spermatocytes undergo the first meiotic division, through the stages of leptotene, zygotene, pachytene, and diplotene to generate the secondary spermatocytes which after the second meiotic division give rise to four haploid round spermatids. During spermiogenesis, the round spermatids elongate and mature into spermatozoa with fully compacted chromatin. Then, they are transported through the lumen of the seminiferous tubules to the epididymis where they acquire motility [33, 34].

Accumulating data have indicated that as spermatogenesis progresses, many changes in telomere dynamics occur and there is an inverse correlation between TL and the expression of telomerase activity from spermatogonial stem cells to terminally differentiated male gametes [34] (Fig. 18.3). Specifically, in spermatogonia,

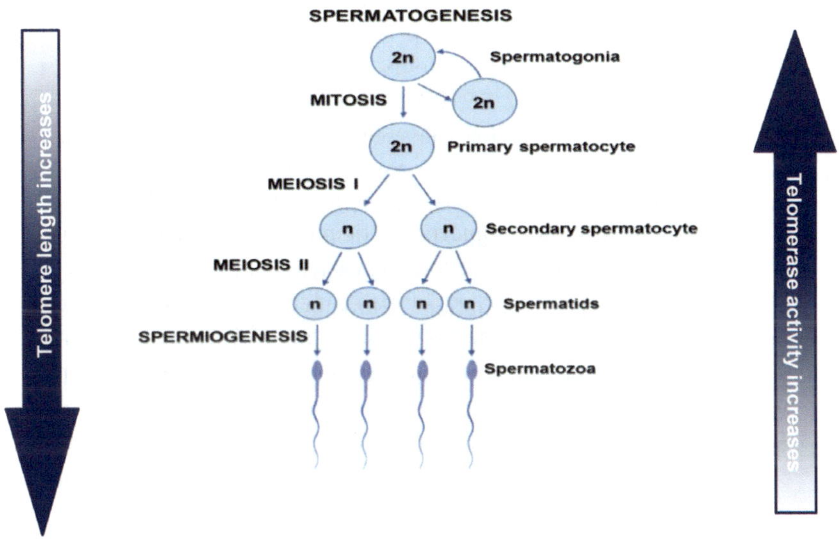

Figure 18.3 Telomere length and telomerase activity in spermatogenesis.

telomere length is short, telomerase is most active, and telomeres are randomly positioned [34, 56]. Following spermatogonial proliferation and differentiation into the pachytene spermatocytes, telomeres are elongated, telomerase levels are high, and they are concentrated in one pole of the nucleus [34]. During the transition of pachytene spermatocytes into the haploid round spermatids, telomere length either remains stable or marginally decreases, telomerase activity has similarly high levels and telomeres redistributed to a more central localization [34, 56]. During spermiogenesis further telomere lengthening happens, there is no telomerase activity, and telomeres are returning to the nuclear periphery. Therefore, they are clustered together and the two telomeric ends of each chromosome are joined into dimers and tetramers, forming a looped chromosome configuration [37, 56, 57]. Consequently, mature spermatozoa have longer telomeres than spermatogonia and absent telomerase activity suggesting a telomerase-independent elongation mechanism has not yet been identified [14, 19]. Additionally, mature spermatozoa have a well-defined nuclear organization of their genome with the telomeric regions found toward the nuclear periphery or bound to the nuclear membrane through a sperm-specific telomere-binding protein complex (hSTBP), which does not contain shelterin proteins but rather a sperm-specific variant of histone H2B [37, 56–58].

It has been suggested that the specific telomere sperm nuclear architecture in mature spermatozoa is necessary because these are the first structures in the sperm nucleus that respond to oocyte signals for male pronucleus development at fertilization [34, 56, 59]. A growing number of reports have demonstrated the importance of STL in pronucleus formation following entry of sperm into oocyte and microtubule-guided movement after fertilization in good blastocyst quality, in apoptosis and implantation rate [39, 41, 60]. Moreover, increased STL is necessary for the maintenance of the species-telomere length in the newborn [34, 56, 59].

STL has been found to have a significant positive correlation with sperm count, motility, vitality, and protamination, and a negative association with DNA fragmentation [51, 60–64]. Several studies have measured STL in both infertile and fertile men and they have shown that STL of infertile men was significantly lower when compared to controls implying that telomere shortening might lead to impaired spermatogenesis [40, 51, 61–64]. A possible explanation is that telomere shortening is triggered by higher levels of oxidative stress in spermatozoa of infertile men [40, 51, 61–64]. On the contrary, Reig-Viader et al. (2014) reported no TL alteration in spermatocytes I of infertile samples compared with controls, and Vecoli et al. (2017) showed a significant increase in STL in areas with high exposure to environmental pollutants. [65, 66].

Recently, Turner et al. (2021) demonstrated for the first time that telomere distribution is altered in the sperm nuclei of infertile males showing an opposite telomere distribution pattern from that of fertile men. Consequently, this would, in turn, alter replication and transcriptional cues that are delivered to the oocyte upon fertilization [67]. Darmishonnejad et al. (2019) compared STL in infertile men with previous failed/low fertilization rates in previous assisted reproductive techniques/intracytoplasmic sperm injection (ART/ICSI) cycles, in comparison with fertile individuals with a high fertilization rate and revealed that in addition to lower sperm parameters in these individuals, STL was also significantly shorter [68]. Another study also found reduced STL in patients who underwent ART compared to fertile men [69].

Only a few studies have examined the correlation between leucocyte telomere length (LTL) and male infertility reporting significantly shorter LTL in infertile men [63, 64, 70–72]. M'kacher et al. (2020) analyzed LTL and chromosomal abnormalities in men with infertility and fertile controls and they demonstrated that the LTL of infertile patients was significantly less than that of healthy donors of similar age and that infertile patients showed significantly more extreme telomere loss and telomere doublet formation than healthy controls, being more pronounced among patients with structural chromosomal aberrations [73].

Taken together, the above findings suggest that telomere length could be used as a novel biomarker of spermatogenic impairment and male fertility, although there are conflicting research results that make difficult their clear connection. Moreover, TL could be used as a parameter for sperm quality during assisted reproductive techniques. Additional studies are needed to confirm the above hypotheses and the combination of an "omics" approach, and the advent of high-throughput technologies are expected to provide new biomarkers and shed additional light on the possible implication of telomeres in diagnosis, prognosis, and treatment of male infertility [22].

18.4 Telomeres and Female Infertility

In developed countries, an increasing proportion of women delay motherhood to advanced age. In Europe, the mean age of women at their first childbirth has gradually increased from 28 years in 2000 to 29.1 years in 2010 and 30.2 years in 2022, while in the USA, the mean age of first-time mothers has increased from 24.9 in 2000 to 25.2 years in 2009 and 26.3 years in 2014 [74]. It is well known, however, that advanced maternal age (AMA $\geq$ 35 years) is strongly associated with infertility, miscarriages, fetal anomalies, pregnancy complications, and adverse perinatal outcomes [32, 75].

Female age-related infertility induces alterations in the endocrine system, the uterus, the ovary, and eggs. Female fertility

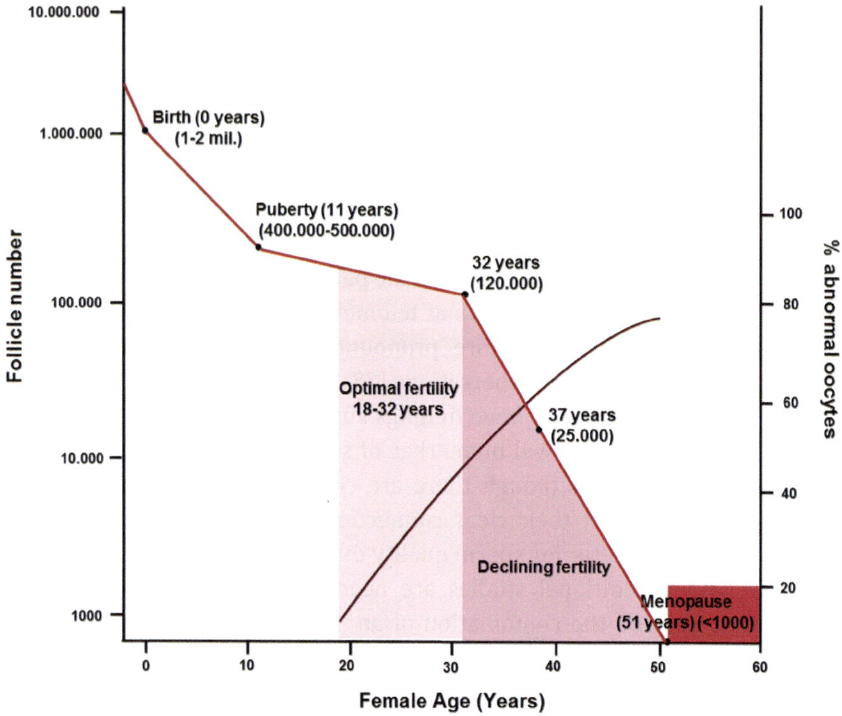

Figure 18.4 Decline in fertility, quality, and quantity of oocytes with increasing female age.

capacity peaks between the late teens and late 20s and begins to decline slowly by 30 years, more rapidly into the late 30s, and accelerated by the mid to late 40s [30–32] (Fig. 18.4). The time decline begins and the rate at which it progresses vary widely in women but always is expected to end 5–10 years before menopause (average age 51 years), where there is no longer ability to become pregnant [36, 76].

It has been evident that ovarian, more specifically, oocyte aging is the cause of age-dependent reproductive failure, because oocyte donation from younger women completely revokes age-dependent infertility in older women [77]. Current knowledge indicates that oogenesis begins during fetal female development and females are born with all the gametes that will produce their lifetime in their ovaries. These gametes are immature and gradually decline with aging [30, 31, 75, 77–79]. The decreasing quantity of oocytes is called "loss of ovarian reserve" and is an inevitable and irreversible process. A female fetal ovary contains about 500–1300 PGCs, called oogonia, during the 5th week of pregnancy which undergoes mitosis and reaches around 6–7 million germ cells by the 2nd trimester of fetal life [75, 78]. Germ cells enter meiosis and stay arrested in the diplotene stage of meiotic prophase I, where many of them are lost through apoptosis. Only 1–2 million primordial follicles remain at birth and finally, approximately 400,000–500,000 primordial follicles survive at puberty [75, 78]. During a normal woman's reproductive lifespan, the majority of follicles are lost by a degenerative process called atresia and only 500 oocytes will mature and release an egg. Around 1000 follicles are lost per month and only 500 oocytes will mature and ovulate [75, 78]. Normally, each month, only 1 follicle will ovulate, and if it is not fertilized, the endometrium sheds from the uterus during a menstrual period. After the age of 37 years, the rate of follicle loss accelerates and by 50 years of age, the number of remaining follicles drops below 1000 indicating the onset of menopause [75] (Figs. 18.4 and 18.5).

Advancing maternal age also diminishes the quality of oocyte, as it has been associated with high embryo fragmentation, apoptosis and cell cycle arrest, and aneuploidy [30, 31, 75, 77–79]. Aberrant recombination and the occurrence of a previous trisomy are other risk factors undoubtedly linked to human aneuploidy. Aneuploidy is the most common chromosomal abnormality in humans, and it is defined as having an abnormal number of chromosomes (trisomy or monosomy), which is not an exact multiple of a haploid number [36]. Most aneuploidies arise from errors in the oocyte and not sperm, due to their prolonged arrest in meiosis I, which begins prenatally and is not completed until the time of ovulation 10–50 years later [80]. Increased maternal age causes aberrant recombination in prophase I and non-disjunction (malsegregation) in anaphase I [80]. Most aneuploid oocytes and embryos undergo apoptosis before implantation causing infertility. However, some escape only to miscarry later during development, which is the main genetic cause of miscarriages, congenital birth defects, and mental retardation [80].

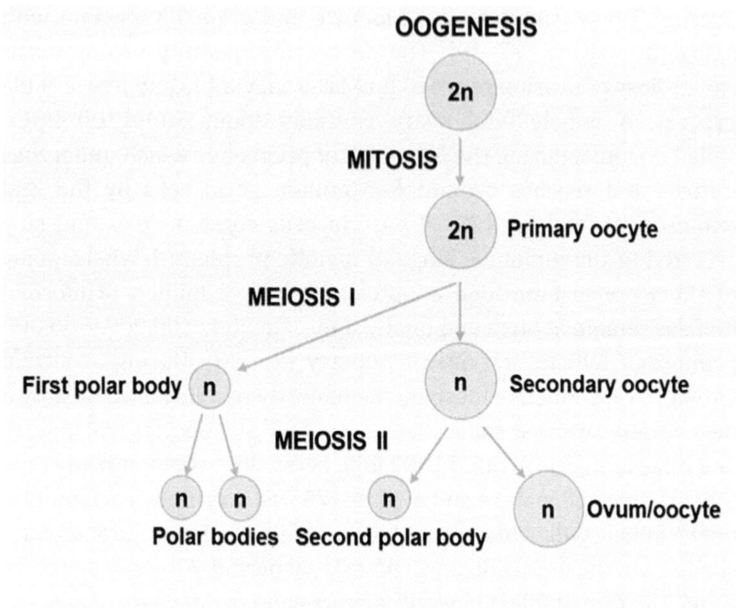

Figure 18.5 Schematic representation of oogenesis.

Currently, there is no reliable biomarker of oocyte aging. Thus, the discovery of new biomarkers useful to identify oocytes with the greatest development competence is very important. Several theories have been proposed to explain age-dependent decreased oocyte quality. According to the production line model, the oocytes that first enter meiosis are the first to ovulate in younger women, and oocytes entering meiosis last are ovulated at the end of the reproductive lifespan [77, 81]. In 2005, Keefe et al. proposed a unifying telomere-based theory of reproductive aging in women, which involves a two-hit hypothesis for oocyte dysfunction: late exit from the production line during oogenesis followed by accumulated exposure to reactive oxygen from prolonged arrest in the adult ovary could explain shorter telomeres in oocytes from older women [77, 81]. Telomeres, due to their high guanine content, are particularly sensitive to oxidative stress caused by excess reactive oxygen species (ROS), which induces telomeric DNA damage and telomere shortening [12, 17, 75]. Consequently, oocytes with shortened telomeres develop a decreased number of chiasmata leading to

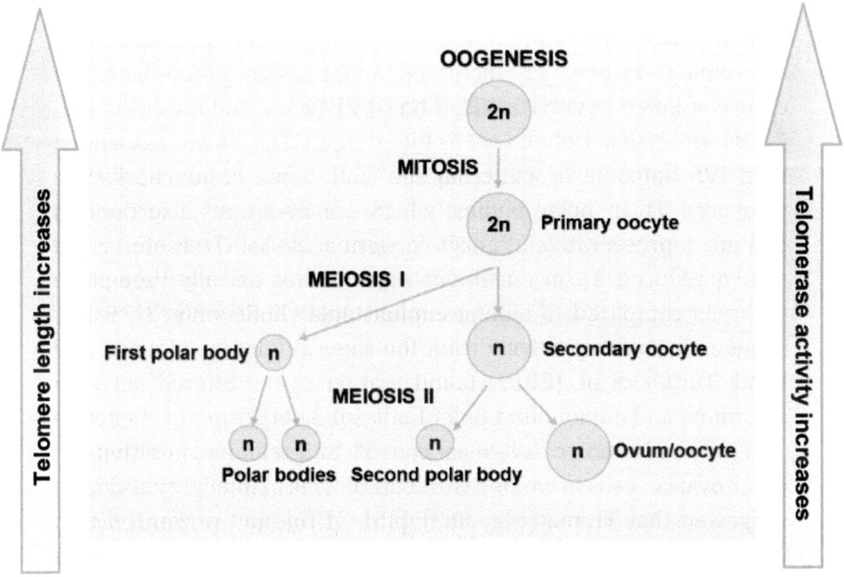

Figure 18.6 Telomere length and telomerase activity in oogenesis.

chromosome non-disjunction, aneuploidy, and diminished oocyte quality [12, 17, 75].

In contrast to the accumulated data concerning telomere dynamics in the male germline, there has been little direct evidence of telomere dynamics in the female germline, mainly due to the difficulty of obtaining human oocytes, technologies used, and ethical concerns regarding their use [19]. Over the past years, there has been some evidence of oocyte telomere length (OTL) implication in female fertility. Average OTL varies from 7.14 kb to 11.4 kb, depending on the developmental stage in which measurement is performed [19]. Telomerase activity and TL undergo marked changes during oogenesis (Fig. 18.6). A peak of telomerase activity is observed in oogonia, then declines during oocyte maturation and remains low or absent in mature oocyte [20, 21, 31, 50]. Also, TL decreases from the phase of prophase I arrest to the metaphase II oocyte [33, 50, 82].

Although the hypothesis of telomere theory of reproductive aging is credible, very few studies have assessed telomere length directly in human oocytes or preimplantation embryos showing conflicting results [50, 81, 83, 84]. Most studies indicate that decreased OTL has been associated with failed implantation, miscarriage, aneuploidy, trisomy 21, increased apoptosis in preimplantation embryos, failed in vitro fertilization (IVF) cycles, and infertility [31, 77, 81, 84]. Turner et al. (2013) found that OTL was not associated with IVF outcome or maternal age [50]. Some researchers have measured TL in polar bodies, which are by-products of meiosis and are representative of oocyte genetic material. Treff et al. have shown reduced TL in aneuploid polar bodies and cleavage-stage embryos compared to sibling euploid polar bodies and cleavage-stage embryos respectively from the same IVF cycle. On the other hand, Turner et al. (2019) found that TL is not altered between aneuploid and euploid first polar bodies [83, 84].

Published reports have measured TL and telomerase activity in other ovarian cells in women with pathologies of infertility and have suggested that TL may play an important role in ovarian function and therefore could be used as a surrogate marker for ovarian aging or infertility. Kinugawa et al. found that telomerase activity is present in the ovaries of fertile women decreasing with age, while it is reduced in women with primary ovarian insufficiency (POI) [85]. Telomerase activity has also been demonstrated in Granulosa cells (GCs) of the ovary, where its expression is linked to their proliferation and differentiation status and is under the control of growth factors and steroid hormones [86]. GCs support oocytes during follicular growth and maturation by supplying them with nutrients and metabolites through gap junctions and regulating their function via hormone secretion [87]. Therefore, GCs are essential for optimal oocyte competence and are considered markers for oocyte quality [87]. Different studies have examined the association of Granulosa cell telomere length (GCTL) with infertility with controversial results. Some have demonstrated that granulosa cell telomeric shortening and diminished telomerase activity are associated with occult ovarian insufficiency in young women, biochemical primary ovarian insufficiency (POI), and polycystic ovary syndrome (PCOS) [87–89]. Another study showed that GCTL did not differ in PCOS, while another one found significantly longer GCTL in PCOS patients [90, 91]. Furthermore, it has been proven that women with high telomerase activity have higher rates of embryo implantation and clinical pregnancy and that telomerase activity is more significant for predicting IVF outcome than telomere length [92, 93]. Two recent studies, however, noted no significant associations between GCTL and any IVF outcomes [94, 95].

Since endometrium is a major factor for successful embryo implantation and the establishment of a pregnancy, some researchers have examined the implication of TL and telomerase activity in endometrial biology. The human endometrium is a highly dynamic, somatic tissue undergoing repetitive monthly cycles of growth, differentiation, shedding, and regeneration throughout a woman's reproductive life, which are regulated by ovarian steroid hormones [96–98]. At menopause, the synthesis of ovarian steroid hormone stops, and the endometrium becomes proliferatively quiescent [97]. However, with the provision of exogenous ovarian steroid hormones, a fully functional endometrium can be regenerated from the remaining thin postmenopausal endometrium making endometrium the only female reproductive organ not showing irreversible age-related changes [96, 97].

Embryo implantation occurs during the window of implantation in the mid-secretory phase, which is defined by the dominant action of progesterone with maximum cell differentiation and is associated with the lowest endometrial TA and the shortest mean TL [96–98]. Studies of TL in pathological endometrium conditions have demonstrated high endometrial telomerase activity and longer TLs in women with endometriosis, reproductive failure, endometrial malignancies, and endometrial hyperplasia [96, 97].

Several reports have investigated the relationship between LTL and reproductive potential and its use as a putative biomarker, with contradictory findings. LTL has been found to be significantly shorter in women with PCOS, with biochemical POI, with recurrent miscarriage, and in women undergoing IVF [88, 99–102]. In contrast, others have shown no difference in leucocyte telomere length (LTL) in PCOS patients and identified significantly longer LTL in PCOS patients and in patients with overt POI [90, 91, 99, 103–105]. In addition, shorter LTL has been associated with higher rates of aneuploidy in women undergoing IVF [94]. A recent study proposed that longer LTL reflects higher oocyte quality, which can compensate for other limiting physiological and behavioral factors and enable successful reproduction [106].

It currently remains unclear whether OTL could be used as a useful tool for predicting female infertility and further research is essential to clarify the molecular pathways involved.

18.5 Telomere Length After Fertilization

After fertilization, telomerase decreases further during the early cleavage stages of embryonic development and then is high again in the blastocyst stages of development [19–21, 31, 50]. The preservation of TL during the early cleavage cycles is performed through the ALT mechanism and from the blastocyst stage onwards, telomerase only maintains the telomere length [31, 41]. Only newly formed embryos originating from germ cells with long TL can preserve TL following fertilization because short or dysfunctional telomeres could cause genetic instability [19, 31, 41]. Average embryo TL varies across the different developmental stages, and it is higher in blastocyst (~11.27 kb).

18.6 TERRA Dynamics

In 2007, it was demonstrated that mammalian telomeres are not transcriptionally silent. On the contrary, they are transcribed into telomeric repeat-containing RNA (TERRA) [104, 107]. TERRA molecules are heterogeneous in length (from 100 bp to 9 kb in mammals) long non-coding RNAs, composed of varying sizes of UUAGGG repeat sequences, and are transcribed from several subtelomeric loci located close to chromosome ends [104, 107]. TERRA molecules localize to telomeres and are involved in the regulation of telomerase activity, telomere length, and heterochromatinization [108]. Consequently, changes in their expression levels are associated with altered telomeric length and promote genome instability and cellular senescence [108, 109].

Recent reports have identified that TERRA is expressed in both male and female germ cells and its colocalization with telomeres and telomerase during all the prophase-I stages is subject to gender-specific features [110]. Interestingly, in spermatogenesis,

TERRA localization at telomeres is maintained throughout the whole process as a structural component without affecting telomere elongation and its expression progressively increases until the beginning of spermiogenesis [65, 108]. Therefore, TERRA has been revealed to be an important structural telomere component contributing to the preservation of telomere stability during the complex chromosome reorganization and movements that take place in gametogenesis [65, 108, 109]. Wang et al. (2017) found that TERRA expression in human peripheral blood leukocytes and LTLs was positively associated with PCOS [104]. Recently, Rocca et al. (2021) found lower TERRA expression in the semen of men who underwent ART/ICSI than in fertile controls [111]. In addition, there was a statistically significant positive correlation between TERRA, STL, and embryo quality suggesting its use as a predictive factor of sperm and embryo quality [111]. Further studies are required to explore the involvement of TERRA in infertility as well as in successful fertilization outcomes [111].

An increasing number of studies in the reproductive field have focused on elucidating the implication of telomere length in male and female infertility, in order to develop a new reliable predictive biomarker that will facilitate personalized fertility counseling and optional infertility treatments. However, the limitations of the methodologies used, and the divergent results observed among studies pose many questions that remain to be fully defined. Further research is required to better understand the underlying biological mechanisms in telomere homeostasis and its association with human infertility before using them in routine clinical practice.

References

1. Moyzis, R. K., Buckingham, J. M., Cram, L. S., Dani, M., Deaven, L. L., Jones, M. D., *et al.* (1988). A highly conserved repetitive DNA sequence, (TTAGGG)n, present at the telomeres of human chromosomes, *Proc. Natl. Acad. Sci. U S A*, **85**, pp. 6622–6626.
2. Griffith, J. D., Comeau, L., Rosenfield, S., Stansel, R. M., Bianchi, A., Moss, H. and de Lange, T. (1999). Mammalian telomeres end in a large duplex loop, *Cell*, **97**, pp. 503–514.

3. Songyang, Z. and Liu, D. (2006). Inside the mammalian telomere interactome: regulation and regulatory activities of telomeres, *Crit. Rev. Eukaryot. Gene. Expr.*, **16**, pp. 03–18.
4. de Lange, T. (2005). Shelterin: the protein complex that shapes and safeguards human telomeres, *Genes. Dev.,* **19**, pp. 2100–2110.
5. de Lange, T. (2018). Shelterin-mediated telomere protection, *Annu. Rev. Genet,* **52**, pp. 223–247.
6. Palm, W. and de Lange, T. (2008). How shelterin protects mammalian telomeres, *Annu. Rev. Genet.*, **42**, pp. 301–334.
7. Hayflick, L. and Moorehead, P.S. (1961). The serial cultivation of human diploid cell strains, *Exp. Cell. Res.*, **25**, pp. 585–621.
8. Harley, C. B., Futcher, A. B. and Greider, C.W. (1990). Telomeres shorten during ageing of human fibroblasts, *Nature*, **345**, pp. 458–460.
9. Olovnikov, A. M. (1971). Principles of marginotomy in template synthesis of polynucleotides, *Dokl. Akad. Nauk. S.S.S.R.,* **201**, pp. 1496–1499.
10. Allsopp, R. C., Vaziri, H., Patterson, C., Goldstein, S., Younglai, E. V., Futcher, A. B., *et al.* (1992). Telomere length predicts replicative capacity of human fibroblasts, *Proc. Natl. Acad. Sci. U S A*, **89**, pp. 10114–10118.
11. Levy, M. Z., Allsopp, R. C., Futcher, A. B., Greider, C. W. and Harley, C. B. (1992). Telomere end-replication problem and cell aging, *J. Mol. Biol,* **225**, pp. 951–960.
12. Shay, J. W. and Wright, W. E. (2011). Role of telomeres and telomerase in cancer, *Semin. Cancer. Biol.,* **21**, pp. 349–353.
13. Greider, C.W. and Blackburn, E.H. (1989). A telomeric sequence in the RNA of Tetrahymena telomerase required for telomere repeat synthesis, *Nature,* **337**, pp. 331–337.
14. Ozturk, S. (2015). Telomerase activity and telomere length in male germ cells, *Biol. Reprod.*, **92**, pp. 53.
15. Herrmann, M., Pusceddu, I., März, W. and Herrmann, W. (2018). Telomere biology and age-related diseases, *Clin. Chem. Lab. Med.*, **56**, pp. 1210–1222.
16. Podlevsky, J. D. and Chen, J. J. (2012). It all comes together at the ends: telomerase structure, function, and biogenesis, *Mutat. Res.,* **730**, pp. 3–11.
17. Srinivas, N., Rachakonda, S. and Kumar, R. (2020). Telomeres and telomere length: a general overview, *Cancers. (Basel),* **12,** pp. 558.

18. Cerone, M. A., Londono-Vallejo, J. A. and Bacchetti, S. (2001). Telomere maintenance by telomerase and by recombination can coexist in human cells, *Hum. Mol. Genet.*, **10**, pp. 1945–1952.

19. Rocca, M. S., Foresta, C. and Ferlin, A. (2019). Telomere length: lights and shadows on their role in human reproduction, *Biol. Reprod.*, **100**, pp. 305–317.

20. Anifandis, G., Samara, M., Simopoulou, M., Messini, C. I., Chatzimeletiou, K., Thodou, E., *et al.* (2021). Insights into the role of telomeres in human embryological parameters, opinions regarding IVF, *J. Dev. Biol.*, **9**, pp. 49.

21. Wright, W. E., Piatyszek, M.A., Rainey, W. E., Byrd, W. and Shay, J. W. (1996). Telomerase activity in human germline and embryonic tissues and cells, *Dev. Genet.*, **18**, pp. 173–179.

22. Balmori, C. and Varela, E. (2018). Should we consider telomere length and telomerase activity in male factor infertility? *Curr. Opin. Obstet. Gynecol.*, **30**, pp. 197–202.

23. Okuda, K., Bardeguez, A., Gardner, J. P., Rodriguez, P., Ganesh, V., Kimura, M., *et al.* (2002). Telomere length in the newborn, *Pediatr. Res.*, **52**, pp. 377–381.

24. Nordfjäll, K., Svenson, U., Norrback, K. F., Adolfsson, R., Lenner, P. and Roos, G. (2009). The individual blood cell telomere attrition rate is telomere length dependent, *PLoS, Genet.*, **5**, pp. e1000375.

25. Gardner, M., Bann, D., Wiley, L., Cooper, R., Hardy, R., Nitsch, *et al.* (2014). Halcyon study team. Gender and telomere length: systematic review and meta-analysis, *Exp. Gerontol.*, **51**, pp. 15–27.

26. Demanelis, K., Jasmine, F., Chen, L. S., Chernoff, M., Tong, L., Delgado, *et al.* (2020). Determinants of telomere length across human tissues, *Science*, **369**, pp. eaaz6876.

27. Mirabello, L., Yu, K., Kraft, P., De Vivo, I., Hunter, D.J., Prescott, J., *et al.* (2010). The association of telomere length and genetic variation in telomere biology genes, *Hum. Mutat.*, **31**, pp. 1050–1058.

28. WHO https://www.who.int/news-room/fact-sheets/detail/infertility.

29. Mallepaly, R., Butler, P.R., Herati, A.S. and Lamb, D.J. (2017). Genetic basis of male and female infertility, *Monogr. Hum. Genet.*, **21**, pp. 1–16.

30. Navot, D., Drews, M. R., Bergh, P. A., Guzman, I., Karstaedt, A., Scott, R. T. Jr., *et al.* (1994). Age-related decline in female fertility is not due to diminished capacity of the uterus to sustain embryo implantation, *Fertil. Steril.*, **61**, pp. 97–101.

31. Keefe, D. L. and Liu, L. (2009). Telomeres and reproductive aging, *Reprod. Fertil. Dev.*, **21**, pp. 10–14.
32. Balasch, J. and Gratacós, E. (2012). Delayed childbearing: effects on fertility and the outcome of pregnancy, *Curr. Opin. Obstet. Gynecol.*, **24**, pp. 187–193.
33. Lopes, A. C., Oliveira, P.F. and Sousa, M. (2019). Shedding light into the relevance of telomeres in human reproduction and male factor infertility, *Biol. Reprod.*, **100**, pp. 318–330.
34. Archi, M. V., Ravindranath, N. and Dym, M. (2000). Telomere length in male germ cells is inversely correlated with telomerase activity, *Biol. Reprod.*, **63,** pp. 591–598.
35. Ozturk, S., Sozen, B. and Demir, N. (2014). Telomere length and telomerase activity during oocyte maturation and early embryo development in mammalian species, *Mol. Hum. Reprod.*, **20**, pp. 15–30.
36. Baird, D. T., Collins, J., Egozcue, J., Evers, L. H., Gianaroli, L., Leridon, H., *et al.* ESHRE Capri Workshop Group. (2005). Fertility and ageing, *Hum. Reprod. Update*, **11**, pp. 261–276.
37. Reig-Viader, R., Garcia-Caldés, M. and Ruiz-Herrera, A. (2016). Telomere homeostasis in mammalian germ cells: a review, *Chromosoma*, **125**, pp. 337–351.
38. Bekaert, S., Derradji, H. and Baatout, S. (2004). Telomere biology in mammalian germ cells and during development, *Dev. Biol.*, **274**, pp. 15–30.
39. Siderakis, M. and Tarsounas, M. (2007). Telomere regulation and function during meiosis, *Chromosome. Res.*, **15**, pp. 667–679.
40. Thilagavathi, J., Kumar, M., Mishra, S. S., Venkatesh, S., Kumar, R. and Dada, R. (2013). Analysis of sperm telomere length in men with idiopathic infertility, *Arch. Gynecol. Obstet.*, **287**, pp. 803–807.
41. Liu, L., Blasco, M., Trimarchi, J. and Keefe, D. (2002). An essential role for functional telomeres in mouse germ cells during fertilization and early development, *Dev. Biol.*, **249**, pp. 74–84.
42. Krausz, C. and Riera-Escamilla, A. (2018). Genetics of male infertility, *Nat. Rev. Urol.*, **15**, pp. 369–384.
43. Harris, I. D., Fronczak, C., Roth, L. and Meacham, R. B. (2011). Fertility and the aging male, *Rev. Urol.*, **13**, pp. e184–90.
44. Gunes, S., Hekim, G. N., Arslan, M. A, and Asci, R. (2016). Effects of aging on the male reproductive system, *J. Assist. Reprod. Genet.*, **33**, pp. 441–454.

45. Aitken, R. J., De Iuliis, G. N. and Nixon, B. (2020). The sins of our forefathers: paternal impacts on De novo mutation rate and development, *Annu. Rev. Genet.*, **54**, pp. 1–24.
46. Kimura, M., Cherkas, L. F., Kato, B. S., Demissie, S., Hjelmborg, J. B., Brimacombe, M., *et al.* (2008). Offspring's leukocyte telomere length, paternal age, and telomere elongation in sperm, *PLoS. Genet.*, **4**, pp. e37.
47. De Meyer, T., Rietzschel, E. R., De Buyzere, M. L., De Bacquer, D., Van Criekinge, W., De Backer, G. G., *et al.* (2007). Paternal age at birth is an important determinant of offspring telomere length, *Hum. Mol. Genet.*, **16**, pp. 3097–3102.
48. Aston, K. I., Hunt, S. C., Susser, E., Kimura, M., Factor-Litvak, P., Carrell, D. and Aviv, A. (2012). Divergence of sperm and leukocyte age-dependent telomere dynamics: implications for male-driven evolution of telomere length in humans, *Mol. Hum. Reprod.*, **18**, pp. 517–522.
49. Antunes, D. M., Kalmbach, K. H., Wang, F., Dracxler, R. C., Seth-Smith, M. L., Kramer, Y., *et al.* (2015). A single cell assay for telomere DNA content shows increasing telomere length heterogeneity, as well as increasing mean telomere length in human spermatozoa with advancing age, *J. Assist. Reprod. Genet.*, **32**, pp. 1685–1690.
50. Turner, S. and Hartshorne, G. M. (2013). Telomere lengths in human pronuclei, oocytes and spermatozoa, *Mol. Hum. Reprod.*, **19**, pp. 510–518.
51. Ferlin, A., Rampazzo, E., Rocca, M. S., Keppel, S., Frigo, A. C., De Rossi, A. and Foresta, C. (2013). In young men sperm telomere length is related to sperm number and parental age, *Hum. Repro.*, **28**, pp. 3370–3376.
52. Eisenberg, D.T., Hayes, M. G. and Kuzawa, C. W. (2012). Delayed paternal age of reproduction in humans is associated with longer telomeres across two generations of descendants, *Proc. Natl. Acad. Sci. U S A*, **109**, pp. 10251–10256.
53. Gentiluomo, M., Luddi, A., Cingolani, A., Fornili, M., Governini, L., Lucenteforte, E., *et al.* (2021). Telomere length and male fertility, *Int. J. Mol. Sci.*, **22**, pp. 3959.
54. Heller, C. G. and Clermont, Y. (1963). Spermatogenesis in man: an estimate of its duration, *Science*, **140**, pp. 184–186.
55. Weinbauer, G. F., Luetjens, C. M., Simoni, M., Nieschlag, E. (2010). Physiology of testicular function. In: Nieschlag, E., Behre, H. M., Nieschlag, S. (eds), *Andrology*, Springer, Berlin, Heidelberg, pp. 11–59.

56. Fice, H. E. and Robaire, B. (2019). Telomere dynamics throughout spermatogenesis, *Genes. (Basel)*, **10**, pp. 525.
57. Zalensky, A.O., Allen, M. J., Kobayashi, A., Zalenskaya, I. A., Balhórn, R. and Bradbury E. M. (1995). Well-defined genome architecture in the human sperm nucleus, *Chromosoma,* **103**, pp. 577–590.
58. Gineitis, A. A., Zalenskaya, I. A., Yau, P. M., Bradbury, E. M. and Zalensky, A. O. (2000). Human sperm telomere-binding complex involves histone H2B and secures telomere membrane attachment, *J. Cell. Biol.*, **151**, pp. 1591–1598.
59. Zalenskaya, I.A., Bradbury, E. M. and Zalensky, A. O. (2000). Chromatin structure of telomere domain in human sperm, *Biochem. Biophys. Res. Commun.*, **279**, pp. 213–218.
60. Yang, Q., Zhao, F., Dai, S., Zhang, N., Zhao, W., Bai, R. and Sun, Y. (2015). Sperm telomere length is positively associated with the quality of early embryonic development, *Hum. Reprod.*, **30**, pp. 1876–1881.
61. Rocca, M. S., Speltra, E., Menegazzo, M., Garolla, A., Foresta, C. and Ferlin, A. (2016). Sperm telomere length as a parameter of sperm quality in normozoospermic men, *Hum. Reprod.*, **31**, pp. 1158–1163.
62. Cariati, F., Jaroudi, S., Alfarawati, S., Raberi, A., Alviggi, C., Pivonello, R. and Wells D. (2016). Investigation of sperm telomere length as a potential marker of paternal genome integrity and semen quality, *Reprod. Biomed. Online*, **33**, pp. 404–411.
63. Darmishonnejad, Z, Zarei-Kheirabadi, F., Tavalaee, M., Zarei-Kheirabadi, M., Zohrabi, D. and Nasr-Esfahani, M. H. (2020). Relationship between sperm telomere length and sperm quality in infertile men, *Andrologia*, **52**, pp. e13546.
64. Amirzadegan, M., Sadeghi, N., Tavalaee, M. and Nasr-Esfahani, M. H. (2021). Analysis of leukocyte and sperm telomere length in oligozoospermic men, *Andrologia*, **53,** pp. e14204.
65. Reig-Viader, R., Capilla, L., Vila-Cejudo, M., Garcia, F., Anguita, B., Garcia-Caldés, M. and Ruiz-Herrera, A. (2014). Telomere homeostasis is compromised in spermatocytes from patients with idiopathic infertility, *Fertil. Steril.*, **102**, pp. 728–738.
66. Vecoli, C., Montano, L., Borghini, A., Notari, T., Guglielmino, A., Mercuri, A., *et al.* (2017). Effects of highly polluted environment on sperm telomere length: a pilot study, *Int. J. Mol. Sci.*, **18**, pp. 1703.
67. Turner, K. J., Watson, E. M., Skinner, B. M. and Griffin, D. K. (2021). Telomere distribution in human sperm heads and its relation to sperm

nuclear morphology: a new marker for male factor infertility? *Int. J. Mol. Sci.*, **22**, pp. 7599.

68. Darmishonnejad, Z., Tavalaee, M., Izadi, T., Tanhaei, S. and Nasr-Esfahani, M. H. (2019). Evaluation of sperm telomere length in infertile men with failed/low fertilization after intracytoplasmic sperm injection, *Reprod. Biomed. Online*, **38**, pp. 579–587.
69. Rocca, M. S., Dusi, L., Di Nisio, A., Alviggi, E., Iussig, B., Bertelle, S., *et al.* (2021). TERRA: a novel biomarker of embryo quality and art outcome, *Genes. (Basel)*, **12**, pp. 475.
70. Kohn, T. P. and Pastuszak, A. W. (2018). Non-obstructive azoospermia and shortened leukocyte telomere length: further evidence linking poor health and infertility, *Fertil. Steril*, **110**, pp. 629–630.
71. Yang, Q., Luo, X., Bai, R., Zhao, F., Dai, S., Li, F., *et al.* (2018). Shorter leukocyte telomere length is associated with risk of non-obstructive azoospermia, *Fertil. Steril.*, **110**, pp. 648–654.
72. Heidary, H., Pouresmaeili, F., Mirfakhraie, R., Omrani, M. D., Ghaedi, H., Fazeli, Z., *et al.* (2018). An association study between longitudinal changes of leukocyte telomere and the risk of azoospermia in a population of Iranian infertile men, *Iran. Biomed. J.*, **22**, pp. 231–236.
73. M'kacher, R., Colicchio, B., Marquet, V., Borie, C., Najar, W., Hempel, W. M., *et al.* (2021). Telomere aberrations, including telomere loss, doublets, and extreme shortening, are increased in patients with infertility, *Fertil. Steril.*, **115**, pp. 164–173.
74. https://www.statista.com/statistics/1251578/average-age-of-mothers-europe.
75. Kalmbach, K. H., Antunes, D. M., Kohlrausch, F. and Keefe, D.L. (2015). Telomeres and female reproductive aging, *Semin. Reprod. Med.*, **33**, pp. 389–395.
76. Velarde, M. C. and Menon, R. (2016). Positive and negative effects of cellular senescence during female reproductive aging and pregnancy, *J. Endocrinol.*, **230**, pp. R59–R76.
77. Keefe, D. L., Marquard, K. and Liu, L. (2006). The telomere theory of reproductive senescence in women, *Curr. Opin. Obstet. Gynecol.*, **18**, pp. 280–285.
78. Broekmans, F. J., Knauff, E. A., te Velde, E. R., Macklon, N. S. and Fauser, B. C. (2007). Female reproductive ageing: current knowledge and future trends, *Trends Endocrinol. Metab.*, **18**, pp. 58–65.

79. Sutherland, J. M. and McLaughlin, E. A. (2021). Ovarian ageing: where are we now? And where to next? *Current Opinion in Endocrine and Metabolic Research,* pp. 1829–1834.
80. Hassold, T. and Hunt, P. (2001). To err (meiotically) is human: the genesis of human aneuploidy, *Nat. Rev. Genet.,* **2**, pp. 280–291.
81. Keefe, D. L., Franco, S., Liu, L., Trimarchi, J., Cao, B., Weitzen, S., *et al.* (2005). Telomere length predicts embryo fragmentation after in vitro fertilization in women: toward a telomere theory of reproductive aging in women, *Am. J. Obstet. Gynecol.,* **192,** pp. 1256–1260.
82. Wright, D. L., Jones, E. L., Mayer, J. F, Oehninger, S., Gibbons, W. E. and Lanzendorf, S. E. (2001). Characterization of telomerase activity in the human oocyte and preimplantation embryo, *Mol. Hum. Reprod.,* **7**, pp. 947–955.
83. Treff, N. R., Su, J., Taylor, D. and Scott R. T. Jr. (2011). Telomere DNA deficiency is associated with the development of human embryonic aneuploidy, *PLoS. Genet.,* **7**, pp. e1002161.
84. Turner, K., Lynch, C., Rouse, H., Vasu, V. and Griffin, D. K. (2019). Direct single-cell analysis of human polar bodies and cleavage-stage embryos reveals no evidence of the telomere theory of reproductive ageing in relation to aneuploidy generation, *Cells,* **8**, pp. 163.
85. Kinugawa, C., Murakami, T., Okamura, K. and Yajima, A. (2000). Telomerase activity in normal ovaries and premature ovarian failure, *Tohoku. J. Exp. Med.,* **190**, pp. 231–238.
86. Chronowska, E. (2012). Regulation of telomerase activity in ovarian granulosa cells, *Indian. J. Exp. Biol.,* **50**, pp. 595–601.
87. Butts, S., Riethman, H., Ratcliffe, S., Shaunik, A., Coutifaris, C. and Barnhart, K. (2009). Correlation of telomere length and telomerase activity with occult ovarian insufficiency, *J. Clin. Endocrinol. Metab.,* **94**, pp. 4835–4843.
88. Xu, X., Chen, X., Zhang, X., Liu, Y., Wang, Z., Wang, P., *et al.* (2017). Impaired telomere length and telomerase activity in peripheral blood leukocytes and granulosa cells in patients with biochemical primary ovarian insufficiency, *Hum. Reprod.,* **32**, pp. 201–207.
89. Li, Y., Deng, B., Ouyang, N., Yuan, P., Zheng, L. and Wang, W. (2017). Telomere length is short in PCOS and oral contraceptive does not affect the telomerase activity in granulosa cells of patients with PCOS, *J. Assist. Reprod. Genet.,* **34**, pp. 849–859.
90. Wei, D., Xie, J., Yin, B., Hao, H., Song, X., Liu, Q., *et al.* (2017). Significantly lengthened telomere in granulosa cells from women with polycystic ovarian syndrome (PCOS), *J. Assist. Reprod. Genet.,* **34**, pp. 861–866.

91. Pedroso, D. C. C., Santana, V. P., Donaires, F. S., Picinato, M. C., Giorgenon, R. C., Santana, B. A., *et al.* (2020). Telomere length and telomerase activity in immature oocytes and cumulus cells of women with polycystic ovary syndrome, *Reprod. Sci.,* **27**, pp. 1293–1303.
92. Chen, H., Wang, W., Mo, Y., Ma, Y., Ouyang, N., Li, R., *et al.* (2011). Women with high telomerase activity in luteinised granulosa cells have a higher pregnancy rate during in vitro fertilisation treatment, *J. Assist. Reprod. Genet.*, **28**, pp. 797–807.
93. Wang, W., Chen, H., Li, R., Ouyang, N., Chen, J., Huang, L., *et al.* (2014). Telomerase activity is more significant for predicting the outcome of IVF treatment than telomere length in granulosa cells, *Reproduction*, **147,** pp. 649–657.
94. Hanson, B.M., Tao, X., Zhan, Y., Kim, J. G., Klimczak, A. M., Herliny, N. S., *et al.* (2021). Shorter telomere length of white blood cells is associated with higher rates of aneuploidy among infertile women undergoing in vitro fertilization, *Fertil. Steril.*, **115**, pp. 957–965.
95. Hao, Y., Lv, M., Peng, J., Zhang, Z., Zhang, Z., Zhang, Z., *et al.* (2021). Predict value of relative telomere length, TERT, and follicular fluid anti-mullerian hormone levels for IVF outcome in infertile women, PREPRINT (Version 1) available at Research Square [https://doi.org/10.21203/rs.3.rs-779338/v1].
96. Valentijn, A. J., Saretzki, G., Tempest, N., Critchley, H. O. and Hapangama, D. K. (2015). Human endometrial epithelial telomerase is important for epithelial proliferation and glandular formation with potential implications in endometriosis, *Hum. Reprod.*, **30**, pp. 2816–2828.
97. Hapangama, D. K., Kamal, A. and Saretzki, G. (2017). Implications of telomeres and telomerase in endometrial pathology, *Hum. Reprod. Update*, **23**, pp. 166–187.
98. Vasilopoulos, E., Fragkiadaki, P., Kalliora, C., Fragou, D., Docea, A. O., Vakonaki, E., *et al.* (2019). The association of female and male infertility with telomere length (review), *Int. J. Mol. Med.*, **44**, pp. 375–389.
99. Hanna, C. W., Bretherick, K. L., Gair, J. L., Fluker, M. R., Stephenson, M. D. and Robinson, W. P. (2009). Telomere length and reproductive aging, *Hum. Reprod.*, **24**, pp. 1206–1211.
100. Li, Q., Du, J., Feng, R., Xu, Y., Wang, H., Sang, Q., *et al.* (2014). A possible new mechanism in the pathophysiology of polycystic ovary syndrome (PCOS): the discovery that leukocyte telomere length is strongly associated with PCOS, *J. Clin. Endocrinol. Metab.*, **99**, pp. E234–240.

101. Czamanski-Cohen, J., Sarid, O., Cwikel, J., Douvdevani, A., Levitas, E., Lunenfeld, E. and Har-Vardi, I. (2015). Cell-free DNA and telomere length among women undergoing in vitro fertilization treatment, *J. Assist. Reprod. Genet.*, **32**, pp. 1697–1703.

102. Miranda-Furtado, C. L., Luchiari, H. R., Chielli Pedroso, D. C., Kogure, G. S., Caetano, L. C., Santana, B. A., *et al.* (2018). Skewed X-chromosome inactivation and shorter telomeres associate with idiopathic premature ovarian insufficiency, *Fertil. Steril.*, **110**, pp. 476–485.e1.

103. Pedroso, D. C., Miranda-Furtado, C. L., Kogure, G. S., Meola, J., Okuka, M., Silva, C., *et al.* (2015). Inflammatory biomarkers and telomere length in women with polycystic ovary syndrome, *Fertil. Steril.*, **103**, pp. 542–547.e2.

104. Wang, C., Shen, F., Zhu, Y., Fang, Y. and Lu, S. (2017). Telomeric repeat-containing RNA (TERRA) is related to polycystic ovary syndrome (PCOS), *Clin. Endocrinol. (Oxf)*, **86**, pp. 552–559.

105. Sayban, S., Mirfakhraie, R., Omrani, M. D., Ghaedi, H., Heidary, H., Yaghoobi, H., *et al.* (2018). Idiopathic premature ovarian failure and its association to the abnormal longitudinal changes of telomere length in a population of Iranian infertile women: a pilot study, *Meta Gene.*, **18**, pp. 58–61.

106. Michaeli, J., Smoom, R., Serruya, N., El Ayoubi, H., Rotshenker-Olshinka, K., Srebnik, N., *et al.* (2022). Leukocyte telomere length correlates with extended female fertility, *Cells*, **11**, pp. 513.

107. Azzalin, C. M., Reichenbach, P., Khoriauli, L., Giulotto, E. and Lingner, J. (2007). Telomeric repeat containing RNA and RNA surveillance factors at mammalian chromosome ends, *Science*, **318**, pp. 798–801.

108. Wang, C., Zhao, L. and Lu, S. (2015). Role of TERRA in the regulation of telomere length, *Int. J. Biol. Sci.*, **11**, pp. 316–323.

109. Reig-Viader, R., Brieño-Enríquez, M. A., Khoriauli, L., Toran, N., Cabero, L., Giulotto, E., *et al.* (2013). Telomeric repeat-containing RNA and telomerase in human fetal oocytes, *Hum. Reprod.*, **28,** pp. 414–422.

110. Reig-Viader, R., Vila-Cejudo, M., Vitelli, V., Buscà, R., Sabaté, M., Giulotto, E., *et al.* (2014). Telomeric repeat-containing RNA (TERRA) and telomerase are components of telomeres during mammalian gametogenesis, *Biol. Reprod.*, **90**, pp. 103.

111. Rocca, M. S., Dusi, L., Di Nisio, A., Alviggi, E., Iussig, B., Bertelle, S., *et al.* (2021). TERRA: a novel biomarker of embryo quality and art outcome, *Genes. (Basel)*, **12**, pp. 475.

Chapter 19

Telomere Length and Human Carcinogenesis: Liable or Random Finding?

Taxiarchis Konstantinos Nikolouzakis,[a] Aristidis Tsatsakis,[b,c] and John Tsiaoussis[a]

[a] *Department of Anatomy, Medical School, University of Crete, Crete, Greece*
[b] *Laboratory of Toxicology, Medical School, University of Crete, Heraklion, Greece*
[c] *Lifeplus S.A., Science & Technological Park of Crete, Vassilika Vouton, Heraklion, Greece*
tknikolouzakis@gmail.com, tsatsaka@uoc.gr, tsiaoussis@uoc.gr

19.1 Introduction

Cancer stands for the most important clinical, social, and economic issue regarding cause-specific disability-adjusted life years (DALYs) among all human pathologies. Exogenous, endogenous, and individual factors, including genetic predisposition, participate in cancer triggering. Telomeres are specific DNA structures positioned at the end of chromosomes and consist of repetitive nucleotide sequences, which, together with shelterin proteins, facilitate the maintenance of chromosomes' stability while protecting them from genomic

Telomeres: Biomarkers of a Healthy Life and Successful Aging
Edited by Aristidis Tsatsakis

ISBN 978-981-5129-49-6 (Hardcover), 978-1-003-56809-4 (eBook)
www.jennystanford.com

erosion. Even though the connection between telomere status and carcinogenesis has been identified, the absence of a universal or even a cancer-specific trend makes consent even more complicated. It is indicative that both short and long telomere lengths have been associated with a high risk of cancer incidence. When evaluating risk associations between cancer and telomere length, a disparity seems to emerge. Even though shorter telomeres have been adopted as a marker of poorer health status and older biological age, longer telomeres due to increased cell growth potential are correlated to the acquiring of cancer-initiating somatic mutations. Therefore, this review aims to comprehensively present the multifaceted pattern of telomere length and cancer incidence association.

19.2 Telomerase Function and Regulation

Telomeres are repetitive DNA sequences (TTAGGG) located at the end of chromosomes, which are associated with the shelterin complex. Among its main functions, telomeres protect chromosomes from end-to-end fusion and DNA degradation. The end replication problem, owing to the inability of DNA polymerase to replicate the 3' end of chromosomes, causes a progressive telomere shortening, which is linked to cell division. When a critical telomere length is reached, cells activate the protective mechanisms, i.e., senescence & apoptosis, to avoid the proliferation of genetically unstable cells.

If these mechanisms fail, cells continue to divide and enter into a crisis stage, which is characterized by massive genomic instability and cell death. Telomerase is a ribonucleoprotein enzyme complex, consisting of two subunits; human telomerase RNA component (hTERC), an RNA sequence pattern on which the synthesis of telomeric parts is based, and a protein called human telomerase reverse transcriptase (hTERT), whose responsible gene is located in chromosome 5 (5p15.33) (Fig. 19.1). TERT gene is 42 kb long and consists of 15 introns and 16 exons with a 260 bp promoter core [1].

The reverse transcriptase domain is encoded by 5–9 exons. The TERT transcript can be spliced into 22 isoforms [2]. While the transcriptional regulation of TERT has been studied extensively, recent work has evaluated the role of alternate splicing of mRNA

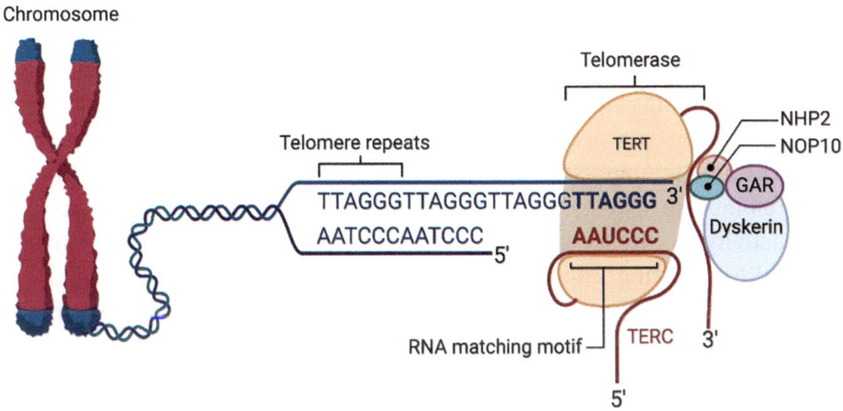

Figure 19.1 Illustration of the telomerase complex. Created with BioRender.com.

transcripts. TERT can be translated from multiple differently spliced transcripts, with only the longest variant having reverse transcriptase enzymatic activity [3]. Breast cancer cell lines with overexpression of transcripts without catalytic function have been shown to have reduced apoptosis conferring a survival advantage [4]. This suggests novel functions of TERT beyond the already described. Such functions are mediated through telomere extension of the TERT promoter (TERTp) region which contains GC boxes that bind the zinc finger transcription factor Sp1, which increases TERT transcription, and E-boxes that bind both transcriptional enhancers and repressors.

TERTp lacks a TATA box but it contains binding sites for many different transcription factors [5]. Two of the six subunits of shelterin, tripeptyl peptidase I (TPP1) and protection of telomeres 1 (POT1), regulate the action of telomerase. hTERT is responsible for the suppression of apoptosis in an early phase before the induction of cytochrome c. Normally, TA is elevated in the early gestation period. hTERC is broadly distributed in the tissues, both present in normal and cancerous cells, while hTERT expression occurs mainly in germ-line cells and most tumor cells. hTERT is required for unrestricted cellular growth, and as a result, it plays a leading role in tumor initiation and further progression.

Telomerase, however, also requires additional enzymes and proteins for its stability and proper function. Dyskerin, functioning as RNA binding protein and enzyme, is a pseudouridine synthetase. Although this function is not of importance for telomerase, it is shown that its presence is obligatory for the enzyme. Moreover, TCBA1 (telomerase Cajal body protein 1) is associated with telomerase activity through dyskerin. Modulation of telomerase activity occurs in several biological tiers, such as transcription, mRNA splicing, sub-cellular localization of each component, and the assemblage of TR and hTERT in an active ribonucleoprotein complex. Transcription of the hTERT gene is most likely the key to the modulation of telomerase activity. The hTERT gene has a length of 35 kb, entailing 16 exons and 15 introns. For the total activation of the hTERT promoter, the concurrent action of MYC and SP1 is deemed essential. TP53, when coming in interplay with SP1, downregulates TERT.

Nuclear factor-kB, hypoxia-inducible factor (HIF-1), and the ETS/MYC complex are also involved in the positive regulation of the hTERT promoter expression. Moreover, the histone methyl-transferase SMYD3 incites TERT expression in healthy as well as malignant cancerous cells. Expression of TERT is constricted by the tumor suppressor genes WT127 and MEN1, and via MAD/MYC and TGF-β/SMAD pathways. TERT expression is also suppressed by the inhibitors p16INK4a and p27KIP1. Post-transcriptionally, regulation of telomerase may take place, mainly, via tissue-specific alternative splicing mechanisms. Notwithstanding that, the telomeres' length is induced in each cell cycle at a lower rate, endorsing cellular senescence [6]. As stated above, loss of DNA sequences can occur due to the end-replication problem that stands upon the dependence of DNA polymerase on promoters (3' telomeric ends), which undergo degeneration and suppression of telomerase. At this point, the activation of telomerase compensates for telomere shortening and allows the cell to successfully exit from the crisis stage.

Telomerase is specifically expressed in immortal cells, such as stem cells, germ tissues, and cancer cells. For the latter, telomerase confers an unlimited replicative potential and has been implicated in immortalization and carcinogenesis (Fig. 19.2a and b).

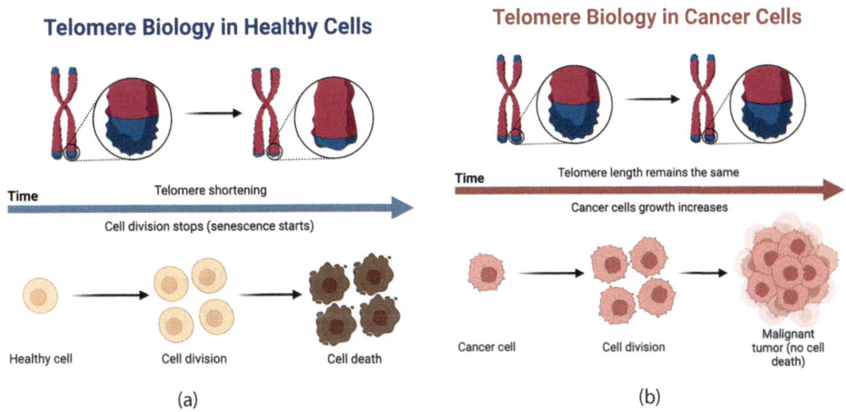

Figure 19.2 Illustration of the differential mechanism of chromosome attrition in (a) normal and (b) cancer cells. Created with BioRender.com.

Telomeres with critical length incite checkpoint signaling mechanisms found in the p53 pathway. The p53 tumor suppressor downregulates the hTERT gene. It was observed that a mutant form of TERT presents the same antiapoptotic activity and that p53-mediates downregulation of hTERT, which is critical for efficient p53-dependent apoptosis. The uncapping of telomeres, instigated by the disruption of TRF2, induces p53 as it represents a signal for breakage (through various mediators, like ataxia-telangiectasia mutated kinase (ATM kinase). In the case protective mechanisms are inactivated, e.g., that of TP53 protein, cells continue with proliferation. In this way, further corrosion of telomeres incites functional impairment regarding telomeric end protection; thus, leading to chromosomal instability.

Consequently, the erosion of telomeres may act as follows: tumor suppression due to induction of senescence, and simultaneously tumor promotion by provoking genomic instability. Brief telomeres could also induce genome-wide DNA methylation, an event that can regulate oncogene and tumor suppressor gene expression.

Overall, the telomere hypothesis supports the notion that shortening of telomeres to a critical length fosters cells to evade further division, whereas protection of telomeres favors proliferation.

When the action of telomerase is inhibited, the result is cellular senescence. On the contrary, the expression of telomerase in ectopic sites permits cellular division, as the length of telomeres remains intact [7, 8].

19.3 Telomerase Independent Elongation

Some cancers are telomerase negative, and their telomere lengths are maintained by a mechanism known as alternative lengthening of telomeres (ALT). This alternative mechanism (ALT) involves the synthesis of new telomeric DNA from a DNA template via homologous recombination (HR) in contrast to the telomerase-dependent elongation. ALT cells can be classified into four different groups according to the recombination mechanism that they use. In human cancer cells where ALT is upregulated, a characteristic telomere phenotype is detected. ALT cells present heterogeneous telomere lengths and longer telomeres than cancer cells, which maintain the telomere status using telomerase.

The ALT mechanism is used less often than telomerase. ALT cells include the promyelocytic leukemia (PML) nuclear bodies that contain telomeric DNA and telomeric binding proteins, and other proteins involved in the recombination process. These ALT-associated PML bodies (APBs) may be used to identify cells, which use the ALT pathway. ALT is characteristic of some tumors, such as neuroepithelial tumors, and osteosarcomas, in some types of soft tissue sarcomas, and occurs in low frequency in some types of carcinomas. In colon carcinogenesis, we suggest this alternative mechanism to maintain TL in case TA is negative [9, 10].

19.4 hTERT Regulation in Cancer Cells

Regulation mechanisms of the hTERT have been a hot topic for the last 20 years. During this time, a number of mechanisms affecting the hTERT gene have been identified. However, recent advances revealed that the hTERT promoter plays a crucial role in regulating its transcription [11].

In fact, hTERT expression was found to be upregulated in tumors via multiple genetic and epigenetic mechanisms including hTERT amplifications (3%), hTERT structural variants (3%), hTERT promoter mutations (31%), and epigenetic modifications through hTERT promoter methylation (53%) [12].

19.5 hTERT Amplifications

Gain or loss of genetic material is a frequent incident in cancer. Gene amplification results from an increase in the number of copies and is associated with overexpression of the amplified gene. Different models have been proposed for the initiation of amplification including DNA replication errors, telomere dysfunction, and the existence of chromosomal fragile sites [13]. Specifically, hTERT gene amplification can result from telomere dysfunction in addition to breakage at fragile sites and the formation of chromosomal fusions [14].

19.6 hTERT Genomic Rearrangements

Another potential mechanism of hTERT upregulation in tumors is the genomic rearrangements affecting the hTERT gene locus (5p15.33). Functionally, these rearrangements bring active enhancers in proximity to the hTERT gene, and the interaction between the promoter and these newly introduced enhancers drives hTERT expression [15].

19.7 Mutation of hTERT Promoter

Mutation of the hTERT promoter represents a frequent but unique genetic alteration that drives hTERT expression and telomerase activation. hTERT core promoter consists of 260 base pairs with multiple transcription-factors binding motifs that regulate gene transcription and telomerase activation [16]. The location of these mutations within the promoter creates additional binding sites for the E-twenty-six (ETS) transcription factor family, thus constituting a novel mechanism of genetic activation in cancer and a possible driver of genomic alteration [17]. Interestingly, mutated hTERT promoter usually occurs in cancers with a low rate of self-renewal, such as brain tumors, liver, melanocytes, and even low-grade bladder cancers, suggesting a role in triggering telomerase activation [18].

19.8 Epigenetic Modification of hTERT

19.8.1 hTERT Promoter Methylation

DNA methylation is catalyzed by a family of DNA methyltransferases (Dnmts) that transfer a methyl group from S-adenyl methionine (SAM) to the fifth carbon of a cytosine residue to form 5-methylcytosine (5mC). Although the brain contains some of the highest levels of DNA methylation of any tissue in the body, 5mC only accounts for ~1% of nucleic acids in the human genome. The majority of DNA methylation occurs on cytosines that precede guanine nucleotide or CpG sites usually located in non-coding regions. DNA methylation is essential for silencing retroviral elements, regulating tissue-specific gene expression, genomic imprinting, and X chromosome inactivation. Importantly, DNA methylation in different genomic regions may exert different influences on gene activities based on the underlying genetic sequence. About 70% of the human gene promoters contain CpG islands. Therefore, DNA methylation has been thought to play an important role in gene expression [19]. Promoter methylation is often associated with gene silencing. However, several studies have shown that methylation of specific regions within the hTERT promoter, particularly, upstream of the hTERT core promoter, is associated with gene activation [20].

There are several explanations as to how hTERT promoter methylation can result in hTERT activation: one explanation is based on the prevention of repressive elements binding caused by DNA methylation at the repressive region [21]. Another possible explanation is a more complex mechanism involving DNA methylation and chromosome structural changes [22]. DNA methylation can contribute to changes in chromatin conformation influencing gene expression by affecting DNA exposure to transcription factor binding [23].

19.8.2 hTERT Regulation Through miRNAs

Different microRNAs or miRNAs have been described as important regulators of hTERT in multiple types of cancer. hTERT-targeting miRNAs negatively regulate its expression, inhibiting tumorigenesis, and are frequently downregulated in cancer [24]. miRNAs can regulate hTERT in either a direct or indirect manner. miRNAs may directly bind to hTERT 3' untranslated region (3'UTR) and interfere with hTERT protein production in cancer cell lines [25]. For example, the downregulation of mir-138 was shown to be associated with hTERT overexpression in anaplastic thyroid carcinoma cells, and the enforced overexpression of mir-138 induced a significant reduction in hTERT expression through interaction with hTERT 3'UTR [26]. miRNAs can also regulate hTERT indirectly by targeting transcription factors involved in hTERT regulation [17]. For example, mir-494 and mir-1294 were reported to downregulate c-Myc, which is a known transcriptional activator of hTERT, in pancreatic cancer and esophageal squamous cell carcinoma [17].

19.9 Example of Colorectal Cancer

The newest advances regarding colorectal cancer suggest that telomere length in tumor tissues is shorter than adjacent mucosa [26, 27]. Furthermore, tumors with a higher number of somatic mutations presented shorter telomeres [27]. Moreover, a correlation between tumor stage and telomere length was identified as lower-stage tumor tissues exhibited shorter telomeres than advanced-stage and metastatic tumors [26]. These studies characterize colorectal cancer tissue with both chromosomal and/or microsatellite instability [26, 27]. Moreover, Piñol-Felis et al. concluded that telomere length could be used as a reliable prognostic factor since telomere shortening was, in their study, correlated to an early stage of tumorigenesis [28].

However, some studies have identified a correlation between colorectal cancer risk and longer telomeres [26, 29]. The two different associations detected in colon cancer patients are suggested to reflect alternative mechanisms of tumorigenesis and specific disease stages [26, 29]. Likewise, studies by Luu et al. and Peacock et al. correlated longer telomeres with an increased risk of colorectal cancer. Specifically, longer telomeres exhibit an elevated risk of accumulating mutations that could lead to transformation and cancer progression [30, 31]. However, a meta-analysis study indicated no association between telomere length and colorectal cancer risk [32].

Furthermore, the analysis of telomere-related protein expression in colorectal cancer tissues showed differences relative to the adjacent mucosa. A positive correlation between the hTERT expression and patients' age in a Saudi Arabian cohort was identified and correlated to the patients' clinicopathological characteristics [33].

Genetic factors affect the association between colorectal cancer risk and telomere length. Thus, Park et al. identified that telomere shortening in cases of tubular adenomas (Tas) was mainly caused by PIK3CA amplification. In contrast, telomere shortening in serrated polyps (SPs) was attributed to BRAF mutations [33, 34]. Furthermore, these authors suggest that tumor genotyping could be a helpful tool to monitor tumor progression [34]. Moreover, a rare P507L variant in TPP1 might increase the risk of colorectal cancer by interrupting TPP1-TIN2 interaction, thus impairing telomerase activity and decreasing telomeres [35].

Epidemiological factors seem to be involved as a study detected shorter telomeres in depressed individuals and identified education and social support as factors toward alterations in telomere length [36]. However, a separate study failed to detect an association between social behavior and telomere length [36].

19.10 Conclusions

Telomeres, chromosome-end DNA-protein structures, are known to shorten progressively over time in most somatic cells. These genome-protecting structures are markers of aging. Notably, short telomeres have been correlated to older age and chronic disease.

A correlation between cancer and telomere length has been suggested with associated uncertainties due to objective difficulties in designing studies of sufficient robustness. A disparity seems to emerge when evaluating risk associations between cancer and telomere length. Even though shorter telomeres have been adopted as a marker of poorer health status and older biological age, longer telomeres due to increased growth potential are correlated to the acquiring of cancer-initiating somatic mutations.

Indeed, the majority of retrospective studies report an increased cancer risk in individuals carrying shorter telomeres; whereas, prospective observational studies detect a weak positive correlation of longer leukocyte telomeres with cancer risk. This association pattern could be partly accounted for by the varying ability of somatic cells to grow; thus, telomere length would exert discrete potential effects.

Moreover, a U-shaped curve of telomere length effects has been detected in various cancers. This suggests that the association with cancer risk would vary among telomere length distribution and not be linear. The pivotal clinical relevance of this knowledge stands on the fact that oncologists who treat these malignancies may seek another tool in their effort to tackle cancer.

Moreover, pathologists may use telomeres, telomerase, hTERT, or any of the implicated proteins as potential biomarkers for cancer prognosis [37, 38]. Furthermore, the cancer-type-specific association is influenced by co-factors, e.g., virus load, inflammatory status, or SNP-disease association. Moreover, the effect of telomere length may differ depending on the disease stage, gender, or even racial belonging.

This is important especially for treatment strategies targeting telomerase since tumors that present long telomeres may be affected but others that exhibit short telomeres may not have the same response [39]. Therefore, telomere length data may give valuable input on cancer development and progression for some types of cancers, but more studies are needed for generalized conclusions.

References

1. Dratwa, M., Wysoczańska, B., Łacina, P., Kubik, T., & Bogunia-Kubik, K. (2020). TERT—regulation and roles in cancer formation, *Frontiers in Immunology*, **11**, pp. 589929.
2. Hrdličková, R., Nehyba, J., & Bose Jr, H. R. (2012). Alternatively spliced telomerase reverse transcriptase variants lacking telomerase activity stimulate cell proliferation, *Molecular and Cellular Biology*, **21**, pp. 4283–4296.
3. Sæbøe-Larssen, S., Fossberg, E., & Gaudernack, G. (2006). Characterization of novel alternative splicing sites in human telomerase reverse transcriptase (hTERT): analysis of expression and mutual correlation in mRNA isoforms from normal and tumour tissues, *BMC Molecular Biology*, **7**, pp. 26.
4. Listerman, I., Sun, J., Gazzaniga, F. S., Lukas, J. L., & Blackburn, E. H. (2013). The major reverse transcriptase-incompetent splice variant of the human telomerase protein inhibits telomerase activity but protects from apoptosis, *Cancer Research*, **73**, pp. 2817–28.
5. Takakura, M., Kyo, S., Kanaya, T., Hirano, H., Takeda, J., Yutsudo, M., *et al.* (1999). Cloning of human telomerase catalytic subunit (hTERT) gene promoter and identification of proximal core promoter sequences essential for transcriptional activation in immortalized and cancer cells, *Cancer Research*, **59**, pp. 551–7.
6. Razgonova, M. P., Zakharenko, A. M., Golokhvast, K. S., Thanasoula, M., Sarandi, E., Nikolouzakis, K., et al. (2020). Telomerase and telomeres in aging theory and chronographic aging theory, *Molecular Medicine Reports*, **3**, pp. 1679–1694.
7. Ayiomamitis, G. D., Notas, G., Zaravinos, A., Zizi-Sermpetzoglou, A., Georgiadou, M., Sfakianaki, O., *et al.* (2014). Differences in telomerase activity between colon and rectal cancer, *Canadian Journal of Surgery*, **3**, pp. 199–208.
8. Bertorelle, R., Rampazzo, E., Pucciarelli, S., Nitti, D., & De Rossi, A. (2014). Telomeres, telomerase and colorectal cancer, *World Journal of Gastroenterology: WJG*, **8**, pp. 1940–1950.
9. Muntoni, A., & Reddel, R. R. (2005). The first molecular details of ALT in human tumor cells, *Human Molecular Genetics*, **14,** Spec No. 2, pp. R191–6.
10. Xu, L., Li, S., & Stohr, B. A. (2013). The role of telomere biology in cancer, *Annual Review of Pathology: Mechanisms of Disease*, **8**, pp. 49–78.

11. Leão, R., Apolónio, J. D., Lee, D., Figueiredo, A., Tabori, U., & Castelo-Branco, P. (2018). Mechanisms of human telomerase reverse transcriptase (h TERT) regulation: clinical impacts in cancer, *Journal of Biomedical Science*, **25**, pp. 1–12.
12. Barthel, F. P., Wei, W., Tang, M., Martinez-Ledesma, E., Hu, X., Amin, S. B., *et al.* (2017). Systematic analysis of telomere length and somatic alterations in 31 cancer types, *Nature Genetics*, **3**, pp. 349–357.
13. Albertson, D. G. (2006). Gene amplification in cancer, *TRENDS in Genetics*, **8**, pp. 447–455.
14. McClintock, B. (1942). The fusion of broken ends of chromosomes following nuclear fusion, *Proceedings of the National Academy of Sciences*, **11**, pp. 458–463.
15. Valentijn, L. J., Koster, J., Zwijnenburg, D. A., Hasselt, N. E., Van Sluis, P., Volckmann, R., *et al.* (2015). TERT rearrangements are frequent in neuroblastoma and identify aggressive tumors, *Nature Genetics*, **47**, pp. 1411–4.
16. Publishing, A, B., Kyo, S., Takakura, M., Fujiwara, T., & Inoue, M. (2008). Understanding and exploiting hTERT promoter regulation for diagnosis and treatment of human cancers, *Cancer Science*, **8**, pp. 1528–1538.
17. Lewis, K. A., & Tollefsbol, T. O. (2016). Regulation of the telomerase reverse transcriptase subunit through epigenetic mechanisms, *Frontiers in Genetics*, **7**, pp. 1–12.
18. Cheng, L., Montironi, R., & Lopez-Beltran, A. (2017). TERT promoter mutations occur frequently in urothelial papilloma and papillary urothelial neoplasm of low malignant potential, *European Urology*, **3**, pp. 497–498.
19. Deaton, A. M., & Bird, A. (2011). CpG islands and the regulation of transcription, *Genes & Development*, **10**, pp. 1010–1022.
20. Castelo-Branco, P., Choufani, S., Mack, S., Gallagher, D., Zhang, C., Lipman, T., *et al.* (2013). Methylation of the TERT promoter and risk stratification of childhood brain tumors: an integrative genomic and molecular study. *The Lancet Oncology*, **6**, pp. 534–542.
21. Castelo-Branco, P., Leão, R., Lipman, T., Campbell, B., Lee, D., Price, A., *et al.* (2016). A cancer specific hypermethylation signature of the TERT promoter predicts biochemical relapse in prostate cancer: a retrospective cohort study, *Oncotarget*, **36**, pp. 57726–57736.
22. Sepehri, Z., Beacon, TH., Osman, FDS., Jahan, S., & Davie, JR. (2019). *Nutritional Epigenomics,* Chapter 2 "DNA methylation and chromatin modifications," Academic Press, Elsevier, **14**, pp. 13–36.

23. Bert, S. A., Robinson, M. D., Strbenac, D., Statham, A. L., Song, J. Z., Hulf, T., *et al.* (2013). Regional activation of the cancer genome by long-range epigenetic remodeling, *Cancer Cell*, **1**, pp. 9–22.
24. Hrdličková, R., Nehyba, J., Bargmann, W., & Bose Jr, H. R. (2014). Multiple tumor suppressor microRNAs regulate telomerase and TCF7, an important transcriptional regulator of the Wnt pathway, *PloS One*, **2**, pp. 86990.
25. Mitomo, S., Maesawa, C., Ogasawara, S., Iwaya, T., Shibazaki, M., Yashima-Abo, A., *et al.* (2008). Downregulation of miR-138 is associated with overexpression of human telomerase reverse transcriptase protein in human anaplastic thyroid carcinoma cell lines, *Cancer Science*, **2**, pp. 280–286.
26. Kroupa, M., Rachakonda, S. K., Liska, V., Srinivas, N., Urbanova, M., Jiraskova, K., *et al.* (2019). Relationship of telomere length in colorectal cancer patients with cancer phenotype and patient prognosis, *British Journal of Cancer*, **4**, pp. 344–350.
27. Lopez-Doriga, A., Valle, L., Alonso, M. H., Ausso, S., Closa, A., Sanjuan, X., *et al.* (2018). Telomere length alterations in microsatellite stable colorectal cancer and association with the immune response, *Biochimica et Biophysica Acta (BBA)-Molecular Basis of Disease*, **9**, pp. 2992–3000.
28. Piñol-Felis, C., Fernández-Marcelo, T., Viñas-Salas, J., & Valls-Bautista, C. (2017). Telomeres and telomerase in the clinical management of colorectal cancer, *Clinical and Translational Oncology*, **19**, pp. 399–408.
29. Le Balc'h, E., Grandin, N., Demattei, M. V., Guyétant, S., Tallet, A., Pagès, J. C., *et al.* (2017). Measurement of telomere length in colorectal cancers for improved molecular diagnosis, *International Journal of Molecular Sciences*, **18**, pp. 1871.
30. Luu, H. N., Qi, M., Wang, R., Adams-Haduch, J., Miljkovic, I., Opresko, P. L., *et al.* (2019). Association between leukocyte telomere length and colorectal cancer risk in the Singapore Chinese Health Study, *Clinical and Translational Gastroenterology*, **10**, pp. 1–9.
31. Peacock, S. D., Massey, T. E., Vanner, S. J., & King, W. D. (2018). Telomere length in the colon is related to colorectal adenoma prevalence, *PloS One*, **13**, pp. e0205697.
32. Naing, C., Aung, K., Lai, P. K., & Mak, J. W. (2017). Association between telomere length and the risk of colorectal cancer: a meta-analysis of observational studies, *BMC Cancer*, **1**, pp. 1–7.
33. Aljarbou, F., Almousa, N., Bazzi, M., Aldaihan, S., Alanazi, M., Alharbi, O., *et al.* (2018). The expression of telomere-related proteins and

DNA damage response and their association with telomere length in colorectal cancer in Saudi patients, *PLoS One*, **13**, pp. e0197154.

34. Jung, S. J., Park, J. H., Hwang, I., & Lee, J. H. (2020). Different TERT expression between colorectal adenoma and serrated polyp, *Medicina*, **9**, pp. 1–5.
35. Li, J., Chang, J., Tian, J., Ke, J., Zhu, Y., Yang, Y., *et al.* (2018). A rare variant P507L in TPP1 interrupts TPP1–TIN2 interaction, influences telomere length, and confers colorectal cancer risk in Chinese population, *Cancer Epidemiology, Biomarkers & Prevention*, **9**, pp. 1029–1035.
36. AlAhwal, M. S., Al Zaben, F., Sehlo, M. G., Khalifa, D. A., Al-Aama, J. Y., Edris, S., *et al.* (2019). Depression and telomere length in colorectal cancer patients in Saudi Arabia, *Asian Journal of Psychiatry*, **40**, pp. 130–131.
37. Nikolouzakis, T. K., Stivaktakis, P. D., Apalaki, P., Kalliantasi, K., Sapsakos, T. M., Spandidos, D. A., *et al.* (2019). Effect of systemic treatment on the micronuclei frequency in the peripheral blood of patients with metastatic colorectal cancer, *Oncology Letters*, **3**, pp. 2703–2712.
38. Nikolouzakis, T. K., Vakonaki, E., Stivaktakis, P. D., Alegakis, A., Berdiaki, A., Razos, N., *et al.* (2021). Novel prognostic biomarkers in metastatic and locally advanced colorectal cancer: micronuclei frequency and telomerase activity in peripheral blood lymphocytes, *Frontiers in Oncology*, **11**, pp. 683605.
39. Guterres, A. N., & Villanueva, J. (2020). Targeting telomerase for cancer therapy, *Oncogene*, **36**, pp. 5811–5824.

Chapter 20

Telomere Length Biology in Blood Disorders and Childhood Cancer

Kleoniki Roka[a] **and Eftichia Stiakaki**[b]

[a]*Division of Pediatric Hematology Oncology, First Department of Pediatrics, National & Kapodistrian University of Athens," Aghia Sophia" Children's Hospital, Athens, Attiki, Greece*

[b]*Department of Pediatric Hematology-Oncology & Autologous Hematopoietic Stem Cell Transplantation Unit, University Hospital of Heraklion & Laboratory of Blood Diseases and Childhood Cancer Biology, School of Medicine, University of Crete, Voutes, Heraklion, Crete, Greece*

nikiroka@med.uoa.gr, efstel@med.uoc.gr

20.1 Introduction

Telomere length (TL) is a dynamic marker affected by both genetic predisposition and environmental conditions [1, 2]. Genetic mutations causing TL shortening result in disorders of premature aging with various manifestations, such as bone marrow failure (BMF),[a] pulmonary fibrosis, liver cirrhosis, premature greying, and

[a]**Bone marrow failure (BMF)**: It refers to the decreased production of one or more major hematopoietic lineages, which leads to diminished or absent hematopoietic precursors in the bone marrow and attendant cytopenia.

Telomeres: Biomarkers of a Healthy Life and Successful Aging
Edited by Aristidis Tsatsakis

ISBN 978-981-5129-49-6 (Hardcover), 978-1-003-56809-4 (eBook)
www.jennystanford.com

increased cancer risk [3, 4]. Moreover, it has been shown that TL is closely related to numerous pathological conditions and aging, although there are differences in children [2, 5].

Telomere length biology has also been associated with human cancer as dysfunctional telomeres participate in genetic instability [2]. Kim et al. made the landmark observation that telomerase activity (TA) is present in 85–90% of human cancers [6]. Since then, the association between telomere length and the risk of cancer has been examined in various epidemiological studies mainly in adults with conflicting findings. However, short telomeres have been linked to a broad spectrum of clinical conditions, which does not necessarily suggest that long telomeres confer an advantage for health and lifespan. Recent studies have shown that longer telomeres appear to increase also the risk of numerous cancer types [5].

It has been reported that, although human somatic cells gradually shorten telomeres to undergo senescence or crisis, cancer cells acquire replicative immortality by activating a telomere maintenance mechanism (TMM) (Fig. 20.1). Similarly to adults, TMMs in children are activated via the enzyme telomerase or the alternative lengthening of telomeres (ALT) mechanism, which, as a consequence, leads to "immortal" cancer cells [7]. Telomerase reverse transcriptase (TERT)[b] plays a principal role in cancer development, ensuring chromosomal stability through TL maintenance and allowing cells to avert senescence [8]. The most important telomerase-mediated TMM are: (a) TERT gene rearrangements, and TERT and TERC gene amplification, (b) TERTp somatic mutations, (c) epigenetic alterations, (d) transcription factor binding, (e) polymorphic variants within TERT gene body and TERTp, and (f) alternative splicing [8]. A study by Barthel et al. showed that cancer cells may arise infrequently without any known TMM activation [9]. This study found that 73% of 6385 tumors with TERT point mutations [10], rearrangements, DNA amplifications, and transcriptional fusions had overexpression of TERT [8]. The alpha thalassemia mental retardation-X-linked

[b]**Telomerase reverse transcriptase (TERT):** It is a catalytic subunit of the enzyme telomerase, which along with the telomerase RNA component (TERC) comprises the most important unit of the telomerase complex, which leads to the extension and replenishment of telomeres.

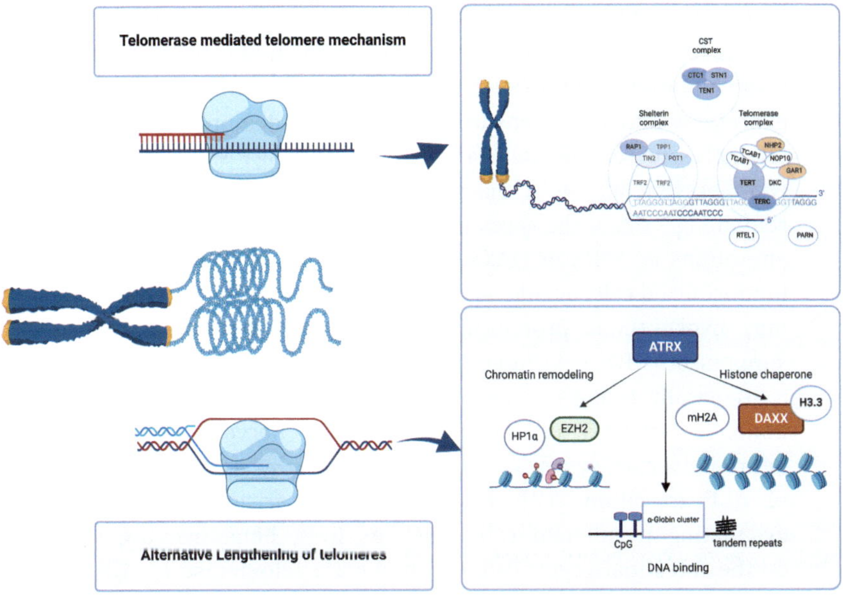

Figure 20.1 Telomere maintenance mechanisms. Created with BioRender.com.

(ATRX) gene [11, 12][c] is one of the most frequently mutated tumor suppressor genes in human cancer-and death-domain associate protein (DAXX)[d] [11, 12] gene together encode a complex that deposits histone variant H3.3 into repetitive heterochromatin.

---

[c]**Alpha thalassemia mental retardation-X-linked (ATRX) gene**: It is named due to its causal role in α-thalassemia with mental impairment, X-linked syndrome, characterized by developmental delay, urogenital abnormalities, distinctive craniofacial features, and α-thalassemia. The ATRX gene, which encodes a SWI/SNF-like chromatin remodeling protein, is frequently mutated in a variety of tumors, including adult lower-grade gliomas, pediatric glioblastoma multiforme, pediatric adrenocortical carcinoma, osteosarcoma, neuroblastoma, and pancreatic neuroendocrine tumors. It is one of the most frequently mutated tumor suppressor genes in human cancers. Recent findings indicate that ATRX plays roles in key molecular pathways, such as the regulation of chromatin state, gene expression, and DNA damage repair, placing ATRX as a central player in the maintenance of genome stability and function.

[d]**Death-domain associate protein (DAXX) gene:** It encodes the death domain-associated protein that was initially identified as a Fas death receptor binding factor inducing apoptosis. DAXX and ATRX genes together encode a complex that deposits histone variant H3.3 into repetitive heterochromatin, thus impacting chromosome stability and telomere maintenance.

Mutations in ATRX and DAXX are often found in tumors especially in pediatrics, suggesting a particular developmental context in which these mutations drive disease [12]. Interestingly, undetectable TERT expression and alterations in ATRX- or DAXX demonstrated longer telomeres, increased telomeric repeat-containing RNA (TERRA), and were present in 5% of the study subjects [8]. Furthermore, the remaining 22% of the cases neither expressed TERT nor harbored alterations in ATRX or DAXX, implying that not all tumors harbor immortalized cells or that additional TMMs exist. Such mechanisms may involve tumor protein p53 (TP53) and retinoblastoma tumor suppressor (RB1) gene alterations [9].

Generally, tumors derived from mesenchymal tissues, including bone, soft tissues, central and peripheral nervous systems, or neuroendocrine systems, are characterized by a high frequency of ALT activation [12]; whereas, tumors arising from tissues originating from stem cells, such as liver, bone marrow, skin, or the intestinal crypt, usually upregulate telomerase [7, 13]. As pediatric tumors are frequently derived from mesenchymal cells, it is estimated, that at least 20% of all pediatric tumors may display the ALT mechanism [7].

Several reports have also suggested that telomere length in cancer is of prognostic value although not all findings are consistent [14].

Despite the limited extent of telomere research in children compared to adults, there has been a substantial number of studies providing the first insights into child telomere biology and determinants.

20.2 Telomeres in Children

In 1998, Frenck et al. reported that telomere attrition rates vary considerably at different ages. Young children lose more than 1 kilobase every year, and this rapid loss is followed by an apparent plateau between the ages of 4 and young adulthood [15]. Researchers have reported no difference in TL among female and male newborns, implying that longer telomeres in women than in men arise from a slower rate of telomeric attrition [16]. Nevertheless, female children possess already longer TL than male children at 4 years of age [15, 17] suggesting that variability in telomere length arises from an early age.

Two genome-wide association studies (GWAS) performed in the pediatric population to look for common adult single nucleotide polymorphisms (SNPs) related to TL failed to replicate results indicating that possibly other genetic variants are involved in the regulation of TL in childhood and adolescence than in adulthood [18, 19].

Data also suggest that apart from sex, several other factors influence TL. Shorter telomeres are observed in children of European ancestry [17], younger maternal age [17], younger paternal age [20], and parents who smoke [21]. Additional factors correlated with shorter TL in children are low socioeconomic status [22], low levels of parental education [22], as well as stress, violence [23], and exposure to institutional care [22, 24].

Furthermore, germline mutations cause dysregulation in telomere homeostasis, resulting in shorter or elongated telomeres and forming a heterogeneous group of diseases called telomere biology disorders (TBDs) [3].

Short telomere syndromes are most frequently caused by inherited mutations in TERT, which account for at least 40% of cases [4, 25, 26].

During the last two decades, highly recurrent somatic mutations in TERT have been reported in numerous cancers, although these alterations occur at a much lower overall frequency compared to adults of about 2.5% in pediatric cancers and tumors of young adults [5]. Data on the age distribution of TERT promoter mutations in pediatric cancer is rare but a few studies suggest a lower frequency in infants as compared to older children [27, 28].

A study analyzing TL using sequencing data from 235 pediatric cancers from the pediatric cancer genome project (PCGP), found telomere lengthening in 32% of solid tumors and 4% of brain tumors, whereas this was not found among hematological malignancies [29]. In 2020, the PCGP updated data from 653 pediatric patients with 23 cancer types showed almost the same results (28.7% of solid tumors and 10.5% of brain tumors had telomere lengthening). Most hematological cancers still showed telomere shortening [30].

Song and colleagues assessed leucocyte TL in 2,427 childhood cancer survivors (median age 7 at diagnosis; age 32 at DNA sampling) and 293 cancer-free controls (median age 35 at DNA sampling) from the St. Jude Lifetime Cohort Study [31, 32]. It was reported that childhood cancer survivors had significantly shorter TL compared to cancer-free controls. In the same study, it was suggested that there was an approximately 11-year reduced telomere reserve among childhood cancer survivors but similar age-dependent telomere attrition when compared with their age-matched pairs. It was also shown that there was an association between early telomere attrition with the occurrence of chronic health conditions [32].

20.3 Cancer in Childhood

Childhood cancer—although relatively rare—is the second leading cause of death in children, following injuries [33].

Cancer development in children has numerous differences compared to adults, with the most obvious being the different age-based incidence rates. In addition, the spectrum of pediatric tumors is different with a trend to develop leukemias more often, embryonal tumors (such as neuroblastoma and Wilms tumor), and sarcomas versus epithelial malignancies. Specifically, leukemia is the most common pediatric malignancy representing almost 28% of childhood cancers, followed by brain tumors (27%), lymphomas (12%), and certain bone cancers (4%). Furthermore, certain types of cancer are almost exclusively observed in children, i.e., neuroblastoma (6%), Wilms tumor (5%), and rhabdomyosarcoma (3%) [33]. It should also be noted that the incidence of different cancer types and the implicated molecular landscape differs with age (Fig. 20.2a and b). Finally, although adult-type tumors are the result of an accumulation of mutations over time, pediatric cancers are thought to be genetically less complex with single mutations being usually the primary oncogenic driver of disease [34].

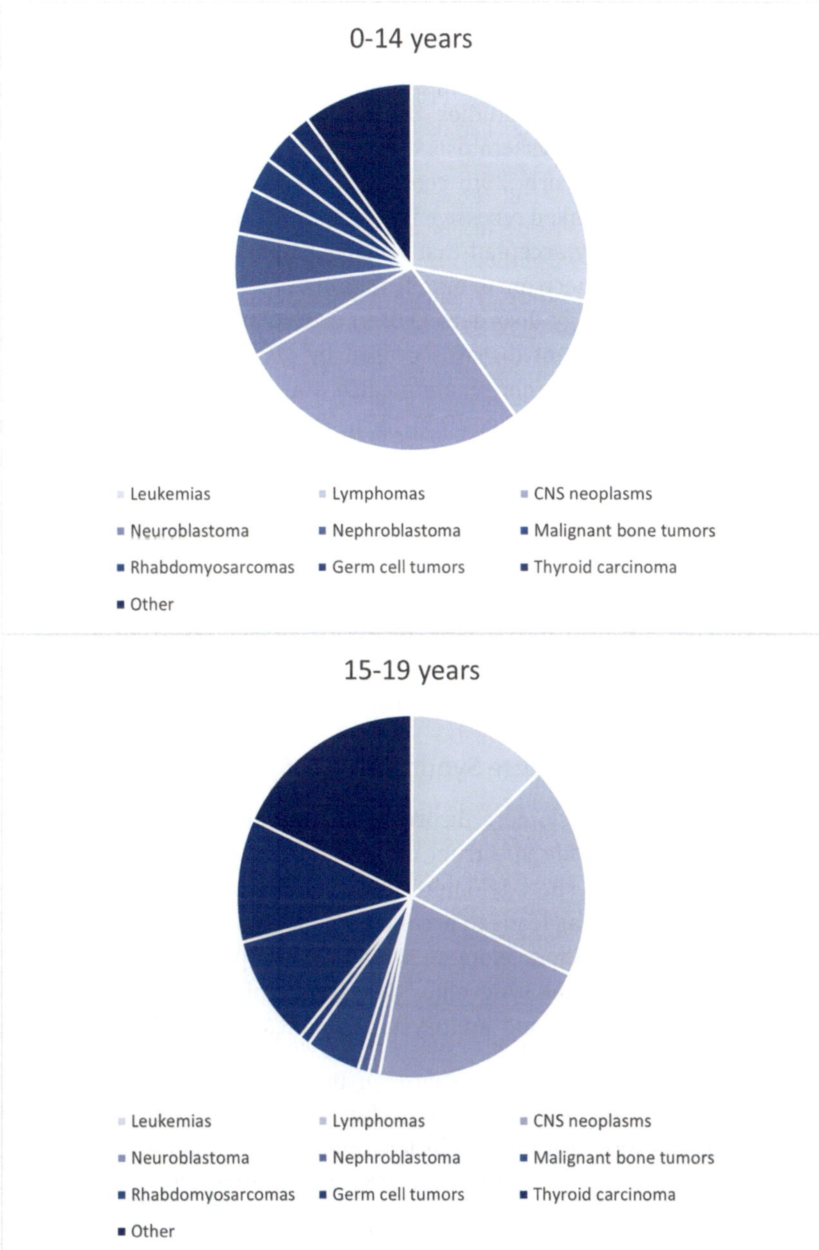

Figure 20.2 Distribution of different cancer types in (a) children 0–14 years and (b) adolescents 15–19 years [33].

20.4 Telomere Biology Disorders

The importance of telomere length maintenance in human disease primarily came from studies of rare monogenic disorders of childhood, initially dyskeratosis congenita (DC). DC was described by Zinnser in the early 20th century and was initially thought to occur through X-linked recessive inheritance (XLR)[e] only [3, 35, 36]. Today, it is widely accepted that females can also be affected and there is a broad spectrum of manifestations.

Telomere biology disorders (TBDs) or telomeropathies encompass a wide range of diseases caused by germline mutations in genes regulating telomere maintenance, thus, usually resulting in very short telomeres (Fig. 20.3) [35]. TBDs may present with a wide spectrum of clinical features affecting multiple organ systems [37].

In the last few years, it has also been shown that longer telomeres not only confer an advantage for health and lifespan but there is growing evidence that mutations responsible for lengthening telomeres are also linked with increased cancer risk (Fig. 20.3) [38, 39].

20.4.1 Short Telomere Syndromes (STS)

The best-studied telomere disorders are the short telomere syndromes, with a wide spectrum of severity that is determined by the extent of the short telomere defect. The resulting premature telomere shortening leads to premature senescence of stem cells in organ reservoirs. Short telomere syndromes are practically accelerated premature aging syndromes that are mainly characterized by genetic anticipation[f] and multisystem manifestations (Table 20.1) [39].

---

[e] **X-linked recessive inheritance:** It manifests only in males. A male with an affected allele on his single X chromosome is homozygous and cannot transmit the disorder to their male offspring, but all his daughters would be carriers. Healthy heterozygous carrier females pass the disorder to affected sons.

[f] **Genetic anticipation:** A genetic phenomenon where the symptoms of a genetic disorder become apparent at an earlier age with each generation.

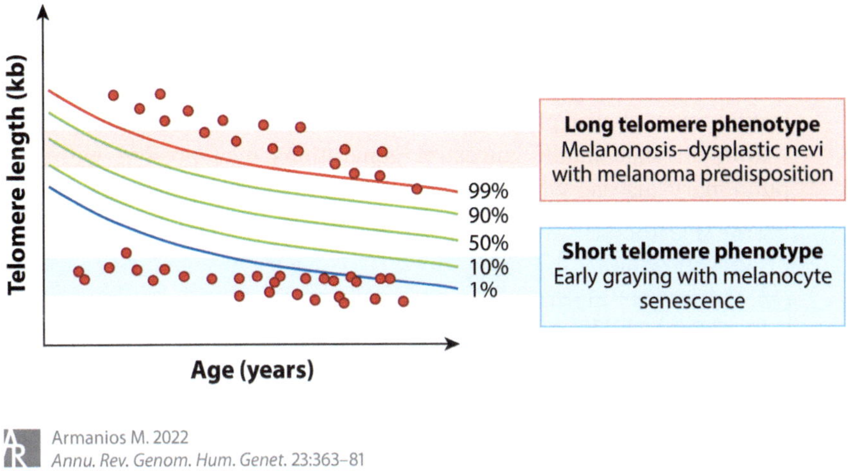

Figure 20.3 Hypothesized long and short telomere syndrome patients with telomeres at extremes of the normal range. Adapted from Armanios M. [2].

Remarkably, in a recent large study with 472432 participants (mean age 57 years), it was shown that reduced TL was associated with a small risk for increased overall mortality, but a higher risk of mortality was associated with specific organs and diseases (cardiovascular, digestive respiratory, musculoskeletal, or hematopoietic diseases) [40].

Table 20.1 Telomere syndrome manifestations that overlap with human age-related phenotypes [41]

High-turnover compartments	Low-turnover compartments
Hair graying	Idiopathic pulmonary fibrosis
Hair loss	Emphysema
Nail ridging	Liver fibrosis and cirrhosis
Periodontal disease	Impaired glucose tolerance
Thrombocytopenia	Defective insulin secretion
Decreased bone marrow cellularity	Insulin resistance
Immunosenescence	Osteoporosis
Gastrointestinal intraepithelial lymphocytosis	
Increased cancer risk	
Chemotherapy intolerance	

One of the main and most interesting characteristics of STS that distinguishes them from other Mendelian disorders is the fact that even though affected patients share a single molecular defect, the predominant clinical phenotypes[g] may appear distinct. For example, within a single family, ancestral generations may present with pulmonary disease whereas their children develop bone marrow failure (BMF).

In general, children and young adults with STS tend to develop the disease in high-turnover tissues such as the bone marrow, whereas adults develop the disease in slow-turnover tissues, especially the lung and liver (Fig. 20.4) [2].

20.4.1.1 Clinical manifestations

Based on the age of the first manifestation, the organ systems involved, the severity of each organ system involvement, as well as the underlying telomere pathophysiology, telomeropathies can be distinguished into three groups-variants [42].

The first group is DC. The classical syndromic form of DC is characterized by the mucocutaneous triad of nail dystrophy, abnormal skin pigmentation, and leukoplakia[h] and often appears in childhood (median age of diagnosis 14 years) [42]. The abnormal skin pigmentation and nail changes appear first and often below the age of 10 years followed by the development of BMF frequently below the age of 20 years [43]. Since the initial report of DC, the spectrum of clinical features has significantly expanded, and diagnostic ages range from infancy to older adults [44].

---

[g]**Phenotype:** The observable characteristics or traits of an organism that are produced by the interaction of the genotype and the environment.

[h]**Leukoplakia:** It is the most common premalignant or "potentially malignant" lesion of the oral mucosa. It is usually a white lesion of the oral mucosa that cannot be clinicopathologically characterized as any other definable lesion.

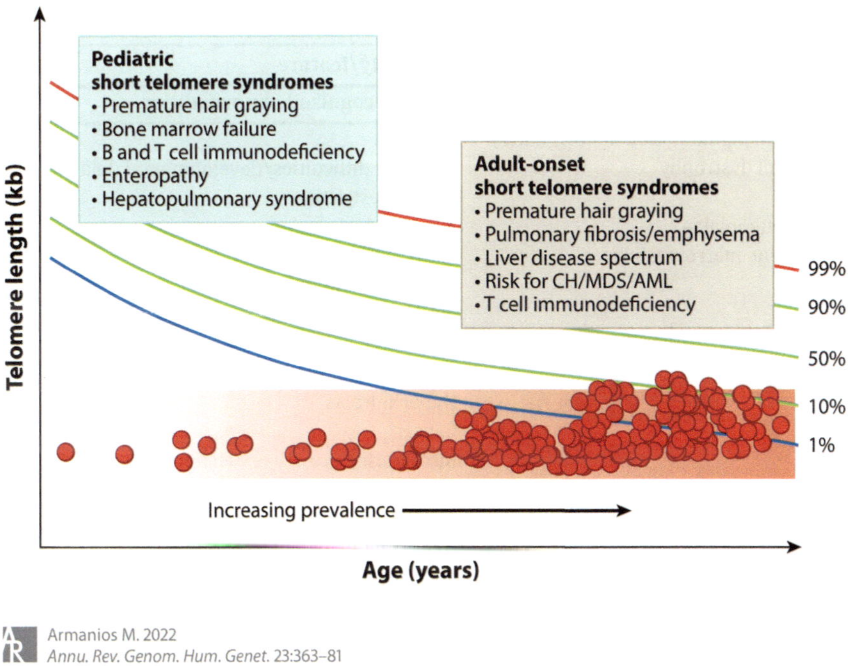

Figure 20.4 Distinct pediatric and adult manifestations of short telomere syndromes and their increasing prevalence with age. Adapted from Armanios M. [2].

Furthermore, with the advances in DC genetics, BMF as the first manifestation besides classic mucocutaneous features is becoming increasingly common [43].

Currently, the minimal clinical criteria for DC diagnosis include the presence of at least two out of the four major features (nail dystrophy, abnormal skin pigmentations, leukoplakia, and BMF and at least two of the other extra-hematopoietic features [45] (Table 20.2).

The second group is characterized by **very early onset severe variants** with extremely short telomeres that manifest very early in life—infancy and childhood—and usually have a poor prognosis. This group comprises [3, 39, 47, 48]:

- **Hoyeraal-Hreidarsson syndrome** (HHS, OMIM#305000): It is a serious and rare variant characterized by cerebellar

Table 20.2 Abnormalities associated with classic DC [46]

Clinical abnormality/feature	
Common/major abnormalities	**Other recognized abnormalities**
Skin pigmentation abnormalities	Epiphora
Nail dystrophy	Learning difficulties/developmental delay/ mental restriction
Leukoplakia	Pulmonary disease
Bone marrow failure	Short stature
	Extensive dental caries/loss
	Esophageal stricture
	Premature hair loss/greying/sparse eyelashes
	Hyperhidrosis
	Cancer
	Intrauterine growth restriction
	Liver disease/enteropathy/peptic ulceration
	Ataxia/cerebellar hypoplasia
	Hypogonadism/undescended testes
	Microcephaly
	Urethral stricture/phimosis
	Osteoporosis/scoliosis/aseptic necrosis
	Deafness

hypoplasia, microcephaly, developmental delay, immunodeficiency, intrauterine growth retardation, and progressive BMF.

- **Revesz syndrome** (RS, OMIM#268130): Patients with RS may additionally present bilateral exudative retinopathy[i] and often cerebral calcifications.
- **Coats-plus syndrome** (CRMCC, OMIM#612199): It is also called cerebroretinal microangiopathy with calcifications and cysts. CRMCC overlaps with RS and is characterized by exudative retinopathy, gastrointestinal vascular ectasia[j],

[i]**Exudative retinopathy:** An idiopathic disorder characterized by retinal telangiectasia with deposition of intraretinal or subretinal exudates potentially leading to retinal detachment and unilateral blindness.

[j]**Vascular ectasia:** An uncommon but often severe cause of upper gastrointestinal bleeding.

gastrointestinal bleeding, osteopenia, bone fractures, poor bone healing, and leukoencephalopathy [49, 50].

It should be noted, that in each of these conditions, additional features of DC may be present.

The last group is the **"cryptic" form**, a late onset of DC with oligosymptomatic manifestations presenting in early adulthood. Patients may present with aplastic anemia (AA)[k], myelodysplastic syndrome (MDS)[l]/acute myeloid leukemia (AML)[m], liver cirrhosis[n], pulmonary fibrosis, or a combination of these [42]. Idiopathic pulmonary fibrosis is considered the primary adult-onset manifestation of STS, diagnosed after the sixth decade [2].

In the last few years, it has become clear that the spectrum of patients who can be considered to have DC has expanded considerably, as shown in Table 20.3 [3, 46].

Other less-known manifestations especially in childhood are:

- **Opportunistic infections** with the absence of mild BMF. It can be the first presenting symptom of an inherited STS.
- **T-cell immunodeficiency.** Recently it was shown that T-cells from STS show a premature aging phenotype and have a distinct molecular program related to the DNA damage response and intrinsic apoptosis [51].
- **Non-infectious enterocolitis** in infancy due to a primarily B-cell immunodeficiency may be also the primary manifestation [4].

---

[k]**Aplastic anemia (AA):** A severe hematologic condition characterized by pancytopenia and a markedly hypocellular or acellular marrow. It can be either inherited or more often acquired.

[l]**Myelodysplastic syndrome (MDS):** It consists of a very heterogeneous group of myeloid disorders characterized by peripheral blood cytopenias and an increased risk of transformation to acute myelogenous leukemia.

[m]**Acute myelogenous leukemia (AML):** A cancer of the myeloid line of blood cells, characterized by the rapid growth of abnormal cells of the bone marrow and interfering with normal blood production.

[n]**Liver cirrhosis:** It is a condition of the liver that develops after a long period of inflammation resulting in the replacement of the healthy liver parenchyma with fibrotic tissue and regenerative nodules and leading to portal hypertension.

Table 20.3 Telomere biology diagnostic criteria [46]

Criteria
1. All three mucocutaneous features:
i. Abnormal skin pigmentation
ii. Nail dystrophy
iii. Leukoplakia
2. At least one out of three mucocutaneous features, combined with bone marrow failure and two other somatic features of DC
3. Aplastic anemia, myelodysplastic syndrome, or pulmonary fibrosis associated with a pathogenic telomerase variant
4. Two or more features seen in DC are associated with very short telomeres that are below 1st centile
5. Four or more features of the Hoyeraal-Hreidarsson syndrome:
i. Growth retardation
ii. Developmental delay
iii. Microcephaly
iv. Bone marrow failure
v. Immunodeficiency
vi. Cerebellar hypoplasia

- **Avascular necrosis (AVN) of the femoral head or humerus** and **minimal trauma fractures (MTF)**. Lately, it has shown 18% of DC/TBDs.
- Patients experience at least one AVN and/or MTF at a median age of 21.9 years. The median age at first MTF was much younger (13.6 years). Importantly, MTF occurred almost exclusively in young patients with severe disease [52].

In conclusion, children and young adults with short telomere syndromes (who have the most severe short telomere defects) tend to develop the disease in high-turnover tissues, such as the bone marrow and skin, with the most common manifestations being bone marrow failure, immunodeficiency, and in some cases enteropathy (Fig. 20.5) [2, 53].

Studies have shown that individuals with TBDs have an increased likelihood of developing organ fibrosis in tissues more susceptible

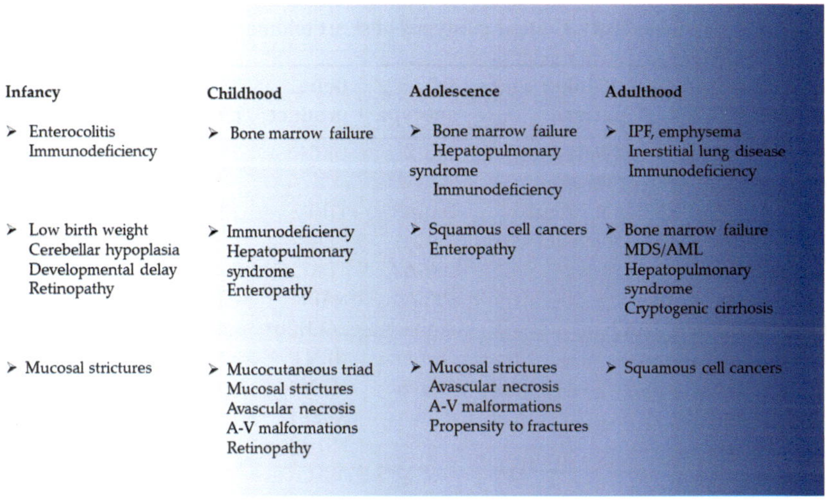

Figure 20.5 Age-dependent manifestations of the short telomere syndromes [4].

to TL shortening, especially after exposure to chemotherapy and radiation [54]. At present, there are no evidence-based recommendations for cancer patients who present greater than the expected therapy-related toxicities. However, it is advised to obtain clinically available TL testing in those patients with developed signs of progressive liver or lung disease or/and grade 3–4 neutropenia or grade 4 mucositis as complications of cytotoxic therapy despite dose reduction [54].

20.4.1.2 Genetic background

The discovery of mutations in dyskerin (DKC1) on the X chromosome causing reduced telomerase activity and short telomeres established the first link between telomere biology and human disease. To date, at least 18 different genes covering all modes of transmission—XLR, autosomal dominant (AD), and autosomal recessive (AR)—have been identified and etiologically associated (Table 20.4) [35, 55].

Consistent with previous reports, diagnosis of TBDs in childhood was more likely with autosomal recessive (AR)/X-linked recessive

Table 20.4 Genetic subtypes of short telomere syndromes

TBD	DC inheritance pattern	DC subtype	Gene product	% of DC patients	Chromosome location
Dyskeratosis congenita	X-linked recessive	DKCX	DKC1	25	Xp28
	Autosomal dominant (AD)	DKCA3	TINF2	12	14q12
		DKCA1	TERC	5	3q26.2
		DKCA2	TERT	3	5p15.33
		DKCA4	NAF1	<1	4q32.2
			ZCCHC8*	<1	12q24.31
			NPM1	<1	5q35.1
			MDM4	<1	1q32.1
			RTEL1		20q13.3
			MDM4		1q32.1
			ACD		16p22.1
			RPA1		17p13.3
	Autosomal recessive (AR)	DKCB5	USB1	2	16q21
		DKCB6	RTEL1	2	20q13.3
		DKCB1	PARN	1	16p13.12
		DKCB4	NOP10	<1	15q14
		DKCB2	TERT	<1	5p15.33
		DKCB3	NHP2	<1	5q35.3
		DKCB7	WRAP53	<1	17p13.1
		DKCB8	CTC1	<1	17p13.1
			ACD/TPP1	<1	16q22.1
			DCLRE1B		1p13.2
			[58]		7q31.33
			POT1		
	Digenic form	DKCD	TYMS [59]		18p11.32
	Uncharacterized			20–25%	?
ReveszS	AD		TINF		14q12
Hoyeraal-Hreidarrson syndrome	AD		TINF2		14q11
	AR		RTEL1		20q13.3
			TERT		5p15.33
Coats plus	AD		STN1		10q24.33
	AR		CTC1		17p13.1

(XLR) disease or TINF2 mutations than autosomal dominant (AD) genotypes[o] (odds ratio [OR] 9.2; $p < 0.01$, adjusted for sex) [56].

20.4.1.3 Telomere length in TBDs

As TL measurement is age-dependent, the clinical and when possible, the genetic findings should be considered. Across the age spectrum, there is not a single threshold applicable to all STS patients.

Generally, children and adolescents with symptomatic short telomere disease usually fall below the first percentile for age, whereas young asymptomatic mutation carriers may have TL between the 1st and 10th percentiles and be at risk of developing late-onset manifestations [4].

Total lymphocyte lengths less than the first percentile for age have a sensitivity and specificity of 97% and 91%, respectively, for differentiating patients with DC from their unaffected relatives [35, 57]. Since 2012, Alter et al. reported that extremely short telomeres were strongly associated with the most severe clinical phenotypes such as HHS and RS. This study also showed a trend toward shorter telomeres in those patients with more features of the diagnostic triad. Finally, patients with mutations in DKC1, TINF2, and unknown genes were found to have shorter telomeres than those with mutations in TERC, TERT, and WRAP53 [57].

It should be noted that telomeres at or below the first percentile rarely occur in patients with other inherited bone marrow failure syndromes, such as Fanconi anemia, Diamond-Blackfan anemia, or Schwachman-Diamond syndrome [60].

20.4.1.4 Propensity to develop blood disorders and malignancies

The most serious clinical complication and the major cause of mortality of TBDs is progressive bone marrow failure (BMF). It is estimated that up to 80–90% of patients develop BMF by the age of 30 years. In the early stages, BMF may involve a single lineage

---

[o] **Genotype:** The genetic makeup of an individual cell or organism that determines or contributes to its phenotype.

(mainly thrombocytopenia), which later evolves into a severe form [43]. The possibility of developing severe BMF with the need for bone marrow transplantation increases with age and reaches a cumulative risk of approximately 50% by the age of 50 years [26]. Rarely, BMF may arise before any sign of mucocutaneous manifestations, thus it could be misinterpreted as idiopathic aplastic anemia.

Apart from BMF, TBD patients have an increased risk of developing both hematological and non-hematological malignancies. In fact, patients with classical DC have also a 40–50% cumulative risk of malignancy by the age of 50 years and an overall median survival of 51 years, which has improved compared to previous studies, mainly due to major advances in supportive treatment and modification of drug regimens or dose reduction [42, 61].

Cancer is an overall rare complication in STSs and affects 10% of patients [26]. Notably, the overall/expected ratio (O/E ratio) for non-transplanted DC patients was 4.2 for any malignancy. Additionally, the O/E ratio for head and neck squamous cell carcinoma (HNSCC) development, especially in the tongue, was extremely high (74 and 216, respectively). Regarding hematological disorders, these patients showed an O/E ratio of 578 and 73 to develop MDS and AML, accordingly. Following the transplant, DC patients had an ever-higher O/E ratio for developing any malignancy, HNSCC in general, and HNSCC in the tongue (30, 432, and 1561, respectively). The transplanted DC patients, also, had an increased possibility to develop Hodgkin (HD) or non-Hodgkin Lymphoma (NHL) [26].

A closer look at the STS solid cancer spectrum reveals an overlap with cancers arising in patients with T-cell immunodeficiency, such as those with acquired immunodeficiency syndromes (AIDS) and those who had undergone solid organ transplantations, thus implying that STS patients may also have defects in T cell-mediated immune surveillance [2].

In conclusion, the clinician, especially the pediatrician should not forget that TBDs are characterized by disease anticipation. This means that an affected individual may have a phenotypically unaffected but mutation-positive parent or siblings at risk. Also, this implies that a carrier offspring may need to be investigated for associated illnesses at a younger age than the presentation of their parent [62].

20.4.2 Long Telomere Syndromes

In the last few years, supporting evidence shows that changes in telomere length causing long telomeres are also associated with disease susceptibility. Studies from cancer-prone families as well as from population-based studies correlate germline variants promoting telomere lengthening to cancer predisposition [63].

In humans, the first study supporting that telomerase upregulation confers a risk of familial cancer was published in 2013. Horn et al. reported a five-generation autosomal dominant family with cutaneous malignant melanoma carrying a mutation in the TERT promoter [64]. Overall, the prevalence of germline TERT promoter mutations in familial melanoma is estimated to be less than 1%. Notably, somatic TERT promoter mutations have also been found in 70% of melanomas [65] as well as numerous other solid tumors [66]. In addition to TERT promoter mutation, additional mutations in four sheltering genes (POT1, TPP1, TERF2IP, and TINF2) have been linked to familial melanoma, glioma, and chronic lymphocytic leukemia, and explain 1–10% of families with these cancers [2, 38].

Finally, in a large population study genetically increased telomere length was associated with higher ORs (95% CIs) of disease for 9 of 22 primary cancers ($p < 0.05$) (Table 20.5) and lower ORs (95% CIs) of disease for 6 of 32 primary non-neoplastic diseases ($p < 0.05$) (Table 20.6) [67].

20.4.3 Paradoxical Effect on Telomere Length

It should be noted that different mutations in identical telomere genes appear to have bidirectional effects on TL implying its delicate regulation [2]. These mutations are found in the same gene, but in a distinct domain, thus mediating a short or long Mendelian telomere phenotype [63]. So far, three genes have been reported to show such a paradoxical effect in TL, namely TERT, POT1, and TPP1 [2, 63].

Table 20.5 Association of genetically longer telomeres with neoplastic diseases [67]

Cancer type	OR	95% CI
Glioma	5.27	3.15–8.81
Endometrial cancer	1.31	1.07–1.61
Kidney cancer	1.55	1.08–2.23
Testicular germ-cell cancer	1.76	1.02–3.04
Melanoma	1.87	1.55–2.26
Bladder cancer	2.19	1.32–3.66
Neuroblastoma	2.98	1.92–4.62
Lung adenocarcinoma	3.19	2.40–4.22
Serous low-malignant-potential ovarian cancer	4.35	2.39–7.94

Table 20.6 Association of genetically longer telomeres with non-neoplastic diseases [67]

Non-neoplastic diseases	OR	95% CI
Coronary heart disease	0.78	0.67–0.90
Abdominal aortic aneurysm	0.63	0.49–0.81
Alzheimer's disease	0.84	0.71–0.98
Celiac disease	0.42	0.28–0.61
Interstitial lung disease	0.09	0.05–0.15
Type 1 diabetes	0.71	0.51–0.98

20.5 Inherited and Acquired Blood Disorders

Studies have shown that in primitive hematopoietic stem cells, there are low levels of telomerase activity (TA). These levels increase in progenitor cells initially and then decrease during differentiation [68]. In hematopoietic cells, TA is sufficient to partially lessen telomere attrition although it cannot prevent telomere shortening, thus telomeres shorten with age [69].

Frenck et al. showed that the rate of telomere attrition in leukocytes varied at different ages. Telomere length from peripheral blood leukocytes shortens at a rate of $>$ 1 kilobase per year in young children, followed by a plateau between age 4 and young adulthood and by gradual attrition later in life [15].

20.5.1 Inherited Bone Marrow Failure Syndromes (IBMFs)

IBMFs comprise a heterogeneous group of disorders with multiorgan manifestations (Table 20.7). The characteristic feature of these patients is a failure in the production of one or more blood lineage. Thus, the clinical spectrum alters in accordance with the type and number of blood cell lines involved [70]. Diagnosis of IBMFs is revealed during evaluation for either the hematologic manifestations often since early childhood or specific congenital anomalies. Therefore, IBMF patients are usually diagnosed by pediatric hematologists or pediatricians [44].

The IBMFs have a tendency to develop myelodysplastic syndrome (MDS) and/or acute myeloid leukemia (AML) despite the phenotypic variability and different underlying pathogenetic mechanisms [70].

Finally, TL is reported as shorter versus normal controls in almost all patients with IBMFs, with the shortest found in DC/TBD patients [60, 71, 72].

20.5.1.1 Fanconi anemia (FA)

FA is a rare, multisystemic, genetic disorder characterized by congenital malformations, BMF, endocrine abnormalities, as well as cancer predisposition, and sensitivity to DNA interstrand crosslinking agents [74].

Cytogenetic analysis using chromosomal breakage assay after exposure to DNA crosslinking agents (mitomycin C or diepoxybutane) is considered the gold standard diagnostic tool [75].

Classical physical abnormalities include those described by the acronyms VACTERL-H (vertebral, anal, cardiac, tracheoesophageal fistula, esophageal atresia, renal, upper limb, and hydrocephalus) or PHENOS (skin pigmentation, small head, small eyes, nervous system, otology, and short stature) [76, 77] and are found in almost 75% of FA patients [78]. At birth and early childhood, only physical signs may be present and range from discreet to extensive. BMF may appear between 5 and 15 years of age and the diagnosis of FA is often made at this stage. Later, during teens or young adulthood, the risk

Table 20.7 Inherited bone marrow failure syndromes [73]

IBMFS	DC	FA	SDS	DBA
Inheritance pattern	AR, XLR	XLR, AR, AD	AR	AD
Non-hematologic features	Classical DC triad Pulmonary fibrosis Liver disease Stenosis of esophagus	Radial ray anomalies VACTERL-H PHENOS	Exocrine pancreatic insufficiency, neurodevelopmental, and skeletal abnormalities	Short stature, craniofacial, and organ abnormalities
Hematological disorders/ malignancies	MDS, AML	MDS, AML	MDS, AML, ALL	MDS, AML, ALL
Solid cancers	HNSCC	HNSCC		Osteo Sarcoma
Underlying biology	Telomere biology	FA/BRCA DDR-pathway	Ribosome biogenesis and processing	Ribosome biogenesis and processing
BMF	AA ($>$ 90%)	AA (~80%)	AA (~20%)	Red cell Aplasia
Telomere length	⇩⇩⇩	⇩⇩	⇩	⇩
Chromosome instability	Yes	Yes	Yes	Yes

of AML and MDS/AML becomes very high [79]. Svahn et al. reported that patients with severe phenotypes are diagnosed at younger ages because of malformations, whereas subjects with mild and moderate phenotypes are diagnosed later usually because of hematological impairment [80]. Notably, it is estimated that approximately one-third of patients have no overt extra hematopoietic abnormalities and can be diagnosed in late adulthood [61].

FA is caused by an inheritable defect in a group of proteins responsible for the DNA repair process. To date, 22 different mutated genes of the FA/breast cancer susceptibility (BRCA) DNA repair pathway have been identified so far in FA patients (Fig. 20.6). The genes are designated as complementation groups FANCA, FANCB, FANCC, FANCD1, FANCD2, FANCE, FANCF, FANCG, FANCI, FANCJ, FANCL, FANCM, FANCN, FANCO, FANCP, FANCQ, FANCR, FANCS, FANCT, FANCU, FANCV, and FANCW, with the most common found in FANCA (59–64%) and FANCC (10–15%) [61, 76, 77, 81, 82]. It is primarily an autosomal recessive disease except for FA due to mutations in the FANCB gene which is X-linked and in the FANCR/RAD51C Paralog C (RAD51) which is an autosomal dominant mutation [77, 83, 84]. It is worth mentioning that several FA genes are also breast and ovarian cancer susceptibility genes, (namely FANCD1/BRCA2, FANCJ/BRCA1 interacting helicase 1(BRIP1), FANCN/partner and localizer of BRCA2 (PALB2), FANCO/RAD51C, and FANCS/BRCA1) [85]. Disruption of the FA/BRCA pathway renders cells sensitive to interstrand-crosslinks-inducing agents.

Eight of the FA proteins (FANC-A, -B, -C, -E, -F, -G, -L, and -M) form the FA core complex, a ubiquitin ligase complex with other associated proteins in the nucleus. FANCM protein and its partners act both as a translocase and a cargo protein and bind DNA in close proximity to the lesion. FA core complex is involved in sensing the DNA lesions and monoubiquitinates FANCD2 and FANCI that form the ID complex. Once the ID complex is monoubiquitinated, FANCD2/FANCI-associated nuclease 1 (FAN1) binds to the ID complex, which localizes with the downstream effector complex, which coordinates the recruitment of proteins to perform interstrand crosslink removal and restart replication. Once the repair is terminated, ubiquitin-specific protease 1 (USP1) and

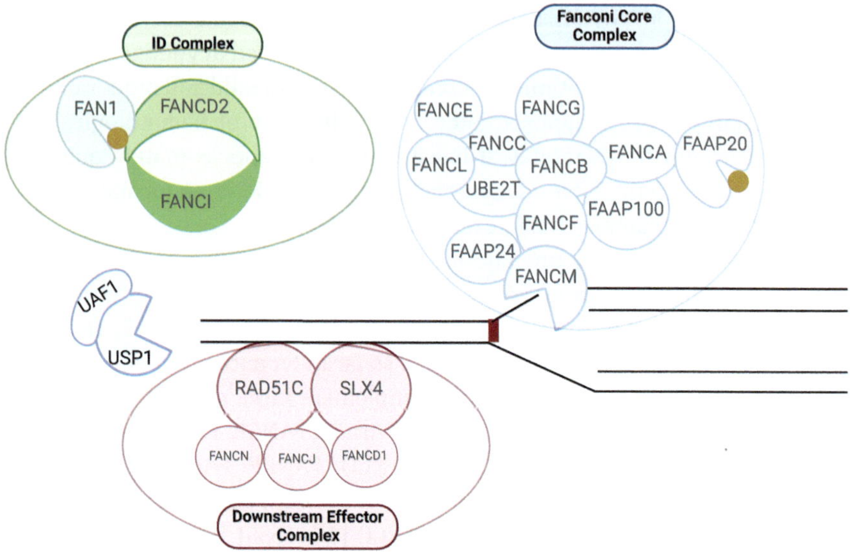

Figure 20.6 The Fanconi anemia repair pathway (Created with Biorender.com).

its partners terminate the reaction by deubiquitinating FANCD2 and FANCI [86].

A recent genotype-phenotype study from the National Cancer Institute cohort showed an association of increased risk of BMF with the PHENOS phenotype [87].

Patients with FA have been reported to present telomere loss/break in peripheral leucocytes, increased end-to-end telomere fusions, and overall shorter telomeres as well as high levels of telomerase activity [88]. In fact, it has been suggested that telomere shortening per year is higher among patients with FA and severe BMF compared to those with non-severe BMF [89]. Recently, Shah et al. reported a high frequency of organ deformities (20%) and severe shortening of TL in the FANCL complementation group compared to the FANCA and FANCG groups [82].

Proposed mechanisms for accelerated telomere shortening in FA include increased chromosomal breakage, excess free radical formation, and/or abnormal regulation of cell proliferation related to the deregulation of apoptosis [82, 84].

BMF remains the major cause of morbidity and probably mortality in FA patients. The risk of full-blown BMF is almost 50% at the age of 40 years and the cumulative incidence of solid malignancies is estimated at 16% at the age of 50 years [70]. Alter et al. reported that the ratio of observed-to-expected cancers (O/E) for any malignancy in non-transplanted FA patients was 19 and was higher compared to other IBMFs. Non-transplanted patients with FA had a higher O/E ratio of developing head and neck squamous cell carcinoma (HNSCC), especially in the tongue (527 and 1054, respectively) as well as esophageal cancer (O/E ratio: 1266). Regarding hematological malignancies, non-transplanted FA patients had an increased O/E ratio of 5669, 213, and 40 for developing MDS, AML, and leukemia, accordingly. Following the transplant, FA patients had an even higher O/E ratio to develop any malignancy, HNSCC in general, and INSCC in the tongue and pharynx of 55, 932, 1451, and 16935, respectively. Transplanted FA patients also had an increased risk of developing NHL [26].

Furthermore, the researchers reported specific early cancers in patients with pathogenic variants in FANCD1/BRCA2 and FANCN/PLAB2 as well as high frequency of solid tumors in patients with one or both FANCA variants within/involving the region of exons 27–30 [87]. It is estimated that approximately 11% of FA patients develop cancer by the age of 18 years [90].

20.5.1.2 Schwachman-Diamond syndrome (SDS)

It is a recessively inherited disorder characterized by exocrine pancreatic dysfunction, bony metaphyseal dysostosis, and impaired hematopoiesis [91]. The majority of patients present early with failure to thrive, malabsorption due to pancreatic insufficiency, and recurrent infections [92].

SDS in most patients (90–95%) results due to mutations in the Schwachman Bodian Diamond syndrome (SBDS) gene located on chromosome 7q11, whereas few patients harbor mutations in SRP54, DNAJC21 of EFL1 genes [26, 70, 93, 94]. Liu et al. showed that SBDS deficiency leads to telomere shortening. Overexpression of disease-associated SBDS mutants or knockdown of SBDS hampered the recruitment of telomerase onto telomeres, while the overall reverse transcriptase activity of telomerase remained unaffected [95].

TL is shorter in SDS patients versus normal controls, but not as short as in patients with DC [60, 91].

Individuals with SDS have an increased risk of BMF, MDS, and AML development. Notably, the incidence of AML ranges from 18% to 36% over 20–30 years. Patients progressing to AML are usually older. The survival of patients with SDS who develop MDS or AML is poor [60, 96]. Alter et al. reported an O/E ratio of 8.5 for developing any malignancy in non-transplanted SDS patients. Solid tumor cumulative incidence was almost 40% by age 45 [26].

20.5.1.3 Diamond-Blackfan anemia (DBA)

DBA is the most common cause of inherited isolated red blood cell production failure. The hallmark of classic DBA is considered a selective decrease in erythroid precursors and normochromic macrocytic anemia associated with various extra hematopoietic manifestations (i.e., craniofacial, thumb, cardiac, and urogenital malformations) [61, 97]. Most patients are diagnosed with transfusion-dependent anemia in the first year of life. Congenital anomalies including dysmorphic facial features, short stature, eye, kidney, and hand abnormalities can be seen in almost half of the patients [92].

It is estimated that spontaneous hematologic remission may occur in almost 25% of DBA patients [98].

Although most cases are sporadic, DBA is considered a genetic disease including autosomal dominant, autosomal recessive, and possibly X-linked type of inheritance. Genes that code for parts of the short 40S or big 60S ribosomal subunits are the main contributors to DBA. RPS19 gene mutations are the most frequent known genetic cause, accounting for about 25% of DBA cases [97, 99].

TL is shorter in Diamond-Blackfan anemia (DBA) when compared to normal controls but not as short as in patients with DC [60, 91].

Few patients with DBA have been reported to have MDS or AML, which suggests a possibility of a higher propensity for malignancy. Some cases have evolved into aplastic anemia [61].

Moreover, DBA patients have an approximately 5-fold higher risk of developing cancer. The relative risks for individual cancers were 45 for colon cancer, 42 for osteogenic sarcoma, and 29 for AML [44, 100]. Alter et al. observed an O/E ratio of 2.5 for developing any malignancy in non-transplanted DBA patients, whereas following transplant an increased O/E ratio of 983 for developing non-Hodgin Lymphoma (NHL). The most frequent cancers in DBA were lung, colon, and cervix [26].

20.5.2 Aplastic Anemia (AA)

Aplastic anemia is a rare hematologic disorder characterized by a marked reduction in the quantity and quality of hematopoietic progenitor and stem cells and an injured, markedly hypocellular, ineffective bone marrow [101, 102]. It usually manifests in the first three decades of life with a median age of 20 years, although a second peak is observed at the age of 60 years [103]. It is estimated that almost 15% of patients with acquired AA undergo the evolution of their disease to myelodysplasia or acute myeloid leukemia (AML) [104].

An immune-mediated pathophysiologic mechanism seems to be implicated in the vast majority of sporadic cases [101]. It has been hypothesized that AA is the outcome of uniform T-cell-mediated autoimmunity and marrow destruction resulting in defective and nearly absent hematopoiesis [102]. This concept is strongly supported by the fact that T-cell immunosuppressive therapy (IST) induces a response in 60–80% of patients with severe aplastic anemia [105, 106].

TL in aplastic anemia (AA) patients is significantly shorter versus age-matched normal controls [88, 107–110]. Initially, the observed short telomeres in aplastic anemia were presumed to be secondary to hematopoietic stress [111]. Currently, the decreased TL is considered a result of increased mitotic demand on a limited pool of stem cells [102, 112].

Loss-of-function mutations in genes of the telomerase complex (TERC and TERT) established a genetic etiology for telomere shortening in marrow failure, although it was later shown that these mutations are not only found in DC patients. Telomerase mutations may also be found in a few patients with acquired aplastic anemia [113].

Calado et al. reported that those patients with severe AA and shorter telomeres have a three-fold higher probability of progressing to myelodysplasia and/or leukemia [113]. The difference was more evident in patients with significant abnormal karyotypes, namely monosomy-7 or complex karyotypes [104]. Specifically, patients with telomeres located in the lower quartile were found to harbor a significant increase in the risk of clonal evolution (24.5%) compared to patients in the other three quartiles. Notably, the proportion of monosomy-7 cells in the bone marrow at diagnosis of AA was inversely correlated with telomere length, years before the emergence of an autonomous and clinically detectable abnormal clone [104].

Since the early 2000s, it has been shown that patients with AA and no response to IST had significantly shorter telomeres compared to normal controls [107–109]. Nevertheless, the NIH group reported that the TL of peripheral blood leukocytes was not related to hematologic response to IST but was associated with an increased risk of hematologic relapse, clonal evolution to myelodysplastic syndrome, and poor overall survival [113].

Children with AA have also significantly shorter telomeres versus healthy-adjusted for age-subjects. Shorter TL appeared to be a significant predictive variable for poor response to T-cell immunosuppressive therapy (IST) in two distinct multivariate analyses [114, 115].

20.5.3 Myelodysplastic Syndromes (MDS)

Myelodysplastic syndromes are clonal hematopoietic disorders characterized by peripheral cytopenia, inefficient hematopoiesis, and an increased risk of progression to AML [116]. They are rare in children accounting for less than 5% of pediatric hematological malignancies and have an annual incidence of 1–4 cases per million [117].

MDS in children is frequently associated with inherited bone marrow failure syndromes (IBMFs) or hereditary predisposition syndromes (Table 20.8) [116]. They have distinct features from

Table 20.8 Classification of syndromes and conditions that predispose children to MDS development [116]

IBMFSs
-Fanconi Anemia
-Diamond-Blackfan anemia
-Schwachman-Diamond syndrome
-Telomere biology disorders
-Congenital amegakaryocytic thrombocytopenia
-Severe congenital neutropenia
Germline predisposition and preexisting platelet disorders
-Myeloid neoplasms with germline RUNX1 mutation
-Myeloid neoplasms with germline ANKRD26 mutation
-Myeloid neoplasms with germline ETV6 mutation
Myeloid neoplasms with germline predisposition and other organ dysfunctions
-Myeloid neoplasms with GATA2 mutation
-MDS with germline SMD9/SAMD9L mutation

adults with different genomic alterations although they have not yet been in-depth studied.

The most frequent pediatric MDS variant is refractory cytopenia of childhood (RCC) with a median age at diagnosis of 7–8 years. Frequently, children may additionally have thrombocytopenia and/or neutropenia, whereas adults usually present with isolated anemia.

Generally, TL shows heterogeneity in MDS [118]. It has mainly been studied in MDS of adulthood showing a progression in telomere shortening. Approximately 50% of MDS patients show a reduction in telomere length (TL) [118–120]. Shorter telomeres in MDS have been correlated with leukemic transformation [118, 119], the presence of complex karyotypic abnormalities [118, 121], and worse overall survival (OS) [121, 122].

In a recent large study of 1514 MDS patients by Myllymäki et al., it was shown that short TL was significantly associated with older age, male sex, somatic mutations that impair DNA damage response, and more severe cytopenia before transplant. Additionally, it was shown that MDS patients with shorter telomeres had inferior survival due to a high risk of non-relapse mortality after transplantation [123].

Based on these results and the same study group, Reilly et al. reported that TERT rare variants without a clinical diagnosis of TBD who underwent allogeneic transplantation accounted for 2.7% of the cases. Notably, those patients with TERT rare variants had significantly shorter TL and younger age at diagnosis. Multivariate analysis further showed that patients with TERT variants showed inferior overall survival due to increased incidence of non-relapse mortality more frequently non-infectious pulmonary cause. These results demonstrate that routine screening for rare TERT variants in MDS patients can identify clinically non-obvious TBDs, regardless of age or clinical suspicion [124].

Data on TL and clinical implications in pediatric MDS patients are scarce. Lately, a study on MDS patients showed shorter TL in pediatric than adult MDS patients, with the shortest TL in patients having childhood BMFs. Furthermore, shorter TL was correlated with a worse prognosis and shorter mean survival time when compared to pediatric MDS with longer telomeres [125].

20.5.4 Leukemias

Several studies mainly in adults have demonstrated that progressive telomere shortening is associated with hematological malignancies. Possible pathophysiologic mechanisms of telomere shortening are considered rapid clonal expansion with different degrees of the contribution of oxidative stress or telomerase dysregulation at least in the early stages of some leukemias [126–128].

20.5.4.1 Acute lymphoblastic leukemia (ALL)

Acute lymphoblastic leukemia is the most common childhood cancer, constituting almost 25% of pediatric cancer diagnoses [129]. Genomic studies promoted the subclassification of pediatric and adult acute lymphoblastic leukemia and outlined the differences among age groups.

Capraro et al. demonstrated that TL is shorter in general in leukemias compared to normal controls. Specifically, TL is significantly shorter in B-cell ALL (B-ALL) vs. T-cell ALL (T-ALL) vs. acute myeloid leukemia (AML), and in patients with abnormal karyotype vs. without cytogenetic abnormality [130].

In addition, the average TL of the blast cell population from both bone marrow and peripheral blood specimens is significantly shorter in childhood acute lymphoblastic leukemia at diagnosis compared to the remission phase [29, 69, 130–132]. It is worth mentioning that in a recent study by Karow et al., TL was suggested as a marker reflecting clonal expansion that could help in the identification of patients with high-risk pediatric ALL [132, 133]. Furthermore, in a study of 38 ALL patients, Vakonaki et al. reported an increase of TL in the remission phase, although there were patients in whom TL remained stable and were the only ones with disease relapse. These findings need further study in larger ALL cohorts, since they may imply that TL could serve as a useful biomarker [134].

In a study of 169 childhood patients, hTERT methylation[p] [135, 136] was more prevalent in T-ALL cases as compared to B-cell precursor[q] (BCP)-ALL (72% vs. 18%). Interestingly, the *t*(12; 21) cases in the BCP group had a much higher methylation rate (63%) than the high hyperdiploid cases (7%). These results strongly indicate that the hTERT promoter methylation status defines specific ALL subgroups and may have a functional relevance [131].

Only recently, the assessment of TL of bone marrow cells from newly diagnosed children with ALL has been proposed as a potential prognostic factor [137].

---

[p]**hTERT methylation:** Human telomerase reverse transcriptase (hTERT) is a functional catalytic protein subunit that together with an RNA component named human telomerase RNA component (hTERC) forms telomerase. Limitless self-renewal is considered one of the hallmarks of cancer and is attained by telomere maintenance through the activation of telomerase. hTERT is required for telomerase activity. It should be underlined that telomerase is activated in germline, hematopoietic, stem, and rapidly renewing cells whereas telomerase activity is very low or absent in somatic cells. hTERT expression is upregulated in tumors via multiple genetic (hTERT promoter mutations) and epigenetic mechanisms (hTERT promoter methylation and miRNAs).

[q]**B-cell precursor acute lymphoblastic leukemia (ALL):** It is a hematologic malignancy characterized by clonal proliferation of abnormal B-cell precursors in the bone marrow. Based on the type of lymphocyte affected as well as other factors ALL is mainly classified as B or T cell ALL.

Regarding TA, it was five times higher in B-ALL than in T-ALL pediatric patients ($p = 0.0057$) and there was a significant positive correlation with hTERT expression [130]. High TA has been reported in leukemia patients and seems to decrease with the attainment of response [133]. Furthermore, high TA was found in patients with elevated WBC, chromosomal abnormalities, and high-risk ALL patients [133]. Apart from short telomeres, in a study by Borssen, it was reported that longer telomeres in low-risk BCP-ALL patients have been also associated with a worse prognosis, although sufficient data to support this observation and explain the underlying pathophysiologic mechanism responsible were not provided [131].

20.5.4.2 Acute myeloid leukemia (AML)

Pediatric acute myeloid leukemia is a heterogeneous malignant disease characterized by abnormal proliferation and impaired differentiation of myeloid cells. It is relatively rare in children and accounts for approximately 20% of childhood leukemias, and despite advances in cytogenetics and molecular profiling, overall survival remains near 70% [138].

TL is shorter in pediatric AML vs. healthy subjects, although longer than in pediatric ALL patients [130, 139]. It has been reported that cells carrying the high-risk molecular aberrations FLT3/ITD or a WT1 mutation and FLT3/ITD had shorter telomeres than did CEBPA-double mutants ($p = 0.0064$ and 0.051, respectively) and NPM1 mutants [139].

Constitutional TERT mutations do not seem to be a risk factor in pediatric AML patients, in contrast to adult AML patients [62, 139, 140]. Moreover, TL was not associated with the number of cytogenetic abnormalities or complex karyotypes. TL does not significantly influence the outcome in terms of five-year overall survival, event-free survival as well as the cumulative incidence of relapse and non-response [139].

It should be noted that patients with acute promyelocytic leukemia (APL) present a significant reduction in TL and a significant positive correlation between short TL and promyelocytic leukemia-retinoic acid receptor-a (PML-RARa)[r] expression [141]. Shortened TL and elevated TA might be indicative of extensive proliferative activity and associated with a higher risk for disease progression and relapse [142].

A large study from the database of the German Study Alliance Leukemia Registry, including 5207 AML patients, supported the need to develop specific screening as well as AML treatment protocols for patients with underlying myeloid neoplasms with germ-line predisposition (MNGLP) and especially the younger <40 years of age, to both reduce toxicity and improve response to therapy [143].

In conclusion, apart from the actual recommendations based solely on family history and clinical findings, age, and aberrant karyotype (perhaps complemented by TL screening for TBD) may provide factors to initiate genetic screening for hereditary neoplasms with germ-line predisposition (MNGLP) [143].

20.5.5 Lymphomas

Hodgkin's lymphoma (HL) is a B-cell malignancy characterized by the presence of Hodgkin and multinucleated Reed-Sternberg cells that affect all age groups.

Studies have shown that HL exhibits telomere dysfunction, telomerase activation, and ALT activation [144, 145]. Newly diagnosed patients with HL show shorter telomeres, although TL was not associated with histologic type, disease stage, and gender [145]. The Hodgkin cells from patients with refractory/relapsing disease contained a significantly higher percentage of very small telomeres ($p = 0.027$) and telomere aggregates ($p = 0.032$) compared with Hodgkin cells of patients entering rapid remission [146].

---

[r] **Promyelocytioc leukemia-retinoic acid receptor-a (PML-RARa):** It is considered the hallmark of acute promyelocytic leukemia. APL is characterized by a reciprocal and balanced translocation involving the retinoic acid receptor α (RARa) on chromosome 17 and the promyelocytic leukemia (PML) gene on chromosome 15 and generates the oncogenic PML-RARα fusion protein. The PML protein plays a role in a number of cellular processes involving homeostasis and tumor suppression mechanisms, including the response to viral infections and stress, senescence, angiogenesis, differentiation, and maintenance of genome stability.

20.6 Solid Tumors

20.6.1 Brain Tumors

Brain tumors exhibit age-based differences in incidence, location, histology, molecular pathology, and outcome [147]. Pediatric brain tumors are the most frequent solid cancers observed. The reported incidence is 5.7 per 100,000 children compared with 29.9 per 100,000 in adult individuals [147]. There is limited data on TL prevalence in pediatric brain tumors.

20.6.1.1 Gliomas

Gliomas, the most frequent brain tumors in childhood, differentiate into low and high grades based on clinical, radiological, histopathological, biological, and molecular aspects.

In pediatric low-grade gliomas, Tabori et al. observed that younger children with more aggressive and frequently recurring tumors had significantly longer telomeres than older ones ($p = 0.00014$). Furthermore, they showed that tumors with a terminal restriction fragment length of < 7.5 did not recur, whereas those with longer telomeres (>8.0) had a high likelihood of late recurrences [148, 149]. Pilocytic astrocytomas[S] have been reported as negative for ALT [148, 150].

Pediatric high-grade gliomas (pHGG) account for almost 11% of central nervous system tumors in subjects less than 14 years and $>$ 50% of cases occur in midline locations. They differ in frequency of isocitrate dehydrogenase (IDH1/2) mutations ($<$ 6%, mostly in adolescents) as well as telomerase reverse transcriptase promoter (TERTp) mutations (5–11% vs. 30–50% in adults) [28, 151]. pHGG usually harbors hotspot mutations in histone H3.3 encoding gene (H3F3A), which are rare in adult gliomas [148].

Abedalthagafi et al. reported that 29.6% of pHGG were positive for ALT and 24.5% immunonegative for ATRX protein, with these two alterations being highly associated with one another

[S] **Pilocytic astrocytoma:** It is the most common childhood brain tumor. The tumor is usually located in the posterior fossa and complete resection if feasible is considered of utmost importance as no other treatment type is needed.

($p < 0.0001$). Moreover, ALT-positive HGG showed more frequent amplification of the platelet-derived growth factor receptor alpha gene (PDGFRA) [150]. Recently, in a study of 579 pediatric brain tumors, it was also shown that ALT is common in pHGG 38.1% vs. < 3% in other pediatric brain tumors and especially in older ages (11.06 vs. 7.9 years, $p = 0.007$) [152]. In addition, all patients with diffuse hemispheric H3G34-mutant pHGG were ALT+ and were usually adolescents or young adults [148, 152]. The G34R-mutant subgroup always used ALT to maintain TL, with either a simultaneous ATRX nuclear loss (63.6%) or a retained ATRX (36.4%). Notably, only 40% of K27M mutant pHGG had elongated telomeres, all of whom retained ATRX expression, whereas the majority of the cases showed telomere shortening [148].

20.6.1.2 Medulloblastoma

It is the most common malignant brain tumor of childhood located in the posterior fossa. Advances in molecular profiling have unraveled a significant heterogeneity among distinct subgroups with differences in both clinical characteristics as well as underlying pathology [153].

Generally, group 3 tumors are usually confined to non-adults, Sonic Hedgehog (SHH[t]) tumors are most frequent in infants and adults, whereas wingless (WNT)[u] and Group 4 are usually diagnosed in children. In a study of 466 medulloblastomas, it was shown that TERT mutations were significantly enriched in SHH tumors compared to the other 3 subgroups ($p < 0.0001$). Furthermore, the 5-year overall survival of SHH tumors with and without TERT mutations was 77.6 ± 7% and 64.1 ± 5.1%, respectively ($p = 0.04$). In addition, TERT mutations defined distinct prognostic factors

[t]**Sonic-Hedgehog medulloblastoma:** It is a medulloblastoma type driven by a pathogenic mutation of SHH signaling. SHH signaling pathway is one of the major trafficking networks that regulate the key events during developmental processes, i.e., growth and patterning of multicellular embryos. Abnormalities in the regulation and transduction of the SHH pathway have been implicated in birth defects, tissue degeneration, stem cell renewal, and cancer growth.

[u]**Wingless medulloblastoma (WNT):** It accounts for 10% of medulloblastoma cases, with the majority of cases harboring CTNNB1 mutations and chromosomal alterations for monosomy-6. Clinically, WNT MBs have the most favorable prognosis with a >95% 5-year survivorship.

conferring good prognosis in SHH and poor prognosis in Group 4 medulloblastoma patients [154].

Hotspot-activating mutations of the hTERT promoter region have been reported in approximately 1/3 of medulloblastoma cases, and are associated with older patients and recurrent tumors [155].

Metastatic MBs activate the ALT pathway with higher incidence compared to non-metastatic cases and those cases with activation of ALT show a worse OS, although the difference was not statistically significant [156].

Finally, activation of ALT was found in 10% of infant MB with high telomere length mainly found in infant SHH-group medulloblastoma [157].

20.6.1.3 Ependymoma

The third most common brain tumor in children ependymoma accounts for up to 10% of childhood CNS tumors and has a high rate of recurrence despite gross total resection [158]. Recently, it has been molecularly characterized, although underlying germline risk factors have not yet been understood. Posterior fossa ependymomas (EPN-PF) are divided into group A (EPN-PF-A), which occurs mainly in young children and has aggressive behavior, and group B (EPN-PF-B), which is more frequent in older children and adults and has a better prognosis [158].

Zhang et al. recently reported that a genetic predisposition to longer telomere length increases the risk of developing ependymoma in adolescents and adults, but not in children younger than 12 years or very young children with EPN-PF-A molecular subtype[v] [159]. It has been proposed that longer telomere length increases cancer risk by augmenting the capacity for sustained cellular replication, allowing pre-malignant cells to accumulate the mutations such as hypermethylation of the TERT promoter

---

[v]**EPN-PF-A molecular subtype:** The term refers to ependymoma occurring in the posterior fossa and molecularly characterized by global reduction of K27me3 in tumor cell nuclei. PF-A typically occurs in young children with a median age of 3 years and has a dismal prognosis with a 10-year overall survival of 56%, and progression-free survival of 24%.

necessary to resist apoptosis and enable replicative immortality [160].

20.6.2 Extracranial Solid Tumors

20.6.2.1 Neuroblastoma

Neuroblastoma (NB) is the most common extracranial solid tumor. Early age of onset, presence of metastatic disease upon diagnosis as well as spontaneous regression of infantile tumors are key features of NB [161]. It is a neural crest-derived malignancy with wide clinical heterogeneity that varies from regression with no need for medical interventions to treatment-resistant tumors with metastatic spread and dismal prognosis [161, 162].

Age at diagnosis inversely correlates with outcome. Infants less than 18 months may present with spontaneously regressing tumors and have an overall survival of 88% [163]. On the contrary, children older than 18 months and younger than 12 years have a 49% overall survival which drops below 10% for adolescents and young adults [161, 164].

Primary tumors can be found anywhere in the sympathetic nervous system, with $>$ 50% occurring in the medulla of the adrenal glands [161]. NB subjects with metastatic disease or older than 18 months or with tumors harboring MYCN amplification are considered as high risk.

NB is one of the most extensively studied pediatric tumors regarding telomere biology. Several reports have reported that TL is highly correlated with prognosis in patients with neuroblastoma. Since 2006, Ohali et al. observed that short telomeres were predictive of a favorable prognosis, whereas long or unchanged telomeres were predictive of a poor outcome in NB patients ($p =$ 0.007). Moreover, in the same study, it was shown that combining TL and TA defined 4 prognostic groups. The one with low TA and short TL had a 100% PFS, whereas the group with high TA and long TL had the worst progression-free survival (PFS) rate (46%). The two intermediate groups had either high TA and short telomeres or low TA and long telomeres and showed a PFS rate of 78 and 67%, respectively [165].

Furthermore, intratumoral diversity of TL in NB patients has been strongly associated with disease progression and death [166].

Based on MYCN gene amplification, TERT gene rearrangements, or ALT, aggressive NB was proposed to be separated into three almost exclusive subgroups [167]. All subgroups are characterized by the activation of a telomere maintenance mechanism (TMM) and correlate with poor outcomes in neuroblastoma [167, 168]. The first two subgroups show high levels of telomere expression. Amplification of MYCN is an established prognostic marker with a known poor prognosis and is observed in almost 20% of the tumors and almost 40% of clinical high-risk NB [167, 169]. A second mechanism of TA in high-risk neuroblastoma is TERT rearrangements that are found in 10–15% of NBs and in almost 23–31% of high-risk NBs [170, 171]. The third mechanism-ALT is a telomerase-independent TMM. This mechanism is present in almost 10–15% and 24% of total and high-risk cases accordingly [167, 172]. ALT positive neuroblastomas show characteristic features. Importantly 55–60% of the ALT-positive neuroblastoma tumors are ATRX mutated [170].

In 2018, Ackermann and colleagues showed that an active TMM (amplified MYCN, TERT rearrangement, TERT outlier expression, or ALT) is a predictor of poor patient prognosis independent of the classical risk stratification system. In the same study, it was also shown that using the current risk stratification, 15.5% of the tumors harboring an active TMM were not classified as high risk, although they had an almost similar poor prognosis with high-risk tumors [168]. Researchers have also shown that 10.9% of the TERT rearranged, as well as $> 30\%$ of ALT-positive NBs were not classified as high-risk, despite their poor prognosis comparable to high-risk tumors [173, 174].

Lastly, Koneru et al. proposed that high-risk neuroblastoma patients can be further classified into three subgroups such as TERT high, ALT^+, and TERT-low/non-ALT. Overall survival was significantly higher in TERT-low/non-ALT patients compared to the other two subgroups [175].

Based on these findings, a revised molecular risk stratification of NB patients has already been proposed, which as a first step will evaluate the presence or not of a TMM and subsequently will include additional prognostic markers like the presence of RAS[W] (Fig. 20.7a) or TP53[X] (Fig. 20.7b) [176] pathway mutation [170]. A stepwise diagnostic workflow for TMM assessment in NB tumor samples that could ultimately guide pediatric oncologists in accurate risk assessment has recently been proposed [177].

20.6.2.2 Sarcomas

Most pediatric sarcomas lack telomerase expression and telomere maintenance is accomplished through ALT activation. It should be noted that sarcomas associated with chromosomal translocation and otherwise stable karyotypes, such as Ewing sarcoma, lack evidence of an ALT mechanism, whereas those with irregular karyotypes like osteosarcoma, use ALT [178].

The most frequent primary bone tumor in children is osteosarcoma [179]. Several studies in osteosarcomas found detectable levels of telomerase in almost 50% of the cases. In the OS series, the predominant TMM is ALT [180, 181]. Ulaner et al. observed both ALT and TA in the same tumors, which is uncommon in other neoplasms. Notably, OS cases with the absence of both TA and ALT were found to strongly correlate with improved survival and accounted for 18% [180, 182]. In addition, it was shown that ATRX mutation[c] and loss of expression were observed in 30% of osteosarcomas [183]. A subsequent study demonstrated that the prevalence of telomerase expression was associated with worse event-free and overall survival [181]. Lately, de Nonnevilee et al. demonstrated TOP3A amplification as the major genomic feature of ALT tumors expressing WT-ATRX [184].

[W]**RAS signaling pathway:** The renin-angiotensin system (RAS) has an essential role in driving normal physiological cellular proliferation, and dysregulation of the pathway commonly occurs during tumorigenesis. P53 pathway function gives cancer cells a survival advantage to bypass the resolution of oncogenic signals and DNA damage to continue abnormal proliferation.

[X]**TP53 pathway:** TP53 is a gene that encodes the p53 tumor suppressor protein commonly referred to as the "Guardian of the Genome". Its main biological function appears to involve the protection of the DNA integrity of the cell. p53 pathway is a complex cellular stress response network with multiple diverse inputs and downstream outputs relevant to its role as a tumor suppressor pathway. Loss of p53 pathway function gives cancer cells a survival advantage to bypass the resolution of oncogenic signals and DNA damage to continue abnormal proliferation.

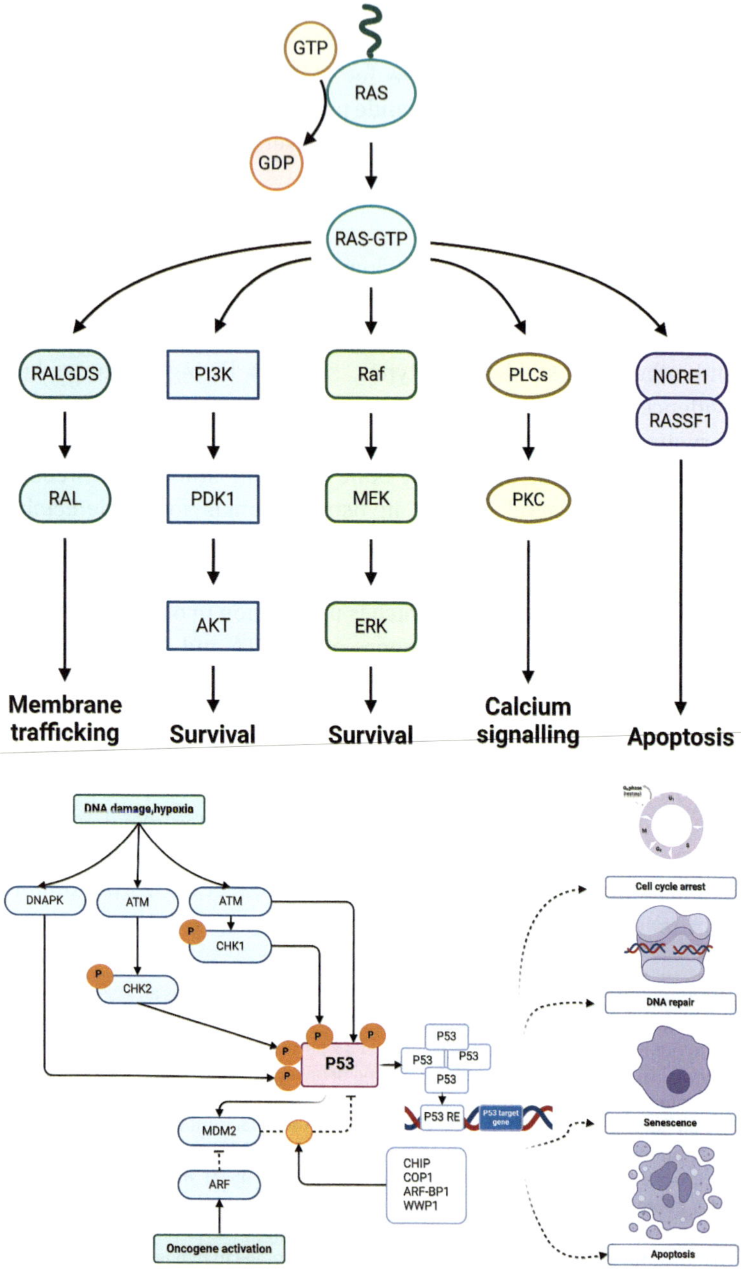

Figure 20.7 (a) The RAS pathway and (b) the p53 pathway (Created with Biorender.com).

Ewing sarcoma (ES) is a primitive bone and soft tissue tumor of children or adolescents composed of small, round cells showing limited neuroectodermal differentiation. In contrast to osteosarcoma, Ewing sarcoma patients do not use the ALT mechanism and are telomerase-positive [182, 185]. ES patients with shorter telomeres [186] or high TA have shown a worse prognosis [185].

The most frequent soft tissue sarcoma in children is rhabdomyosarcoma. It consists of two major histological subtypes:

- Alveolar type that harbors a translocation between FOXO1A gene at 13q and PAX3 at 1p36.
- Embryonal type that harbors no translocation but exhibits loss of heterozygosity (LOH) at 11p15 [187].

Rhabdomyosarcomas seem to have distinct TMM according to histological type. Alveolar RMS exhibits no ALT phenotype and the majority presented TA, whereas in embryonal RMS, both telomerase and ALT may play a role. Of notice 7/31 tumors presented no evidence of TMM. Finally, Ohali et al. found significantly longer telomeres in embryonal RMS vs. alveolar. Furthermore, TL shorter than 7.1 kb in alveolar RMS had a significantly better outcome than TL > 7.1 kb (69% vs. 25%, respectively) [188].

20.6.2.3 Wilms tumor (WT)

It is the most common renal tumor in infants and young children. Telomerase expression has been investigated in different studies, and high expression levels of the TERT[y] [189] or TERC were proposed as adverse prognostic factors [178]. WT were found mostly TA-positive [190]. Venturini et al. observed the presence of at least one TTM in 82% of WTs. Of them, activation of ALT was found in 32% of the cases, and in approximately 15% of cases, ALT was the

---

[y]**Telomerase activity:** It is upregulated in <70% of human cancers by TERT point mutations, rearrangements, DNA amplifications, and transcript fusions. Mutations in the promotor of TERT are one of the most frequent noncoding mutations in cancer, that increase TERT expression and replicative potential of cells. Limits to cell proliferation imposed by progressive telomere erosion are avoided in cells with corrupted DNA damage responses such as p53. Once p53 is lost, tumor progression accelerates the s chromosome without telomeres showing instability and propensity to genetic rearrangements.

sole TMM mechanism [191]. Notably, 18% of the WT cases seemed to possess no known TMM.

In a study of 244 WTs, cases with high levels of TER expression had twice the risk of recurrence compared to tumors with low levels. The prognostic significance of TER expression persisted in a multivariate analysis including tumor stage and patient age [192].

20.6.2.4 Hepatoblastoma (HBL)

Hepatoblastoma is the most common liver tumor in children, usually presenting before the first three years of age. Most HBLs are usually sporadic, although there is an association with constitutional genetic abnormalities, such as Beckwith-Wiedemann syndrome and familial adenomatous polyposis [193]. Over 90% of primary HBLs have detectable TERT mRNA expression. High TERT mRNA expression or telomerase activity was associated with a 10-year event-free survival estimate (EFS) of approximately 40%, whereas low or absent expression was associated with a 10-year EFS of about 90%. TERT mRNA level was an independent prognostic factor in a multivariate model including histology, stage, gender, age, and completeness of resection [178, 194].

20.6.2.5 Retinoblastoma (RB)

Studies on telomere biology in retinoblastoma are rare. Gupta et al. reported telomerase activity is observed in 50% of RBs and the presence of significantly longer telomeres in patients with telomerase-positive tumors [195].

20.7 Telomere Length Biology and Future Challenges

It is evident that our current knowledge of telomere length biology and maintenance mechanisms in pediatric oncology is still limited. An in-depth study of pediatric cancers that show so many differences compared to adults is essential in understanding the biological behavior of cancer types, risk estimation, and group stratification in the future. In addition, understanding the implicating mechanisms within each cancer type and subtype may allow the implementation of appropriate therapeutic strategies targeting telomere maintenance mechanisms.

References

1. Gorenjak, V., *et al.* (2020) Telomere length determinants in childhood, *Clin Chem Lab Med*, **58,** pp. 162–177.
2. Armanios, M. (2022). The role of telomeres in human disease. *Annu Rev Genomics Hum Genet*, **23**, pp. 363–381.
3. Kam, M.L.W., T.T.T. Nguyen, and Ngeow, J.Y.Y. (2021). Telomere biology disorders. *NPJ Genom Med*, **6**, pp. 36.
4. Schratz, K.E. (2020). Extrahematopoietic manifestations of the short telomere syndromes, *Hematology Am Soc Hematol Educ Program*, **2020**, pp. 115–122.
5. Ackermann, S. and Fischer, M. (2019). Telomere maintenance in pediatric cancer, *Int J Mol Sci*, **20**(23), pp. 5836.
6. Kim, N.W., *et al.* (1994). Specific association of human telomerase activity with immortal cells and cancer, *Science*, **266,** pp. 2011–5.
7. Claude, E. and Decottignies, A. (2020). Telomere maintenance mechanisms in cancer: telomerase, ALT or lack thereof, *Curr Opin Genet Dev*, **60**, pp. 1–8.
8. Dratwa, M., *et al.* (2020). TERT-regulation and roles in cancer formation, *Front Immunol*, **11,** pp. 589929.
9. Barthel, F.P., *et al.* (2017). Systematic analysis of telomere length and somatic alterations in 31 cancer types. *Nat Genet*, **49**, pp. 349–357.
10. Colebatch, A.J., A. Dobrovic, and Cooper, W.A. (2019). TERT gene: its function and dysregulation in cancer, *J Clin Pathol*, **72,** pp. 281–284.
11. Clatterbuck Soper, S.F. and Meltzer, P.S. (2023). ATRX/DAXX: guarding the genome against the hazards of ALT, *Genes*, **14**, pp. 790.
12. Dyer, M.A., *et al.* (2017). ATRX and DAXX: mechanisms and mutations, *Cold Spring Harb Perspect Med*, **7**, pp. a026567.
13. Heaphy, C.M., *et al.* (2011). Prevalence of the alternative lengthening of telomeres telomere maintenance mechanism in human cancer subtypes, *The American Journal of Pathology*, **179**, pp. 1608–1615.

14. Adam, R., *et al.* (2017). Prognostic role of telomere length in malignancies: a meta-analysis and meta-regression, *Exp Mol Pathol,* **102**, pp. 455–474.
15. Frenck, R.W., Jr., E.H. Blackburn, and Shannon, K.M. (1998). The rate of telomere sequence loss in human leukocytes varies with age, *Proc Natl Acad Sci U S A,* **95**, pp. 5607–10.
16. Okuda, K., *et al.* (2002). Telomere length in the newborn, *Pediatr Res,* **52**, pp. 377–81.
17. Ly, K., *et al.* (2019). Telomere length in early childhood is associated with sex and ethnicity. *Scientific Reports,* **9**, pp. 10359.
18. Zeiger, A.M., *et al.* (2018). Genetic determinants of telomere length in African American youth, *Scientific Reports,* **8**, pp. 13265.
19. Stathopoulou, M.G., *et al.* (2015). Genetic determinants of leucocyte telomere length in children: a neglected and challenging field, *Paediatr Perinat Epidemiol,* **29**, pp. 146–50.
20. Chen, L., *et al.* (2022). Variability in newborn telomere length is explained by inheritance and intrauterine environment, *BMC Med,* **20**, pp. 20.
21. Andreu-Sánchez, S., *et al.* (2022). Genetic, parental and lifestyle factors influence telomere length, *Commun Biol,* **5**, pp. 565.
22. Coimbra, B.M., *et al.* (2017). Stress-related telomere length in children: a systematic review, *J Psychiatr Res,* **92**, pp. 47–54.
23. Chen, X.Y., *et al.* (2022). Association between childhood exposure to family violence and telomere length: a meta-analysis, *Int J Environ Res Public Health,* **19,** pp. 12151.
24. Drury, S.S., *et al.*. (2014). The association of telomere length with family violence and disruption, *Pediatrics,* **134**, pp. e128–37.
25. Schratz, K.E., *et al.* (2020). Cancer spectrum and outcomes in the Mendelian short telomere syndromes, *Blood,* **135**, pp. 1946–1956.
26. Alter, B.P., *et al.* (2018). Cancer in the National Cancer Institute inherited bone marrow failure syndrome cohort after fifteen years of follow-up, *Haematologica,* **103**, pp. 30–39.
27. Koelsche, C., *et al.* (2013). Distribution of TERT promoter mutations in pediatric and adult tumors of the nervous system, *Acta Neuropathol,* **126**, pp. 907–15.
28. Gielen, G.H., *et al.* (2015). Genetic analysis of diffuse high-grade astrocytomas in infancy defines a novel molecular entity, *Brain Pathol,* **25**, pp. 409–17.

29. Parker, M., *et al.* (2012). Assessing telomeric DNA content in pediatric cancers using whole-genome sequencing data, *Genome Biol*, **13**, pp. R113.
30. Wang, Z., *et al.* (2020). Molecular mechanism of telomere length dynamics and its prognostic value in pediatric cancers, *J Natl Cancer Inst*, **112**, pp. 756–764.
31. Walsh, K.M. (2020). Telomere attrition in childhood cancer survivors, *Clinical Cancer Research*, **26**, pp. 2281–2283.
32. Song, N., *et al.* (2020). Shortened leukocyte telomere length associates with an increased prevalence of chronic health conditions among survivors of childhood cancer: a report from the St. Jude Lifetime Cohort, *Clin Cancer Res*, **26**, pp. 2362–2371.
33. Siegel, R.L., *et al.* (2021). Cancer statistics, *CA Cancer J Clin*, **71**, pp. 7–33.
34. Braun, B.S. and Lessnick, S.L. (2009). Pediatric malignancies: update on sarcomas and leukemia development in children, *Current Opinion in Genetics & Development*, **19**, pp. 92–96.
35. Savage, S.A. (2022). Dyskeratosis congenita and telomere biology disorders, *Hematology Am Soc Hematol Educ Program*, **2022**, pp. 637–648.
36. Zinsser, F. (1906). Atrophia cutis reticularis cum pigmentatione dystrophia unguium et leukoplakia oris, *Ikongr Dermatol*, **5**, pp. 219–223.
37. Niewisch, M.R. and Savage, S.A. (2019). An update on the biology and management of dyskeratosis congenita and related telomere biology disorders, *Expert Rev Hematol*, **12**, pp. 1037–1052.
38. Stanley, S.E. and Armanios, M. (2015). The short and long telomere syndromes: paired paradigms for molecular medicine, *Curr Opin Genet Dev*, **33**, pp. 1–9.
39. Armanios, M. and Blackburn, E.H. (2012). The telomere syndromes, *Nat Rev Genet*, **13**, pp. 693–704.
40. Schneider, C.V., *et al.* (2022). Association of telomere length with risk of disease and mortality, *JAMA Intern Med*, **182**, pp. 291–300.
41. Armanios, M. (2013). Telomeres and age-related disease: how telomere biology informs clinical paradigms, *J Clin Invest*, **123**, pp. 996–1002.
42. Vieri, M., T.H. Brümmendorf, and Beier, F. (2021). Treatment of telomeropathies, *Best Pract Res Clin Haematol*, **34**, pp. 101282.

43. Dokal, I. (2011). Dyskeratosis congenita, *Hematology Am Soc Hematol Educ Program*, **2011**, pp. 480–6.
44. Alter, B.P. (2017). Inherited bone marrow failure syndromes: considerations pre- and posttransplant, *Blood,* **130**, pp. 2257–2264.
45. Tummala, H., A. Walne, and Dokal, I. (2022). The biology and management of dyskeratosis congenita and related disorders of telomeres, *Expert Rev Hematol*, **15**, pp. 685–696.
46. Dokal, I., *et al.* (2015). Clinical utility gene card for: dyskeratosis congenita - update 2015, *Eur J Hum Genet*, **23**(4), pp. e1–e4.
47. Armando, R.G., *et al.* (2019). Telomeropathies: etiology, diagnosis, treatment and follow-up, ethical and legal considerations, *Clin Genet,* **96**, pp. 3–16.
48. Bertuch, A.A. (2016). The molecular genetics of the telomere biology disorders, *RNA Biol*, **13**, pp. 696–706.
49. Dorgaleleh, S., *et al.* (2022). Molecular insight of dyskeratosis congenita: defects in telomere length homeostasis, *J Clin Transl Res,* **8**, pp. 20–30.
50. Callea, M., *et al.* (2022). Multisystemic manifestations in rare diseases: the experience of dyskeratosis congenita, *Genes (Basel)*, **13**, pp. 496.
51. Wagner, C.L., *et al.* (2018). Short telomere syndromes cause a primary T cell immunodeficiency, *J Clin Invest*, **128**, pp. 5222–5234.
52. Niknafs, A.M., *et al.* (2022). Avascular necrosis and minimal trauma bone fractures in patients with dyskeratosis congenita, *Blood*, **140**(Supplement 1), pp. 2947–2948.
53. Jonassaint, N.L., *et al.* (2013). The gastrointestinal manifestations of telomere-mediated disease, *Aging Cell*, **12**, pp. 319–23.
54. Agrusa, J.E., *et al.* (2019). Severe therapy-related toxicities after treatment for Hodgkin lymphoma due to a pathogenic TERT variant and shortened telomeres, *Pediatr Blood Cancer*, **66**, pp. e27779.
55. Adam, S., *et al.* (2017). Concise review: getting to the core of inherited bone marrow failures, *Stem Cells*, **35**, pp. 284–298.
56. Shimamura, A. (2022). Telomere biology disorders: ends and (genetic) means, *Blood*, **139**, pp. 1776–1777.
57. Alter, B.P., *et al.* (2012). Telomere length is associated with disease severity and declines with age in dyskeratosis congenita, *Haematologica,* **97**, pp. 353–9.
58. Kermasson, L., *et al.* (2022). Inherited human Apollo deficiency causes severe bone marrow failure and developmental defects, *Blood,* **139**, pp. 2427–2440.

59. Tummala, H., *et al.* (2022). Germline thymidylate synthase deficiency impacts nucleotide metabolism and causes dyskeratosis congenita, *Am J Hum Genet*, **109**, pp. 1472–1483.

60. Alter, B.P., *et al.* (2015). Telomere length in inherited bone marrow failure syndromes, *Haematologica*, **100**, pp. 49–54.

61. Dokal, I., H. Tummala, and Vulliamy, T. (2022). Inherited bone marrow failure in the pediatric patient, *Blood*, **140**, pp. 556–570.

62. Allegra, A., *et al.* (2017). Telomerase and telomere biology in hematological diseases: a new therapeutic target, *Leuk Res*, **56**, pp. 60–74.

63. McNally, E.J., Luncsford, P.J., and Armanios, M. (2019). Long telomeres and cancer risk: the price of cellular immortality, *J Clin Invest*, **129**, pp. 3474–3481.

64. Horn, S., *et al.* (2013). TERT promoter mutations in familial and sporadic melanoma, *Science*, **339**, pp. 959–61.

65. Huang, F.W., *et al.* (2013). Highly recurrent TERT promoter mutations in human melanoma, *Science*, **339**, pp. 957–9.

66. Heidenreich, B., *et al.* (2014). TERT promoter mutations in cancer development, *Curr Opin Genet Dev*, **24**, pp. 30–7.

67. Haycock, P.C., *et al.* (2017). Association between telomere length and risk of cancer and non-neoplastic diseases: a Mendelian randomization study, *JAMA Oncol*, **3**, pp. 636–651.

68. Counter, C.M., *et al.* (1995). Telomerase activity in normal leukocytes and in hematologic malignancies, *Blood*, **85**, pp. 2315–20.

69. Polychronopoulou, S. and Koutroumba, P. (2004). Telomere length variation and telomerase activity expression in patients with congenital and acquired aplastic anemia, *Acta Haematol*, **111**, pp. 125–31.

70. Savage, S.A. and Dufour, C. (2017). Classical inherited bone marrow failure syndromes with high risk for myelodysplastic syndrome and acute myelogenous leukemia, *Semin Hematol*, **54**, pp. 105–114.

71. Miwata, S., *et al.* (2021). Clinical diagnostic value of telomere length measurement in inherited bone marrow failure syndromes, *Haematologica*, **106**, pp. 2511–2515.

72. Gadalla, S.M., *et al.* (2010). Telomere length in blood, buccal cells, and fibroblasts from patients with inherited bone marrow failure syndromes, *Aging (Albany NY)*, **2**, pp. 867–74.

73. Choijilsuren, H.B., Y. Park, and Jung, M. (2021). Mechanisms of somatic transformation in inherited bone marrow failure syndromes, *Hematology*, **2021**, pp. 390–398.

74. Dufour, C. (2017). How I manage patients with Fanconi anaemia, *Br J Haematol*, **178**, pp. 32–47.
75. Dufour, C. and Pierri, F. (2022). Modern management of Fanconi anemia, *Hematology*, **2022**, pp. 649–657.
76. Fiesco-Roa, M., *et al.* (2022). Fanconi anemia and dyskeratosis congenita/telomere biology disorders: two inherited bone marrow failure syndromes with genomic instability, *Front Oncol*, **12**, pp. 949435.
77. Merfort, L.W., *et al.* (2022). Cytogenetics in Fanconi anemia: the importance of follow-up and the search for new biomarkers of genomic instability, *Int J Mol Sci*, **23**, pp. 14119.
78. Alter, B.P. (2002). Bone marrow failure syndromes in children, *Pediatr Clin North Am*, **49**, pp. 973–88.
79. Soulier, J. (2011). Fanconi anemia, *Hematology*, **2011**, pp. 492–497.
80. Svahn, J., *et al.* (2016). Somatic, hematologic phenotype, long-term outcome, and effect of hematopoietic stem cell transplantation. An analysis of 97 Fanconi anemia patients from the Italian national database on behalf of the Marrow Failure Study Group of the AIEOP (Italian Association of Pediatric Hematology-Oncology), *Am J Hematol*, **91**, pp. 666–71.
81. Kutler, D.I., *et al.* (2003). A 20-year perspective on the International Fanconi Anemia Registry (IFAR), *Blood*, **101**, pp. 1249–56.
82. Shah, A., *et al.* (2021). Severe telomere shortening in Fanconi anemia complementation group L, *Mol Biol Rep*, **48**, pp. 585–593.
83. Alter, B.P. (2014). Fanconi anemia and the development of leukemia, *Best Pract Res Clin Haematol*, **27**, pp. 214–21.
84. Savage, S.A. and Alter, B.P. (2008). The role of telomere biology in bone marrow failure and other disorders, *Mech Ageing Dev*, **129**, pp. 35–47.
85. Casari, E., *et al.* (2022). To fix or not to fix: maintenance of chromosome ends versus repair of DNA double-strand breaks, *Cells*, **11**, pp. 3224.
86. Renaudin, X. and Rosselli, F. (2020). The FANC/BRCA pathway releases replication blockades by eliminating DNA interstrand cross-links, *Genes (Basel)*, **11**, pp. 585.
87. Altintas, B., *et al.* (2023). Genotype-phenotype and outcome associations in patients with Fanconi anemia: the National Cancer Institute cohort, *Haematologica*, **108**, pp. 69–82.
88. Ball, S.E., *et al.* (1998). Progressive telomere shortening in aplastic anemia, *Blood*, **91**, pp. 3582–92.
89. Li, X., *et al.* (2003). Abnormal telomere metabolism in Fanconi's anaemia correlates with genomic instability and the probability of

developing severe aplastic anaemia, *British Journal of Haematology*, **120**, pp. 836–845.

90. Dutzmann, C.M., *et al.* (2022). Cancer in children with Fanconi anemia and ataxia-telangiectasia: a nationwide register-based cohort study in Germany, *J Clin Oncol*, **40**, pp. 32–39.
91. Thornley, I., *et al.* (2002). Abnormal telomere shortening in leucocytes of children with Shwachman-Diamond syndrome, *Br J Haematol*, **117**, pp. 189–92.
92. Cantu, C. and Proytcheva, M.A. (2015). Bone marrow failure syndromes: a practical approach to diagnosis, *Journal of Hematopathology*, **8**, pp. 101–112.
93. Myers, K.C., *et al.* (2014). Variable clinical presentation of Shwachman-Diamond syndrome: update from the North American Shwachman-Diamond syndrome registry, *J Pediatr*, **164**, pp. 866–70.
94. Myers, K.C., *et al.* (2020). Clinical features and outcomes of patients with Shwachman-Diamond syndrome and myelodysplastic syndrome or acute myeloid leukaemia: a multicentre, retrospective, cohort study, *Lancet Haematol*, **7**, pp. e238–e246.
95. Liu, Y., *et al.* (2018). Shwachman-Diamond syndrome protein SBDS maintains human telomeres by regulating telomerase recruitment, *Cell Rep*, **22**, pp. 1849–1860.
96. Kennedy, A.L., *et al.* (2021). Distinct genetic pathways define pre-malignant versus compensatory clonal hematopoiesis in Shwachman-Diamond syndrome, *Nat Commun*, **12**, pp. 1334.
97. Da Costa, L.M., Marie, I., and Leblanc, T.M. (2021). Diamond-Blackfan anemia, *Hematology*, **2021**, pp. 353–360.
98. West, A.H. and Churpek, J.E. (2017). Old and new tools in the clinical diagnosis of inherited bone marrow failure syndromes, *Hematology Am Soc Hematol Educ Program*, **2017**, pp. 79–87.
99. Wegman-Ostrosky, T. and Savage, S.A. (2017). The genomics of inherited bone marrow failure: from mechanism to the clinic, *British Journal of Haematology*, **177**, pp. 526–542.
100. Vlachos, A., *et al.* (2008). Diagnosing and treating Diamond-Blackfan anaemia: results of an international clinical consensus conference, *Br J Haematol*, **142**, pp. 859–76.
101. Shallis, R.M., R. Ahmad, and Zeidan, A.M. (2018). Aplastic anemia: etiology, molecular pathogenesis, and emerging concepts, *Eur J Haematol*, **101**, pp. 711–720.

102. Young, N.S. (2018). Aplastic anemia, *N Engl J Med*, **379**, pp. 1643–1656.

103. Eva, M., *et al.* (2008). Epidemiology of aplastic anemia: a prospective multicenter study, *Haematologica*, **93**, pp. 518–523.

104. Calado, R.T., *et al.* (2012). Short telomeres result in chromosomal instability in hematopoietic cells and precede malignant evolution in human aplastic anemia, *Leukemia*, **26**, pp. 700–707.

105. Rosenfeld, S.J., *et al.* (1995). Intensive immunosuppression with antithymocyte globulin and cyclosporine as treatment for severe acquired aplastic anemia, *Blood*, **85**, pp. 3058–65.

106. Young, N.S., Calado, R.T. and Scheinberg, P. (2006). Current concepts in the pathophysiology and treatment of aplastic anemia, *Blood*, **108**, pp. 2509–19.

107. Lee, J.J., *et al.* (2001). Telomere length changes in patients with aplastic anaemia, *Br J Haematol*, **112**, pp. 1025–30.

108. Brümmendorf, T.H., *et al.* (2001). Telomere length in leukocyte subpopulations of patients with aplastic anemia, *Blood*, **97**, pp. 895–900.

109. Brümmendorf, T.H., *et al.* (2001). Telomere length dynamics in normal individuals and in patients with hematopoietic stem cell-associated disorders, *Ann N Y Acad Sci*, **938**, pp. 293–303; discussion 303–4.

110. Edison, E.S., *et al.* (2017). Telomere length is significantly reduced in patients with aplastic anemia and is not influenced by gender and severity, *Blood*, **130**(Supplement 1), pp. 4964–4964.

111. Calado, R.T. and Young, N.S. (2008). Telomere maintenance and human bone marrow failure, *Blood*, **111**, pp. 4446–55.

112. Townsley, D.M., Dumitriu, B., and Young, N.S. (2014). Bone marrow failure and the telomeropathies, *Blood*, **124**, pp. 2775–83.

113. Scheinberg, P., *et al.* (2010). Association of telomere length of peripheral blood leukocytes with hematopoietic relapse, malignant transformation, and survival in severe aplastic anemia, *Jama*, **304**, pp. 1358–64.

114. Sakaguchi, H., *et al.* (2014). Peripheral blood lymphocyte telomere length as a predictor of response to immunosuppressive therapy in childhood aplastic anemia, *Haematologica*, **99**, pp. 1312–6.

115. Narita, A., *et al.* (2015). Paroxysmal nocturnal hemoglobinuria and telomere length predicts response to immunosuppressive therapy in pediatric aplastic anemia, *Haematologica*, **100**, pp. 1546–52.

116. Locatelli, F. and Strahm, B. (2018). How I treat myelodysplastic syndromes of childhood, *Blood*, **131**, pp. 1406–1414.

117. Galaverna, F., Ruggeri, A., and Locatelli, F. (2018). Myelodysplastic syndromes in children, *Curr Opin Oncol*, **30**, pp. 402–408.

118. Boultwood, J., *et al.* (1997). Telomere length in myelodysplastic syndromes, *Am J Hematol*, **56**, pp. 266–71.

119. Ohyashiki, K., *et al.* (2001). Telomere dynamics in myelodysplastic syndromes and acute leukemic transformation, *Leuk Lymphoma*, **42**, pp. 291–9.

120. Rollison, D.E., *et al.* (2011). Telomere length in myelodysplastic syndromes, *Leukemia & Lymphoma*, **52**, pp. 1528–1536.

121. Hwang, S.M., *et al.* (2016). Short telomere length and its correlation with gene mutations in myelodysplastic syndrome, *J Hematol Oncol*, **9**, pp. 62.

122. Williams, J., *et al.* (2017). Telomere length is an independent prognostic marker in MDS but not in de novo AML, *British Journal of Haematology*, **178**, pp. 240–249.

123. Myllymäki, M., *et al.* (2020). Short telomere length predicts nonrelapse mortality after stem cell transplantation for myelodysplastic syndrome, *Blood*, **136**, pp. 3070–3081.

124. Reilly, C.R., *et al.* (2021). The clinical and functional effects of TERT variants in myelodysplastic syndrome, *Blood*, **138**, pp. 898–911.

125. Im, K., *et al.* (2015). Profiles of telomere length adult and childhood myelodysplastic syndromes: a comparison with hematologic diseases, *Blood*, **126**, pp. 5231–5231.

126. Kawauchi, K., Akiyama, M., and Yamada, O. (2013). The mechanisms of telomere and telomerase regulation in hematologic malignancies, **1**, pp. 115–183.

127. Drummond, M.W., *et al.* (2005). Dysregulated expression of the major telomerase components in leukaemic stem cells, *Leukemia*, **19**, pp. 381–9.

128. Oikawa, S. and Kawanishi, S. (1999). Site-specific DNA damage at GGG sequence by oxidative stress may accelerate telomere shortening, *FEBS Lett*, **453**, pp. 365–8.

129. Brady, S.W., *et al.* (2022). The genomic landscape of pediatric acute lymphoblastic leukemia, *Nat Genet*, **54**, pp. 1376–1389.

130. Capraro, V., *et al.* (2011). Telomere deregulations possess cytogenetic, phenotype, and prognostic specificities in acute leukemias, *Exp Hematol*, **39**, pp. 195–202.e2.

131. Borssén, M., *et al.* (2011). hTERT promoter methylation and telomere length in childhood acute lymphoblastic leukemia: associations with immunophenotype and cytogenetic subgroup, *Exp Hematol,* **39**, pp. 1144–51.

132. Karow, A., *et al.* (2021). Targeting telomere biology in acute lymphoblastic leukemia, *Int J Mol Sci*, **22**, pp. 6653.

133. Engelhardt, M., *et al.* (1998). Telomerase activity and telomere length in pediatric patients with malignancies undergoing chemotherapy, *Leukemia*, **12**, pp. 13–24.

134. Vakonaki, E., *et al.* (2022). PB1754: telomere length in childhood acute lymphoblastic leukemia, *Hemasphere*, **6**(Suppl), pp. 1635–1636.

135. Leão, R., *et al.* (2018). Mechanisms of human telomerase reverse transcriptase (hTERT) regulation: clinical impacts in cancer, *Journal of Biomedical Science*, **25**, pp. 22.

136. Roka, K., Solomou, E.E., and Kattamis, A. (2023). Telomere biology: from disorders to hematological diseases, *Front Oncol*, **13**, pp. 1167848.

137. Galati, P.C., *et al.* (2022). Relative telomeric length of bone marrow cells at diagnosis and its association with minimal residual disease in juvenile acute lymphoblastic leukemia, *Blood*, **140**(Supplement 1), pp. 11849–11849.

138. Elgarten, C.W. and Aplenc, R. (2020). Pediatric acute myeloid leukemia: updates on biology, risk stratification, and therapy, *Curr Opin Pediatr*, **32**, pp. 57–66.

139. Aalbers, A.M., *et al.* (2013). Telomere length and telomerase complex mutations in pediatric acute myeloid leukemia, *Leukemia*, **27**, pp. 1786–9.

140. Calado, R.T., *et al.* (2009). Constitutional hypomorphic telomerase mutations in patients with acute myeloid leukemia, *Proc Natl Acad Sci U S A*, **106**, pp. 1187–92.

141. Noguera, N.I., *et al.* (2019). Acute promyelocytic leukemia: update on the mechanisms of leukemogenesis, resistance and on innovative treatment strategies, *Cancers (Basel)*, **11**, pp. 1591.

142. Ghaffari, S.H., *et al.* (2008). Telomerase activity and telomere length in patients with acute promyelocytic leukemia: indicative of proliferative activity, disease progression, and overall survival, *Ann Oncol*, **19**, pp. 1927–34.

143. Kirschner, M., *et al.* (2022). Impaired overall survival in young patients with acute myeloid leukemia and variants in genes predisposing for myeloid malignancies, *Hemisphere*, **6**, pp. e787.

144. Lima, M.F., *et al.* (2022). Consecutive inhibition of telomerase and alternative lengthening pathway promotes Hodgkin's lymphoma cell death, *Biomedicines*, **10**, pp. 2299.

145. M'Kacher, R., *et al.* (2007). Telomere shortening and associated chromosomal instability in peripheral blood lymphocytes of patients with Hodgkin's lymphoma prior to any treatment are predictive of second cancers, *Int J Radiat Oncol Biol Phys*, **68**, pp. 465–71.

146. Knecht, H., *et al.* (2012). Three-dimensional telomere signatures of Hodgkin- and Reed-Sternberg cells at diagnosis identify patients with poor response to conventional chemotherapy, *Transl Oncol*, **5**, pp. 269–77.

147. Ostrom, Q.T., *et al.* (2018). CBTRUS statistical report: primary brain and other central nervous system tumors diagnosed in the United States in 2011–2015, *Neuro Oncol*, **20**(suppl. 4), pp. iv1–iv86.

148. Minasi, S., *et al.* (2021). Alternative lengthening of telomeres in molecular subgroups of paediatric high-grade glioma, *Childs Nerv Syst*, **37**, pp. 809–818.

149. Tabori, U., *et al.* (2006). The role of telomere maintenance in the spontaneous growth arrest of pediatric low-grade gliomas, *Neoplasia*, **8**, pp. 136–42.

150. Abedalthagafi, M., *et al.* (2013). The alternative lengthening of telomere phenotype is significantly associated with loss of ATRX expression in high-grade pediatric and adult astrocytomas: a multi-institutional study of 214 astrocytomas, *Mod Pathol*, **26**, pp. 1425–32.

151. Killela, P.J., *et al.* (2013). TERT promoter mutations occur frequently in gliomas and a subset of tumors derived from cells with low rates of self-renewal, *Proc Natl Acad Sci U S A*, **110**, pp. 6021–6.

152. Stundon, J.L., *et al.* (2022). ALT in pediatric high-grade gliomas can occur without ATRX mutation and is enriched in patients with pathogenic germline MMR variants, *Neuro Oncol*, **25**, pp. 1331–1342.

153. Juraschka, K. and Taylor, M.D. (2019). Medulloblastoma in the age of molecular subgroups: a review, *J Neurosurg Pediatr*, **24**, pp. 353–363.

154. Remke, M., *et al.* (2013). TERT promoter mutations are highly recurrent in SHH subgroup medulloblastoma, *Acta Neuropathol*, **126**, pp. 917–29.

155. Viana-Pereira, M., *et al.* (2017). Study of hTERT and histone 3 mutations in medulloblastoma, *Pathobiology*, **84**, pp. 108–113.

156. Minasi, S., *et al.* (2019). Telomere elongation via alternative lengthening of telomeres (ALT) and telomerase activation in primary metastatic medulloblastoma of childhood, *J Neurooncol*, **142**, pp. 435–444.

157. Buttarelli, F.R., *et al.* (2022). MEDB-68: analysis of telomeres length and alternative lengthening of telomeres (ALT) in molecular subgroups of infant medulloblastoma, *Neuro-Oncology*, **24**(Supplement 1), pp. i122–i122.
158. Gojo, J., *et al.* (2017). Telomerase activation in posterior fossa group A ependymomas is associated with dismal prognosis and chromosome 1q gain, *Neuro Oncol*, **19**, pp. 1183–1194.
159. Zhang, C., *et al.* (2020). Genetic predisposition to longer telomere length and risk of childhood, adolescent and adult-onset ependymoma, *Acta Neuropathol Commun*, **8**, pp. 173.
160. Walsh, K.M., *et al.* (2013). Genetic variants in telomerase-related genes are associated with an older age at diagnosis in glioma patients: evidence for distinct pathways of gliomagenesis, *Neuro-Oncology*, **15**, pp. 1041–1047.
161. Matthay, K.K., *et al.* (2016). Neuroblastoma, *Nature Reviews Disease Primers*, **2**, pp. 16078.
162. Johnsen, J.I., Dyberg, C., and Wickström, M. (2019). Neuroblastoma: a neural crest derived embryonal malignancy, *Front Mol Neurosci*, **12**, pp. 9.
163. Kawano, A., *et al.* (2021). Stage 4S neuroblastoma: molecular, histologic, and immunohistochemical characteristics and presence of 2 distinct patterns of MYCN protein overexpression, a report from the children's oncology group, *Am J Surg Pathol*, **45**, pp. 1075–1081.
164. Zeineldin, M., Patel, A.G. and Dyer, M.A. (2022). Neuroblastoma: when differentiation goes awry, *Neuron*, **110**, pp. 2916–2928.
165. Ohali, A., *et al.* (2006). Telomere length is a prognostic factor in neuroblastoma, *Cancer*, **107**, pp. 1391–1399.
166. Pezzolo, A., *et al.* (2015). Intratumoral diversity of telomere length in individual neuroblastoma tumors, *Oncotarget*, **6**, pp. 7493–503.
167. George, S.L., *et al.* (2020). Novel therapeutic strategies targeting telomere maintenance mechanisms in high-risk neuroblastoma, *J Exp Clin Cancer Res*, **39**, pp. 78.
168. Ackermann, S., *et al.* (2018). A mechanistic classification of clinical phenotypes in neuroblastoma, *Science*, **362**, pp. 1165–1170.
169. Lee, J.W., *et al.* (2018). Clinical significance of MYCN amplification in patients with high-risk neuroblastoma, *Pediatr Blood Cancer*, **65**, pp. e27257.
170. Stainczyk, S.A. and Westermann, F. (2022). Neuroblastoma—telomere maintenance, deregulated signaling transduction and beyond, *International Journal of Cancer*, **150**, pp. 903–915.

171. Valentijn, L.J., *et al.* (2015). TERT rearrangements are frequent in neuroblastoma and identify aggressive tumors, *Nat Genet*, **47**, pp. 1411–4.

172. Dagg, R.A., *et al.* (2017). Extensive proliferation of human cancer cells with ever-shorter telomeres, *Cell Rep*, **19**, pp. 2544–2556.

173. Roderwieser, A., *et al.* (2019). Telomerase is a prognostic marker of poor outcome and a therapeutic target in neuroblastoma, *JCO Precis Oncol*, **3,** pp. 1–20.

174. Hartlieb, S.A., *et al.* (2021). Alternative lengthening of telomeres in childhood neuroblastoma from genome to proteome, *Nature Communications*, **12**, pp. 1269.

175. Koneru, B., *et al.* (2020). Telomere maintenance mechanisms define clinical outcome in high-risk neuroblastoma, *Cancer Research*, **80**, pp. 2663–2675.

176. Hernández Borrero, L.J. and El-Deiry, W.S. (2021). Tumor suppressor p53: Biology, signaling pathways, and therapeutic targeting, *Biochim Biophys Acta Rev Cancer*, **1876**, pp. 188556.

177. Meeser, A., *et al.* (2022). Reliable assessment of telomere maintenance mechanisms in neuroblastoma, *Cell Biosci*, **12**, pp. 160.

178. Tabori, U. and Dome, J.S. (2007). Telomere biology of pediatric cancer, *Cancer Invest*, **25**, pp. 197–208.

179. Sanders, R.P., *et al.* (2004). Telomerase expression predicts unfavorable outcome in osteosarcoma, *Journal of Clinical Oncology*, **22**, pp. 3790–3797.

180. Ulaner, G.A., *et al.* (2003). Absence of a telomere maintenance mechanism as a favorable prognostic factor in patients with osteosarcoma, *Cancer Res*, **63**, pp. 1759–63.

181. Sanders, R.P., *et al.* (2004). Telomerase expression predicts unfavorable outcome in osteosarcoma, *J Clin Oncol*, **22**, pp. 3790–7.

182. Ulaner, G.A., *et al.* (2004). Divergent patterns of telomere maintenance mechanisms among human sarcomas: sharply contrasting prevalence of the alternative lengthening of telomeres mechanism in Ewing's sarcomas and osteosarcomas, *Genes Chromosomes Cancer*, **41**, pp. 155–62.

183. Liau, J.Y., *et al.* (2015). Comprehensive screening of alternative lengthening of telomeres phenotype and loss of ATRX expression in sarcomas, *Mod Pathol*, **28**, pp. 1545–54.

184. de Nonneville, A., *et al.* (2022). TOP3A amplification and ATRX inactivation are mutually exclusive events in pediatric osteosarcomas using ALT, *EMBO Mol Med*, **14**, pp. e15859.

185. Ohali, A., *et al.* (2003). Association between telomerase activity and outcome in patients with nonmetastatic Ewing family of tumors, *J Clin Oncol*, **21**, pp. 3836–43.

186. Avigad, S., *et al.* (2007). Short telomeres: a novel potential predictor of relapse in Ewing sarcoma, *Clinical Cancer Research*, **13**, pp. 5777–5783.

187. Leiner, J. and Le Loarer, F. (2020). The current landscape of rhabdomyosarcomas: an update, *Virchows Arch*, **476**, pp. 97–108.

188. Ohali, A., *et al.* (2008). Different telomere maintenance mechanisms in alveolar and embryonal rhabdomyosarcoma, *Genes, Chromosomes and Cancer*, **47**, pp. 965–970.

189. Lansdorp, P.M. (2022). Telomeres, aging, and cancer: the big picture, *Blood*, **139**, pp. 813–821.

190. Dome, J.S., *et al.* (1999). High telomerase reverse transcriptase (hTERT) messenger RNA level correlates with tumor recurrence in patients with favorable histology Wilms' tumor, *Cancer Res*, **59**, pp. 4301–7.

191. Venturini, L., *et al.* (2011). Telomere maintenance in wilms tumors: first evidence for the presence of alternative lengthening of telomeres mechanism, *Genes, Chromosomes and Cancer*, **50**, pp. 823–829.

192. Yashima, K., *et al.* (1998). Expression of the RNA component of telomerase in Wilms tumor and nephrogenic rest recapitulates renal embryogenesis, *Hum Pathol*, **29**, pp. 536–42.

193. Hiyama, E. (2014). Pediatric hepatoblastoma: diagnosis and treatment, *Translational Pediatrics*, **3**, pp. 293–299.

194. Hiyama, E., Yamaoka, H., Matsunaga, T., Hayashi, Y., Ando, H., Suita, S., *et al.* (2004). High expression of telomerase is an independent prognostic indicator of poor outcome in hepatoblastoma, *British Journal of Cancer*, **91**, pp. 972–979.

195. Gupta, J., Han, L. P., Wang, P., Gallie, B. L., Bacchetti, S. (1996). Development of retinoblastoma in the absence of telomerase activity, *JNCI: Journal of the National Cancer Institute*, **88**, pp. 1152–1157.

Chapter 21

Skin Aging

Maria Sifaki,[a] Stella Baliou,[b,c] Sabine Kruger-Krasagakis,[d] Polytimi Sidiropoulou,[e,f] Dimitra Nikolopoulou,[b,c] and Aristidis Tsatsakis[b,c]

[a]*Skin Clinic, Heraklion, Crete, Greece*
[b]*Laboratory of Toxicology, Medical School, University of Crete, Heraklion, Greece*
[c]*Lifeplus S.A., Science & Technological Park of Crete, Vassilika Vouton, Heraklion, Greece*
[d]*Department of Dermatology & Venereology, General University Hospital of Heraklion, Faculty of Medicine, University of Crete, Greece*
[e]*1st Department of Dermatology-Venereology, Faculty of Medicine, "A. Sygros" Hospital, National and Kapodistrian University of Athens, Athens, Greece*
[f]*Research Group of Clinical Pharmacology and Pharmacogenomics, Faculty of Pharmacy, School of Health Sciences, National and Kapodistrian University of Athens, Athens, Greece*
stelllabaliou@gmail.com

21.1 Introduction

Skin's primary role is to act as a shield, providing protection against external insults, such as microbial pathogens, chemicals, and physical stressors, maintaining internal homeostasis, with the stratum corneum playing a crucial role in this context [1].

Telomeres: Biomarkers of a Healthy Life and Successful Aging
Edited by Aristidis Tsatsakis

ISBN 978-981-5129-49-6 (Hardcover), 978-1-003-56809-4 (eBook)
www.jennystanford.com

From a structural perspective, the skin is a complex organ divided into three layers: epidermis, dermis, and hypodermis [2]. The skin comprises different cell types and compartments with distinct functions. The outermost skin layer, the epidermis, is divided into four compartments (stratum basale, spinosum, granulosum, and corneum with the terminally differentiated, nonviable corneocytes). The epidermis contains mainly keratinocytes (90–95%) accompanied by melanocytes, Langerhans, and Merkel cells at rates below 5% [3]. Keratinocytes serve as reservoirs of keratin contributing to the skin's rigidity and water resistance. Another cell type in the basal layer of the epidermis is the melanocyte, which produces the melanin that plays a crucial role in conferring protection against ultraviolet (UV) radiation [4]. Melanocytes also exhibit immune-modulatory functions by expressing major histocompatibility complex II (MHC II) antigens. Merkel cells, found in the lower epidermis, express mechanoreceptors allowing interactions with cutaneous neurons and skin sensation [5]. Moreover, the epidermis contains bone marrow-derived Langerhans cells (LCs) and dendritic cells (DCs), which act as antigen-presenting cells [6].

The epidermis is divided from the dermis through the basement membrane at the dermal-epidermal junction. The dermis is responsible for the nutrition and structural support of the epidermis [7]. The dermal compartment is a connective tissue comprising different cell types, proteins (i.e., collagen and elastin), glycosaminoglycans (i.e., hyaluronan, chondroitin-sulfate, heparin-sulfate), and proteoglycans (i.e., aggrecan, versican, neurocan). It is known that different immune cell types (lymphocytes, macrophages, mast cells, DCs, natural killer cells) reside in the dermis [8]. In addition to immune cells, the dermis primarily consists of fibroblasts that produce an intricate extracellular matrix (ECM) essential for the dermis' properties. Fibroblasts also play a role in regulating the immune response to invading pathogens [5]. Sweat glands may be found in certain body areas within the dermis, surrounded by nerves, blood, and lymphatic vessels embedded in the ECM. Changes in the ECM can impact the regenerative capacity and differentiation of mesenchymal stem cells (MSCs) within the dermal compartment [9].

The hypodermis, the layer beneath the dermis, mainly consists of adipose tissue containing adipocytes embedded in collagen fibers. This layer ensures thermal insulation and energy storage [10]. Adipocytes are present both in dermal and subcutaneous adipose tissue and play a crucial role in skin photoaging [11].

Special consideration has been given to skin cell types and telomere length dynamics. In particular, epidermal cells, such as keratinocytes, melanocytes, and LCs, demonstrate elevated expression of the human telomerase reverse transcriptase (hTERT) gene and telomerase. Conversely, cells in deeper layers, including mast cells, dermal stem cells, and the bulge component of hair follicle units in the dermis, and hypodermal adipocytes, exhibit lower relative levels of hTERT and telomerase expression. Notably, hair follicle stem cells display heightened expression, while fibroblasts appear to lack both hTERT and telomerase expression [12].

21.2 Skin Aging

Aging is a complex multifactorial process characterized by accumulated DNA damage that drives cells into apoptosis or senescence, leading to functional decline in every tissue and organ [13]. On a cellular level, aging was initially introduced by Hayflick and Moorhead, who demonstrated that cells enter a state of irreversible growth arrest after several divisions, termed replicative senescence [14]. Then, Watson and Olovnikov suggested the inefficient DNA replication at the very ends of the chromosomes in a process called "end replication problem" [15]. The critically shortened telomeres are tightly linked to cellular senescence through the accumulation of DNA damage that cannot be repaired [16]. Current knowledge indicates that senescent cells are increasingly deposited in aging tissues and organs, thereby contributing to tissue degeneration and malignant transformation [17].

Skin aging is a gradual process caused by both intrinsic and extrinsic factors, leading to a progressive age-related decline in the functional and structural integrity of the skin [18]. Research findings have shown that intrinsic or chronological aging is mainly associated with genetic and metabolic alterations, while extrinsic aging results from exposure to external factors such as solar radiation [19]. It should also be noted that only 3% of skin aging has intrinsic background [20].

As the skin ages, structural alterations begin to arise compromising its functionality [21]. Notably, significant histological changes include the flattening of the dermal-epidermal junction accompanied by the degradation of ECM components, especially collagen and elastic fibers [22]. This results in a reduction in both epidermal and dermal surfaces and decreased exchange of nutrients and metabolites between these skin layers [23]. Studies have also supported a decline in fibroblast proliferative activity and a nearly 1.0–1.5% annual reduction in collagen production since early adulthood [24, 25].

21.3 Hallmarks of Skin Aging

Incredible progress has been made in the field of aging. Skin aging is characterized by the following hallmarks: genome instability, telomere shortening, cellular senescence, altered nutrient-sensing, reprogramming of epigenetic landscape, loss of proteostasis, impaired mitochondrial function, and stem cell elimination. [26]. Indeed, senescent cells exhibit numerous features that make them metabolically active and unable to replicate [26].

The major driving force for skin aging is the accumulation of DNA damage that causes premature telomere shortening, which eventually leads to cellular senescence [27]. When DNA injury occurs, the telomeres located at the chromosomal ends are the most vulnerable regions [28]. Telomeres consist of specific DNA repeat sequences (5′ TTAGGG 3′), which are surrounded by proteins from the shelterin complex [29]. After several cell divisions, telomeres shorten by destabilizing the T-loop, which then exposes the chromosomal ends as double-stranded breaks, ultimately triggering cell senescence [30]. Notably, oxidative stress can accelerate the rate of telomere shortening resulting in greater cellular senescence [30]. The telomere shortening can be reversed through the action of telomerase. Telomerase combats telomere erosion by adding new telomeric repeats via a process that involves the telomerase RNA component (TERC), which acts as the template for synthesizing new repeats, and the catalytic element (hTERT) [31].

Regarding genome instability in skin aging, telomere shortening has been observed in dermal fibroblasts derived from systemic sclerosis patients and in combination with DNA damage led to fibroblast senescence [32]. In line with this, it has been supported that senescence plays a significant role in the layers of the epidermis and dermis as individuals age [33].

Moreover, the connection between telomeres and skin aging has attracted attention. For example, defects in the shelterin protein complex have been associated with dyskeratosis congenita (DC) and its cutaneous manifestations [34].

Apart from the impact of genome instability on skin aging, research has indicated that epigenetic changes are also associated with the aging process of the skin. To support this, distinct hypermethylation patterns in the skin of older individuals have been observed, which corresponded to a decline of specific transcriptional networks [35]. The decline in proteasome function observed in older dermal fibroblasts confirmed the significant role of proteostasis loss in skin aging [35]. Similarly, aging dermal fibroblasts, keratinocytes, melanocytes, and epidermal stem cells showed increased ECM degradation and decreased autophagy [36].

21.4 Clinical Perspectives of Skin Aging

In general, the clinical signs of skin aging include wrinkle formation, decreased elasticity, dryness, pigmentary lesions, hair greying, and impaired wound healing [10, 37]. Skin aging involves various changes that result in skin atrophy. As skin ages, its ability to act as a protective barrier against external factors weakens, making it more prone to environmental insults [26].

From a histological viewpoint, the key change in intrinsic skin aging is cutaneous atrophy [38]. Intrinsic skin aging can be triggered by telomere shortening, cellular senescence, redox imbalance, and hormonal changes [38, 39]. The decrease in sex hormones with age seems to contribute to skin dysfunction [23].

Extrinsic skin aging manifests as coarse wrinkles, skin laxity, rough skin texture, uneven pigmentation, and telangiectatic blood vessels in photo-exposed skin areas [40]. Various external factors interfere with the skin balance accelerating the aging process. Major contributors to extrinsic aging, such as sun exposure, air pollution, smoking, inadequate nutrition, stress, sleep deprivation, and alcohol consumption, lead to irreversible skin damage [41]. The duration and intensity of such external factors are crucial in determining the rate at which skin ages.

Research indicates that over 80% of skin aging is linked to over-exposure to UV radiation [42]. Following prolonged UV exposure, the epidermis thickens in contrast to the epidermal thinning occurring during normal aging [43]. The histological presence of epidermal hyperplasia and thickening during extrinsic photo-aging results from an accumulation of corneocytes in the stratum corneum, the outermost layer of the epidermis [43]. Moreover, exposure to external factors like tobacco use has been shown to accelerate skin aging, leading to more wrinkle formation and elastosis due to higher matrix metalloproteinases (MMPs) expression and ECM degradation [44].

21.5 Molecular Mechanisms of Skin Aging

21.5.1 Senescence

Growing evidence suggests that senescent melanocytes, keratinocytes, and fibroblasts can accumulate in aging skin. The permanent cell cycle arrest in aged skin can be triggered by telomere shortening, mitochondrial dysfunction, oxidative stress, DNA damage, and/or inflammation (Fig. 21.1) [46, 47]. Cellular senescence is closely related to telomere dysfunction and DNA damage, which are perpetuated by impaired mitochondrial function and accumulation of free radicals [16, 45], Additionally, senescent cells have been found to produce various mediators involved in the senescence-associated secretory phenotype (SASP) orchestrating changes in the epigenetic landscape and metabolic changes by regulating catabolic pathways [48–51].

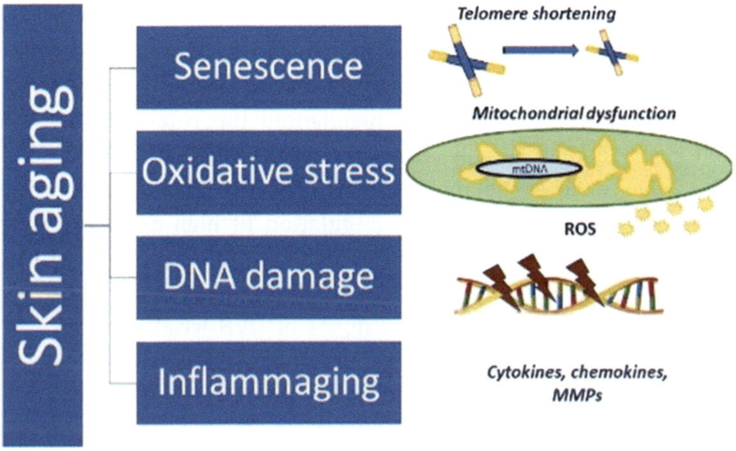

Figure 21.1 The four underlying mechanisms that drive skin aging. Genome instability, with the principal characteristic of telomere shortening, induces senescence. Oxidative stress can accelerate senescence, leading to skin aging. Besides, most ROS production arises from mitochondrial dysfunction in cells. DNA damage and inflammaging (chronic low-grade inflammation) are additional mechanisms involved in skin aging. Abbreviations: ROS, reactive oxygen species; mtDNA, mitochondrial DNA; and MMPs, matrix metalloproteinases.

Senescent cells have been shown to accumulate in all layers of aged skin in response to intrinsic or extrinsic stimuli [48, 49] with the majority of studies focusing on dermal fibroblasts [40, 48, 50–52]. Accordingly, the role of senescence has been confirmed in the case of skin exposome to photoaging [40, 48, 50, 51]. Besides, aged fibroblasts in the dermis were more susceptible to senescence than keratinocytes due to increased accumulation of protein and DNA damage accounting for weaker repair mechanisms and lower oxidative defense [52–55].

The role of senescence in extrinsic skin aging has been thoroughly examined after UV radiation. An increased number of senescent cells were found in the skin after UVB exposure [60, 61]. In particular, fibroblasts and keratinocytes were cell-cycle arrested showing upregulated activity of p53 transcription factor, cell cycle regulators (p16INK4A, p21Waf-1), and senescence-associated β-galactosidase (SA-β-Gal) [60, 61]. In UVB-irradiated melanocytes, the expression of cell cycle regulators p16INK4A and p53 was also increased, indicating the induction of senescence in the epidermis, especially in melanocytes, after repeated UVB exposure [57]. Notably, Victorelli et al. highlighted the role of p16INK4A cell cycle regulators only in melanocytes during skin aging [58]. The senescence of melanocytes was driven by the disturbance in telomeric sequences and downregulation of high-mobility group box 1 (HMGB1) [58]. The senescence in melanocytes was unexpected since fully differentiated melanocytes are characterized by low cell turnover [59]. Low doses of UVB irradiation also induced stress-induced premature senescence (SIPS) in keratinocytes [60].

Further, keratinocytes and fibroblasts became senescent via different DNA damage pathways [61]. In particular, keratinocytes became senescent through the activation of the p38 mitogen-activated protein kinases (MAPK) signaling pathway, whereas fibroblasts through telomere shortening [62].

Telomere shortening is a significant indicator of cellular senescence, contributing to the aging process and the development of age-related diseases [63]. With this respect, evaluation of telomere length (TL) within the skin has demonstrated more accelerated telomere shortening in the dermis compared to the epidermis. Interestingly, no differences in the TL between these two skin layers were observed after sun exposure [64]. In other skin cell types, telomere erosion seemed to mediate the negative effects of UV radiation. For example, basal cells in UV-exposed skin exhibit more pronounced telomere shortening compared to sun-protected areas, possibly due to the increased susceptibility of telomeres to UV-induced oxidative stress. [65]. Notably, telomere shortening was not detected in sun-protected human epidermis [58]. Keratinocytes appear to counteract telomere attrition through the activity of telomerase [66]. In addition to TL investigations, human studies have revealed that keratinocytes and melanocytes exhibit DNA damage in telomere-associated foci (TAF), leading to cellular senescence [58]. Notably, skin disorders associated with telomere dysfunction, such as xeroderma pigmentosum (XP) and dyskeratosis congenita (DC), are characterized by increased senescence [67].

21.5.2 Oxidative Stress

The free radical theory prevails in the molecular layout of skin aging [23]. In this context, mitochondrial dysfunction seems to induce a shift to the redox balance toward increased production of free radicals, thus driving senescence in aged skin cells [33]. Indeed, dysfunctional mitochondria can produce increased amounts of reactive oxygen species (ROS) in senescent cells, which is also an essential characteristic of cellular senescence [68].

Several intrinsic factors have also been involved in ROS overproduction. Indeed, hormones can enhance age-related dysfunction by compromising the redox balance, leading to the accumulation of free radicals [69]. From a molecular perspective, the alterations in cellular redox status can result from mitochondrial dysfunction, endoplasmic reticulum stress, and activation of nicotinamide adenine dinucleotide phosphate (NADPH) oxidases and cyclooxygenases (COXs) [70]. In addition, external stimuli, like UV radiation, air pollution, and tobacco use, also contribute to redox imbalance and senescence (Fig. 21.2) [33].

For example, UV exposure contributes to skin aging through induction of oxidative stress. UV radiation seems to cause a redox imbalance in epidermal cells, leading to cellular damage. This can trigger a recruitment of macrophages releasing pro-inflammatory mediators, in order to eliminate the damaged cells eventually, leading to a redox disequilibrium that disrupts the dermal-epidermal junction and collagen production [71]. After repeated UV exposure, the photo-damaged skin was characterized by a 10-fold rise in mitochondrial DNA mutations that were linked to elevated MMP levels that degraded the ECM [72]. UV radiation has emerged as a crucial environmental factor resulting in oxidative damage or stress in aged fibroblasts and keratinocytes [73].

After UV exposure, several molecular alterations have been reported during skin aging. Receptor tyrosine kinases (RTKs) became more phosphorylated triggering the MAPK signaling pathway and the subsequent transcription nuclear factor-kappa B (NF-kB) and activator protein-1 (AP-1). In the case of photodamaged skin, accelerated collagen degradations was observed through increased expression of MMPs [21]. The mechanism underlying

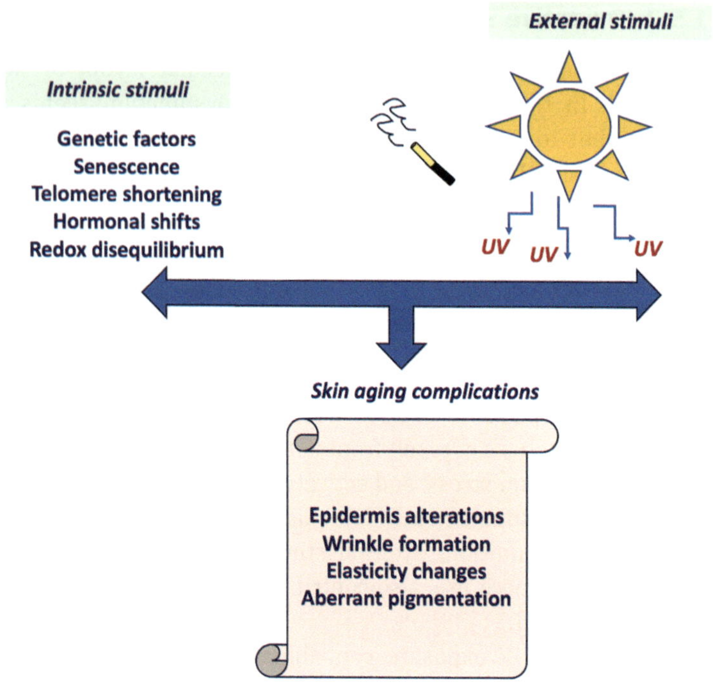

Figure 21.2 Types of skin aging stimuli and their effects. Skin aging can be intrinsic or extrinsic. Genetic factors, senescence, telomere shortening, hormonal shifts, and redox disequilibrium account for intrinsic aging, while UV exposure, smoking, and air pollution are crucial factors driving extrinsic skin aging. Skin aging manifests with epidermis alterations, wrinkle formation, elasticity changes, and aberrant pigmentation.

the increased ROS generation was also based on the induction of the MAPK cascade, leading to AP-1 transcriptional transactivation. Taken together, skin aging was driven by MAPK-mediated ECM degradation in a ROS-dependent manner [74]. In the case of UV exposure, the elevated ECM degradation in dermal fibroblasts was also attributed to the activation of MAPK and transforming growth factor-beta1 (TGF-β1) [75].

In line with this, metabolites in senescent cells have been implicated in the regulation of catabolic pathways. The increase in adenosine monophosphate/adenosine triphosphate (AMP/ATP) and ADP/ATP ratios was attributed to the activation of adenosine monophosphate-activated protein kinase (AMPK) signaling, which was related to the downregulation of catabolic pathways. To confirm this, mitochondrial complexes I-V were found to be significantly downregulated in dermal samples after UV exposure [76]. Moreover, the dermis of older individuals showed a reduction in mitophagy by 77% compared to young people [76]. During skin aging, the epidermis indicated a reduced expression of hexokinase 2 (HK2) and downregulation of the pentose-phosphate pathway, which was consistent with a rise in glucose levels [77]. In addition, senescent human skin fibroblasts and melanocytes also had an altered choline metabolism [78]. Indeed, senescent melanocytes demonstrated reduced phosphocholine expression, whereas senescent fibroblasts showed increased expression of glycerol-phosphocholine [78].

21.5.3 DNA Damage

Several theories suggest that skin aging is associated with DNA damage accumulation [79]. Research supports that prolonged DNA damage, caused by defects in DNA replication or TL maintenance, can lead to permanent cell-cycle arrest known as senescence [80]. This persistent DNA damage is often characterized by double-strand breaks, which activate the ataxia-telangiectasia mutated (ATM) kinase [81], triggering the phosphorylation of the p53 transcription factor and the formation of γ-H2AX nuclear foci [88, 89]. While DNA damage itself is not a definitive marker of senescence, the presence of DNA damage in TAF can be used to identify senescent cells [82]. Therefore, persistent DNA damage acts as a catalyst for cell senescence accelerating skin aging.

A characteristic example of DNA damage driving skin aging is UV radiation. In particular, UV radiation is the main factor responsible for skin changes during extrinsic aging accounting for approximately 80% of the whole process [18]. UV radiation is categorized into two types: UVA and UVB, with wavelengths ranging between 320–400 nm and 290–320 nm, respectively [23]. The harmful effects of UVA are significantly greater than those of UVB impacting both the dermal and epidermal layers through oxidative stress and inflammation [23]. For instance, UVA exposure has been linked to telomere shortening in photoaged human skin [83]. On the other hand, UVB is considered a more potent mutagen than UVA due to its ability to increase the production of pyrimidines during DNA replication [56, 84].

Regarding the molecular effects of UVB radiation, it has been supported that UVB exposure leads to oxidative stress-induced DNA damage, resulting in cellular senescence [85]. Specifically, UVB radiation triggers the rearrangement of nucleotides within DNA strands disrupting DNA replication [86]. This radiation also causes the formation of covalent bonds between two thymidines creating thymidine dimers that can persist through DNA replication. As a result, the damaging impact of UVB radiation on DNA is exacerbated by insufficient nucleotide excision repair mechanisms [87]. This leads to the accumulation of DNA mutations ultimately impairing the structure and function of the skin [88]. Notably, UVB-induced DNA damage primarily affects keratinocytes and melanocytes altering the secretion of proteolytic enzymes and the soluble epidermal factor (ESF) [23].

From a structural standpoint, UV exposure has emerged as the major factor responsible for connective tissue alterations, impairing the skin's structure [23]. The key components affected by this disorganization are collagens and elastin. The structural integrity of the skin is compromised by the elevated presence of MMPs, which weakens the connection between the dermis and epidermis ultimately contributing to skin laxity and wrinkle formation [89]. MMPs are known to degrade dermal collagens, with MMP-1 cleaving type I, II, and III collagen, and MMP-9 type IV and V collagen [23]. A striking example of the impact of UV radiation is the abnormal expression and disarray of fragmented collagen type I fibers in UV-exposed skin areas [90]. Additionally, the accumulation of proteases after UV exposure results in increased formation of truncated elastin, leading to the characteristic feature of solar elastosis in photoaged skin [91].

21.5.4 Inflammaging

The aging process is characterized by persistent low-level inflammation, a phenomenon known as inflammaging [92, 93]. In skin aging, senescent cells play a key role in driving this inflammatory process. The close connection between inflammation and senescence is evidenced by the SASP, which consists of growth factors, chemokines, and cytokines. Senescent cells have a negative impact on neighboring cells inducing senescence through the paracrine effect mediated by SASP factors [33]. Additionally, several studies have shown that senescent cells can induce cell death in surrounding cells by releasing free radicals or SASP factors [94].

In skin aging, recent studies have shown that melanocytes secrete SASP mediators in neighboring cells [58]. Immunofluorescence in situ hybridization (immunoFISH) experiments showed that senescent melanocytes have an increased number of TAF due to persistent DNA damage. Indeed, keratinocytes and fibroblasts exhibited telomere damage and reduced replicative capacity due to their proximity to senescent melanocytes, and this interaction is believed to disrupt epidermal turnover. Of note, the paracrine telomere damage caused by the senescent melanocytes is dependent on the cell-surface CXCR3 receptor and the presence of free radicals [58].

Elucidating the inflammation underlying skin aging, various factors, including the insulin-like growth factor binding protein 7 (IGFBP7), MMPs, cytokines (such as IL-6 and IL-8), and chemokine receptors (such as CXCR2) were detected in senescent melanocytes and dermal fibroblasts [95, 96]. Additionally, in vivo studies supported that the inflammatory responses sustained due to high collagen degradation, which was affected by ROS generation [97]. The mechanism behind this involves the translocation of HMGB1 to the nucleus, leading to increased expression of pro-inflammatory mediators and MMPs [98]. Furthermore, other transcription factors like GATA binding protein 4 (GATA4) and CCAAT/enhancer-binding protein beta (C/EBPβ) were found to be involved in promoting the SASP during skin aging [99]. At a post-translational level, the inactivation of SirT1 histone deacetylase appeared to be crucial in enhancing the acetylation and subsequent activation of pro-inflammatory mediators related to SASP [100]. The mTOR signaling cascade has also been implicated in regulating SASP components by stabilizing SASP transcriptome, thereby influencing age-associated inflammation [101].

Additionally, it is important to note that SASP can arise from active interactions between different immunocompetent cells and other cell types, such as keratinocytes or fibroblasts, involved in acquired immune responses. Following UV exposure, the expression of SASP components was found to increase in both keratinocytes and fibroblasts, leading to disruption in collagen balance and compromised skin function [102]. Specifically, UVA radiation seems to trigger the expression of IL-6 promoting collagen degradation, while UVB-induced collagen breakdown through DNA damage or inflammation [103].

Moreover, senescent cells can negatively affect the skin-resident immune cells, impairing their immunosurveillance ability. Studies have shown that the accumulation of immunosuppressive cells, such as T regulatory (Treg) cells, can disrupt the functionality of macrophages during the aging process [104]. Also, reduced recruitment of antigen-presenting LCs has been observed in the aged epidermis [92]. This can compromise the host defense mechanism deteriorating the skin's function over time.

In line with this, the presence of persistent chronic inflammation has been associated with an imbalance in inflammatory and anti-inflammatory macrophages (M1/M2). Recent research showed a negative correlation between the M1-type macrophages and abnormal collagen formation, while the induction of M2 macrophages is crucial in maintaining skin homeostasis influencing not only the quantity but also the quality of the collagen matrix in skin tissue [105, 106].

Last, a noticeable characteristic of photoaging is the progressive buildup of advanced glycation end (AGE) products in the dermis, which impedes skin elasticity and promotes collagen degradation [107]. Targeting these AGE products could thus pave the way toward delaying skin aging.

21.6 Role of Telomeres in Skin Aging

As the skin ages, a number of visible and histological changes begin to appear as a result of both intrinsic and extrinsic stressors. This aging process is characterized by changes in skin cells as well as structural and functional alterations in ECM components, such as collagens and elastin [108].

The primary molecular characteristics of aging include telomere attrition, epigenetic and mitochondrial malfunction, and DNA damage [12]. Telomeres, acting as protective caps at the chromosomal ends, play a critical role in the aging process by sustaining genomic integrity and stability during cell division. As normal cells replicate, telomeres gradually shorten, which eventually leads to a state of irreversible growth arrest known as cellular senescence. Of note, although telomere shortening accelerates skin aging, it also acts as a "mitotic clock", preventing abnormal proliferation in cancer [109, 110].

In the context of skin aging, the progressive shortening of telomeres impairs the regenerative capacity of skin cells resulting in reduced collagen production, loss of skin elasticity, cellular dysfunction, and even, carcinogenesis. Notably, the telomerase enzyme complex, which preserves the TL, can be found in the basal epidermal keratinocytes but is almost undetectable in the dermal fibroblasts. As a result, UV-induced ROS, a major cause of oxidative stress in the skin, may have distinct toxic effects on skin fibroblasts compared to keratinocytes. In fact, keratinocytes seem to be more resistant to UVB-induced DNA damage and are more prone to undergo apoptosis compared to fibroblasts. Thus, while defective keratinocytes are removed by apoptosis, fibroblasts with shortened telomeres may remain in the dermis layer and become senescent [111]. Moreover, previous studies have indicated that telomeres were significantly shorter in fibroblasts exposed to UVA than in unirradiated controls [110].

21.7 Telomerase- and Telomere-Based Skin Anti-Aging Approaches

Recent research is increasingly focused on the mechanisms of aging and potential strategies to delay genomic instability, telomere attrition, and cellular senescence. Since telomere shortening is involved in the aging process, skin might be an accessible tissue for manipulation of telomerase and telomere dysfunction opening new perspectives in the prevention, delay, or even reversal of cutaneous aging through dietary interventions and/or topically applied preparations [12]. As the effects of oxidative stress may in part be mediated by telomere-associated cell senescence, decreasing ROS or increasing antioxidants in cells would thus provide a means to control skin aging [111].

In this regard, antioxidant and anti-inflammatory agents have already emerged as key anti-aging compounds. Indeed, several bioactive substances can affect telomere biology, partially due to their antioxidant and anti-inflammatory capacities. Essential micronutrients capable of guarding and enhancing the antioxidant status in our cells include vitamins A, C, E, and D [12, 112].

The vitamin E complex (tocopherols) is the primary antioxidant in the skin [113]. Previous studies have indicated that vitamin E, the most potent and abundant lipophilic radical scavenger in vivo, can significantly reduce free radical-induced DNA damage [114, 115]. Moreover, Makpol et al. investigating the effects of alpha-tocopherol on normal human skin fibroblasts have shown that vitamin E could have the potential to maintain the TL by restoring the activity of telomerase [115].

Several lines of evidence have also shown that vitamin C (ascorbic acid) has skin anti-aging effects due to its high radical-scavenging activity offering protection from oxidative stress and telomere attrition. In fact, experimental models have already demonstrated that treatment with vitamin C can delay telomere loss in epidermal keratinocytes [116, 117]. In addition, a cross-sectional study including 7.094 individuals has recently supported that greater vitamin C intake is correlated with longer human telomeres [118].

Of note, retinoic acid, the biologically active metabolite of vitamin A, has been shown to decrease telomerase function in cancer cells, while in low concentrations it induced telomerase activity in normal human oral keratinocytes [12, 119]. Further, a positive association between vitamin A intake and TL in female young adults has recently been supported by Mizuno et al. [120].

Although the exact role of vitamin D (cholecalciferol) in cellular senescence has yet to be determined, emerging evidence supports the implication of vitamin D signaling pathway in genomic stability and telomere biology. In this respect, serum vitamin D levels have positively been correlated with both longer telomeres and increased telomerase action in humans, but the current data are not consistent [121].

In total, topically applied or orally supplemented polyphenols are among the most studied phytochemicals with known antioxidant and anti-inflammatory properties [12, 122]. In recent years, several biomolecules of the polyphenolic group, such as green tea catechins, grape seed resveratrol, flavonoids, procyanidins, and curcumin, have been extensively investigated in the context of aging and seem to be promising anti-senescence agents [122, 123].

At this point, available data have indicated that polyphenols could enhance TERT gene expression in both human and murine skin cells, thus preventing cell membrane and DNA damage by oxidative stress [12]. It has also been suggested that polyphenols are able to increase telomerase activity and preserve telomere length, contributing to increased longevity and prevention of age-related diseases [123, 124].

Skin lipids are a principal component of the epidermal barrier, protecting against water and mineral loss, as well as the penetration of harmful environmental factors [125, 126]. Since skin aging may alter the lipid profile in cutaneous and body tissues, fatty acids could thus be a modifiable factor in navigating our aging [12].

Unsaturated omega-6 and omega-3 fatty acids are important regulators of redox balance and inflammation by inhibiting pro-inflammatory cytokines, leucocyte chemotaxis, and eicosanoid production [12, 126]. Interestingly, fermented fish oil has been shown to reduce ROS production and suppress MMPs (MMP-1/2/9) in human keratinocytes [12, 127]. Despite limited evidence, a beneficial effect of polyunsaturated omega-3 fatty acids on telomere maintenance has already been reported [12, 127]. Indeed, both animal and human studies have indicated that omega-3 fatty acids may slow down accelerated telomere shortening and subsequent premature cellular senescence [127, 129]. Notably, a randomized controlled trial has demonstrated that it is not omega-3 itself, but rather the ratio between omega-3 and omega-6 fatty acids that is important. As the plasma omega 6/omega-3 ratio decreases, TL increases [12].

Polysaccharides are a major group of naturally derived antioxidant, anti-inflammatory, and immunomodulatory carbohydrate molecules with low cytotoxicity, classified as plant-based, animal-based, and fungal polysaccharides [129–131]. Multiple polysaccharides have been found to exert unique anti-aging effects in different animal and cell models [12, 129].

In fact, it has been demonstrated that polysaccharides found in marine algae could not only reduce intracellular ROS levels but also prevent photo-aging by regulating the NF-κB, ap-1, and MAPK signaling pathways [63]. These polysaccharides have also shown potential in counteracting aging by reducing oxidation- and inflammation-related damage increasing telomerase activity, and inhibiting telomere shortening in animal models [130]. The anti-aging effect of polysaccharides isolated from turmeric may partly be mediated by the upregulation of the TERT function [130]. In clinical studies, dietary supplementation with the polysaccharide extract of Astragalus seemed to enhance TL in healthy subjects [130].

Notably, some polysaccharides have also been reported to impair the telomeric regions or inhibit telomerase enzyme activity in cancer cells to exert antitumor effects suggesting a different mode of action depending on specific disease states [12, 130].

Although the results observed in animal and cell models are not always applicable to humans, current evidence supports the potential of the above-mentioned compounds for use in anti-aging strategies to promote skin youth and improve overall well-being and longevity.

21.8 Conclusions

Overall, this chapter provides an overview of skin aging, its molecular mechanisms, and potential therapeutic approaches. Cutaneous aging is driven by both intrinsic and extrinsic factors. Intrinsic aging is mainly determined by telomere shortening and hormonal changes, while external factors, such as UV radiation, air pollution, and tobacco use, contribute to extrinsic aging. The most prevalent hypothesis on skin aging focuses on cellular senescence and its related processes, including oxidative stress, low-grade inflammation (inflammaging), telomere shortening, and DNA damage. Senescent fibroblasts play a crucial role in skin aging by inducing DNA damage and senescence in neighboring cells, ultimately compromising skin regeneration and structure. While keratinocytes possess telomerase to counteract telomere attrition, they also contribute to skin aging through the release of cytokines. Further research is clearly needed to understand the senescence processes in order to identify targeted therapeutic interventions for controlling skin aging.

Abbreviations

Activator protein-1 (AP-1)
Adenosine monophosphate/adenosine triphosphate (AMP/ATP)
Adenosine monophosphate-activated protein kinase (AMPK)
Advanced glycation end (AGE)
CCAAT/enhancer-binding protein beta (C/EBPβ)
C-X-C motif chemokine receptor 3 (CXCR3)
Cyclooxygenases (COXs)
Dendritic cells (DCs)
Dyskeratosis congenita (DC)
Extracellular matrix (ECM)
Hexokinase 2 (HK2)
High-mobility group box 1 (HMGB1)
Human telomerase reverse transcriptase (hTERT)
Immunofluorescence in situ hybridization (immunoFISH)
Langerhans cells (LHCs)
Major histocompatibility complex II (MHC II)
Mesenchymal stem cells (MSCs)
Nicotinamide adenine dinucleotide phosphate (NADPH)
Nuclear factor-kappa B (NF-kB)
p38 mitogen-activated protein kinases (MAPK)
Receptor tyrosine kinases (RTKs)
Senescence-associated secretory phenotype (SASP)
Senescence-associated β-galactosidase (SA-β-Gal)
Soluble epidermal factor (ESF)
Stress-induced premature senescence (SIPS)
T regulatory (Treg)

Telomerase RNA component (TERC)
Telomere length (TL)
Telomere-associated foci (TAF)
Transforming growth factor-beta1 (TGF-β1)
Ultraviolet (UV)
Xeroderma pigmentosum (XP)

References

1. Choi, E. H. (2019). Aging of the skin barrier, *Clin Dermatol*, **37**, pp. 336–345.
2. d'Adda di Fagagna, F. (2008). Living on a break: cellular senescence as a DNA-damage response, *Nat Rev Cancer*, **8**, pp. 512–522.
3. Stalder, J. F., Tennstedt, D., Deleuran, M., Fabbrocini, G., de Lucas, R., Haftek, M., Cottin, K., Saint Aroman, M. (2014). Fragility of epidermis and its consequence in dermatology, *J Eur Acad Dermatol Venereol*, **28**, pp. 1–18.
4. Nielsen, K. P., Zhao, L., Stamnes, J. J., Stamnes, K. and Moan, J. (2006). The importance of the depth distribution of melanin in skin for DNA protection and other photobiological processes, *J Photochem Photobiol B*, **82**, pp. 194–198.
5. Richmond, J. M., & Harris, J. E. (2014). Immunology and skin in health and disease, *Cold Spring Harb Perspect Med*, **4**, pp. a015339.
6. Sarin, K. Y., Cheung, P., Gilison, D., Lee, E., Tennen, R. I., Wang, E., Artandi, M. K., Oro, A. E., Artandi, S. E. (2005). Conditional telomerase induction causes proliferation of hair follicle stem cells, *Nature*, **436**, pp. 1048–1052.
7. Krishnan, R., Rajeswari, R., Venugopal, J., Sundarrajan, S., Sridhar, R., Shayanti, M., & Ramakrishna, S. (2012). Polysaccharide nanofibrous scaffolds as a model for in vitro skin tissue regeneration, *J Mater Sci Mater Med*, **23**, pp. 1511–1519.
8. Tsepkolenko, A., Tsepkolenko, V., Dash, S., Mishra, A., Bader, A., Melerzanov, A. and Giri, S. (2019). The regenerative potential of skin and the immune system, *Clin Cosmet Investig Dermatol*, **12**, pp. 519–532.
9. Gerasymchuk, M., Cherkasova, V., Kovalchuk, O. and Kovalchuk, I. (2020). The role of microRNAs in organismal and skin aging, *Int J Mol Sci*, **21**, pp. 5281.

10. Khavkin, J. and Ellis, D. A. F. (2011). Aging skin: histology, physiology, and pathology, *Facial Plast Surg Clin North Am*, **19**, pp. 229–234.
11. Geng, R., Kang, S.-G., Huang, K. and Tong, T. (2021). Boosting the photoaged skin: the potential role of dietary components, *Nutrients*, **13**, pp. 1691.
12. Jacczak, B., Rubiś, B. and Totoń, E. (2021). Potential of naturally derived compounds in telomerase and telomere modulation in skin senescence and aging, *Int J Mol Sci*, **22**, pp. 6381.
13. Höhn, A., Weber, D., Jung, T., Ott, C., Hugo, M., Kochlik, B., Kehm, R., König, J., Grune, T., Castro, J. P. (2017). Happily (n)ever after: aging in the context of oxidative stress, proteostasis loss and cellular senescence, *Redox Biol*, **11**, pp. 482–501.
14. Hayflick, L. and Moorhead, P. S. (1961). The serial cultivation of human diploid cell strains, *Experimental Cell Research*, **25**, pp. 585–621.
15. Blackburn, E. H. and Challoner, P. B. (1984). Identification of a telomeric DNA sequence in Trypanosoma brucei, *Cell*, **36**, pp. 447–457.
16. Fagagna, F. d'Adda di, Reaper, P. M., Clay-Farrace, L., Fiegler, H., Carr, P., von Zglinicki, T., Saretzki, G., Carter, N. P., Jackson, S. P. (2003). A DNA damage checkpoint response in telomere-initiated senescence, *Nature*, **426**, pp. 194–198.
17. Jeyapalan, J. C., Ferreira, M., Sedivy, J. M. and Herbig, U. (2007). Accumulation of senescent cells in mitotic tissue of aging primates, *Mech Ageing Dev*, **128**, pp. 36–44.
18. Friedman, O. (2005). Changes associated with the aging face, *Facial Plast Surg Clin North Am*, **13**, pp. 371–380.
19. Mancini, M., Lena, A. M., Saintigny, G., Mahé, C., Di Daniele, N., Melino, G. and Candi, E. (2014). MicroRNAs in human skin ageing, *Ageing Res Rev*, **17**, pp. 9–15.
20. Poljšak, B., Dahmane, R. G. and Godić, A. (2012). Intrinsic skin aging: the role of oxidative stress, *Acta Dermatovenerol Alp Pannonica Adriat*, **21**, pp. 33–36.
21. Kammeyer, A. and Luiten, R. M. (2015). Oxidation events and skin aging, *Ageing Res Rev*, **21**, pp. 16–29.
22. Farage, M. A., Miller, K. W., Elsner, P. and Maibach, H. I. (2007). Structural characteristics of the aging skin: a review, *Cutan Ocul Toxicol*, **26**, pp. 343–357.
23. Puizina-Ivić, N. (2008). Skin aging, *Acta Dermatovenerol Alp Pannonica Adriat*, **17**, pp. 47–54.

24. Tobin, D. J. (2017). Introduction to skin aging, *J Tissue Viability*, **26**, pp. 37–46.

25. Oikarinen, A. (1990). The aging of skin: chronoaging versus photoaging, *Photodermatol Photoimmunol Photomed*, **7**, pp. 3–4.

26. Jin, S., Li, K., Zong, X., Eun, S., Morimoto, N. and Guo, S. (2023). Hallmarks of skin aging: update, *Aging Dis*, **14**, pp. 2167–2176.

27. Moskalev, A. A., Shaposhnikov, M. V., Plyusnina, E. N., Zhavoronkov, A., Budovsky, A., Yanai, H. and Fraifeld, V. E. (2013). The role of DNA damage and repair in aging through the prism of Koch-like criteria, *Ageing Res Rev*, **12**, pp. 661–684.

28. Blackburn, E. H., Greider, C. W. and Szostak, J. W. (2006). Telomeres and telomerase: the path from maize, Tetrahymena and yeast to human cancer and aging, *Nat Med*, **12**, pp. 1133–1138.

29. Palm, W. and de Lange, T. (2008). How shelterin protects mammalian telomeres? *Annu Rev Genet*, **42**, pp. 301–334.

30. Takai, H., Smogorzewska, A. and de Lange, T. (2003). DNA damage foci at dysfunctional telomeres, *Current Biology*, **13**, no. 17, pp. 1549–1556.

31. Shay, J. W. (2018). Telomeres and aging, *Current Opinion in Cell Biology*, **52**, pp. 1–7.

32. Usategui, A., Municio, C., Arias-Salgado, E. G., Martín, M., Fernández-Varas, B., Del Rey, M. J., Carreira, P., González, A., Criado, G., Perona, R., Pablos, J. L. (2022). Evidence of telomere attrition and a potential role for DNA damage in systemic sclerosis, *Immun Ageing*, **19**, pp. 7.

33. Papaccio, F., D Arino, A., Caputo, S. and Bellei, B. (2022). Focus on the contribution of oxidative stress in skin aging, *Antioxidants (Basel)*, **11**, pp. 1121.

34. Dorgaleleh, S., Naghipoor, K., Hajimohammadi, Z., Dastaviz, F. and Oladnabi, M. (2022). Molecular insight of dyskeratosis congenita: defects in telomere length homeostasis, *J Clin Transl Res*, **8**, pp. 20–30.

35. Grönniger, E., Weber, B., Heil, O., Peters, N., Stäb, F., Wenck, H., Korn, B., Winnefeld, M., Lyko, F. (2010). Aging and chronic sun exposure cause distinct epigenetic changes in human skin, *PLoS Genet*, **6**, pp. e1000971.

36. Kim, H. S., Park, S.-Y., Moon, S. H., Lee, J. D. and Kim, S. (2018). Autophagy in human skin fibroblasts: impact of age, *Int J Mol Sci*, **19**, pp. 2254.

37. Waller, J. M. and Maibach, H. I. (2005). Age and skin structure and function, a quantitative approach (I): blood flow, pH, thickness, and ultrasound echogenicity, *Skin Res Technol*, **11**, pp. 221–235.

38. Farage, M. A., Miller, K. W., Elsner, P. and Maibach, H. I. (2007). Structural characteristics of the aging skin: a review, *Cutan Ocul Toxicol*, **26**, pp. 343–357.

39. Lee, H., Hong, Y. and Kim, M. (2021). Structural and functional changes and possible molecular mechanisms in aged skin, *Int J Mol Sci*, **22**, pp. 12489.

40. Wlaschek, M., Tantcheva-Poór, I., Naderi, L., Ma, W., Schneider, L. A., Razi-Wolf, Z., Scharffetter-Kochanek, K. (2001). Solar UV irradiation and dermal photoaging, *J Photochem Photobiol B*, **63**, pp. 41–51.

41. Krutmann, J., Bouloc, A., Sore, G., Bernard, B. A. and Passeron, T. (2017). The skin aging exposome, *J Dermatol Sci*, **85**, pp. 152–161.

42. Young, A. R. (2006). Acute effects of UVR on human eyes and skin, *Prog Biophys Mol Biol*, **92**, pp. 80–85.

43. Kligman, L. H. (1989). Photoaging, manifestations, prevention, and treatment, *Clin Geriatr Med*, **5**, pp. 235–251.

44. Morita, A. (2007). Tobacco smoke causes premature skin aging, *J Dermatol Sci*, **48**, pp. 169–175.

45. Passos, J. F., Nelson, G., Wang, C., Richter, T., Simillion, C., Proctor, C. J., Miwa, S., Olijslagers, S., Hallinan, J., Wipat, A., Saretzki, G., Rudolph, K. L., Kirkwood, T. B., von Zglinicki, T. (2010). Feedback between p21 and reactive oxygen production is necessary for cell senescence, *Mol Syst Biol*, **6**, pp. 347.

46. Korolchuk, V. I., Miwa, S., Carroll, B. and von Zglinicki, T. (2017). Mitochondria in cell senescence: is mitophagy the weakest link? *EBioMedicine*, **21**, pp. 7–13.

47. Gorgoulis, V., Adams, P. D., Alimonti, A., Bennett, D. C., Bischof, O., Bishop, C., Bishop, C., Campisi, J., Collado, M., Evangelou, K., Ferbeyre, G., Gil, J., Hara, E., Krizhanovsky, V., Jurk, D., Maier, A. B., Narita, M., Niedernhofer, L., Passos, J. F., Robbins, P. D., Schmitt, C. A., Demaria, M. (2019). Cellular senescence: defining a path forward, *Cell*, **179**, pp. 813–827.

48. Fitsiou, E., Pulido, T., Campisi, J., Alimirah, F. and Demaria, M. (2021). Cellular senescence and the senescence-associated secretory phenotype as drivers of skin photoaging, *J Invest Dermatol*, **141**, pp. 1119–1126.

49. Tuttle, C. S. L., Waaijer, M. E. C., Slee-Valentijn, M. S., Stijnen, T., Westendorp, R. and Maier, A. B. (2020). Cellular senescence and chronological age in various human tissues: a systematic review and meta-analysis, *Aging Cell*, **19**, pp. e13083.

50. Toutfaire, M., Bauwens, E. and Debacq-Chainiaux, F. (2017). The impact of cellular senescence in skin ageing: a notion of mosaic and therapeutic strategies, *Biochem Pharmacol*, **142**, pp. 1–12.
51. Velarde, M. C. and Demaria, M. (2016). Targeting senescent cells: possible implications for delaying skin aging: a mini-review, *Gerontology*, **62**, pp. 513–518.
52. Zhang, J., Yu, H., Man, M.-Q. and Hu, L. (2024). Aging in the dermis: fibroblast senescence and its significance, *Aging Cell*, **23**, pp. e14054.
53. D'Errico, M., Lemma, T., Calcagnile, A., Santis, L. P. D. and Dogliotti, E. (2007). Cell type and DNA damage specific response of human skin cells to environmental agents, *Mutation Research/Fundamental and Molecular Mechanisms of Mutagenesis*, **614**, pp. 37–47.
54. Rodier, F., Coppé, J.-P., Patil, C. K., Hoeijmakers, W. A. M., Muñoz, D. P., Raza, S. R., Freund, A., Campeau, E., Davalos, A. R., Campisi, J. (2009). Persistent DNA damage signalling triggers senescence-associated inflammatory cytokine secretion, *Nat Cell Biol*, **11**, pp. 973–979.
55. Collado, M. and Serrano, M. (2010). Senescence in tumours: evidence from mice and humans, *Nat Rev Cancer*, **10**, pp. 51–57.
56. Chen, W., Kang, J., Xia, J., Li, Y., Yang, B., Chen, B., Sun, W., Song, X., Xiang, W., Wang, X., Wang, F., Wan, Y., Bi, Z. (2008). p53-related apoptosis resistance and tumor suppression activity in UVB-induced premature senescent human skin fibroblasts, *Int J Mol Med*, **21**, pp. 645–653.
57. Wang, A. S., Ong, P. F., Chojnowski, A., Clavel, C. and Dreesen, O. (2017). Loss of lamin B1 is a biomarker to quantify cellular senescence in photoaged skin, *Sci Rep*, **7**, pp. 15678.
58. Victorelli, S., Lagnado, A., Halim, J., Moore, W., Talbot, D., Barrett, K., Chapman, J., Birch, J., Ogrodnik, M., Meves, A., Pawlikowski, J. S., Jurk, D., Adams, P. D., van Heemst, D., Beekman, M., Slagboom, P. E., Gunn, D. A., Passos, J. F. (2019). Senescent human melanocytes drive skin ageing via paracrine telomere dysfunction, *EMBO J*, **38**, pp. e101982.
59. Taylor, K. L., Lister, J. A., Zeng, Z., Ishizaki, H., Anderson, C., Kelsh, R. N., Jackson, I. J., Patton, E. E. (2011). Differentiated melanocyte cell division occurs in vivo and is promoted by mutations in Mitf, *Development*, **138**, pp. 3579–3589.
60. Lewis, D. A., Yi, Q., Travers, J. B. and Spandau, D. F. (2008). UVB-induced senescence in human keratinocytes requires a functional insulin-like growth factor-1 receptor and p53, *Mol Biol Cell*, **19**, pp. 1346–1353.

61. Nassour, J. and Abbadie, C. (2016). A novel role for DNA single-strand breaks in senescence and neoplastic escape of epithelial cells, *Mol Cell Oncol*, **3**, pp. e1190885.
62. Ryu, Y. S., Kang, K. A., Piao, M. J., Ahn, M. J., Yi, J. M., Bossis, G., Hyun, Y. M., Park, C. O., Hyun, J. W. (2019). Particulate matter-induced senescence of skin keratinocytes involves oxidative stress-dependent epigenetic modifications, *Exp Mol Med*, **51**, pp. 1–14.
63. Vaiserman, A. and Krasnienkov, D. (2021). Telomere length as a marker of biological age: state-of-the-art, open issues, and future perspectives, *Front. Genet.*, **11**, pp. 630186.
64. Sugimoto, M., Yamashita, R. and Ueda, M. (2006). Telomere length of the skin in association with chronological aging and photoaging, *J Dermatol Sci*, **43**, pp. 43–47.
65. Oikawa, S., Tada-Oikawa, S. and Kawanishi, S. (2001). Site-specific DNA damage at the GGG sequence by UVA involves acceleration of telomere shortening, *Biochemistry*, **40**, pp. 4763–4768.
66. Krunic, D., Moshir, S., Greulich-Bode, K. M., Figueroa, R., Cerezo, A., Stammer, H., Stark, H. J., Gray, S. G., Nielsen, K. V., Hartschuh, W., Boukamp, P. (2009). Tissue context-activated telomerase in human epidermis correlates with little age-dependent telomere loss, *Biochim Biophys Acta*, **1792**, pp. 297–308.
67. Demaria, M., Desprez, P. Y., Campisi, J. and Velarde, M. C. (2015). Cell autonomous and non-autonomous effects of senescent cells in the skin, *J Invest Dermatol*, **135**, pp. 1722–1726.
68. Salma, F., Yassire, O., Youssef, B., Corinne, D. and Ameziane El Hassani, R. (2024). Methods for detection of mitochondrial reactive oxygen species in senescent cells, *Methods Cell Biol*, **181**, pp. 33–41.
69. Hensley, K. and Floyd, R. A. (2002). Reactive oxygen species and protein oxidation in aging: a look back, a look ahead, *Arch Biochem Biophys*, **397**, pp. 377–383.
70. Rinnerthaler, M., Bischof, J., Streubel, M. K., Trost, A. and Richter, K. (2015). Oxidative stress in aging human skin, *Biomolecules*, **5**, pp. 545–589.
71. Takahara, M., Kang, K., Liu, L., Yoshida, Y., McCormick, T. S. and Cooper, K. D. (2003). iC3b arrests monocytic cell differentiation into CD1c-expressing dendritic cell precursors: a mechanism for transiently decreased dendritic cells in vivo after human skin injury by ultraviolet B, *J Invest Dermatol*, **120**, pp. 802–809.

72. Berneburg, M., Plettenberg, H., Medve-König, K., Pfahlberg, A., Gers-Barlag, H., Gefeller, O. and Krutmann, J. (2004). Induction of the photoaging-associated mitochondrial common deletion in vivo in normal human skin, *J Invest Dermatol*, **122**, pp. 1277–1283.
73. Hwang, J. S., Hwang, J. S., Chang, I. and Kim, S. (2007). Age-associated decrease in proteasome content and activities in human dermal fibroblasts: restoration of normal level of proteasome subunits reduces aging markers in fibroblasts from elderly persons, *J Gerontol A Biol Sci Med Sci*, **62**, pp. 490–499.
74. Fisher, G. J. and Voorhees, J. J. (1998). Molecular mechanisms of photoaging and its prevention by retinoic acid: ultraviolet irradiation induces MAP kinase signal transduction cascades that induce Ap-1-regulated matrix metalloproteinases that degrade human skin in vivo, *J Investigative Dermatol Symp. Proc.*, **3**, pp. 61–68.
75. Quan, T., Shao, Y., He, T., Voorhees, J. J. and Fisher, G. J. (2010). Reduced expression of connective tissue growth factor (CTGF/CCN2) mediates collagen loss in chronologically aged human skin, *J Invest Dermatol*, **130**, pp. 415–424.
76. Oblong, J. E., Bowman, A., Rovito, H. A., Jarrold, B. B., Sherrill, J. D., Black, M. R., Nelson, G., Kimball, A. B., Birch-Machin, M. A. (2020). Metabolic dysfunction in human skin: restoration of mitochondrial integrity and metabolic output by nicotinamide (niacinamide) in primary dermal fibroblasts from older aged donors, *Aging Cell*, **19**, pp. e13248.
77. Kuehne, A., Hildebrand, J., Soehle, J., Wenck, H., Terstegen, L., Gallinat, S., Knott, A., Winnefeld, M., Zamboni, N. (2017). An integrative metabolomics and transcriptomics study to identify metabolic alterations in aged skin of humans in vivo, *BMC Genomics*, **18**, pp. 169.
78. Windler, C., Gey, C. and Seeger, K. (2017). Skin melanocytes and fibroblasts show different changes in choline metabolism during cellular senescence, *Mech Ageing Dev*, **164**, pp. 82–90.
79. Haendeler, J., Dröse, S., Büchner, N., Jakob, S., Altschmied, J., Goy, C., Spyridopoulos, I., Zeiher, A. M., Brandt, U., Dimmeler, S. (2009). Mitochondrial telomerase reverse transcriptase binds to and protects mitochondrial DNA and function from damage, *Arterioscler Thromb Vasc Biol*, **29**, pp. 929–935.
80. Carrero, D., Soria-Valles, C. and López-Otín, C. (2016). Hallmarks of progeroid syndromes: lessons from mice and reprogrammed cells, *Dis Model Mech*, **9**, pp. 719–735.
81. Turenne, G. A., Paul, P., Laflair, L. and Price, B. D. (2001). Activation of p53 transcriptional activity requires ATM's kinase domain and

multiple N-terminal serine residues of p53, *Oncogene*, **20**, pp. 5100–5110.

82. Hewitt, G., Jurk, D., Marques, F. D. M., Correia-Melo, C., Hardy, T., Gackowska, A., Anderson, R., Taschuk, M., Mann, J., Passos, J. F. (2012). Telomeres are favoured targets of a persistent DNA damage response in ageing and stress-induced senescence, *Nat Commun*, **3**, pp. 708.
83. Henle, E. S., Han, Z., Tang, N., Rai, P., Luo, Y. and Linn, S. (1999). Sequence-specific DNA cleavage by Fe2+-mediated fenton reactions has possible biological implications, *J Biol Chem*, **274**, pp. 962–971.
84. You, Y. H., Lee, D. H., Yoon, J. H., Nakajima, S., Yasui, A. and Pfeifer, G. P. (2001). Cyclobutane pyrimidine dimers are responsible for the vast majority of mutations induced by UVB irradiation in mammalian cells, *J Biol Chem*, **276**, pp. 44688–44694.
85. Farage, M. A., Miller, K. W., Elsner, P. and Maibach, H. I. (2008). Intrinsic and extrinsic factors in skin ageing: a review, *Int J Cosmet Sci*, **30**, pp. 87–95.
86. Ravanat, J. L., Douki, T. and Cadet, J. (2001). Direct and indirect effects of UV radiation on DNA and its components, *J Photochem Photobiol B*, **63**, pp. 88–102.
87. Panich, U., Sittithumcharee, G., Rathviboon, N. and Jirawatnotai, S. (2016). Ultraviolet radiation-induced skin aging: the role of DNA damage and oxidative stress in epidermal stem cell damage mediated skin aging, *Stem Cells Int*, **2016**, pp. 7370642.
88. Kamenisch, Y. and Berneburg, M. (2009). Progeroid syndromes and UV-induced oxidative DNA damage, *J Investig Dermatol Symp Proc*, **14**, pp. 8–14.
89. Contet-Audonneau, J. L., Jeanmaire, C. and Pauly, G. (1999). A histological study of human wrinkle structures: comparison between sun-exposed areas of the face, with or without wrinkles, and sun-protected areas, *Br J Dermatol*, **140**, pp. 1038–1047.
90. Trautinger, F., Mazzucco, K., Knobler, R. M., Trenz, A. and Kokoschka, E. M. (1994). UVA- and UVB-induced changes in hairless mouse skin collagen, *Arch Dermatol Res*, **286**, pp. 490–494.
91. Bonta, M., Daina, L. and Muţiu, G. (2013). The process of ageing reflected by histological changes in the skin, *Rom J Morphol Embryol*, **54**, pp. 797–804.
92. Pilkington, S. M., Bulfone-Paus, S., Griffiths, C. E. M. and Watson, R. E. B. (2021). Inflammaging and the skin, *J Invest Dermatol*, **141**, pp. 1087–1095.

93. Franceschi, C., Bonafè, M., Valensin, S., Olivieri, F., De Luca, M., Ottaviani, E. and De Benedictis, G. (2000). Inflammaging: an evolutionary perspective on immunosenescence, *Ann N Y Acad Sci*, **908**, pp. 244–254.

94. Nelson, G., Wordsworth, J., Wang, C., Jurk, D., Lawless, C., Martin-Ruiz, C. and von Zglinicki, T. (2012). A senescent cell bystander effect: senescence-induced senescence, *Aging Cell*, **11**, pp. 345–349.

95. Acosta, J. C., Banito, A., Wuestefeld, T., Georgilis, A., Janich, P., Morton, J. P., Athineos, D., Kang, T. W., Lasitschka, F., Andrulis, M., Pascual, G., Morris, K. J., Khan, S., Jin, H., Dharmalingam, G., Snijders, A. P., Carroll, T., Capper, D., Pritchard, C., Inman, G. J., Longerich, T., Sansom, O. J., Benitah, S. A., Zender, L., Gil, J. (2013). A complex secretory program orchestrated by the inflammasome controls paracrine senescence, *Nat Cell Biol*, **15**, pp. 978–990.

96. Wajapeyee, N., Serra, R. W., Zhu, X., Mahalingam, M. and Green, M. R. (2008). Oncogenic BRAF induces senescence and apoptosis through pathways mediated by the secreted protein IGFBP7, *Cell*, **132**, pp. 363–374.

97. Ezure, T., Sugahara, M. and Amano, S. (2019). Senescent dermal fibroblasts negatively influence fibroblast extracellular matrix-related gene expression partly via secretion of complement factor D, *Biofactors*, **45**, pp. 556–562.

98. Biran, A., Zada, L., Abou Karam, P., Vadai, E., Roitman, L., Ovadya, Y., Porat, Z., Krizhanovsky, V. (2017). Quantitative identification of senescent cells in aging and disease, *Aging Cell*, **16**, pp. 661–671.

99. Kang, C., Xu, Q., Martin, T. D., Li, M. Z., Demaria, M., Aron, L., Lu, T., Yankner, B. A., Campisi, J., Elledge, S. J. (2015). The DNA damage response induces inflammation and senescence by inhibiting autophagy of GATA4, *Science*, **349**, pp. aaa5612.

100. Hayakawa, T., Iwai, M., Aoki, S., Takimoto, K., Maruyama, M., Maruyama, W. and Motoyama, N. (2015). SIRT1 suppresses the senescence-associated secretory phenotype through epigenetic gene regulation, *PLoS One*, **10**, pp. e0116480.

101. Kuilman, T., Michaloglou, C., Vredeveld, L. C. W., Douma, S., van Doorn, R., Desmet, C. J., Aarden, L. A., Mooi, W. J., Peeper, D. S. (2008). Oncogene-induced senescence relayed by an interleukin-dependent inflammatory network, *Cell*, **133**, pp. 1019–1031.

102. Waldera Lupa, D. M., Kalfalah, F., Safferling, K., Boukamp, P., Poschmann, G., Volpi, E., Götz-Rösch, C., Bernerd, F., Haag, L., Hueben-

thal, U., Fritsche, E., Boege, F., Grabe, N., Tigges, J., Stühler, K., Krutmann, J. (2015). Characterization of skin aging-associated secreted proteins (SAASP) produced by dermal fibroblasts isolated from intrinsically aged human skin, *J Invest Dermatol*, **135**, pp. 1954–1968.

103. Bierman, J. C., Laughlin, T., Tamura, M., Hulette, B. C., Mack, C. E., Sherrill, J. D., Tan, C. Y. R., Morenc, M., Bellanger, S., Oblong, J. E. (2020). Niacinamide mitigates SASP-related inflammation induced by environmental stressors in human epidermal keratinocytes and skin, *Int J Cosmet Sci*, **42**, pp. 501–511.
104. Tiemessen, M. M., Jagger, A. L., Evans, H. G., van Herwijnen, M. J. C., John, S. and Taams, L. S. (2007). CD4+CD25+Foxp3+ regulatory T cells induce alternative activation of human monocytes/macrophages, *Proc Natl Acad Sci U S A*, **104**, pp. 19446–19451.
105. Horiba, S., Kawamoto, M., Tobita, R., Kami, R., Ogura, Y. and Hosoi, J. (2023). M1/M2 macrophage skewing is related to reduction in types I, V, and VI collagens with aging in sun-exposed human skin, *JID Innov*, **3**, pp. 100222.
106. Guimarães, G. R., Almeida, P. P., de Oliveira Santos, L., Rodrigues, L. P., de Carvalho, J. L. and Boroni, M. (2021). Hallmarks of Aging in macrophages: consequences to skin inflammaging, *Cells*, **10**, pp. 1323.
107. Farrar, M. D. (2016). Advanced glycation end products in skin ageing and photoageing: what are the implications for epidermal function? *Exp Dermatol*, **25**, pp. 947–948.
108. Zhang, S. and Duan, E. (2018). Fighting against skin aging: the way from bench to bedside, *Cell Transplant*, **27**, pp. 729–738.
109. Jin, S., Li, K., Zong, X., Eun, S., Morimoto, N. and Guo, S. (2023). Hallmarks of skin aging: update, *Aging Dis*, **14**, pp. 2167–2176.
110. Son, N., Cui, Y. and Xi, W. (2022). Association between telomere length and skin cancer and aging: a mendelian randomization analysis, *Front Genet*, **13**, pp. 931785.
111. Buckingham, E. M. and Klingelhutz, A. J. (2011). The role of telomeres in the ageing of human skin, *Exp Dermatol*, **20**, pp. 297–302.
112. Fenech, M. F., Bull, C. F. and Van Klinken, B. J.-W. (2023). Protective effects of micronutrient supplements, phytochemicals and phytochemical-rich beverages and foods against DNA damage in humans: a systematic review of randomized controlled trials and prospective studies, *Adv Nutr*, **14**, pp. 1337–1358.
113. Solway, J., McBride, M., Haq, F., Abdul, W. and Miller, R. (2020). Diet and dermatology: the role of a whole-food, plant-based diet in preventing

and reversing skin aging - a review, *J Clin Aesthet Dermatol*, **13**, pp. 38–43.

114. Factor, V. M., Laskowska, D., Jensen, M. R., Woitach, J. T., Popescu, N. C. and Thorgeirsson, S. S. (2000). Vitamin E reduces chromosomal damage and inhibits hepatic tumor formation in a transgenic mouse model, *Proc Natl Acad Sci U S A*, **97**, pp. 2196–2201.
115. Makpol, S., Zainuddin, A., Rahim, N. A., Yusof, Y. A. and Ngah, W. Z. (2010). Alpha-tocopherol modulates hydrogen peroxide-induced DNA damage and telomere shortening of human skin fibroblasts derived from differently aged individuals, *Planta Med*, **76**, pp. 869–875.
116. Buckingham, E. M. and Klingelhutz, A. J. (2011). The role of telomeres in the ageing of human skin, *Exp Dermatol*, **20**, pp. 297–302.
117. Yokoo, S., Furumoto, K., Hiyama, E. and Miwa, N. (2004). Slow-down of age-dependent telomere shortening is executed in human skin keratinocytes by hormesis-like-effects of trace hydrogen peroxide or by anti-oxidative effects of pro-vitamin C in common concurrently with reduction of intracellular oxidative stress, *J Cell Biochem*, **93**, pp. 588–597.
118. Cai, Y., Zhong, Y., Zhang, H., Lu, P.-L., Liang, Y.-Y., Hu, B. and Wu, H. (2023). Association between dietary vitamin C and telomere length: a cross-sectional study, *Front Nutr*, **10**, pp. 1025936.
119. You, Y. O., Lee, G. and Min, B. M. (2000). Retinoic acid extends the in vitro life span of normal human oral keratinocytes by decreasing p16(INK4A) expression and maintaining telomerase activity, *Biochem Biophys Res Commun*, **268**, pp. 268–274.
120. Mizuno, Y., Konishi, S., Goto, C., Yoshinaga, J., Hidaka, M. and Imai, H. (2021). Association between nutrient intake and telomere length in Japanese female university students, *Biomarkers*, **26**, pp. 138–145.
121. Pusceddu, I., Farrell, C.-J. L., Di Pierro, A. M., Jani, E., Herrmann, W. and Herrmann, M. (2015). The role of telomeres and vitamin D in cellular aging and age-related diseases, *Clin Chem Lab Med*, **53**, pp. 1661–1678.
122. Csekes, E. and Račková, L. (2021). Skin aging, cellular senescence and natural polyphenols, *Int J Mol Sci*, **22**, pp. 12641.
123. D'Angelo, S. (2023). Diet and aging: the role of polyphenol-rich diets in slow down the shortening of telomeres: a review, *Antioxidants (Basel)*, **12**, pp. 2086.
124. Pereira, Q. C., Dos Santos, T. W., Fortunato, I. M. and Ribeiro, M. L. (2023). The molecular mechanism of polyphenols in the regulation of ageing hallmarks, *Int J Mol Sci*, **24**, pp. 5508.

125. Bouwstra, J. A., Nădăban, A., Bras, W., McCabe, C., Bunge, A. and Gooris, G. S. (2023). The skin barrier: an extraordinary interface with an exceptional lipid organization, *Prog Lipid Res*, **92**, pp. 101252.

126. Ali, S., Scapagnini, G. and Davinelli, S. (2022). Effect of omega-3 fatty acids on the telomere length: a mini meta-analysis of clinical trials, *Biomol Concepts*, **13**, pp. 25–33.

127. Hyun, Y. J., Piao, M. J., Kang, K. A., Zhen, A. X., Madushan Fernando, P. D. S., Kang, H. K., Ahn, Y. S., Hyun, J. W. (2019). Effect of fermented fish oil on fine particulate matter-induced skin aging, *Mar Drugs*, **17**, pp. 61.

128. Ogłuszka, M., Lipiński, P. and Starzyński, R. R. (2022). Effect of omega-3 fatty acids on telomeres: are they the elixir of youth? *Nutrients*, **14**, pp. 3723.

129. Guo, X., Luo, J., Qi, J., Zhao, X., An, P., Luo, Y. and Wang, G. (2022). The role and mechanism of polysaccharides in anti-aging, *Nutrients*, **14**, pp. 5330.

130. Xu, W., Han, S., Huang, M., Yin, J., Yang, F. and Luo, F. (2022). Antiaging effects of dietary polysaccharides: advance and mechanisms, *Oxid Med Cell Longev*, **2022**, pp. 4362479.

131. Yu, Y., Shen, M., Song, Q. and Xie, J. (2018). Biological activities and pharmaceutical applications of polysaccharide from natural resources: a review, *Carbohydr Polym*, **183**, pp. 91–101.

Part V

Therapeutic Approaches

Chapter 22

Telomeres, Telomerase, and Shelterin Complex: Promising Drug Targets for Longevity, Age-Related Diseases, and Cancer

Marios Spanakis[a,b] **and Aristidis Tsatsakis**[a,b]

[a] *Department of Forensic Sciences and Toxicology, School of Medicine, University of Crete, Heraklion, Greece*

[b] *Computational Bio-Medicine Laboratory, Institute of Computer Science, Foundation for Research and Technology—Hellas, Heraklion, Crete, Greece*

mspanakis@ics.forth.gr, tsatsaka@uoc.gr

22.1 Introduction

Telomeres are protective nucleotide sequences -(TTAGGG)n- located at the ends of eukaryotic chromosomes. Telomeres are associated with specific proteins to form loop structures called telomere loops (T-Loop and D-Loop) (Fig. 22.1). Due to the nature of DNA replication, the lagging strand in the replication process cannot completely replicate the chromosome ends leaving 3′ single-stranded overhang chain of unpaired nucleotides in the end of chromosomes. Thus, telomere T-loops form a loop structure with a 3' overhanging chain.

Telomeres: Biomarkers of a Healthy Life and Successful Aging
Edited by Aristidis Tsatsakis

ISBN 978-981-5129-49-6 (Hardcover), 978-1-003-56809-4 (eBook)
www.jennystanford.com

D-loop or displacement loop, seen in genetic recombination, forms when a single-stranded DNA invades homologous double-stranded DNA, aiding in genetic information exchange, repair, and recombination, fostering genome diversity, and maintenance [1]. While telomeres do not have translational value, they play a pivotal role in maintaining genomic integrity and cellular viability. Their primary function is to preserve genetic information shielding chromosomes from degradation, recombination, or fusion. Telomere loops are formed from telomeres in conjunction with specific proteins known as the shelterin complex [2]. This complex safeguards telomeres from degradation and incorrect repair, while also regulating access by preventing telomeres from being recognized as double-strand breaks that could activate DNA damage repair mechanisms [3]. Under normal conditions, during each cell division, telomeres undergo a natural shortening process resulting in a reduction in chromosome length as part of the replication process. This shortening continues until the strand's length reaches a certain limit known as the Hayflick limit. At this point, DNA mechanisms are activated leading to cellular senescence or apoptosis [4, 5]. To counteract this process and ensure the stability of essential genetic information, DNA mechanisms preserve telomeres after each replication process through a specialized ribonucleoprotein enzyme called telomerase, which is tasked with replenishing telomeric ends. Telomerase, by elongating telomeres, maintains cellular replicative capacity and counteracts the effects of telomere shortening.

Overall, a delicate equilibrium exists in considering the dynamics and regulation of telomeres, shelterins, and telomerase activity [6]. Any dysregulation can contribute to uncontrolled cell proliferation or cellular senescence. Telomere dynamics have been extensively studied in cancer, where the reactivation of telomerase or alternative telomere maintenance mechanisms often confers immortalization to cancer cells enabling uncontrolled cell proliferation and tumor progression [7–9]. Additionally, disruptions in the shelterin complex can lead to telomere dysfunction promoting genomic instability and providing a conducive environment for oncogenesis [3, 10, 11].

Regarding aging, the gradual attrition of telomeres due to limited telomerase activity in most somatic cells contributes to

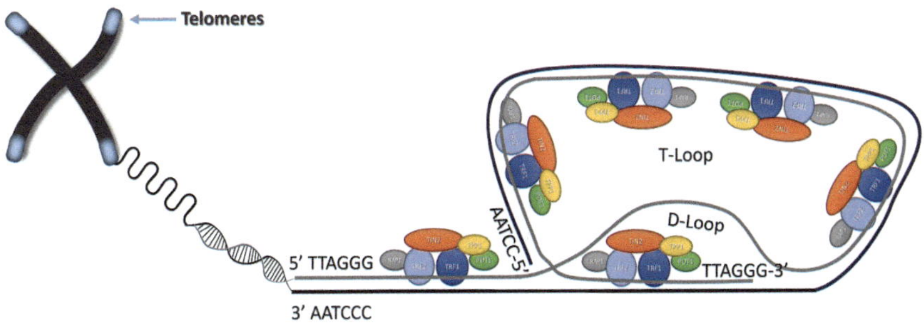

Figure 22.1 Representation of telomeres at the end of linear chromosomes representing the loop structures (T-Loop & D-Loop) and the shelterin complex.

replicative senescence and age-related decline in tissue function. Notably, the rate of telomere shortening, rather than the initial telomere length, can be associated with the aging process [12]. This phenomenon may have broader implications for overall tissue and organ deterioration observed with advancing age. Telomere shortening can disrupt chromosomal stability, induce DNA damage responses, and trigger cellular stress pathways, collectively enhancing susceptibility to age-related diseases and accelerating the aging process.

This chapter aims to explore the multifaceted relationship between telomeres, telomerase, and the shelterin complex as to their properties and basic biological functions, and their impact on aging, age-related diseases, and cancer. Moreover, it will briefly explore their potential role as emerging drug targets for interventions regarding cancer, and to improve longevity, well-being, and overall health.

22.2 Shelterin Complex Components and Role in Cell Function

The shelterin (or telosome) is a protein complex consisting of six proteins, each of which contributes specific functions to the preservation of telomere integrity (Fig. 22.2). As described earlier, telomeric DNA is formed from repetitive double-stranded sequences

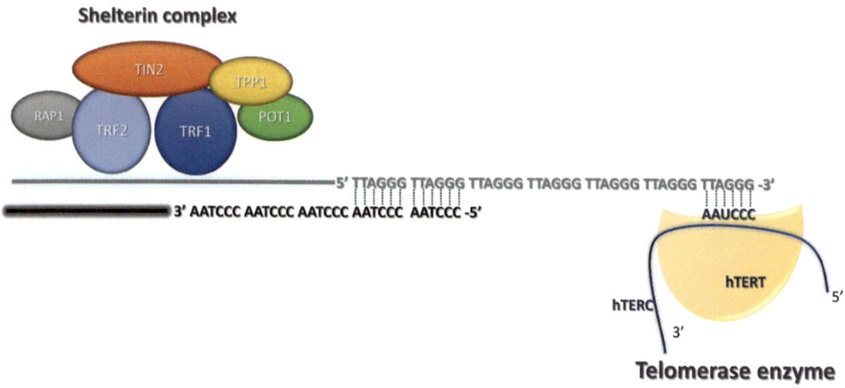

Figure 22.2 Representation of shelterin complex and telomerase during elongation in telomere edges in human chromosomes.

of 5'-TTAGGG-3' (G-strand) (2–15 kilobases in humans) coupled with the complementary 3'-AATCCC-5' (C-strand), with an overhanging 3' chain of 50–400 nucleotides at the end. A portion of the telomere's last double-stranded stretch produces a T-loop structure (telomere-loop), which is subsequently invaded by the overhanging 3' G-strand to generate a D-loop structure (displacement-loop) (Fig. 22.1). Shelterin deficiency or dysregulation can result in telomere uncapping, activating damage-signaling pathways that can lead to apoptosis, senescence, end-to-end fusions, homology-directed repair, non-homologous end joining, or genomic instability [11, 13].

I. Telomere Repeat Binding Factor 1 (TRF1)

TRF1 is a homodimeric protein that specifically recognizes and binds to the double-stranded TTAGGG region of the telomeres [14, 15]. By promoting the formation of a protective loop structure known as the T-loop, TRF1 prevents the exposure of the chromosome's ends and minimizes the chances of telomeric fusions. TRF1 employs helicase and tankyrase proteins to facilitate TL lengthening and the PIN2/TERF1-interacting telomerase inhibitor 1 (PINX1) to regulate telomere elongation by telomerase [16]. TRF1 is highly expressed in stem cells and contributes to the generation of induced pluripotent stem cells [17]. TRF1 levels seem to decrease with aging and current data associate increased TRF1 with improved memory and health span in several experimental models [18]. Considering cancer, studies suggest an upregulation of TRF1 in cancer stem cells (CSCs) such as in cases of brain tumors (i.e., glioblastoma multiforme, GBM) marking TRF1 as a potential drug target [19, 20].

II. Telomere Repeat Binding Factor 2 (TRF2)

TRF2 is structurally related to TRF1 homodimeric protein binding to the double-stranded TTAGGG region of telomeres like TRF1 [21, 22]. Its primary function is to protect telomeres from the activation of DNA damage response mechanisms. Under normal conditions, TRF2 prevents the recognition of double-strand DNA breaks, and its loss is associated with the activation of p53 and other DNA repair mechanisms whereas its overexpression leads to TL shortening. TRF1 and TRF2 recruit the rest of the proteins to form the telosome. They both prevent telomerase from adding more units to telomeres regulating their replication and the exposure to replication stress [23].

III. Repressor/Activator Protein 1 (RAP1)

RAP1 is a stabilizing protein inhibiting DNA repair mechanism. It binds to the duplex telomeric DNA and participates in regulating TL length and telomerase activity. Additionally, RAP1 interacts with TRF2 contributing to the protection of telomeres from DNA damage responses [24].

IV. Protection of Telomere 1 (POT1)

POT1 recognizes and binds to the single-stranded G-rich overhang at the 3' end of telomeres. Its role in protecting the telomeric overhang from degradation is essential for maintaining telomere length and preventing unwanted DNA repair activities. POT1 stabilizes the D-loop sheltering the 3'G overhang part and prevents nucleases from degrading DNA and thus regulating the length of the single-stranded part of telomeres [25].

V. POT1 and TIN2-Interacting Protein 1 or Adrenocortical Dysplasia Protein Homolog (TPP1)

TPP1 forms a critical subcomplex with POT1 and TIN2. Together with POT1, it binds to the single-stranded G-rich telomeric overhang. This interaction shields the single-stranded DNA from being recognized as a DNA damage signal preventing undesirable activation of DNA repair pathways. Lack of TPP1 leads to reduced levels of POT1 at telomeres, reduced telomerase processivity, ATR-dependent DNA damage response, and p53-dependent cell growth arrest.

VI. TRF1-Interacting Nuclear Factor 2 (TIN2)

TIN2 acts as a bridge, facilitating the interaction between TRF1 and TRF2 with other shelterin components. This essential role in mediating protein-protein interactions helps stabilize the shelterin complex and coordinate its functions in telomere maintenance. TIN2 links units attached to the double-stranded DNA (TRF1 and TRF2) and attached to the single-stranded DNA units (TPP1-POT1 complex) [26].

The significant coordination of the shelterin complex and its precise binding to telomeric DNA forms a protective shield around chromosome ends, effectively preventing telomere dysfunction and cellular senescence [3, 10, 27, 28]. Till today it is presumed that the shelterin complex contributes to the following processes:

- **Telomere Length Regulation**: Shelterin controls telomerase access to telomeres. Shelterin's inhibition of telomerase activity in most somatic cells helps maintain telomeres at a stable length throughout the lifespan of these cells, preventing uncontrolled telomere elongation.
- **Protection against DNA Damage Responses**: By preventing telomeres from being recognized as DNA double-strand breaks, shelterin averts the activation of DNA repair mechanisms that could lead to genomic instability and cellular dysfunction. This protective function helps maintain chromosomal integrity and prevents unwanted cellular outcomes.
- **Preserving Telomeric Chromatin Structure**: Shelterin's role in forming and stabilizing the T-loop structure at telomeres is crucial for maintaining the specialized chromatin environment unique to telomeric regions. This compact structure prevents the exposure of vulnerable chromosome ends and reduces the risk of telomeric fusions and other chromosomal abnormalities.

- **Cellular Senescence Regulation**: Shelterin dysfunction or disruption of its components can lead to telomere shortening and subsequent cellular senescence, a state of irreversible growth arrest. Cellular senescence contributes to aging and age-related diseases. The proper functioning of shelterin helps delay the onset of cellular senescence and supports cellular health and longevity.

Overall, the shelterin complex plays an important role in maintaining the stability and functionality of telomeres. Through its coordination of telomeric DNA binding, regulation of telomere length, and protection against DNA damage responses, shelterin ensures the preservation of genomic integrity and cellular viability.

22.3 Telomerase: Structure, Function, and Regulation

Telomerase is a ribonucleoprotein enzyme that plays a key role in maintaining telomere length and function ensuring genome stability and prolonging cellular replication capacity (Fig. 22.2). The core of telomerase consists of two subunits: the catalytic protein subunit identified as telomerase reverse transcriptase (TERT or hTERT for humans) and the RNA component, telomerase RNA (TERC or TR, or hTERC for humans). Together, TERT and TERC form an active holoenzyme complex that elongates telomere.

The mechanism of action of telomerase is based on a distinct and complicated enzymatic process [29]. When a cell divides, the conventional DNA replication procedure is unable to fully replicate the outer ends of the linear chromosomes. This leads to a progressive shortening of telomeres with each cell division. Telomerase restores telomeres by using its integrated RNA component (TERC) as a template. TERC contains a repetitive sequence that serves as a template for the synthesis of telomeric DNA. During telomere elongation, telomerase binds to the telomere overhang (3'-G-rich single-stranded overhang), and the TERC RNA uses its template region to direct the synthesis of new telomeric DNA sequences and elongate the telomere. This enzymatic process takes the form of reverse transcription, in which telomerase synthesizes DNA using RNA as a template. The newly synthesized telomeric DNA is then integrated into the telomeric region, replacing the lost telomeric repeats that occurred during previous replications.

Telomerase activity is tightly regulated to prevent uncontrolled elongation of telomeres, which could lead to cell immortality, which although sounds good is not, as it can lead to tumorigenesis [6]. The activity of telomerase is regulated by several mechanisms, such as:

- **Cell Cycle:** telomerase activity is usually restricted to specific stages of the cell cycle. In most somatic cells, telomerase is active only during embryonic development and is subsequently downregulated in adult tissues, except in certain regenerative cell populations (e.g., stem cells). This tight regulation helps prevent excessive telomere elongation during somatic cell division.
- **Shelterin-Mediated Regulation:** Shelterin proteins bind to telomeres and control telomerase accessibility to these regions. In its inactive state, shelterin prevents telomerase from accessing and extending telomeres, thus preventing uncontrolled telomere maintenance.
- **Epigenetic Regulation:** DNA methylation and histone modifications may affect the expression of telomerase components resulting in altered telomerase activity and telomere maintenance.
- **Alternative Lengthening of Telomeres (ALT):** A telomerase-independent mechanism known as ALT allows telomeres to be maintained. This mechanism involves homologous recombination-based processes to maintain telomere length bypassing the need for telomerase. This mechanism has been observed in cancer cells and in some rare cases in non-cancer cells.
- **Telomerase Regulation by Non-Coding RNAs:** Recent research suggests that several non-coding RNAs can interact with telomerase components and modulate their activity. These non-coding RNAs could function as regulators or effectors in the telomerase complex and contribute to fine-tuning its function.

22.4 Telomere Role in Aging and Disease

Telomerase activity and telomere length play a crucial role in the aging process as a "biological clock" for the human body [29, 30]. As cells divide and telomeres undergo natural shortening with each replication cycle, a limit is reached (Hayflick limit) at which cell division can no longer be sustained leading to a growth halt, a phenomenon called cellular senescence [4, 5, 27]. At this point, critical cellular functions decline, and the affected cells are less and less able to renew the body's tissues and organs. Telomerase, by elongating telomeres provides a way to counteract telomere shortening delaying senescence, and extending cell life. In certain cell types, such as embryonic stem cells and some immune cells, telomerase is highly active, allowing these cells to divide and maintain their function for longer periods of time. However, in most somatic cells, telomerase activity is either absent or significantly reduced after early development leading to progressive shortening of telomeres as cells divide repeatedly. This gradual loss of telomeric DNA contributes to cellular aging and is associated with age-related decline in tissue function and increased susceptibility to various diseases.

Telomeropathies or telomere biology disorders (TBD) are a group of syndromes that are usually inherited and characterized by abnormalities in genes associated directly or indirectly with telomere length or function [31–33]. These conditions often lead to premature aging, increased susceptibility to various diseases, and an elevated risk of organ failure due to impaired cellular renewal caused by dysfunctional telomeres [34, 35]. In most cases, TBDs lead to syndromes that cause dysfunction or abnormalities in the lungs, bone marrow, or neuron cells. For example, idiopathic pulmonary fibrosis (IPF) has been linked to shortened telomeres due to mutations within the shelterin complex. Aplastic anemia is a bone marrow disorder associated with mutations that alter telomere maintenance and result in reduced red blood cell production. Another well-described disorder is dyskeratosis congenita (DC), a rare inherited disease characterized by abnormalities in the skin, nails, and mucous membranes. DC patients often experience bone marrow failure, an increased risk of cancer, and other health issues due to mutations affecting telomere maintenance. Another syndrome is Hoyeraal-Hreidarsson Syndrome (HHS), a severe multisystem disorder involving developmental delay, bone marrow failure, immune deficiency, and other health problems. Lastly, the Coats Plus Syndrome (CPS) leads to abnormalities in bones, the brain, and eyes (such as retinal telangiectasia) [36–38].

Beyond the cases of TBDs where telomere dysfunctions are linked with specific syndromes, cellular senescence and telomere characteristics have increasingly been associated with various chronic diseases broadening the role of telomere dynamics in the physiology of the human body. Shortened telomeres have been associated with an increased risk of cardiovascular diseases, such as coronary heart disease and stroke. Telomere dysfunction in vascular cells can contribute to impaired endothelial function as a result of chronic inflammation, oxidative stress, and atherosclerosis, all of which are key factors in cardiovascular pathogenesis [39, 40]. In addition, cardiovascular complications often occur at a young age in patients with premature aging syndromes characterized by telomerase dysfunction [33]. In the nervous system, shortened telomeres have been observed in neurodegenerative disorders including Alzheimer's and Parkinson's diseases. Telomere dysfunction may exacerbate neuroinflammation and oxidative stress, which are hallmarks of neurodegenerative disorders [41]. This association suggests that telomere attrition may contribute to the progressive loss of neuronal function and cognitive decline observed in these conditions [42–44]. Moreover, accelerated cellular aging in neuron cells can expand also in neurological disorders (i.e., depression) potentially introducing new drug targets and maybe, quantifiable biomarkers for these conditions [45]. As for metabolic syndromes, an increased rate of telomere shortening has been implicated in the development and progression of type 2 diabetes. Shorter telomeres in pancreatic beta cells and peripheral blood cells have been associated with insulin resistance and impaired glucose metabolism. Telomerase dysfunction in beta cells may contribute to their dysfunction and reduced insulin secretion[46, 47]. As we further realize the role of telomere function, we further reveal patterns across other chronic disorders related to autoimmune diseases or loss of homeostatic mechanisms. These observations provide another dimension of molecular mechanisms that define the connection between persistent immune activation and the gradual aging of the immune system (i.e., in rheumatoid arthritis) or the decline in homeostasis mechanisms (i.e., osteoporosis) [48–50].

Apart from chronic diseases, as individuals age, another significant concern arises—infertility. Naturally, reproductive potential decreases with age and there's emerging consideration that telomere characteristics could serve as an infertility biomarker [51]. Except for the natural decline in reproductive ability, studies suggest that shortened telomeres in ovarian cells may influence ovarian aging, potentially affecting both egg quality and quantity for conception. Similarly, shorter telomeres in sperm cells have been associated with reduced motility and increased DNA damage [52]. Early data also suggest a potential link between shorter telomeres and the risk of gestational diabetes or preeclampsia [53]. Nevertheless, as infertility involves a mix of somatic and psychological factors, further research is needed in this area to solidify any significant correlations [52].

Regardless of TBDs, chronic diseases, age, or lifestyle-related disorders, the unraveling of telomeres' role in cell homeostasis quickly gained attention in cancer research [54, 55]. Dysfunctional telomere maintenance, often due to telomerase activation, is a hallmark of cancer cells enabling their replicative immortality [56]. Although short telomeres in normal somatic cells contribute to cellular aging, cancer cells often activate telomerase to maintain telomere length and achieve unlimited replicative potential [7, 9]. In some cancer types, telomerase reactivation occurs through mechanisms, such as gene mutations or epigenetic changes enabling uncontrolled cell proliferation and tumor growth [57]. This activation can lead to oncogenic chromosomal rearrangements promoting tumorigenesis. Telomerase activation is a hallmark across nearly all cancer types exhibiting expression intensity unmatched by any other known tumor marker [58–61].

For all the above chronic conditions (including cancer), it is well understood that apart from the genetic predisposition, lifestyle and epigenetic regulations play an important role. Hence, within this notion, continuously emerging evidence suggests that telomere characteristics are often associated with the onset of chronic or age-related diseases where lifestyle may contribute. This marks telomere dynamics as a biomarker of effect as to exposome analysis considering a person's genetic background, environmental exposure, and lifestyle.

22.5 Targeting, Telomerase, and the Shelterin Complex

Telomeres, telomerase, and the shelterin complex have gained attraction as potential therapeutic targets notably in cancer and age-related disorders due to their crucial roles in cellular biology [57, 62]. The significance of these structures, especially in cancer, provides a promising landscape for innovative drug development aiming to revolutionize healthcare and longevity [63]. However, results are mainly on the preclinical level due to the complex role of telomeres in cellular homeostasis. Generally, the efforts focus on either targeting telomerase or proteins participating in the shelterin complex.

I. **Targeting Telomerase**

- **Telomerase Inhibitors:** Telomerase inhibitors are small-molecule compounds designed to block telomerase activity leading to telomere shortening and impaired cellular replication in cancer cells [54]. Several telomerase inhibitors have been developed and are being evaluated in preclinical and clinical studies. G-quadruplex stabilizers, such as imetelstat (GRN163L), show promise in inhibiting telomerase activity by interfering with the telomerase RNA template and disrupting the telomerase-telomeric DNA interaction. Although several efforts for developing telomerase inhibitors have been made, till 2023, imeltestat was the first telomerase inhibitor to go from preclinical level to clinical trials for various cancer types and was in the phases II or III [61, 64]. In addition, several tyrosine kinases and Wnt/β-catenin signaling inhibitors seem to have inhibitory action against telomerase [61]. Apart from conventional medicines, secondary metabolites of natural products, such as polyphenols, terpenoids, sesquiterpene, xanthones, and even alkaloids have been studied for potential telomerase inhibition toward novel compounds in cancer research. Some well-documented compounds to be mentioned are epigallocatechin gallate, curcumin, genistein, gingerol, diosgenin, sulforaphane, resveratrol, indole-3-carbinol, oleanane, pristimerin, several phenolic acids, ginsenosides, silybin, silymarin, and berberine [65].

- **Telomerase Activators:** Telomerase activators continue to attract attention as emerging anti-aging agents that promote longevity and delay the onset of age-related diseases [39, 54]. Metformin represents the most recent example of a drug with anti-aging properties engaging mechanisms that involve both direct and indirect activation of telomerase [66]. Furthermore, given the process of cellular senescence resulting from cellular attrition, inflammation, and oxidative stress, several studies are endeavoring to elucidate the role of compounds with antioxidant or anti-inflammatory properties as potential telomerase activators [67, 68].
- **Immunotherapeutic Vaccines:** Therapeutic cancer vaccines (TCV) targeting human telomerase (hTERT) have been developed to stimulate an immune response against telomerase-expressing cancer cells. These vaccines aim to stimulate T cells and antibodies to recognize and attack cancer cells with high hTERT expression. Although the research dates back 20 years and met several successes and pitfalls the emergence of DNA/RNA technologies in vaccine development renewed the interest and the perspectives for development of effective vaccines [69, 70]. Till today, several TCVs for hTERT are being investigated in clinical trials alone or in combination therapies for their potential efficacy in treating various cancers [71]. GV1001 is one of the most known examples and the first TCV for hTERT that is in several clinical trials not only in cancer but also for Alzheimer's [71, 72]. Similarly, UV1 is a TCV hTERT

candidate that has entered phase I clinical trials [70]. As for the novel vaccine platforms, INVAC-1 is a DNA-based vaccine currently under phase I trials to investigate the safety, tolerability, clinical response, and immunogenicity in patients with solid tumors [73].

- **Telomerase Gene Silencing:** RNA interference (RNAi) or antisense oligonucleotides can be used to selectively downregulate the expression of telomerase components, such as hTERT, in cancer cells. By silencing hTERT, cancer cells lose telomerase activity, leading to telomere shortening and growth inhibition. This approach is being explored as a novel strategy for targeted cancer therapy [74].
- **Telomerase Gene Therapy:** Gene therapy approaches involve the introduction of functional telomerase genes into cancer cells with deficient telomerase activity. Gene therapy for telomerase has shown promise in preclinical studies, but further research is needed to address safety concerns and ensure targeted delivery [75].

II. **Targeting the Shelterin Complex**

- **Shelterin Disruptors:** Researchers are exploring the development of small molecules that disrupt interactions within the shelterin complex leading to telomere dysfunction and cell death in cancer cells. Targeting proteins like TIN2 or TPP1 could potentially destabilize the shelterin complex disrupting its protective functions and promoting telomere shortening. For example, mepacrine, an antiprotozoal and immunomodulatory agent, and anticancer drugs, such as anthracyclines (e.g., doxorubicin), etoposide, and bortezomib, disrupt shelterins directly by targeting TRF1 and POT1 or indirectly through tankyrase TNKS1 [76–79].
- **T-Loop Stabilization:** The shelterin complex plays a critical role in forming the T-loop structure, which protects telomeres from being recognized as double-strand breaks. Novel interventions that stabilize the T-loop could enhance telomere protection and potentially limit telomerase ac-

cess to telomeres providing a promising target for drug research [80].

- **Epigenetic Modulators:** Epigenetic regulation plays a role in shelterin complex function. Modulating the epigenetic landscape through targeted drugs may influence shelterin activity and impact telomere maintenance. Epigenetic therapies may offer new approaches to modulate shelterin functions and affect telomere biology [81].
- **Alternative Lengthening of Telomere (ALT) Pathway Inhibitors:** ALT is a type of homologous recombination that serves as an alternative mechanism for tumors to maintain their telomeres independently of telomerase expression. Tumors that utilize the ALT pathway for telomere maintenance could be targeted by inhibiting the specific components involved in this alternative mechanism. By disrupting ALT-mediated telomere lengthening, these interventions could lead to telomere dysfunction and cancer cell death [82, 83].
- **Synthetic Lethality Approaches:** Synthetic lethality targets vulnerabilities in cancer cells by exploiting specific genetic or molecular features. Combining drugs that target shelterin components with other agents that impact DNA repair or replication pathways may result in synergistic effects selectively killing cancer cells [82].

As biomedical research evolves, emerging technologies provide innovative tools to exploit the telomere system as a potential drug target. These methods include targeting the shelterin complex using the CRISPR/Cas9 system utilizing advanced drug delivery systems and nanomedicine technologies and tailoring treatments for specific tumor types with or without combination therapies [61, 84, 85]. It is important to state that while the therapeutic potential of targeting telomerase and the shelterin complex is promising, challenges remain in achieving selective and effective treatments. Considering anti-aging factors, the scientific pursuit is to maintain a delicate balance: enhancing telomerase activity without compromising cellular homeostasis or risking tumorigenesis [86]. Careful consideration of potential off-target effects and resistance mechanisms is essential in the development of these interventions. Additionally, personalized approaches considering the specific molecular characteristics of individual patients and their tumors may further enhance the success of these novel therapeutic strategies. Continued research and clinical trials will be crucial in translating these drug targets into safe and effective treatments for various diseases, including cancer and age-related disorders.

22.6 Conclusions

Telomeres are a key element for maintaining cellular homeostasis and longevity, influencing cellular viability, genomic integrity, and critical biological processes. Dysregulation of any of the participating elements leads to telomeropathies, premature aging, and increased susceptibility to diseases. Shortened telomeres and shelterin disturbances are implicated in various age-related disorders impacting tissue function and overall cellular health. Apart from genetics, telomere characteristics and the shortening rate can serve as novel biomarkers for conditions like cardiovascular complications, neurodegenerative disorders, metabolic syndromes, autoimmune diseases, and even infertility, reflecting lifestyle's impact on health and aging. In cancer, targeting telomerase and shelterin complex seem promising as new targets against uncontrolled cancer cell proliferation. However, challenges remain in developing precise, effective treatments, while considering potential side effects and resistance mechanisms. Ongoing research and clinical trials are crucial to harnessing these discoveries for improved treatments, potentially revolutionizing healthcare and human longevity.

References

1. Greider, C.W. (1999). Telomeres Do D-Loop-T-Loop, *Cell,* **97**, pp. 419–422.
2. Srinivas, N., Rachakonda, S., Kumar, R. (2020). Telomeres and telomere length: a general overview, *Cancers (Basel)*, **12**, pp. 558.

3. Shiekh, S. A., Jack, A., Mustafa, G., Kodikara, S. G., Gyawali, P., Hoque, M. E., *et al.* (2023). Impact of shelterin complex on telomere accessibility, *Biophys. J.*, **122**, pp. 73.
4. Shay, J. W., Wright, W. E. (2000). Hayflick, his limit, and cellular ageing, *Nat. Rev. Mol. Cell Biol.*, **1**, pp. 72–76.
5. Hayflick, L. (1965). The limited in vitro lifetime of human diploid cell strains, *Exp. Cell Res.*, **37**, pp. 614–636.
6. Bianchi, A., Shore, D. (2008). Molecular cell review how telomerase reaches its end: mechanism of telomerase regulation by the telomeric complex, *Mol. Cell*, **31**, pp. 153–65.
7. Khodadadi, E., Mir, S. M., Memar, M. Y., Sadeghi, H., Kashiri, M., Faeghiniya, M., *et al.* (2021). Shelterin complex at telomeres: Roles in cancers, *Gene Reports*, **23**, pp. 101174.
8. Lu, R., Pickett HA. (2022). Telomeric replication stress: the beginning and the end for alternative lengthening of telomeres cancers, *Open Biology*, **12**, pp. 220011.
9. Okamoto, K., Seimiya, H. (2019). Revisiting telomere shortening in cancer, *Cells*, **8**, pp. 107.
10. De Lange, T. (2005). Shelterin: the protein complex that shapes and safeguards human telomeres, genes and development, **19**, pp. 2100–10.
11. De Lange, T. (2018). Shelterin-mediated telomere protection, *Annu. Rev. Genet.*, **52**, pp. 223–247.
12. Whittemore, K., Vera, E., Martínez-Nevado, E., Sanpera, C., Blasco, M.A. (2019). Telomere shortening rate predicts species life span, *Proc. Natl. Acad. Sci. USA*, **116**, pp. 15122–15127.
13. Xin, H., Liu, D., Songyang, Z. (2008). The telosome/shelterin complex and its functions, *Genome Biol.*, **9**, pp. 232.
14. Broccoli, D., Smogorzewska, A., Chong, L., de Lange, T. (1997). Human telomeres contain two distinct Myb-related proteins, TRF1 and TRF2, *Nat. Genet.*, **17**, pp. 235.
15. Bianchi, A., Smith, S., Chong, L., Elias, P., De Lange, T. (1997). TRF1 is a dimer and bends telomeric DNA, *EMBO J.*, **16**, pp. 1785–94.
16. Soohoo, C. Y., Shi, R., Lee, T. H., Huang, P., Lu, K. P., Zhou, X. Z. (2011). Telomerase inhibitor PinX1 provides a link between TRF1 and telomerase to prevent telomere elongation, *J. Biol. Chem.*, **286**, pp. 3894.
17. Schneider, R. P., Garrobo, I., Foronda, M., Palacios, J. A., Marión, R. M., Flores, I., *et al.* (2013). TRF1 is a stem cell marker and is essential for the generation of induced pluripotent stem cells, *Nat. Commun.*, **4**, pp. 1946.

18. Derevyanko, A., Whittemore, K., Schneider, R. P., Jiménez, V., Bosch, F., Blasco, M. A. (2017). Gene therapy with the TRF1 telomere gene rescues decreased TRF1 levels with aging and prolongs mouse health span, *Aging Cell*, **16**, pp. 1353–68.
19. Bejarano, L., Schuhmacher, A. J., Squatrito, M., Blasco, M. A. (2017). Inhibition of TRF1 telomere protein impairs tumor initiation and progression in glioblastoma mouse models and patient-derived xenografts, *Cancer Cell*, **32**, pp. 590–607.
20. Cherfils-Vicini, J., Gilson, E. (2019). Inhibiting TRF1 upstream signaling pathways to target telomeres in cancer cells, *EMBO Mol. Med.*, **11**, pp. e10845.
21. Chen, Y., Yang, Y., Van Overbeek, M., Donigian, J. R., Baciu, P., De Lange, T., *et al.* (2008). A shared docking motif in TRF1 and TRF2 used for differential recruitment of telomeric proteins, *Science*, **319**, pp. 1092–6.
22. Fairall, L., Chapman, L., Moss, H., De Lange, T., Rhodes, D. (2001). Structure of the TRFH dimerization domain of the human telomeric proteins TRF1 and TRF2, Mol. *Cell*, **8**, pp. 351–61.
23. Lin, J., Countryman, P., Buncher, N., Kaur, P., Longjiang, E., Zhang, Y., *et al.* (2014). TRF1 and TRF2 use different mechanisms to find telomeric DNA but share a novel mechanism to search for protein partners at telomeres, *Nucleic Acids Res.*, **42**, pp. 2493.
24. Nandakumar, J., Cech, T. R. (2013). Finding the end: recruitment of telomerase to telomeres, *Nat. Rev. Mol. Cell Biol.*, **14**, pp. 69–82.
25. Aramburu, T., Plucinsky, S., Skordalakes, E. (2020). POT1-TPP1 telomere length regulation and disease, *Comput. Struct. Biotechnol. J.*, **18**, pp. 1939.
26. Takai, K. K., Hooper, S., Blackwood, S., Gandhi, R., de Lange, T. (2010). In vivo stoichiometry of shelterin components, *J. Biol. Chem.*, **285**, pp. 1457–67.
27. Diotti, R., Loayza, D. (2011). Shelterin complex and associated factors at human telomeres, *Nucleus*, **2**, pp. 119–35.
28. Lim, C. J., Cech, T. R. (2021). Shaping human telomeres: from shelterin and CST complexes to telomeric chromatin organization, *Nat. Rev. Mol. Cell Biol.*, **22**, pp. 283–98.
29. Hayflick, L. (1998). How and why we age, *Exp. Gerontol.*, **33**, pp. 639–53.
30. Razgonova, M. P., Zakharenko, A. M., Golokhvast, K. S., Thanasoula, M., Sarandi, E., Nikolouzakis, K., *et al.* (2022). Telomerase and telomeres in

aging theory and chronographic aging theory (review), *Mol. Med. Rep.*, **22**, pp. 1679–94.

31. Grill, S., Nandakumar, J. (2021). Molecular mechanisms of telomere biology disorders, *J. Biol. Chem.*, **296**, pp. 100064.
32. Calado, R. T., Young, N. S. (2009). Telomere diseases, *New England Journal of Medicine*, **361**, pp. 2353–65.
33. Rossiello, F., Jurk, D., Passos, J. F., d'Adda di Fagagna, F. (2022). Telomere dysfunction in ageing and age-related diseases, *Nat. Cell Biol.*, **24**, pp. 135.
34. Opresko, P. L., Shay, J. W. (2017). Telomere-associated aging disorders, *Ageing Res. Rev.*, **33**, pp. 52.
35. Carvalho, V. S., Gomes, W. R., Calado, R. T. (2022). Recent advances in understanding telomere diseases, *Fac. Rev.*, **11**, pp. 31.
36. Armanios, M., Blackburn, E. H. (2012). The telomere syndromes, *Nat. Rev. Genet.*, **13**, pp. 693–704.
37. Holohan, B., Wright, W. E., Shay, J. W. (2014). Cell biology of disease: telomeropathies: an emerging spectrum disorder, *J. Cell Biol.*, **205**, pp. 289–99.
38. Glousker, G., Touzot, F., Revy, P., Tzfati, Y., Savage, S. A. (2015). Unraveling the pathogenesis of Hoyeraal-Hreidarsson syndrome, a complex telomere biology disorder, *Br. J. Haematol.*, **170**, pp. 457.
39. Yeh, J. K., Wang, C. Y. (2016). Telomeres and telomerase in cardiovascular diseases, *Genes (Basel)*, **7**, pp. 58.
40. Yeh, J. K., Lin, M. H., Wang, C. Y. (2019). Telomeres as therapeutic targets in heart disease, *JACC Basic Transl. Sci.*, **4**, pp. 855–65.
41. Martínez-Cué, C., Rueda, N. (2020). Cellular senescence in neurodegenerative diseases, *Front. Cell Neurosci.*, **14**, pp. 16.
42. Vakonaki, E., Tsiminikaki, K., Plaitis, S., Fragkiadaki, P., Tsoukalas, D., Katsikantami, I., *et al.* (2018). Common mental disorders and association with telomere length, *Biomed. Rep.*, **8**, pp. 111–6.
43. Anitha, A., Thanseem, I., Vasu, M. M., Viswambharan, V., Poovathinal, S. A. (2019). Telomeres in neurological disorders, *Adv. Clin. Chem.*, **90**, pp. 81–132.
44. Levstek, T., Kozjek, E., Dolžan, V., Trebušak Podkrajšek, K. (2020). Telomere attrition in neurodegenerative disorders, *Front. Cell Neurosci.*, **14**, pp. 219.
45. Verhoeven, J. E., Révész, D., Wolkowitz, O. M., Penninx, B. W. J. H. (2014). Cellular aging in depression: permanent imprint or reversible process:

an overview of the current evidence, mechanistic pathways, and targets for interventions, *Bioessays*, **36**, pp. 968–78.

46. Kuhlow, D., Florian, S., von Figura, G., Weimer, S., Schulz, N., Petzke, K. J., *et al.* (2010). Telomerase deficiency impairs glucose metabolism and insulin secretion, *Aging (Albany NY)*, **2**, pp. 650.
47. Wang, J., Dong, X., Cao, L., Sun, Y., Qiu, Y., Zhang, Y., *et al.* (2016). Association between telomere length and diabetes mellitus: a meta-analysis, *J. Int. Med. Res.*, **44**, pp. 1156–73.
48. Hohensinner, P. J., Goronzy, J. J., Weyand, C. M. (2011). Telomere dysfunction, autoimmunity and aging, *Aging Dis.*, **2**, pp. 524.
49. Kakridonis, F., Pneumatikos, S. G., Vakonaki, E., Berdiaki, A., Tzatzarakis, M. N., Fragkiadaki, P., *et al.* (2023). Telomere length as a predictive biomarker in osteoporosis (review), *Biomed. Rep.*, **19**, pp. 87.
50. Fragkiadaki, P., Nikitovic, D., Kalliantasi, K., Sarandi, E., Thanasoula, M., Stivaktakis, P., *et al.* (2020). Telomere length and telomerase activity in osteoporosis and osteoarthritis, *Exp. Ther. Med.*, **19**, pp. 1626–1632.
51. Vasilopoulos, E., Fragkiadaki, P., Kalliora, C., Fragou, D., Docea, A. O., Vakonaki, E., *et al.* (2019). The association of female and male infertility with telomere length (review), *Int. J. Mol. Med.*, **44**, pp. 375–89.
52. Rocca, M. S., Foresta, C., Ferlin, A. (2019). Telomere length: lights and shadows on their role in human reproduction, *Biol. Reprod.*, **100**, pp. 305–17.
53. Harville, E. W., Williams, M. A., Qiu, C. F., Mejia, J., Risques, R. A. (2010). Telomere length, pre-eclampsia, and gestational diabetes, *BMC Res. Notes*, **3**, pp. 113.
54. Fragkiadaki, P., Renieri, E., Kalliantasi, K., Kouvidi, E., Apalaki, E., Vakonaki, E., *et al.* (2022). Telomerase inhibitors and activators in aging and cancer: a systematic review, *Mol. Med. Rep.*, **25**, pp. 158.
55. Granger, M. P., Wright, W. E., Shay, J. W. (2002). Telomerase in cancer and aging, *Crit. Rev. Oncol. Hematol.*, **41**, pp. 29–40.
56. Low, K. C., Tergaonkar, V. (2013). Telomerase: central regulator of all of the hallmarks of cancer, *Trends Biochem. Sci.*, **38**, pp. 426–34.
57. Bilsland, A. E., Cairney, C. J., Nicol Keith W. (2011). Targeting the telomere and shelterin complex for cancer therapy: current views and future perspectives, *Journal of Cellular and Molecular Medicine*, **15**, pp. 179–86.
58. Akincilar, S. C., Unal, B., Tergaonkar, V. (2016). Reactivation of telomerase in cancer, *Cell Mol. Life Sci.*, **73**, pp. 1659–70.

59. Jafri, M. A., Ansari, S. A., Alqahtani, M. H., Shay, J.W. (2016). Roles of telomeres and telomerase in cancer, and advances in telomerase-targeted therapies, *Genome Medicine*, **8**, pp. 1–18.
60. Trybek, T., Kowalik, A., Góźdź, S., Kowalska, A. (2020). Telomeres and telomerase in oncogenesis, *Oncol. Lett.*, **20**, pp. 1015–27.
61. Ali, J. H., Walter, M. (2023). Combining old and new concepts in targeting telomerase for cancer therapy: transient, immediate, complete and combinatory attack (TICCA), *Cancer Cell. Int.*, **23**, pp. 197.
62. Jäger, K., Walter, M. (2016). Therapeutic targeting of telomerase, *Genes (Basel)*, **7**, pp. 39.
63. Smith-Sonneborn, J. (2020). Telomerase biology associations offer keys to cancer and aging therapeutics, *Curr. Aging Sci.*, **13**, pp. 11–21.
64. Platzbecker, U., Santini, V., Fenaux, P., Sekeres, M.A., Savona, M.R., Madanat, Y.F., *et al.* (2023). Imetelstat in patients with lower-risk myelodysplastic syndromes who have relapsed or are refractory to erythropoiesis-stimulating agents (IMerge): a multinational, randomised, double-blind, placebo-controlled, phase 3 trial, *Lancet*, **403**.
65. Ganesan, K., Xu, B. (2018). Telomerase inhibitors from natural products and their anticancer potential, *Int. J. Mol. Sci.*, **19**, pp. 13.
66. Hu, D., Xie, F., Xiao, Y., Lu, C., Zhong, J., Huang, D., *et al.* (2021). Metformin: a potential candidate for targeting aging mechanisms, *Aging Dis.*, **12**, pp. 480.
67. Tsoukalas, D., Fragkiadaki, P., Docea, A. O., Alegakis, A. K., Sarandi, E., Thanasoula, M., *et al.* (2019). Discovery of potent telomerase activators: unfolding new therapeutic and anti-aging perspectives, *Mol. Med. Rep.*, **20**, pp. 3701.
68. de Jesus, B. B., Schneeberger, K., Vera, E., Tejera, A., Harley, C. B., Blasco, M. A. (2011). The telomerase activator TA-65 elongates short telomeres and increases health span of adult/old mice without increasing cancer incidence, *Aging Cell*, **10**, pp. 604–21.
69. Mizukoshi, E., Kaneko, S. (2019). Telomerase-targeted cancer immunotherapy, *Int. J. Mol. Sci.*, **20**, pp. 1823.
70. Ellingsen, E. B., Mangsbo, S. M., Hovig, E., Gaudernack, G. (2021). Telomerase as a target for therapeutic cancer vaccines and considerations for optimizing their clinical potential, *Front. Immunol.*, **12**, pp. 682492.
71. Jo, J. H., Kim, Y. T., Choi, H. S., Kim, H. G., Lee, H. S., Choi, Y. W., *et al.* (2023). Efficacy of GV1001 with gemcitabine/capecitabine in previously untreated patients with advanced pancreatic ductal

adenocarcinoma having high serum eotaxin levels (KG4/2015): an open-label, randomised, phase 3 trial, *Br. J. Cancer*, **130**, pp. 43–52.

72. Koh, S. H., Kwon, H. S., Choi, S. H., Jeong, J. H., Na, H. R., Lee, C.N., *et al.* Efficacy and safety of GV1001 in patients with moderate-to-severe Alzheimer's disease already receiving donepezil: a phase 2 randomized, double-blind, placebo-controlled, multicenter clinical trial, *Alzheimer's Res. Ther.*, **13**, pp. 66.
73. Teixeira, L., Medioni, J., Garibal, J., Adotevi, O., Doucet, L., Durey, M. A. D., *et al.* (2020). A first-in-human phase i study of INVAC-1, an optimized human telomerase DNA vaccine in patients with advanced solid tumors, *Clin. Cancer Res.*, **26**, pp. 588–97.
74. Laudadio, I., Carissimi, C., Fulci, V. (2019). How RNAi machinery enters the world of telomerase? *Cell Cycle*, **8**, pp. 1056.
75. Hong, J., Yun, C. O. (2019). Telomere gene therapy: polarizing therapeutic goals for treatment of various diseases, *Cells*, **8**, pp. 392.
76. Ci, X., Li, B., Ma, X., Kong, F., Zheng, C., Björkholm, M., *et al.* (2015). Bortezomib-mediated down-regulation of telomerase and disruption of telomere homeostasis contributes to apoptosis of malignant cells, *Oncotarget*, **6**, pp. 38079–92.
77. Kato, M., Nakayama, M., Agata, M., Yoshida, K. (2013). Gene expression levels of human shelterin complex and shelterin-associated factors regulated by the topoisomerase II inhibitors doxorubicin and etoposide in human cultured cells, *Tumour Biol.*, **34**, pp. 723–33.
78. Zhang, B., Qian, D., Ma, H. H., Jin, R., Yang, P. X., Cai, M. Y., *et al.* (2012). Anthracyclines disrupt telomere maintenance by telomerase through inducing PinX1 ubiquitination and degradation, *Oncogene*, **31**, pp. 1–12.
79. Sun, H., Xiang, J., Li, Q., Liu, Y., Li, L., Shang, Q., *et al.* (2012). Recognize three different human telomeric G-quadruplex conformations by quinacrine, *Analyst*, **137**, pp. 862–7.
80. Folini, M., Gandellini, P., Zaffaroni, N. (2009). Targeting the telosome: therapeutic implications, *Biochim. Biophys. Acta*, **1792**, pp. 309–16.
81. Dogan, F., Forsyth, N. R. (2021). Telomerase regulation: a role for epigenetics, *Cancers (Basel)*, **13**, pp. 1–24.
82. Zhang, J. M., Zou, L. (2020). Alternative lengthening of telomeres: from molecular mechanisms to therapeutic outlooks, *Cell Biosci.*, **10**, pp. 1–9.
83. O'Rourke, J. J., Bythell-Douglas, R., Dunn, E. A., Deans, A. J. (2019). ALT control, delete: FANCM as an anti-cancer target in alternative lengthening of telomeres, *Nucleus*, **10**, pp. 221–30.

84. Porika, M., Tippani, R., Saretzki, G. C. (2022). CRISPR/Cas: a new tool in the research of telomeres and telomerase as well as a novel form of cancer therapy, *Int. J. Mol. Sci.*, **23**, pp. 3002.

85. Philippi, C., Loretz, B., Schaefer, U. F., Lehr, C.M. (2010). Telomerase as an emerging target to fight cancer: opportunities and challenges for nanomedicine, *J. Control Release*, **146**, pp. 228–40.

86. Ait-Aissa, K., Ebben, J. D., Kadlec, A. O., Beyer, A. M. (2016). Friend or foe? telomerase as a pharmacological target in cancer and cardiovascular disease, *Pharmacol. Res.*, **111**, pp. 422–433.

Chapter 23

Therapeutic Targeting of Telomerase

Eren Ozcagli,[a] Esma Söylemez Yeşilçimen,[b] Çiğdem Sevim,[c] Mehtap Kara,[a] and Aristidis Tsatsakis[d]

[a] *Department of Pharmaceutical Toxicology, Faculty of Pharmacy, Istanbul University, Beyazıt, Istanbul, Turkey*
[b] *Department of Pharmaceutical Toxicology, School of Pharmacy, University of Istanbul Medipol, Istanbul, Turkey*
[c] *Department of Medical Pharmacology, Faculty of Medicine, University of Kastamonu, Kastamonu, Turkey*
[d] *Department of Toxicology and Forensic Sciences, Medical School, University of Crete, Heraklion, Greece*
eren.ozcagli@istanbul.edu.tr, tsatsaka@uoc.gr

23.1 Introduction

Telomeres, comprised of DNA and protein complexes, are situated at the termini of eukaryotic chromosomes shielding against factors that induce instability in the genome. Telomerase is an enzyme that plays a crucial role in maintaining the length and integrity of telomeres. Telomere research is a complex and multifaceted field that involves investigating various aspects of telomere biology, including their structure, function, regulation, and implications for health and disease. Therapeutic targeting of telomerase is a strategy

Telomeres: Biomarkers of a Healthy Life and Successful Aging
Edited by Aristidis Tsatsakis

ISBN 978-981-5129-49-6 (Hardcover), 978-1-003-56809-4 (eBook)
www.jennystanford.com

that has been explored for various medical purposes primarily in the context of cancer treatment and potentially in age-related diseases. Future approaches for therapeutic applications involve designing therapies that modulate telomerase activity to maintain telomere length within a healthy range exploring the potential of drugs that target senescent cells and investigating novel drugs that specifically target the molecular pathways involved in telomere maintenance. The goal of targeting telomerase is to either inhibit its activity to prevent cancer cell proliferation or activate it to promote tissue regeneration and to struggle with certain aspects of aging. The complexity of telomere biology highlights the need for careful consideration when exploring therapeutic interventions that target telomeres or telomerase. Before adopting any therapeutic intervention, rigorous testing and evaluation will be necessary to ensure the safety and effectiveness of the approach.

23.2 Telomeres

Telomeres protect the integrity of linear chromosomes by consisting of repetitive sequences located at the chromosome ends. Telomeric DNA, which consists of a repetitive pattern (GGTTAG/CCAATC in humans), primarily exists as a double-stranded form. However, it terminates with a brief single-stranded counterpart that possesses a G-rich 3′ overhang (Fig. 23.1) [1]. The ends of linear chromosomes face two main biological obstacles: the issue of end replicating and safeguarding them [2].

Differentiating these ends of chromosomes from other forms of linear DNA such as damaged DNA ends that necessitate repair plays a crucial role. In order to achieve this, a cluster of proteins known as the shelterin complex specifically attaches to telomeric sequences [3]. Shelterin, alternatively recognized as the telosome, constitutes a protein complex acknowledged for safeguarding telomeres against DNA repair processes and overseeing the activity of telomerase in the majority of eukaryotic organisms. By doing so, the shelterin complex effectively tackles the issue of safeguarding the ends of chromosomes, effectively averting DNA repair reactions triggered by loose DNA ends.

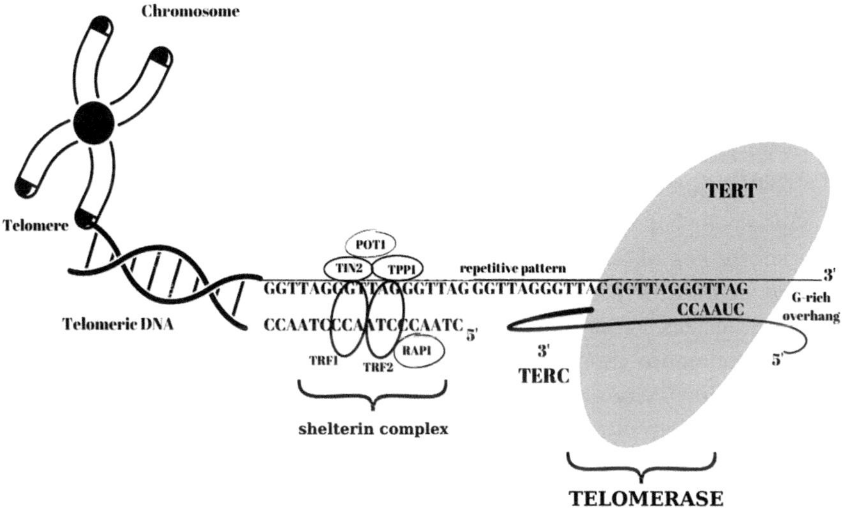

Figure 23.1 Schematic presentation of telomere, shelterin complex, and telomerase.

It also plays an important role in maintaining the integrity and stability of the genetic material during cell division consisting of repetitive DNA sequences and associated proteins [4]. If telomere instability occurs with dysfunction or disruption of shelterin components, this may result in cellular aging, genomic instability, and the potential of developing certain diseases, including cancer. It has been reported that these proteins are highly expressed in various cancers [5].

The shelterin complex is comprised of six proteins known as TRF1, TRF2, RAP1, TIN2, TPP1, and POT1, which work together to selectively bind telomeric sequences. The functions of the shelterin complex address the challenge of end-protection by obstructing the DNA repair signals that result from exposed DNA termini. These signals consist of the initiation of DNA damage response and the application of DNA repair mechanisms like non-homologous end-joining, alternative end-joining, and homologous recombination [1, 6–9].

Biological aging is a natural and time-dependent process of physical and functional changes that occur in living organisms over time. It is a complex, multifaceted phenomenon that affects all biological systems, from individual cells to entire organisms. As cells replicate, human telomeres naturally become shorter by losing approximately 50–250 bp after each mitosis, contributing to the process of cellular aging and the limited lifespan of many types of cells. Therefore, the length of telomeric DNA determines the lifespan of a cell [10]. A critical issue that arises at chromosome ends is the shortening of telomeres. This shortening occurs due to incomplete replication of the lagging strand by the DNA polymerase, which synthesizes DNA in the 5'–3' direction. The end-replication problem and telomere shortening have important implications for cellular aging, longevity, and the development of age-related diseases [11]. The problem of end-replication was effectively addressed through the advent of an RNP complex called telomerase. Telomerase comprises an enzymatic reverse transcriptase (TERT), the non-coding human telomerase RNA (hTR), and additional cofactors that serve as a template for adding telomeric repeats to the ends of the chromosome resolving the issue [12, 13].

23.3 Telomerase Activity

Telomerase is an enzyme that contains a built-in RNA template that complements the telomeric DNA sequence and it is responsible for extending the telomeric DNA by adding repetitive sequences to the ends of chromosomes. This helps prevent the loss of essential genetic information during each round of DNA replication [14].

In each cell division, chromosomes undergo a shortening phenomenon called the "end-replication problem." The inability of DNA polymerases to fully replicate the 3' end of linear duplex DNA results in this phenomenon. Telomerase utilizes its RNA subunit as a template to elongate the ends of chromosomes by synthesizing single-stranded telomeric repeats, thus providing a solution to the "end-replication problem" [15, 16]. Initially observed in protozoan models, telomeres and telomerase have also been confirmed to exist in various organisms including humans, yeast, and plants [16]. At present, the exact mechanism for recruiting telomerase remains unclear. The basic components of the human telomerase holoenzyme consist of a catalytic reverse transcriptase known as human telomerase reverse transcriptase (hTERT) and a basic RNA containing human telomerase RNA (hTR) [17, 18]. Telomerase shares several characteristics with conventional reverse transcriptases, while also exhibiting distinct properties. Notably, the enzymatic activity of telomerase can be influenced by ribonuclease and protease treatment indicating the involvement of both RNA and protein in its enzymatic function [16].

Telomerase utilizes the RNA template to attach itself to the unpaired 3′ end of a chromosome. The 3′ end of the DNA associates with the RNA template, forming a hybrid structure. Telomerase facilitates the elongation process of the 3′ end of the RNA molecule towards the end of the template region, adding six nucleotides (GGTTAG) one at a time. This sequential addition, in turn, causes the telomerase enzyme complex to move along the recently synthesized strand and further lengthen the telomere. This movement is repeated in multiple cycles, relocating the newly formed 3' end of the DNA strand within the template preparing it for the subsequent round of telomere synthesis. Telomerase continues to add multiple repeats by moving to fresh binding sites along the recently synthesized strand [16]. After the initial identification of telomerase in Tetrahymena extracts, scientists identified a comparable enzymatic activity in HeLa cells obtained from malignant tumors [19].

Since then, the scientific community has displayed significant interest in investigating the relationship between telomerase activity and tumors. Even though research has indicated the widespread presence of telomerase activity in human cancer cells, with roughly 85–90% of primary tumors demonstrating this characteristic, the majority of somatic cells generally lack telomerase activity [20]. However, adult pluripotent stem cells, which actively contribute to tissue regeneration, represent an exception in this regard. The correlation between telomerase activity and cancer has prompted researchers to view telomerase as a potential target for both cancer diagnosis and treatment, thus driving the focus of numerous studies. Telomerase activity has been the subject of significant scientific interest due to its potential implications for treating age-related diseases and extending a healthy lifespan [21]. The potential applications of manipulating telomerase activity are an active area of research and hold promise for various medical and biological purposes.

23.4 Telomerase Activity and Health

Telomere biology disorders (TBD) can have a wide range of clinical manifestations and can affect multiple organ systems. They are typically inherited depending on the specific genetic mutation in an autosomal dominant or recessive manner [22]. Management of these disorders often involves regular monitoring, supportive care, and, in some cases, treatments like hematopoietic stem cell transplantation. Early diagnosis and genetic counseling are crucial for individuals with TBD. Additionally, ongoing research into these disorders is helping to improve our understanding and management of these rare conditions.

TBD are characterized by abnormalities in telomere maintenance and function. Telomere biology disorders are typically caused by mutations in genes involved in telomere maintenance, and they can lead to a wide range of health problems. Some of the most common TBD include:

- **Aplastic Anemia (AA), Myelodysplastic Syndrome (MDS), or Acute Myeloid Leukemia (AML):** AA is a condition in which the bone marrow fails to produce enough blood cells. Some cases of AA are caused by mutations in telomere-related genes leading to shortened telomeres in blood-forming cells [23]. MDS is a group of bone marrow disorders characterized by abnormal and ineffective production of blood cells including red blood cells, white blood cells, and platelets. These disorders have complex pathogenesis as they have also been associated with abnormalities in telomere biology [24]. AML is characterized by the rapid growth of abnormal white blood cells. AML cells may have altered telomere length maintenance mechanisms because of mutations in telomerase reverse transcriptase (TERT) or telomerase RNA (TERC) [25].

- **Idiopathic Pulmonary Fibrosis (IPF):** IPF is the most common manifestation of TBD resulting in progressive lung fibrosis with a deteriorating course and an average survival time of three years.
  IPF represents a lung condition marked by the gradual stiffening of the lungs, due to the formation of scar tissue leading to an escalating challenge for the patient to breathe. While it advances at a slow pace for certain individuals, in the majority of cases, the rapid progression of breathlessness results in respiratory failure for the patient. It primarily affects males over the age of 60 who are smokers, and in clinical settings, it can be identified by the presence of typical interstitial pneumonia (UIP) patterns on high-resolution computed tomography (HRCT) or lung biopsy [26]. Approximately 30% of individuals diagnosed with sporadic or familial pulmonary fibrosis possess certain genetic factors that make them more susceptible to developing this condition. TERT and TERC mutations are responsible for 8–15% of familial cases and 1–3% of sporadic cases of IPF. In addition to these, other telomere mutations including PARN, RTEL1, ZCCHC8, TINF2, NAF1, and DKC1 account for approximately 1–3% of familial cases. These genetic mutations are associated with the development of pulmonary fibrosis [26–28].
- **Dyskeratosis Congenita (DC):** DC is a rare inherited disorder characterized by a triad of symptoms, including skin abnormalities, bone marrow failure, and pulmonary fibrosis (scarring of the lung tissue). Mutations in several genes, including TERC, TERT, and DKC1, have been associated with DC [29, 30].

Severe DC variants, such as Hoyeraal-Hreidarsson Syndrome (HHS) and Coats Plus Syndrome (CPS), have been also studied to examine the relationship between syndromes and telomeres. HHS is a severe disorder that includes symptoms like developmental delay, immune deficiency, bone marrow failure, and cerebellar hypoplasia. Mutations in genes associated with telomere maintenance, such as DKC1 and TINF2, have been linked to this syndrome [31, 32].

CPS is a disorder characterized by retinal telangiectasia (abnormal blood vessels in the retina), brain malformations, gastrointestinal bleeding, and other symptoms. Mutations in the CTC1 gene, which is involved in telomere maintenance, have been identified in individuals with this syndrome [33].

23.5 Telomerase Activation for Regenerative Medicine

23.5.1 Aging and Longevity

Some of the health conditions tend to occur more frequently as individuals grow older.

Aging is a complex biological process associated with various changes in the body including cellular, physiological, and structural changes. These age-related changes can contribute to the development of certain diseases and conditions. Some common age-related diseases include cancer, cardiovascular diseases, neurodegenerative diseases, etc. It is important to note that, while these diseases are more common in older individuals, they are not an inevitable part of aging. Biological indicators of aging are measurable characteristics or changes in the human body that reflect the aging process. These indicators provide insight into the biological age of an individual, which may differ from their chronological age. Biological aging can vary from person to person, and these indicators help scientists and healthcare professionals assess an individual's overall health and susceptibility to age-related diseases. Some common biological indicators of aging include epigenetic changes, hormone levels, transcriptomic-, proteomic-, metabolomics-based, and composite biomarker predictors. Recently measuring telomere length has become a common method used to assess cellular aging and is often utilized as a biological indicator of aging as well [34].

Telomere length measurements can provide valuable insights into the aging process and age-related diseases, as shorter telomeres are often associated with cellular senescence and increased susceptibility to age-related health issues [35].

As telomeres shorten, cells eventually reach a point where their telomeres become critically short. At this stage, cells may enter a state of replicative senescence, where they can no longer divide and function properly. One of the most intriguing possibilities is using telomerase to extend the lifespan of cells and potentially slow down the aging process, which is composed of a variety of mechanisms. From the perspective of telomere biology, safely increasing telomerase activity in somatic cells has the potential to delay the onset of replicative senescence and extend the functional lifespan of these cells. This phenomenon contributes to the aging process and is thought to be a key factor in the decline of organ function, tissue integrity, and overall aging-associated health. It has been known that many age-related diseases are associated with cellular senescence and telomere shortening. Modulating telomerase activity might provide a way to delay or mitigate the onset and progression of these diseases potentially improving overall health in the aging population [36]. However, it is important to approach with caution. There are potential risks associated with artificially increasing telomerase activity including the possibility of promoting uncontrolled cell growth and an increased risk of cancer [37]. Additionally, the aging process is influenced by a multitude of factors including genetics, hormones, lifestyle, and environmental exposures [38]. Telomerase is just one piece of the puzzle. However, an alteration of that piece can change the whole stability and result in serious health consequences.

23.5.2 Tissue Regeneration

Tissue regeneration is the natural process by which living organisms repair or replace damaged or lost tissues, restoring their function and structure. This process is essential for maintaining the health and functionality of organs, tissues and cells throughout the life of an organism. Tissue regeneration and telomerase are interconnected in the context of aging and the potential for extending a healthy lifespan. Telomere length plays a crucial role in enabling high rates of cell proliferation during the intricate process of regeneration. Consequently, in order to support this heightened proliferation, the activity of telomerase is essential for the maintenance of telomere length [39]. Telomerase activity could be harnessed to improve tissue regeneration by enhancing the longevity and division capacity of stem cells having higher telomerase activity. This approach might be able to improve damaged tissue and organ regeneration by providing new approaches in the field of regenerative medicine [40, 41].

In the process of aging, the initial steps of wound healing exhibit a similar proinflammatory reaction observed in dermal fibroblasts. Senescent cells release a combination of cytokines and chemokines into their surroundings, triggering the activation of immune cells. Furthermore, the breakdown of fibrin clots and the dermal matrix is influenced significantly by proteolytic activities [42]. The aspect requiring investigation regarding cellular aging is the degree to which this process triggers or contributes to disease development particularly those linked to human aging. The conducted experiments revealed an escalation in the count of cells positive for senescence-associated beta-galactosidase in the dermis samples obtained from volunteers, which suggests a potential contribution of the aging phenotype to pathological conditions. In a study conducted using a reconstructed skin model with enhanced telomerase expression, the dermal integrity of in vitro aged fibroblasts was successfully restored. The findings from studies on rejuvenating skin suggest that tissues containing an abundance of aged or nearly senescent cells exhibit a hindered ability to heal wounds. This is further backed by the observation of an elevated presence of senescent fibroblasts in biopsies of chronic wounds [43–45].

Additionally, when examining mouse strains that have been bred within the same genetic pool, it becomes apparent that they possess long telomeres and display active telomerase function. However, if the RNA component responsible for telomerase is removed in a manner that aligns with the original genetic makeup, the telomeres in these mice will gradually shorten after approximately 6–7 generations. Consequently, at a certain stage, the mice may become sterile due to this significant reduction in telomere length [46, 47]. As researchers delve further into the intricate system of mice, studies on the dynamics of telomeres and the role of telomerase have expanded to explore various aquatic vertebrates [48, 49].

23.6 Using Telomerase Targeting in Treatment Strategies

In many cancer cells, telomerase is activated allowing them to divide and proliferate continuously. Therefore, telomerase is highly active in many cancer cells, which contributes to their uncontrolled growth and immortality. Developing treatments that selectively inhibit telomerase activity in cancer cells could provide a new approach to cancer therapy. These treatments, known as telomerase inhibitors, are being investigated as potential ways to target and kill cancer cells while sparing healthy cells. Several telomerase inhibitors have been studied in preclinical and clinical trials for their potential in cancer treatment. Some of these trials have shown promising results in terms of inhibiting cancer cell growth particularly in certain types of cancer [50]. Inhibition of human telomerase reverse transcriptase (hTERT) activity through hTERT promoter suppression is an important approach for telomerase inhibition [51].

23.6.1 Telomerase Regulators

23.6.1.1 Synthetic direct telomerase inhibitors

Several synthetic compounds have been developed to directly target and decrease the activity of the telomerase enzyme. Epigallocatechin gallate, a component found in tea, has been utilized to synthesize MST-312 and MST-199, which have demonstrated a reduction in telomerase activity. The U937 cell line was subjected to prolonged treatment with MST resulting in the inhibition of cell growth and subsequent telomere shortening. Furthermore, the presence of MST-312 in treated cells was linked to an increased number of senescent cells as indicated by senescence-associated-β-galactosidase staining. Additional research has highlighted MST-312 as a potent inhibitor of hepatocellular carcinoma cells. However, the specific mechanisms through which MST inhibits telomerase activity remain unclear [52, 53].

Small molecule inhibitors are compounds designed to inhibit telomerase activity by targeting the telomerase enzyme's active site or disrupting its interaction with telomeres. In the context of telomerase inhibition, small molecules are of particular interest because they can be more easily developed into drugs for clinical use and one of them is BIBR1532. This small molecule inhibitor targets the active site of the TERT enzyme disrupting its ability to elongate telomeres. By blocking this essential function, it inhibits the replicative potential of cancer cells potentially limiting their ability to divide and grow. While it has shown promise in preclinical models for various cancers, further research and clinical trials are needed to determine its efficacy and safety in larger populations [54, 55].

BIBR1532, a selective telomerase inhibitor that is not nucleosidic, hampers the reassembly of telomerase from hTR and recombinant hTERT by directly targeting the fundamental components of telomerase, akin to the native enzyme found in tumor cells. Results from an in vitro study have demonstrated the synergistic effect of BIBR1532 when combined with anticancer treatments, such as chemotherapy or radiotherapy. However, it is important to acknowledge that this inhibitor exhibits considerable toxicity across various cell types. Furthermore, there is evidence suggesting that it lacks efficacy in targeting telomerase activity at low, non-toxic dosages [54].

Imetelstat is a synthetic oligonucleotide that binds to the RNA component (TERC) of telomerase preventing its interaction with TERT. TERC is essential for the assembly and function of the telomerase complex. By binding to TERC, Imetelstat disrupts the interaction between TERC and TERT preventing the telomerase enzyme from accessing telomeres and elongating them. This leads to telomere shortening and limits the replicative potential of cancer cells. Imetelstat has been investigated for various cancers, such as non-small cell lung cancer, osteosarcoma, and hematologic malignancies including myelodysplastic syndromes (MDS) and myelofibrosis [56–58]. Both, BIBR1532 and Imetelstat (GRN163L), are promising in the context of telomerase inhibition, but challenges remain. One challenge is achieving specificity for cancer cells while sparing normal cells as telomerase is also active in some healthy tissues particularly stem cells.

Research has demonstrated that modified dihydropyrazole compounds effectively hinder the functioning of telomerase and exhibit potent anti-tumor properties against a range of cancers (such as those affecting the stomach, breast, prostate, and hepatoma). Moreover, these derivatives exhibit favorable selectivity toward tumor cells when compared to somatic cells [59]. Silibinin, a flavonoid with polyphenolic properties, serves as an effective prostate epithelium-specific androgen receptor and an anticancer medication. It successfully decreases the activity of telomerase and prostate-specific antigen (PSA) playing a crucial role in combating cancer [60]. Moreover, the combination of silibinin and curcuminoids has shown promising results in reducing hTERT gene expression within breast cancer cells. This highlights the potential of silibinin as a valuable anti-proliferative agent for treating prostate cancer [60]. Structure-oriented designs of derivatives containing ethanesulfonyl fluoride are a distinct category of chemical compounds that exhibit potential as synthetic inhibitors of telomerase, thereby amplifying their anticancer efficacy. Small interfering RNAs (siRNAs), a newly developed method for inhibiting hTERT expression, are anticipated to have promising potential for treating ovarian cancer when used alongside magnetic nanoparticles [61].

Resistance to telomerase inhibitors can develop over time limiting their long-term effectiveness [62]. Ongoing research focuses on improving the efficacy, safety, and specificity of small molecule inhibitors for telomerase inhibition in cancer therapy. It is prioritized to inhibit the telomerase enzyme in the target cancer cells without damaging healthy cells in the organism. Clinical trials and further research are essential to fully understand the potential benefits and limitations of using these small molecule inhibitors in treating cancer by inhibiting telomerase activity.

23.6.1.2 Synthetic indirect telomerase inhibitors

There are synthetic compounds that indirectly influence telomerase activity by stimulating cellular pathways. Acridine compounds including geldanamycin, GA alkyne, and bis-amido chloroacridine, do not directly attach to telomerase but instead bind to the heat shock protein HSP90 chaperone and create acridine-HSP90 inhibitory ligands. To elicit effective anticancer effects, HSP90 telomerase activity necessitates the presence of acridine compounds. Consequently, acridine binding to HSP90 hampers telomerase activity and reduces telomerase expression. Thus, acridine compounds hold the potential of powerful agents in the fight against cancer [63].

There are additional synthetic compounds aside from telomerase inhibitors that incorporate coumarins in platinum complexes. Among these eight complexes, three of them were found to trigger cell death (apoptosis) in Sloan-Kettering ovarian cancer cells that have developed resistance to the drug cisplatin. Apoptosis was induced through signaling pathways associated with mitochondrial dysfunction. Furthermore, one of these complexes specifically acts as a telomerase inhibitor that targets the c-myc promoter [64].

23.6.1.3 Synthetic telomerase activators

The occurrence of age-related ailments or diseases associated with the dysfunction or shortening of telomeres, such as AIDS, AA, and pulmonary fibrosis, has drawn attention toward the research and creation of substances that activate telomerase. GRN510, a new activator in the form of a small molecule, is currently under experimentation as a potential medication to restrict fibrosis induced by bleomycin in mice with heterozygous characteristics. This activator has also shown a roughly four-fold increase in telomerase activity in both laboratory settings and living organisms. Because these small molecule activators have been shown to delay the development of lung fibrosis and hinder the accumulation of senescent cells, it is predicted that they can be beneficial in treating pulmonary fibrosis [65].

23.6.1.4 Non-synthetic-natural direct telomerase activators

Certain genetic products play a regulatory role in telomerase function either during transcription or post-transcription. These particular products have the potential to serve as therapeutic targets for the treatment of cancer and various diseases. The activation of telomerase can be linked to somatic mutations occurring in the hTERT promoter. Researchers have identified the Prospero homeobox protein 1 (PROX1) as a newly discovered TERT transcription activator that exhibits high affinity binding to the mutant hTERT promoter. In hepatocellular carcinoma cells expressing

PROX1, TERT promoter mutations can enhance promoter activity. Furthermore, PROX1 has been found to be essential for the upregulation of TERT in both Hep3B and HepG2 cells. Therefore, PROX1 represents a promising target for potential therapies aimed at treating hepatocellular carcinoma [66]. The cell division cycle 5-like (CDC5L) protein is an additional protein that functions as a telomerase activator by attaching to the hTERT promoter. Encoded by the CDC5L gene, this protein exhibits high levels of expression in specific cancer cells, particularly in colorectal cancer [67]. As the contributor to the upregulation of hTERT, leading to the growth of tumors, the suppressor of Ty homolog-5 (SPT5) gene holds potential as a valid target for therapy and a fresh biomarker for colon cancer. The gene suppressing the Ty 5 homolog-5 (SUPT5H) gene could be considered a potent therapeutic target and an innovative biomarker for colon cancer [68]. Researchers have observed a correlation between the hormone leptin and the expression of hTERT suggesting that leptin could play a crucial role in regulating hepatocellular carcinoma (Fig. 23.2) [69].

23.6.1.5 Non-synthetic-natural telomerase inhibitors

Various naturally occurring substances with telomerase inhibitory properties are utilized as effective medications for cancer treatment. One such compound is oxoisoaporphine derived from *Menispermum dauricum*, which exhibits notable antitumoral capabilities. The activity of oxoisoaporphine is attributed to its robust affinity for G-quadruplexes when forming metal complexes. This interaction leads to the stabilization of the telomeric structure, ultimately hindering telomerase from replicating telomeres [70].

A different compound employed as an anti-cancer medication in HCC is sulforaphane, which can be extracted from broccoli. This compound possesses the potential for cancer treatment both in laboratory settings (in vitro) and within living organisms (in vivo). The primary mechanism of action for sulforaphane involves its rapid conversion into a metabolite known as 4-methylthiobutyl isothiocyanate (MTBITC). Researchers have documented MTBITC's ability to trigger apoptosis (cell death) in HCC cells. Moreover, MTBITC has shown effectiveness against telomerase operating independently from TP53, a suppressor of telomerase activity [71].

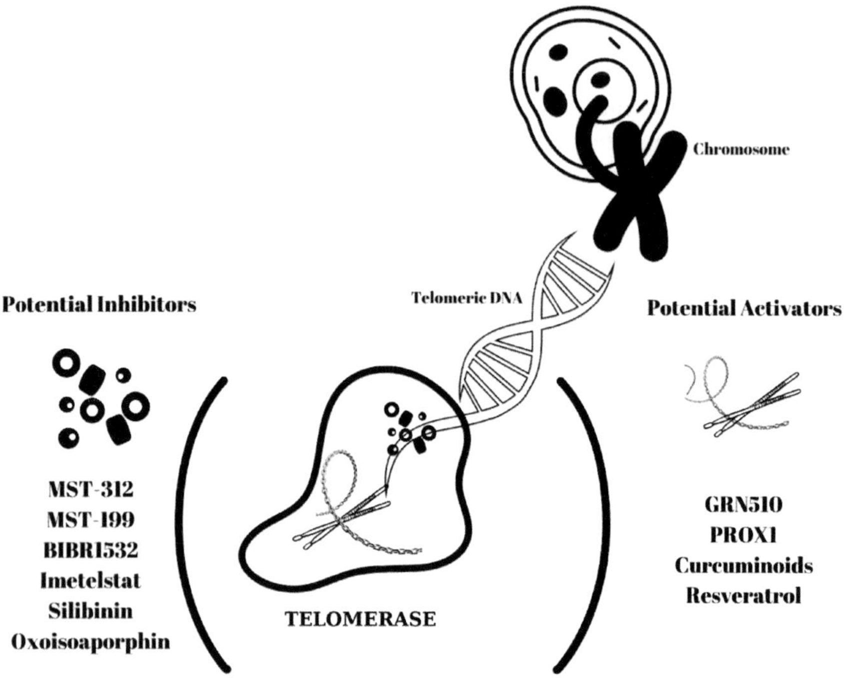

Figure 23.2 Potential telomerase activators and inhibitors.

Cruciferous vegetables contain a natural compound called indole-3-carbinol (I3C), which acts as a telomerase inhibitor and is employed in the management of prostate cancer. By treating a prostate cancer cell line with I3C, the activity of telomerase and the expression of hTERT mRNA are significantly suppressed. It has been observed that combining I3C with diethylstilbestrol (DES) enhances the inhibitory effects on telomerase activity, gene expression, and cell viability. These findings indicate that a combination therapy approach might prove beneficial in the treatment of prostate cancer [72].

23.6.1.6 Non-synthetic-natural indirect telomerase activators

Curcuminoids, which are natural polyphenol compounds derived from turmeric, have been identified as a category of limited natural compounds that demonstrate positive regulation of telomerase in diseases linked to telomerase dysfunction. Research suggests that curcuminoids have the ability to enhance telomerase activity, despite not being directly bound to the telomerase enzyme. Instead, they contribute significantly to the interaction between telomerase and telomeric DNA [73]. Resveratrol, a naturally occurring polyphenol, is utilized in the management of Werner syndrome (WS), a condition characterized by early aging and chromosomal instability resulting from WRN[a] gene mutations. Resveratrol's capacity to sustain telomere length without compromising cell viability has propelled its prominence in WS therapy [74].

23.6.1.7 Oligonucleotide-based inhibitors

Oligonucleotide-based inhibitors represent a promising approach to target telomerase activity via inhibition in cancer cells. These inhibitors are designed to target the RNA component or the mRNA of the TERT gene, both of which are essential for telomerase function. Antisense oligonucleotides (ASOs) are designed to bind to the mRNA of TERT preventing its translation into protein. By reducing TERT protein levels, ASOs can inhibit telomerase activity [75]. Targeting different subunits of telomerase with siRNA with high efficiency and selectivity is attracting increasing attention as innovative drugs, which are promising in cancer treatment. siRNA molecules can be used to specifically target and degrade TERT mRNA reducing TERT protein expression [76].

23.6.2 Gene Editing Techniques

Gene editing techniques are promising approaches for cancer treatment that target specific genetic mutations or alterations that enable cancer cells to grow and spread. These techniques aim to target genes that play a crucial role in cancer development and to treat disease by making changes in these genes. These treatment approaches hold significant potential for precision medicine and personalized cancer treatments. CRISPR-Cas9 technology is a revolutionary and versatile tool for gene editing and genome

[a]The WRN gene is responsible for the production of the Werner protein, which plays a critical role in repairing damaged DNA.

manipulation, and it can be used to generate rapid and specific genomic changes in living organisms. Gene editing using the CRISPR-Cas9 system can be used to disrupt the TERT gene in cancer cells and inactivate TERT expression [77]. Transcription activator-like effector nucleases (TALENs) and zinc-finger nucleases (ZFNs) can be used to create single or double-strand breaks in the TERT gene at specific locations leading to gene disruption. However, the applicability of both methods is limited due to their high cost and time-consuming nature [78].

23.6.3 G-Quadruplex Stabilizers

G-quadruplexes (G4) are non-canonical, four-stranded, nucleic acid secondary structures formed in guanine-rich sequences, in which guanine nucleotides bond with each other via Hoogsteen hydrogen bonding. The imbalance of G4 by various carcinogenic agents causes overexpression of the oncogene and dysregulation of oncogenesis, which promotes cellular growth by allowing telomeric ends to elongate. G-quadruplex stabilizers are specific small molecules that stabilize G4 structures. G-quadruplex stabilizers, potential anti-cancer therapeutics, play a role in telomere targeting in cancer therapy. G-quadruplexes play a role in regulating telomere length and function, inhibit telomerase activity by binding to and stabilizing the G-quadruplexes at the telomeric ends, and stimulate telomere shortening in cancer cells. G-quadruplex inhibits telomerase activity by targeting the G-rich telomeric DNA and prevents telomeric elongation [79].

23.6.4 Therapeutic Vaccines

Immunotherapy strategies targeting telomerase aim to harness the immune system's natural ability to recognize and eliminate cancer cells by targeting telomerase-expressing cells. Therapeutic vaccines targeting telomerase are a novel approach to cancer treatment. These vaccines are designed to stimulate the patient's immune system to recognize and attack cancer cells that overexpress telomerase. By targeting telomerase, therapeutic vaccines aim to induce a specific immune response against cancer cells, potentially slowing or halting disease progression as a part of immunotherapy approaches.

TERT inhibition is often considered a part of combination therapies. Combining TERT inhibitors with other cancer treatments can enhance their effectiveness by targeting multiple aspects of cancer cell growth and survival. Therefore, telomerase vaccines are often used in combination with other cancer treatments, such as checkpoint inhibitors (CPIs), targeted therapies, or chemotherapy. Combination therapies may improve treatment outcomes by increasing the overall anti-tumor immune response. Therefore, telomerase-targeting therapeutic vaccines are considered promising components in combination therapies [80]. Clinical trials are conducted to assess the safety and efficacy of these vaccines in various cancer types, such as malignant melanoma, ovarian cancer, acute myelogenous leukemia (AML), hepatocellular carcinoma, and metastatic castration-resistant prostate cancer. TERT vaccines hold promise as a potential addition to cancer treatment options. However, further clinical data is needed [81–83].

23.6.5 Epigenetic Modulators

Some compounds that modulate epigenetic processes can indirectly affect TERT expression. Targeting telomerase through epigenetic modulation is an area of interest in medical research due to its potential implications for treating various diseases. Some studies have explored the use of epigenetic drugs in cancer, such as DNA methyltransferase inhibitors and histone deacetylase inhibitors, to downregulate telomerase expression in cancer cells [84]. Epigenetic modulation of telomerase expression or activity could be investigated as a potential therapeutic approach for cardiovascular conditions, such as atherosclerosis and heart failure, or cellular aging-associated neurological disorders, like Alzheimer's and Parkinson's. Exploring the role of telomerase and its epigenetic regulation in these diseases may provide insights into potential treatments [85].

23.6.6 Stem Cell Therapies

Telomerase activity is present in most adult stem cell types, though at significantly lower levels. However, telomerase activity is in high concentration in stem cells, which are capable of infinite self-replication and differentiation into various cell types. Maintaining and enhancing telomerase activity in stem cells is crucial for improving their therapeutic potential. Epigenetic modulation of telomerase may play a role in enhancing the regenerative potential of stem cell therapies [86].

23.6.7 RNA-Based Therapies

RNA-based approaches encompass a diverse set of techniques and technologies that leverage the unique properties of RNA molecules for various applications including therapeutic interventions. Modulating telomerase activity through RNA-based approaches is being explored for various medical purposes. RNA-based therapies, such as RNA interference (RNAi) and small RNA molecules, can be designed to specifically target and degrade TERT RNA or inhibit its translation [87].

23.6.8 Therapeutic Targeting

Telomeres and health are closely linked due to their role in cellular aging, longevity, and the development of various age-related diseases. As we know telomerase activity is primarily a potential target for aging process treatments. Aging-related circumstances, such as bone loss, metabolic slowdown, neuronal action speed loss, etc., could be improved via telomerase targeting strategies with no cancer initiation risk. By using some non-integrating adeno-associated (AAV) vectors, AAV9121, for this purpose, telomerase activity can be increased without clonal proliferation. Although various genomic instability situations have been observed in studies aimed at increasing telomerase activity in aging studies, no signs of cancer have been found. As studies on regulating and improving telomerase activity increase, more reliable strategies may be discovered in the future. Many different working models for regulating telomerase activity are available in the literature. The G4TERT-ER model is one of these models [88]. Telomerase is also a target structure, especially in cancer treatment strategies. Immunotherapy is a new treatment model that has been on the agenda in the treatment of various cancers in recent years, and some immunotherapy strategies also include telomerase. GV1001, an anticancer peptide vaccine composed of 16 amino acids and originating from human telomerase reverse transcriptase (hTERT), has been created for the purpose of addressing advanced pancreatic cancer, non-small cell lung cancer, melanoma, and various other forms of cancer. G1001 targeted the hTERT causing a reduction in cellular heat shock protein levels and exerting antitumor effects. It has been shown that GV1001 induces cell death in renal cell cancers, pancreatic, and non-small cell lung cancer types. In the GV1001 vaccine, immune system cells acquire the ability to specifically recognize those with hTERT activation in cancer cells, thus exerting a specific targeted effect on tumor cells. In some studies, it has been reported that adding GV1001 as a supplement to the applied treatment contributes to more tumor regression. Methods developed and still being studied for cancer treatment as an immunotherapy strategy are GX301, UV1, and Vx001.

Another immunotherapy method that is on the agenda is the use of dendritic cells. GRNVAC1 is one of these strategies. hTERT and lysosomal associated membrane protein 1 (LAMP1) derived from cancer patients' dendritic cell-based immunotherapy GRNVAC1 was seen as very effective against acute myeloid leukemia. It has also been seen that this therapy was well tolerated by patients. GRNVAC2 also uses the same pathway but it is derived from stem cells. It has also been reported that these treatment strategies reduce the risk of metastasis. TERT572Y is another experimental model against pancreatic cancer. This is another dendritic cell-based therapy. It has been shown that 50% of patients responded to the therapy with slight side effects. Promoters of the human telomerase reverse transcriptase gene (phTERT) and INVAC-1 are called DNA immunotherapeutic vaccines against tumors. These two strategies affect the CD-8 T cells [80].

23.7 Conclusion

The future of telomerase research holds significant promise and potential implications in various areas of medicine and biology. In addition to being a genetic biomarker, telomeres are also considered metabolic biomarkers. Telomere research is a promising biomarker both in monitoring aging processes and in evaluating various exposures and diseases that affect whole metabolism. While it is challenging to predict the future with certainty, several avenues of exploration and development can be anticipated including therapeutic targeting of telomerase. It is important to note that while the potential benefits of telomerase-related therapies are exciting, there are challenges and risks associated with manipulating such a fundamental aspect of cellular biology. Unintended consequences, including the potential for increased cancer risk, must be carefully evaluated. In summary, the future of telomerase research holds promise for advancing our understanding of aging, cancer, and regenerative medicine. Continued research, ethical considerations, and clinical trials will shape the development and application of telomerase-related interventions in the coming years.

References

1. Palm, W. and de Lange, T. (2008). How shelterin protects mammalian telomeres, *Annual Review of Genetics*, **42**, pp. 301–334.
2. Levy, M. Z., *et al.* (1992). Telomere end-replication problem and cell aging, *Journal of Molecular Biology*, **225**, pp. 951–960.
3. Roake, C. M., and Artandi, S. E. (2020). Regulation of human telomerase in homeostasis and disease, *Nature Reviews Molecular Cell Biology*, **21**, pp. 384–397.
4. Stewart, J. A., *et al.* (2012). Maintaining the end: roles of telomere proteins in end-protection, telomere replication and length regulation, *Mutation Research/Fundamental and Molecular Mechanisms of Mutagenesis*, **730**, pp. 12–19.
5. Wolf, S. E., and Shalev, I. (2023). The shelterin protein expansion of telomere dynamics: linking early life adversity, life history, and

the hallmarks of aging, *Neuroscience & Biobehavioral Reviews*, **152**, pp. 105261.

6. Lazzerini-Denchi, E. and Sfeir, A. (2016). Stop pulling my strings—what telomeres taught us about the DNA damage response, *Nature Reviews Molecular Cell Biology*, **17**, pp. 364–378.
7. de Lange, T. (2018). Shelterin-mediated telomere protection, *Annual Review of Genetics*, **52**, pp. 223–247.
8. Bianchi, M. S., *et al.* (2000). Telomeres, telomerase activity and gene amplification, *Journal of Genetics and Molecular Biology*, **11**, pp. 47–54.
9. Smith, E. M., D.F. Pendlebury, D. F., and J. Nandakumar, J. (2020). Structural biology of telomeres and telomerase, *Cellular and Molecular Life Sciences*, **77**, pp. 61–79.
10. Shammas, M. A. (2011). Telomeres, lifestyle, cancer, and aging, *Current Opinion in Clinical Nutrition and Metabolic Care*, **14**, pp. 28.
11. Srinivas, N., Rachakonda, S., and Kumar, R. (2020). Telomeres and telomere length: a general overview, *Cancers*, **12**, pp. 558.
12. Maestroni, L., Matmati, S., and Coulon, S. (2017). Solving the telomere replication problem, *Genes*, **8**, pp. 55.
13. Bonnell, E., Pasquier, E., and Wellinger, R. J. (2021). Telomere replication: solving multiple end replication problems, *Frontiers in Cell and Developmental Biology*, **9**, pp. 668171.
14. Wang, Y., Sušac, L., and Feigon, J. (2019). Structural biology of telomerase, *Cold Spring Harbor Perspectives in Biology*, **11**, pp. a032383.
15. Greider, C. W. and Blackburn, E. H. (1985). Identification of a specific telomere terminal transferase activity in Tetrahymena extracts, *Cell*, **43**, pp. 405–413.
16. Zhou, X. and Xing, D. (2012). Assays for human telomerase activity: progress and prospects, *Chemical Society Reviews*, **41**, pp. 4643–4656.
17. Wyatt, H. D., West, S. C., and Beattie, T. L. (2010). In TERT preting telomerase structure and function, *Nucleic Acids Research*, **38**, pp. 5609–5622.
18. Autexier, C. and Lue, N. F. (2006). The structure and function of telomerase reverse transcriptase, *Annu. Rev. Biochem.*, **75**, pp. 493–517.
19. Morin, G. B. (1989). The human telomere terminal transferase enzyme is a ribonucleoprotein that synthesizes TTAGGG repeats, *Cell*, **59**, pp. 521–529.
20. Shay, J. W. and Bacchetti, S. (1997). A survey of telomerase activity in human cancer, *European Journal of Cancer*, **33**, pp. 787–791.

21. Criscuolo, F., *et al.* (2018). Experimental manipulation of telomere length: does it reveal a corner-stone role for telomerase in the natural variability of individual fitness? *Philosophical Transactions of the Royal Society B: Biological Sciences*, **373**, pp. 20160440.
22. Armanios, M. (2013). Telomeres and age-related disease: how telomere biology informs clinical paradigms, *The Journal of Clinical Investigation*, **123**, pp. 996–1002.
23. Calado, R. T. and Young, N. S. (2008). Telomere maintenance and human bone marrow failure, *Blood, The Journal of the American Society of Hematology,* 111, pp. 4446–4455.
24. Zahid, M. F., *et al.* (2016). Insight into the molecular pathophysiology of myelodysplastic syndromes: targets for novel therapy, *European Journal of Haematology*, **97**, pp. 313–320.
25. Lansdorp, P. M. (2017). Maintenance of telomere length in AML, *Blood Advances*, **1**, pp. 2467–2472.
26. Byrjalsen, A., *et al.* (2022). Telomere biology disorders, *Ugeskr Laeger*, **184**, pp. V03220220.
27. van Batenburg, A. A., *et al.* (2020). From organ to cell: multi-level telomere length assessment in patients with idiopathic pulmonary fibrosis, *PLoS One*, **15**, pp. e0226785.
28. Wang, H., *et al.* (2022). KLF4 regulates TERT expression in alveolar epithelial cells in pulmonary fibrosis, *Cell Death & Disease*, **13**, pp. 435.
29. Nelson, N. D. and Bertuch, A. A. (2012). Dyskeratosis congenita as a disorder of telomere maintenance, *Mutation Research/Fundamental and Molecular Mechanisms of Mutagenesis*, **730**, pp. 43–51.
30. Savage, S. A. (2022). Dyskeratosis congenita and telomere biology disorders, *Hematology*, **2022**, pp. 637–648.
31. Gramatges, M. M., *et al.* (2013). A homozygous telomerase T-motif variant resulting in markedly reduced repeat addition processivity in siblings with Hoyeraal-Hreidarsson syndrome, *Blood, The Journal of the American Society of Hematology*, **121**, pp. 3586–3593.
32. Glousker, G., *et al.* (2015). Unraveling the pathogenesis of Hoyeraal-Hreidarsson syndrome, a complex telomere biology disorder, *British Journal of Haematology*, **170**, pp. 457–471.
33. Savage, S. A. and Niewisch, M. R. (2022). Dyskeratosis congenita and related telomere biology disorders, *GeneReviews® [Internet].* (University of Washington, Seattle. GeneReviews is a registered trademark of the University of Washington, Seattle).

34. Jylhävä, J., Pedersen, N. L. and Hägg, S. (2017). Biological age predictors, *EBioMedicine*, **21**, pp. 29–36.

35. Vaiserman, A. and Krasnienkov, D. (2021). Telomere length as a marker of biological age: state-of-the-art, open issues, and future perspectives, *Frontiers in Genetics*, **11**, pp. 630186.

36. Semeraro, M. D., *et al.* (2020). Physical activity, a modulator of aging through effects on telomere biology, *Aging (Albany NY)*, **12**, pp. 13803.

37. Ghareghomi, S., *et al.* (2021). Fundamental insights into the interaction between telomerase/TERT and intracellular signaling pathways, *Biochimie*, **181**, pp. 12–24.

38. Mather, K. A. (2022). Genetic and environmental factors in ageing and age-related disease, *MDPI*, **13**, pp. 396.

39. Martínez-Balsalobre, E., *et al.* (2021). Telomerase and alternative lengthening of telomeres coexist in the regenerating zebrafish caudal fins, *bioRxiv*. doi: https://doi.org/10.1101/2021.11.15.468592.

40. Nalobin, D., *et al.* (2020). Telomeres and telomerase in heart ontogenesis, aging and regeneration, *Cells*, **9**, pp. 503.

41. Wei, F., *et al.* (2012). Vitamin C treatment promotes mesenchymal stem cell sheet formation and tissue regeneration by elevating telomerase activity, *Journal of Cellular Physiology*, **227**, pp. 3216–3224.

42. Luger, T. and Lotti, T. (1998). Neuropeptides: role in inflammatory skin diseases, *Journal of the European Academy of Dermatology and Venereology*, **10**, pp. 207–211.

43. Bizot-Foulon, V., *et al.* (1995). Uncoordinate expressions of type I and III collagens, collagenase and tissue inhibitor of matrix metalloproteinase 1 along in vitro proliferative life span of human skin fibroblasts: regulation by all-trans retinoic acid, *Cell Biology International*, **19**, pp. 129–136.

44. Vande Berg, J. S., *et al.* (1998). Fibroblast senescence in pressure ulcers, *Wound Repair and Regeneration*, **6**, pp. 38–49.

45. Funk, W. D., *et al.* (2000). Telomerase expression restores dermal integrity to in vitro-aged fibroblasts in a reconstituted skin model, *Experimental Cell Research*, **258**, pp. 270–278.

46. Blasco, M. A., *et al.* (1997). Telomere shortening and tumor formation by mouse cells lacking telomerase RNA, *Cell*, **91**, pp. 25–34.

47. Lee, H.-W., *et al.* (1998). Essential role of mouse telomerase in highly proliferative organs, *Nature*, **392**, pp. 569–574.

48. McChesney, P. A., Elmore, L. W., and Holt, S. E. (2005). Vertebrate marine species as model systems for studying telomeres and telomerase, *Zebrafish*, **1**, pp. 349–355.
49. Elmore, L. W., *et al.* (2008). Upregulation of telomerase function during tissue regeneration, *Experimental Biology and Medicine*, **233**, pp. 958–967.
50. Vertecchi, E., Rizzo, A., and Salvati, E. (2022). Telomere targeting approaches in cancer: beyond length maintenance, *International Journal of Molecular Sciences*, **23**, pp. 3784.
51. Bajaj, S., *et al.* (2020). Targeting telomerase for its advent in cancer therapeutics, *Medicinal Research Reviews*, **40**, pp. 1871–1919.
52. Fragkiadaki, P., *et al.* (2022). Telomerase inhibitors and activators in aging and cancer: a systematic review, *Molecular Medicine Reports*, **25**, pp. 1–11.
53. Seimiya, H., *et al.* (2002). Telomere shortening and growth inhibition of human cancer cells by novel synthetic telomerase inhibitors MST-312, MST-295, and MST-199, *Molecular Cancer Therapeutics*, **1**, pp. 657–665.
54. Pascolo, E., *et al.* (2002). Mechanism of human telomerase inhibition by BIBR1532, a synthetic, non-nucleosidic drug candidate, *Journal of Biological Chemistry*, **277**, pp. 15566–15572.
55. Altamura, G., *et al.* (2021). The small molecule BIBR1532 exerts potential anti-cancer activities in preclinical models of feline oral squamous cell carcinoma through inhibition of telomerase activity and down-regulation of TERT, *Frontiers in Veterinary Science*, **7**, pp. 620776.
56. Frink, R.E., *et al.* (2016). Telomerase inhibitor imetelstat has preclinical activity across the spectrum of non-small cell lung cancer oncogenotypes in a telomere length dependent manner, *Oncotarget*, **7**, pp. 31639.
57. Bruedigam, C. and Lane, S. W. (2016). Telomerase in hematologic malignancies, *Current Opinion in Hematology*, **23**, pp. 346–353.
58. Hu, Y., *et al.* (2015). The HSP90 inhibitor alvespimycin enhances the potency of telomerase inhibition by imetelstat in human osteosarcoma, *Cancer Biology & Therapy*, **16**, pp. 949–957.
59. Wang, Y., *et al.* (2016). Dihydropyrazole derivatives as telomerase inhibitors: structure-based design, synthesis, SAR and anticancer evaluation in vitro and in vivo, *European Journal of Medicinal Chemistry*, **112**, pp. 231–251.

60. Thelen, P., *et al.* (2004). Inhibition of telomerase activity and secretion of prostate specific antigen by silibinin in prostate cancer cells, *The Journal of Urology*, **171**, pp. 1934–1938.

61. Chen, X., *et al.* (2018). Ethenesulfonyl fluoride derivatives as telomerase inhibitors: structure-based design, SAR, and anticancer evaluation in vitro, *Journal of Enzyme Inhibition and Medicinal Chemistry*, **33**, pp. 1266–1270.

62. Guterres, A. N. and Villanueva, J. (2020). Targeting telomerase for cancer therapy, *Oncogene*, **39**, pp. 5811–5824.

63. Roe, S., *et al.* (2015). Synthesis and biological evaluation of hybrid acridine-HSP90 ligand conjugates as telomerase inhibitors, *Organic & Biomolecular Chemistry*, **13**, pp. 8500–8504.

64. Meng, T., *et al.* (2018). Synthesis and biological evaluation of substituted 3-(2'-benzimidazolyl) coumarin platinum (II) complexes as new telomerase inhibitors, *Journal of Inorganic Biochemistry*, **189**, pp. 143–150.

65. Le Saux, C. J., *et al.* (2013). A novel telomerase activator suppresses lung damage in a murine model of idiopathic pulmonary fibrosis, *PloS One*, **8**, pp. e58423.

66. Kim, Y. J., *et al.* (2018). Suppression of PROX1-mediated TERT expression in hepatitis B viral hepatocellular carcinoma, *International Journal of Cancer*, **143**, pp. 3155–3168.

67. Li, J., *et al.* (2017). CDC5L promotes hTERT expression and colorectal tumor growth, *Cellular Physiology and Biochemistry*, **41**, pp. 2475–2488.

68. Chen, R., *et al.* (2015). Suppressor of Ty homolog-5, a novel tumor-specific human telomerase reverse transcriptase promoter-binding protein and activator in colon cancer cells, *Oncotarget*, **6**, pp. 32841.

69. Stefanou, N., *et al.* (2010). Leptin as a critical regulator of hepatocellular carcinoma development through modulation of human telomerase reverse transcriptase, *BMC Cancer*, **10**, pp. 1–10.

70. Wei, Z.-Z., *et al.* (2016). Oxoisoaporphine as potent telomerase inhibitor, *Molecules*, **21**, pp. 1534.

71. Herz, C., *et al.* (2014). The isothiocyanate erucin abrogates telomerase in hepatocellular carcinoma cells in vitro and in an orthotopic xenograft tumour model of HCC, *Journal of Cellular and Molecular Medicine*, **18**, pp. 2393–2403.

72. Adler, S., Rashid, G. and Klein, A. (2011). Indole-3-carbinol inhibits telomerase activity and gene expression in prostate cancer cell lines, *Anticancer Research*, **31**, pp. 3733–3737.
73. Taka, T., *et al.* (2014). Curcuminoid derivatives enhance telomerase activity in an in vitro TRAP assay, *Bioorganic & Medicinal Chemistry Letters*, **24**, pp. 5242–5246.
74. Uchiumi, F., *et al.* (2011). The effect of resveratrol on the Werner syndrome RecQ helicase gene and telomerase activity, *Current Aging Science*, **4**, pp. 1–7.
75. Eckburg, A., *et al.* (2020). Oligonucleotides and microRNAs targeting telomerase subunits in cancer therapy, *Cancers*, **12**, pp. 2337.
76. Sasaki, S. (2019). Development of novel functional molecules targeting DNA and RNA, *Chemical and Pharmaceutical Bulletin*, **67**, pp. 505–518.
77. Brane, A. C. and Tollefsbol, T. O. (2019). Targeting telomeres and telomerase: studies in aging and disease utilizing CRISPR/Cas9 technology, *Cells*, **8**, pp. 186.
78. Balon, K., *et al.* (2022). Targeting cancer with CRISPR/Cas9-based therapy, *International Journal of Molecular Sciences*, **23**, pp. 573.
79. Ivancich, M., *et al.* (2017). Treating cancer by targeting telomeres and telomerase, *Antioxidants*, **6**, pp. 15.
80. Mizukoshi, E. and Kaneko, S. (2019). Telomerase-targeted cancer immunotherapy, *International Journal of Molecular Sciences*, **20**, pp. 1823.
81. Filaci, G., *et al.* (2021). Telomerase-based GX301 cancer vaccine in patients with metastatic castration-resistant prostate cancer: a randomized phase II trial, *Cancer Immunology, Immunotherapy*, **70**, pp. 3679–3692.
82. Vienot, A., *et al.* (2023). Evaluation of the interest to combine a CD4 Th1-inducer cancer vaccine derived from telomerase and atezolizumab plus bevacizumab in unresectable hepatocellular carcinoma: a randomized non-comparative phase II study (TERTIO–PRODIGE 82), *BMC Cancer*, **23**, pp. 710.
83. Ellingsen, E. B., Bjørheim, J. and Gaudernack, G. (2023). Therapeutic cancer vaccination against telomerase: clinical developments in melanoma, *Current Opinion in Oncology*, **35**, pp. 100.
84. Zhang, X., *et al.* (2015). The DNA methylation inhibitor induces telomere dysfunction and apoptosis of leukemia cells that is attenuated by telomerase over-expression, *Oncotarget*, **6**, pp. 4888.

85. Lee, H.-S., *et al.* (2018). Systematic analysis of compounds specifically targeting telomeres and telomerase for clinical implications in cancer therapy, *Cancer Research*, **78**, pp. 6282–6296.

86. Saraswat, K. and Rizvi, S.I. (2017). Novel strategies for anti-aging drug discovery, *Expert Opinion on Drug Discovery*, **12**, pp. 955–966.

87. Wu, X., *et al.* (2023). Targeting proteins in nucleus through dual-regulatory pathways acting in cytoplasm, *Nano Letters*, **23**, pp. 5811–5821.

88. de Jesus, B. B. and Blasco, M. A. (2013). Telomerase at the intersection of cancer and aging, *Trends in Genetics*, **29**, pp. 513–520.

Index

For Product Safety Concerns and Information please contact our EU representative GPSR@taylorandfrancis.com Taylor & Francis Verlag GmbH, Kaufingerstraße 24, 80331 München, Germany

Batch number: 10726505

Printed by Printforce, the Netherlands